Sign up for eAlerts today!

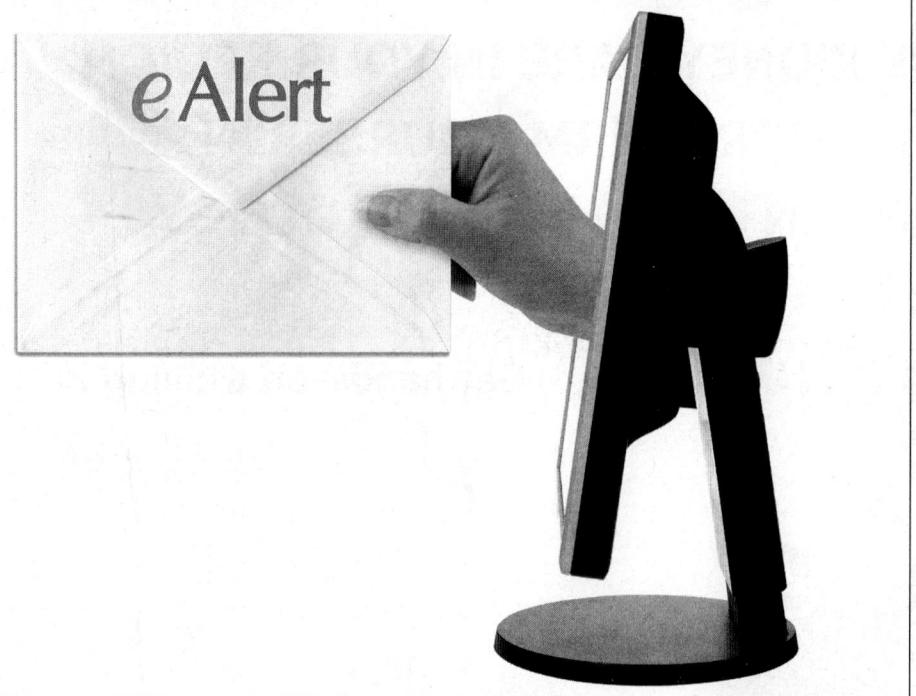

Elsevier publishes the **most respected, influential information sources** in every medical and scientific field. Our **eAlerts** let you know about new products, special offers, and promotions in your specialty. You'll also get occasional surveys to help us better meet your information needs.

It's the **best way to stay connected** with **the latest resources** in your field!

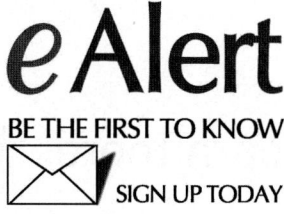

www.us.elsevierhealth.com

*We respect your privacy and do not disclose, rent, or sell your personal information to any non-affiliated third party without your consent, except as may be stated in the Elsevier Privacy Policy. For additional information, please visit **www.us.elsevierhealth.com**.*

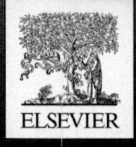

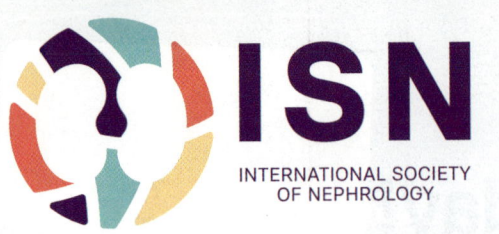 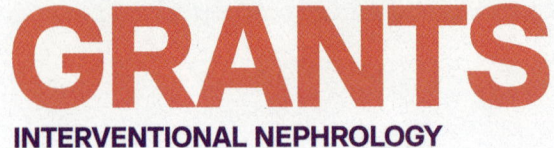 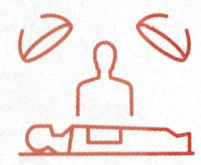

ADVANCE KIDNEY CARE IN YOUR REGION WITH SHORT-TERM COURSES IN INTERVENTIONAL NEPHROLOGY

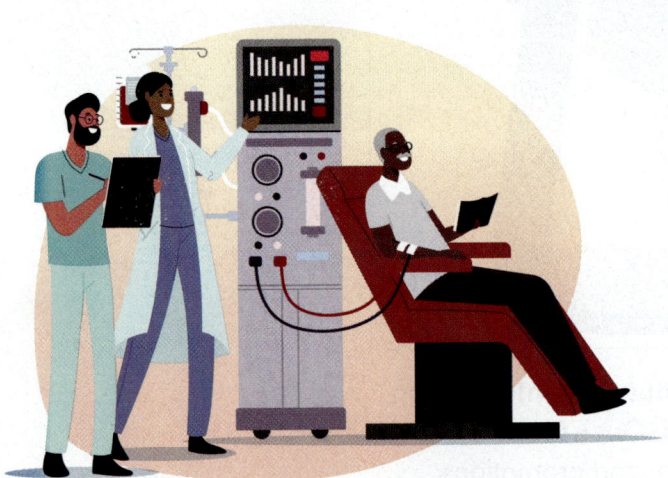

Get **hands-on training** in

- kidney biopsy,
- CVC placement,
- PD catheter insertion,
- endovascular procedures,
- nephrology POCUS

at one of **17 Interventional Nephrology Training Centers**.

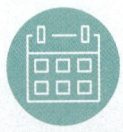 Apply by **JUNE 1**

→ for a **1–4-week foundation course**
→ or a **3-month advanced course**.

Learn more: **theisn.org/in**

Or contact us at **fellowship@theisn.org**.

Open to all ISN members from LIC, LMIC, UMIC

Join/Renew › theisn.org/membership   theisn.org

kidney INTERNATIONAL

EDITOR
Pierre Ronco, Paris
Clinical Investigation, Glomerulonephritis, Renal Immunopathology

DEPUTY EDITOR
Brad Rovin, Columbus
Clinical Trials, Translational Nephrology, Clinical and Experimental Autoimmunity

PAST EDITORS
Detlef Schlöndorff, New York
Qais Al-Awqati, New York
Saulo Klahr, St. Louis
Thomas E. Andreoli, Little Rock
Roscoe R. Robinson, Durham

NEPHROLOGY DIGEST EDITOR
Johannes Schlöndorff, Columbus
Podocyte Biology

KI EDITORIAL FELLOWS
Isabelle Ayoub, Columbus
Eugene Chan, Hong Kong
Muzamil Olamide Hassan, Ile-Ife
Christoph Kuppe, Aachen
Veronica Miguel, Madrid
Griffith B. Perkins, Adelaide

STATISTICIANS
Vernon Chinchilli, Hershey
Monique Elseviers, Antwerp
Vic Hasselblad, Jacksonville
Georg Heinze, Vienna
Susan Hogan, Chapel Hill
Zhezhen Jin, New York
Eiichiro Kanda, Okayama
Joseph Kim, Toronto
Lan Kong, Hershey
Yi-Ju Li, Durham
Jennie Ma, Charlottesville
Rajasekhar Ramakrishnan, New York
Jesse Schold, Cleveland
Peter Song, Ann Arbor
Elani Streja, Orange
Natasha Wiebe, Edmonton

ASSOCIATE EDITORS
Olivier Devuyst, Zurich
Physiology, Genetics, Translational Nephrology
Tilman B. Drueke, Paris
CKD, Hypertension, Nephrolithiasis
Iain Drummond, Salisbury Cove
Kidney Organogenesis and Congenital Defects, Kidney Injury and Regeneration, Kidney Genetic Model Systems
Jürgen Floege, Aachen
Glomerulonephritis, CKD-MBD
Agnes B. Fogo, Nashville
Clinical and Experimental Renal Pathology, Experimental CKD, Diabetic Nephropathy
John (Cijiang) He, New York
Clinical and Experimental Diabetic Kidney Disease, Glomerular Cell Biology, Kidney Fibrosis
T. Alp Ikizler, Nashville
Dialysis, Clinical CKD, Acute Kidney Injury, Nutrition, Metabolism
Reiko Inagi, Tokyo
Experimental AKI and CKD, CKD Pathophysiology, Cell Signaling

Krzysztof Kiryluk, New York
Genetic Epidemiology, Precision Medicine and Systems Biology
Maarten Naesens, Leuven
Transplant; Immunology
Jai Radhakrishnan, New York
Editor of KIR, Clinical Studies, Glomerular Disease, Educational Content
Germaine Wong, Sydney
Life Course Epidemiology, Health Economics and Onconephrology
Yun Xia, Singapore
Kidney Organoid, Pluripotent Stem Cell, Differentiation, Disease Modelling

CONSULTING EDITORS
Amélie Bernier-Jean, Montreal
Epidemiology and Clinical Biostatistics, Lifestyle Medicine, Chronic Kidney Disease
Letizia De Chiara, Firenze
Experimental AKI and CKD, AKI-CKD Transition, Kidney Injury and Regeneration

EDITORIAL BOARD

Dwomoa Adu, Accra
Evren Azeloglu, New York
Sean Barbour, Vancouver
Jonathan Barratt, Leicester
John Bertram, Clayton
Peter Boor, Aachen
Frank Bridoux, Poitiers
Kirk Campbell, New York
Daniel Cattran, Toronto
Christos Chatziantoniou, Paris
Philip Clayton, Adelaide
P. Toby Coates, Adelaide
Steven Coca, New York
Terence Cook, London
Vivette D'Agati, New York
Ilse S. Daehn, New York
Farhad Danesh, Chicago
John Daugirdas, Chicago
Andrew Davenport, London
Vikas Dharnidharka, St. Louis
Kent Doi, Tokyo
Jie Dong, Beijing
Zheng Dong, Augusta
Kai-Uwe Eckardt, Berlin
Somchai Eiam-Ong, Bangkok
Roger Evans, Melbourne
Pieter Evenepoel, Leuven
Robert Fairchild, Cleveland
Sarah Faubel, Denver
Christian Faul, Birmingham
Fernando Fervenza, Rochester
Danilo Fliser, Homburg
Josephine Forbes, Brisbane
Alessia Fornoni, Miami
Anna Francis, Brisbane
Barry Freedman, Winston-Salem

Masafumi Fukagawa, Isehara
Amit Garg, London, Ontario
Vesna Garovic, Rochester
Rasheed Adebayo Gbadegesin, Durham
Richard Glassock, Laguna Niguel
David S. Goldfarb, New York
Mark Haas, Los Angeles
Volker Haase, Nashville
Jan Halbritter, Leipzig
Peter C. Harris, Rochester
Sho Hasegawa, Bunkyo-Ku
Michelle Hladunewich, Toronto
Fan Fan Hou, Guangzhou
Pascal Houillier, Paris
Chi-yuan Hsu, San Francisco
Tobias B. Huber, Hamburg
Benjamin Humphreys, St. Louis
Masao Iwagami, Tsukuba
Vivekanand Jha, New Delhi
Kenar Jhaveri, Great Neck
Jaap Joles, Utrecht
Kamyar Kalantar-Zadeh, Orange
Keizo Kanasaki, Izumo
Frederick Kaskel, New York
A. Richard Kitching, Clayton
Anna Koettgen, Freiburg
Jeffrey Kopp, Bethesda
Matthias Kretzler, Ann Arbor
Christian Kurts, Bonn
Gérard Lambeau, Valbonne
David Leaf, Boston
Christophe Legendre, Paris
Kevin Lemley, Los Angeles
Emmanuel Letavernier, Paris
Adeera Levin, Vancouver
Philip K.T. Li, Hong Kong

Christoph Licht, Toronto
John Lieske, Rochester
Adrian Liew, Singapore
Melissa Little, Brisbane
Wai Lim, Perth
Kathleen Liu, San Francisco
Youhua Liu, Pittsburgh
Alexandre Loupy, Paris
Friedrich Luft, Berlin
Magdalena Madero, Mexico City
Sethu Madhavan, Columbus
Johannes Mann, München
Peter J. Margetts, Hamilton
Glen Markowitz, New York
Ziad Massy, Paris
Kunihiro Matsushita, Baltimore
Mignon McCulloch, Cape Town
Juan Manuel Mejia-Vilet, Mexico City
Timothy W. Meyer, Palo Alto
Imari Mimura, Tokyo
Jeffrey Miner, St. Louis
Marcus Moeller, Aachen
Jeremiah Morrissey, St. Louis
Rosa Moysés, São Paulo
Masaomi Nangaku, Tokyo
David Nikolic-Paterson, Clayton
Marina Noris, Ranica
Ikechi Okpechi, Cape Town
Cristian Pattaro, Bolzano
Aldo Peixoto, West Haven
Mark Perazella, New Haven
Giorgina B. Piccoli, Torino
Janos Peti-Peterdi, Los Angeles
Martin Pollak, Boston
Ambra Pozzi, Nashville
Susan Quaggin, Chicago

W. Brian Reeves, San Antonio
Heather Reich, Toronto
Giuseppe Remuzzi, Bergamo
Connie Rhee, Orange
Mariano Rodriguez, Cordoba
Paola Romagnani, Firenze
Avi Rosenberg, Bethesda
Michael Ross, New York
Lubka Roumenina, Paris
Mario Schiffer, Erlangen
Kai Schmidt-Ott, New York
Stephan Segerer, Aarau
Kumar Sharma, La Jolla
Natalie Staplin, Oxford
Katalin Susztak, Philadelphia
Yoshio Terada, Nankoku
Tetsuhiro Tanaka, Tokyo
Sydney C.W. Tang, Hong Kong
Pierre-Louis Tharaux, Paris
Joshua Thurman, Denver
Jens Titze, Singapore
Marcello Tonelli, Edmonton
Hernan Trimarchi, Buenos Aires
Frank van der Sande, Maastricht
Marc Vervloet, Amsterdam
Marina Vivarelli, Rome
Carsten Wagner, Zurich
Angela Wang, Hong Kong
Jack Wetzels, Nijmegen
Keng-Thye Woo, Singapore
Christina Wyatt, Durham
Motoko Yanagita, Kyoto
Xueqing Yu, Guangzhou
Suzuki Yusuke, Tokyo
Elena V. Zakharova, Moscow
Hong Zhang, Beijing

www.kidney-international.org

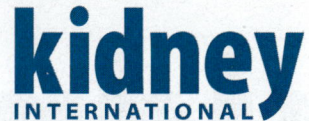

Kidney International (ISSN: 0085-2538; EISSN: 1523-1755) is the official publication of the International Society of Nephrology (ISN) and is published monthly for the ISN by Elsevier, 230 Park Avenue, Suite 800, New York, NY 10169, USA. **BUSINESS OFFICE:** 1600 John F. Kennedy Boulevard, Suite 1800, Philadelphia, PA 19103-2899. Accounting and Circulation Offices: 3251 Riverport Lane, Maryland Heights, MO 63043.

Periodicals postage paid at New York, NY and additional mailing offices (not valid for journal supplements).

Scope

Kidney International is devoted to kidney research. It aims to inform the researcher, the clinical investigator, and the practicing nephrologist on all aspects of kidney research. These include the latest clinical studies on emerging developments in nephrology and the highest level of original research studies in clinical and basic kidney research. The journal reflects the field through critical reviews, commentaries, original articles, remarkable images, news features, guidelines, and problem-focused articles for the diagnosis and treatment of kidney patients.

This journal is covered by BIOSIS, Chemical Abstracts, EMBASE/Excerpta Medica, Index Medicus/Medline, Science Citation Index, Current Contents/Life Sciences, Current Contents/Clinical Medicine, SciSearch, Reference Update, CABS, Biological Abstracts, Global Health, EBSCO, Adonis, and PASCAL.

Editorial

Manuscripts should be submitted online at http://mc.manuscriptcentral.com/ki. Detailed instructions for authors submitting online are available at the above website address. For online submission problems, consult the help section on the submission site or call +1 434 817 2040 x167.

Executive Editor, *Kidney International*: Patricia Morrissey. Tel: +1 314 454 8919. E-mail: pmorriss@wustl.edu

Managing Editor, *Kidney International*: Betsy Lueg. E-mail: lueg@wustl.edu

Managing Editor and Social Media Editor, *Kidney International*: Susan L. Small. E-mail: small_s@wustl.edu

Managing Editor, *Kidney International Supplements*; Assistant Managing Editor, *Kidney International*: Christine Burgos-Clavel. E-mail: christine.burgos@krctnn.com (questions regarding *Kidney International Supplements* should be addressed to Christine)

USA POSTMASTER: Send change of address to *Kidney International*, Elsevier, Journal Returns, 450 Fame Avenue, Hanover, PA 17331, USA.

Customer Service

Please visit our Support Hub page https://service.elsevier.com for assistance or contact: United States and Canada: Telephone (800) 654-2452. E-mail: JournalsCustomerService-usa@elsevier.com (for print support); journalsonlinesupport-usa@elsevier.com (for online support). Europe, Africa, Middle East: Telephone 44 (0) 1865 843434; E-mail: JournalsCustomerServiceEMEA@elsevier.com. Asia and Australia: Telephone 65 6349-0222; E-mail: asiainfo@elsevier.com.

ANNUAL SUBSCRIPTION RATES:

Kidney International is published in 12 issues per year. Personal subscription prices for 2024 are: US Print & Online: $1,571; International Print & Online: $1,736.

For institutional and other pricing options, including access information and terms and conditions, please visit https://www.elsevier.com/books-and-journals/journal-pricing. Personal and institutional subscriptions include *Kidney International Supplements*, Volume 13, 2024.

Current prices are in effect for back volumes and back issues.

Further information on this journal is available from the Publisher or from this journal's website (www.kidney-international.org). Information on other Elsevier products is available through Elsevier's website (http://www.elsevier.com).

Society

All members of ISN receive *Kidney International* as part of their membership. For information about membership and the society, address correspondence to: International Society of Nephrology, Global Operations Center, Avenue des Arts 1-2, B-1210 Brussels, Belgium. Tel: +32 2 808 0420, Fax: +32 2 808 4454. E-mail: info@theisn.org, www.theisn.org

CONTACT INFORMATION
ISN Members

Please direct queries about print issue orders or online journal access to the ISN (see above for address).

Advertising

Inquiries concerning display advertising should be addressed to: USA/Canada: Jane Liss, Tel: +1 732-890-9812, E-mail: jliss@triplethreatmedia.com and Jen Callow, Tel: +1 732-580-8884, E-mail: jcallow@triplethreatmedia.com; International: Robert Bayliss, Tel: 44 20 7424 4454, E-mail: r.bayliss@elsevier.com.

Inquiries concerning recruitment/classified advertising should be addressed to: USA/Canada: Rob Issler, Tel: +1 321-400-8279, E-mail: robert.isslerjr@therapeuticsol.com; International: Elsevier Classified, Tel: 44 1425 462 736, E-mail: elsevierclassified@elsevier.dbfactory.co.uk.

Supplements

Inquiries concerning *Kidney International Supplements* should be addressed to: Craig Smith. Tel:+1 212-462-1933, E-mail: c.smith@elsevier.com

© **2024 International Society of Nephrology.**

This journal and the individual contributions contained in it are protected under copyright by the International Society of Nephrology, and the following terms and conditions apply to their use in addition to the terms of any Creative Commons or other use license that has been applied by the publisher to an individual article:

Photocopying

Single photocopies of single articles may be made for personal use as allowed by national copyright laws. Permission is not required for photocopying of articles published under the CC BY license nor for photocopying for noncommercial purposes in accordance with any other user license applied by the publisher. Permission of the publisher and payment of a fee is required for all other photocopying, including multiple or systematic copying, copying for advertising or promotional purposes, resale, and all forms of document delivery. Special rates are available for educational institutions that wish to make photocopies for nonprofit educational classroom use.

Derivative Works

Users may reproduce tables of contents or prepare lists of articles including abstracts for internal circulation within their institutions or companies. Other than for articles published under the CC BY license, permission of the publisher is required for resale or distribution outside the subscribing institution or company. For any subscribed articles or articles published under a CC BY-NC-ND license, permission of the publisher is required for all other derivative works, including compilations and translations.

Storage or Usage

Except as outlined above or as set out in the relevant user license, no part of this publication may be reproduced, stored in a retrieval system, or transmitted in any form or by any means, electronic, mechanical, photocopying, recording, or otherwise, without prior written permission of the publisher.

Permissions

For information on how to seek permission visit www.elsevier.com/permissions or call: (+1) 800-523-4069 x 3808.

AUTHOR RIGHTS

Author(s) may have additional rights in their articles as set out in their agreement with the publisher (more information at http://www.elsevier.com/authorsrights).

REPRINTS: For queries about author offprints, e-mail authorsupport@elsevier.com. To order 100 or more reprints for educational, commercial, or promotional use, contact Derrick Imasa at 212-633-3874, Elsevier Inc., 230 Park Avenue, Suite 800, New York, NY 10169-0901, USA. Fax: 212-462-1935; e-mail: reprints@elsevier.com.

NOTICE

Practitioners and researchers must always rely on their own experience and knowledge in evaluating and using any information, methods, compounds or experiments described herein. Because of rapid advances in the medical sciences, in particular, independent verification of diagnoses and drug dosages should be made. To the fullest extent of the law, no responsibility is assumed by the publisher and the International Society of Nephrology for any injury and/or damage to persons or property as a matter of products liability, negligence or otherwise, or from any use or operation of any methods, products, instructions or ideas contained in the material herein.

Although all advertising material is expected to conform to ethical (medical) standards, inclusion in this publication does not constitute a guarantee or endorsement of the quality or value of such product or of the claims made of it by its manufacturer.

Printed on acid-free paper, effective with Volume 69, Issue 1, 2006. Printed and bound in the USA by Sheridan Warehouse, Hanover, PA, USA.

contents

VOL 105 | ISSUE 3 | MARCH 2024

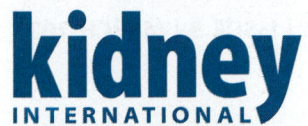

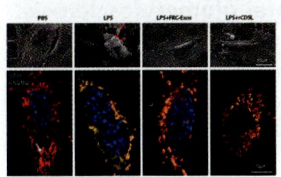

FRC-Exos improves septic kidney injury through CD5L. In the top row, after LPS treatment for 24 hours, SEM was used to observe the membrane morphology of PKTCs. Shown in the bottom row, MitoTracker Red CMXRos was used to label mitochondria, and staining with GSDMD antibodies was performed (green). (Images are from the article by Li et al., found on page 508.)

399 **in this issue**

obituaries

400 **In remembrance of Eberhard Ritz, MD (1938–2023)**
Kai-Uwe Eckardt and Kerstin Amann

403 **A tribute to Edmund J Lewis, MD**
Stephen M. Korbet

editorial: special report

406 **Mind the gap in kidney care: translating what we know into what we do**
Valerie A. Luyckx, Katherine R. Tuttle, Dina Abdellatif, Ricardo Correa-Rotter, Winston W.S. Fung, Agnès Haris, Li-Li Hsiao, Makram Khalife, Latha A. Kumaraswami, Fiona Loud, Vasundhara Raghavan, Stefanos Roumeliotis, Marianella Sierra, Ifeoma Ulasi, Bill Wang, Siu-Fai Lui, Vassilios Liakopoulos and Alessandro Balducci; for the World Kidney Day Joint Steering Committee OPEN

418 **journal club**

nephrology digest

421 **Secrets and myths between tubules—new insights on erythropoietin production from single-cell technology**
Kai-Uwe Eckardt and Armin Kurtz

423 **Reconstructing the interface between the human intestine and immune system: potential to advance mechanistic studies in IgA nephropathy**
Huamin Wang, James Zuiani, P. Toby Coates AO and Yun Xia

commentaries

427 **Mining the amyloid-plaque proteome to uncover disease mechanisms in renal amyloidoses**
Mario Nuvolone and Giampaolo Merlini

430 **Gene editing: a near future for the treatment of genetic kidney diseases**
Fernando Gómez-García and Miguel A. Garcia-Gonzalez

433 **Advancing parathyroid anatomy understanding through single-cell RNA sequencing in uremic secondary hyperparathyroidism**
Iddo Z. Ben-Dov

435 **Refining GFR estimation: a quest for the unobservable truth?**
Tariq Shafi

437 **APOL1-mediated and Mendelian forms of "heretofore" idiopathic collapsing glomerulopathy: lessons from Brazil**
Nicholette D. Palmer and Barry I. Freedman

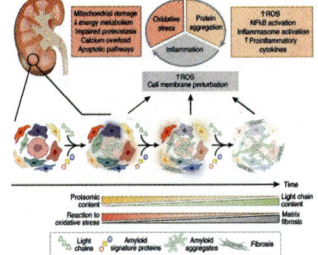

See page 427

Kidney International (ISSN: 0085-2538; EISSN: 1523-1755) is the official publication of the International Society of Nephrology (ISN) and is published monthly for the ISN by Elsevier, 230 Park Avenue, Suite 800, New York, NY 10169-0901, USA. BUSINESS OFFICE: 1600 John F. Kennedy Boulevard, Suite 1800, Philadelphia, PA 19103-2899. Accounting and Circulation Offices: 3251 Riverport Lane, Maryland Heights, MO 63043. Periodicals postage paid at New York, NY and at additional mailing offices. **USA POSTMASTER:** Send change of address to Kidney International, Elsevier, Journal Returns, 450 Fame Avenue, Hanover, PA 17331, USA.

contents

VOL 105 | ISSUE 3 | MARCH 2024

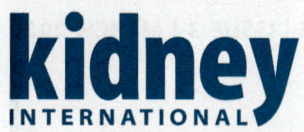

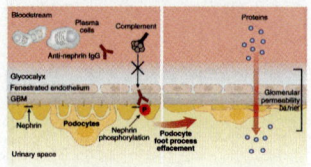

See page 440

440 **Anti-nephrin antibodies in recurrence of focal segmental glomerulosclerosis: closer to discovering the Holy Grail?**
Marina Vivarelli and Manuela Colucci

442 **Exploring nontraditional cardiorenal advantages of SGLT-2 inhibitors and GLP-1 receptor agonists**
Jia-Jin Chen, Tao-Han Lee and Huang-Yu Yang

445 **Alternative creatinine-based GFR estimates in United States populations—similar performance, same gaps—is it time to move on?**
June Fabian

KDIGO executive conclusions

447 **Executive summary of the KDIGO 2024 Clinical Practice Guideline for the Management of ANCA–Associated Vasculitis**
Jürgen Floege, David R.W. Jayne, Jan-Stephan F. Sanders, Vladimír Tesar, Ethan M. Balk, Craig E. Gordon, Gaelen Adam, Marcello A. Tonelli, Michael Cheung, Amy Earley and Brad H. Rovin OPEN

meeting report

450 **Post-transplant recurrence of focal segmental glomerular sclerosis: consensus statements**
Rupesh Raina, Swathi Jothi, Dieter Haffner, Michael Somers, Guido Filler, Prabhav Vasistha, Ronith Chakraborty, Ron Shapiro, Parmjeet S. Randhawa, Rulan Parekh, Christopher Licht, Timothy Bunchman, Sidharth Sethi, Guneive Mangat, Joshua Zaritsky, Franz Schaefer, Bradley Warady, Sharon Bartosh, Mignon McCulloch, Khalid Alhasan, Agnieszka Swiatecka-Urban, William E. Smoyer, Anil Chandraker, Hui Kim Yap, Vivekanand Jha, Arvind Bagga and Jai Radhakrishnan

policy forum

464 **Kidney biopsies among persons living in hotspots of CKDu: a position statement from the International Society of Nephrology's Consortium of Collaborators on CKDu**
Eranga Wijewickrama, Suman Behera, Pablo Garcia, Carmen Avila-Casado, Ben Caplin, Vicente Sanchez Paolo, Karen Courville, David Friedman, Magdalena Madero, Vivekanand Jha, Neeraja Kambham, Adeera Levin and Shuchi Anand; on behalf of the International Society of Nephrology's International Consortium of Collaborators on CKDu

mini review

470 **Pretransplant screening for coronary artery disease: data are required before practice change**
John S. Gill and Steven J. Chadban

review

473 **Complement activation and effector pathways in membranous nephropathy**
Andreas D. Kistler and David J. Salant

basic research

484 **A proteomic atlas of kidney amyloidosis provides insights into disease pathogenesis**
Charalampos Charalampous, Surendra Dasari, Ellen McPhail, Jason D. Theis, Julie A. Vrana, Angela Dispenzieri, Nelson Leung, Eli Muchtar, Morie Gertz, Marina Ramirez-Alvarado and Taxiarchis Kourelis

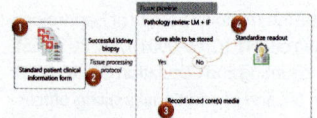

See page 464

contents

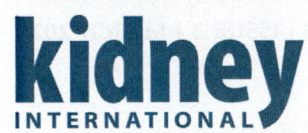

VOL 105 | ISSUE 3 | MARCH 2024

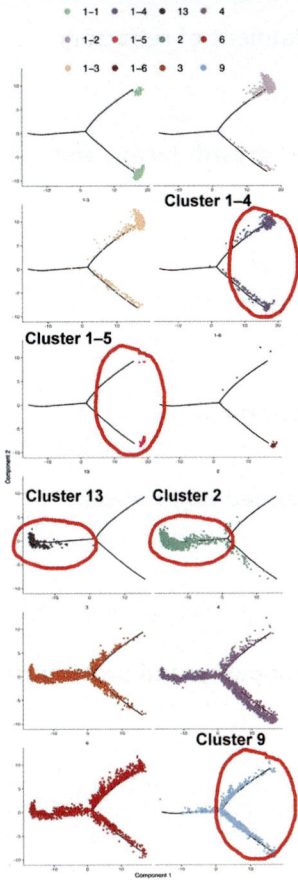

See page 562

496 **In vivo base editing rescues primary hyperoxaluria type 1 in rats**
Zhoutong Chen, Dexin Zhang, Rui Zheng, Lei Yang, Yanan Huo, Dan Zhang, Xiaoliang Fang, Yueyan Li, Guofeng Xu, Dali Li and Hongquan Geng

508 **Fibroblastic reticular cell-derived exosomes are a promising therapeutic approach for septic acute kidney injury**
Yiming Li, Chang Hu, Pan Zhai, Jing Zhang, Jun Jiang, Jinmeng Suo, Bo Hu, Jing Wang, Xiaocheng Weng, Xiang Zhou, Timothy R. Billiar, John A. Kellum, Meihong Deng and Zhiyong Peng OPEN

524 **Collectin 11 has a pivotal role in host defense against kidney and bladder infection in mice**
Kun-Yi Wu, Bo Cao, Wan-Bing Chen, Weiju Wu, Shujuan Zhao, Xiao-Yun Min, Jurong Yang, Jin Han, Xia Dong, Na Wang, Yi Wu, Peter Garred, Steven H. Sacks, Wuding Zhou and Ke Li

540 **Chronic kidney disease in a murine model of non-alcoholic steatohepatitis (NASH)**
Xuezhu Li, Dipankar Bhattacharya, Yue Yuan, Chengguo Wei, Fang Zhong, Feng Ding, Vivette D. D'Agati, Kyung Lee, Scott L. Friedman and John Cijiang He

clinical investigation

562 **Single-cell RNA sequencing reveals transdifferentiation of parathyroid chief cells into oxyphil cells in patients with uremic secondary hyperparathyroidism**
Jianping Mao, Huaizhou You, Mengjing Wang, Yongbing Ba, Jing Qian, Ping Cheng, Chuhan Lu and Jing Chen

582 **Evaluation of novel candidate filtration markers from a global metabolomic discovery for glomerular filtration rate estimation**
Nora F. Fino, Ogechi M. Adingwupu, Josef Coresh, Tom Greene, Ben Haaland, Michael G. Shlipak, Veronica T. Costa e Silva, Roberto Kalil, Ayse L. Mindikoglu, Susan L. Furth, Jesse C. Seegmiller, Andrew S. Levey and Lesley A. Inker

593 **Idiopathic collapsing glomerulopathy is associated with *APOL1* high-risk genotypes or Mendelian variants in most affected individuals in a highly admixed population**
Precil D. Neves, Andreia Watanabe, Elieser H. Watanabe, Amanda M. Narcizo, Kelly Nunes, Antonio M. Lerario, Frederico M. Ferreira, Lívia B. Cavalcante, Janewit Wongboonsin, Denise M. Malheiros, Lectícia B. Jorge, Matthew G. Sampson, Irene L. Noronha and Luiz F. Onuchic

608 **A multi-institutional study found a possible role of anti-nephrin antibodies in post-transplant focal segmental glomerulosclerosis recurrence**
Yoko Shirai, Kenichiro Miura, Kiyonobu Ishizuka, Taro Ando, Shoichiro Kanda, Junya Hashimoto, Yuko Hamasaki, Kiyohiko Hotta, Naoko Ito, Kazuho Honda, Kenji Tanabe, Tomoko Takano and Motoshi Hattori

618 **A population-based cohort defined risk of hyperkalemia after initiating SGLT-2 inhibitors, GLP1 receptor agonists or DPP-4 inhibitors to patients with chronic kidney disease and type 2 diabetes**
Edouard L. Fu, Julianna Mastrorilli, Katsiaryna Bykov, Deborah J. Wexler, Alexander Cervone, Kueiyu Joshua Lin, Elisabetta Patorno and Julie M. Paik

629 **Performance of the European Kidney Function Consortium (EKFC) creatinine-based equation in United States cohorts**
Pierre Delanaye, Andrew D. Rule, Elke Schaeffner, Etienne Cavalier, Junyan Shi, Andrew N. Hoofnagle, Ulf Nyman, Jonas Björk and Hans Pottel

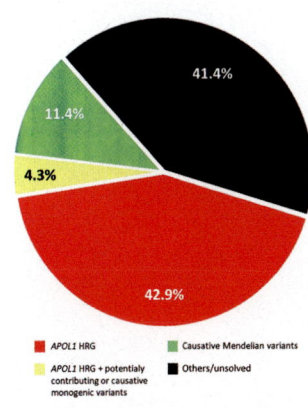

See page 593

contents

VOL 105 | ISSUE 3 | MARCH 2024

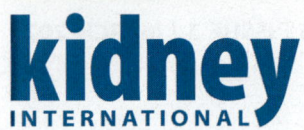

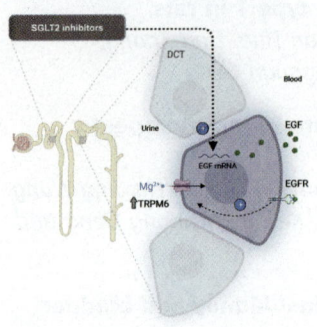

See page 638

letters to the editor

638 **Sodium-glucose cotransporter 2 inhibitors in the treatment of refractory hypomagnesemia**
Armando Luis Negri

638 **Sodium-glucose cotransporter 2 inhibition, epidermal growth factor, and magnesium homeostasis: is there a link?**
Chintan V. Shah

639 **The authors reply**
Wenjun Ju, Hiddo J.L. Heerspink, Matthias Kretzler and Petter Bjornstad

nephrology image

640 **Bile cast nephropathy after sinusoidal obstruction syndrome**
Toshiki Terao, Kyosuke Horikawa and Ken-ichi Matsuoka

641 **Cardiac tamponade diagnosed on nephrologist-performed point-of-care ultrasonography**
Aisha Batool and Abhilash Koratala

make your diagnosis

643 **The Case | A patient with skin rash, monoclonal gammopathy, and proteinuria**
Justyna Fryc and Beata Naumnik

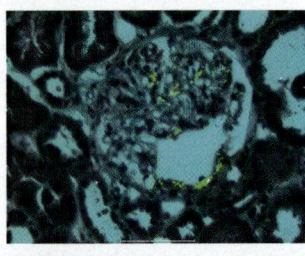

See page 643

A multi-institutional study found a possible role of anti-nephrin antibodies in post-transplant focal segmental glomerulosclerosis recurrence

Shirai *et al.* measured the levels of anti-nephrin antibodies in 22 Japanese children who received kidney transplants for kidney failure due to focal segmental glomerulosclerosis (FSGS). The children who had a genetic cause of FSGS and those who had no recurrence of FSGS after transplant had anti-nephrin antibody levels that were comparable to healthy individuals. All 11 patients who had post-transplant recurrence of FSGS had very high levels of anti-nephrin antibodies in serum before transplantation or after recurrence. Transplant biopsies showed punctate IgG colocalized with nephrin, and nephrin tyrosine phosphorylation was increased. Anti-nephrin antibody levels decreased significantly in patients who achieved remission of recurrent FSGS but remained high in those who did not remit. These data are suggestive of a causal link between anti-nephrin antibodies and FSGS recurrence after transplant. These findings will need to be confirmed in a diverse patient population. **See page 608**

Idiopathic collapsing glomerulopathy is associated with *APOL1* high-risk genotypes or Mendelian variants in most affected individuals in a highly admixed population

The incidence of collapsing glomerulopathy (CG) with progression to kidney failure seems to be higher in Brazil than other countries. To investigate this, Neves *et al.* looked at the genetics of a highly admixed Brazilian cohort of 70 adult and pediatric patients with CG. A causative genetic basis for CG was found in approximately 60% of these patients. Of these patients, 80.5% had a high-risk *APOL1* genotype and 19.5% had causative Mendelian variants. The Mendelian variants included several previously associated genes (*MYH9*, *TRPC6*, *COQ2*, *COL4A3*, *and TTC21B*), as well as novel gene variants in *COL4A5*, *COQ2*, and *PLCE1*. These data suggest that genetic causes account for the high level of idiopathic CG in Brazil. **See page 593**

A proteomic atlas of kidney amyloidosis provides insights into disease pathogenesis

Charalampos *et al.* characterized the amyloid plaque proteomes laser microdissected from kidney tissues from over 2500 patients with amyloidosis. The investigation included cases of light chain (AL), heavy chain (AH), leukocyte chemotactic factor 2 type (ALECT2), secondary (AA), fibrinogen (AFib), apo AIV (AApoAIV), and apo CII (AApoCII) amyloidosis. The impetus for this study was to determine if the proteins within amyloid plaques could identify the mechanisms by which amyloid deposition damages the kidney. Although each type of amyloid displayed unique and common proteins, and although the proteomes of some types of amyloid clustered near each other, and others were far more distinct, complement proteins seemed to be a common element in all of the plaques. These data beg the question of whether complement activation may be a common mechanism of tissue injury in amyloidosis. Given the large number of complement therapeutics available now, the implications are clear. **See page 484**

Chronic kidney disease in a murine model of non-alcoholic steatohepatitis (NASH)

Nonalcoholic steatohepatitis (NASH) has been considered clinically to be a risk factor for chronic kidney disease, but a direct link has not been established. Li *et al.* undertook an investigation to demonstrate a causal relationship using a well-characterized murine model of NASH. They studied the kidneys of NASH mice and noted that the animals developed proteinuria, glomerulosclerosis, interstitial fibrosis, and an accumulation of intrarenal lipid. Transcriptomic analysis of kidney cortices from NASH mice demonstrated a dysregulated metabolic signature, whereas metabolomic studies demonstrated that phospho- and sphingolipids were the most prominently dysregulated renal lipids. Proving causality, liver transplantation was found to attenuate kidney dysfunction, fibrosis, and proteinuria. **See page 540**

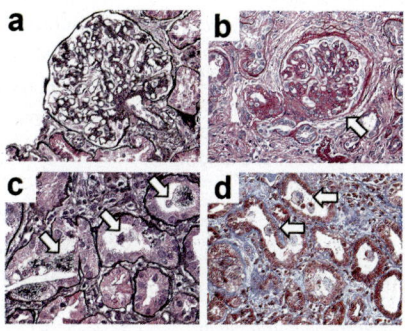

In remembrance of Eberhard Ritz, MD (1938–2023)

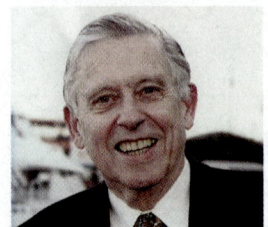

Eberhard Ritz

Kai-Uwe Eckardt[1] and Kerstin Amann[2]

[1]Department of Nephrology and Medical Intensive Care, Charité–Universitätsmedizin Berlin, Berlin, Germany; and [2]Institute of Nephropathology, University Hospital Erlangen, Erlangen, Germany

Correspondence: Kai-Uwe Eckardt, Department of Nephrology and Medical Intensive Care, Charité – Universitätsmedizin Berlin, Charitéplatz 1, Berlin 10117, Germany. E-mail: kai-uwe.eckardt@charite.de

Eberhard Ritz, one of the most prominent nephrologists to date and a past president of the International Society of the Nephrology (ISN) died on October 29, 2023, at the age of 85 years. He was a polymath and a cosmopolitan whose exceptional talents and aspiration have left a deep impact on clinical nephrology.

Eberhard was born in Heidelberg, Germany, where he spent most of his life. Despite the difficult circumstances under which he grew up during and after the war, his multiple talents and broad interests in natural sciences, languages, history, and music soon became obvious. When he decided to study medicine, some of his teachers felt this was a waste of talent and that he was better suited to philosophy or history. Nevertheless, he attained his goal at the universities of Heidelberg, Montpellier (France), and Munich. Subsequently, in 1964, he started his clinical training in Zurich (Switzerland) under the supervision of Walter Siegenthaler, one of the leading internists at that time, whom Eberhard Ritz had long admired. In 1966, he moved to JE Kirk's lab at Washington University in St. Louis, Missouri, as a National Institutes of Health (NIH) postdoctoral fellow, to study the pentose cycle and the metabolism of acid mucopolysaccharides in experimental and human atherosclerosis.

When he returned to Germany, Eberhard Ritz wanted to pursue his interest in vascular biology and disease in the Department of Medicine at Heidelberg University. To his dismay, the department chief had other plans. A talented doctor was urgently required to establish a dialysis unit, as the local urologist wanted to start a transplant program, which he could not do without a dialysis facility. Eberhard strongly protested against being given this assignment, but eventually, he relented, and nephrology became his second love. He successfully built the dialysis unit and expanded it into an independent kidney center, affiliated with the university hospital, and he directed it as Professor of Nephrology from 1974 until his retirement in 2003. He led the center, with its 20 beds, 20 dialysis stations, a large outpatient unit, and research facilities, with great passion and skill, taking responsibility for an increasing number of patients and junior doctors entering the new field.

His early publications, which reflected his interest in basic vascular biology, were soon augmented with clinically relevant publications related to the many health problems and comorbidities of those affected by kidney disease. This work was the foundation of an amazing legacy of close to 1500 publications listed in PubMed, spanning an unusually broad scope of topics. His genuine scientific curiosity, exceptional intellectual capacity, readiness of mind, and remarkable memory allowed him to pursue many different areas of research. Clinical need, careful observation, and interventional studies form the backbone of this work, supplemented whenever possible with experimental approaches. He thereby developed a keen sense for the importance of topics, and he chose to focus on several areas that subsequently proved to have lasting relevance.

He was always interested in the role of hypertension in the development and progression of kidney disease. Early on, he proposed that blood pressure in patients with chronic kidney disease should be lowered as far as possible, provided this did not cause fainting—a stance that was highly controversial at the time. The dominant role of diabetes in the global epidemiology of kidney disease had also been strongly underestimated; Eberhard and others sounded the alert to the nephrology community regarding this rising tide. He not only provided a warning, but also was instrumental in conducting important treatment trials with renin–angiotensin system inhibitors, or statins.[1,2]

An additional, related area of focus allowed Eberhard Ritz to pursue his early interest in vascular pathophysiology even more directly— the importance of cardiovascular comorbidities associated with kidney disease. Again, what is now common knowledge had not been established when Eberhard started studying this interdisciplinary area, and with his coworkers, made the observation that a marked cardiomyopathy in rodents followed subtotal nephrectomy.[3] Also, his interest in antenatal priming for arterial hypertension and kidney disease in adulthood was visionary. The 2003 *New England Journal of Medicine* autopsy study of accident victims was an extraordinary example of his ambition to derive important conclusions from clinical observations.[4] This study showed that young adults with hypertension have half the number of glomeruli as nonhypertensive individuals, but a more than twofold higher average glomerular volume.

Beyond his delivery of patient care and making original scientific contributions, his third passion was medical education in a broad sense. "I love teaching" was a motto Eberhard followed during his career in many ways,[5] and he was always proud of the large number of students and fellows who benefited from their connection with him. Beyond training individuals, he also set standards for postgraduate education in nephrology, be it through his publications or his contributions to symposia and courses. A particular focus of his activities was Middle and Eastern Europe. He praised the end of the Cold War and supported nephrologists from these areas by offering fellowships in his kidney center, remaining for most a dedicated partner and mentor.

In 1976, Eberhard Ritz founded the Heidelberger Seminar, an annual meeting to discuss hot topics and the latest developments in nephrology. The program was structured into 3 main areas—advances in renal physiology, problems in clinical nephrology, and case discussions—reflecting his systematic approach to the field and his broad oversight. During the discussions following the presentations, he was frequently able to establish unexpected connections and add recently discovered details to the diverse topics. Although addressing primarily a national audience of practicing nephrologists, Eberhard took the opportunity to invite international colleagues to all of these meetings. The list of these guest speakers reads like a "who's who" of nephrology during these decades. For several of them, the invitation to Heidelberg was one of their first contacts with nephrology in Germany. Eberhard's high aspiration for innovation and in-depth understanding, in combination with his warm hospitality and strong foundation in history and culture, shaped their perceptions and created long-lasting memories. In his recognition, the Heidelberger Seminar continues, organized by a group of his former coworkers, who are already looking forward to its upcoming 50th anniversary in 3 years.

Eberhard not only brought kidney disease knowledge to Heidelberg, but also exported it, serving as an ambassador of the field worldwide. He was an esteemed speaker at countless international meetings, symposia, and congresses, and a lecturer at many foreign institutions. His language skills and the ability to address audiences in not only English, but also French, Italian, Spanish, Dutch, Polish, and Russian, certainly contributed to his enormous international recognition.

Eberhard's passion for medical education also encompassed his engagement on editorial boards of kidney journals. Most prominent in this context was his responsibility as the second Editor-in-Chief of *Nephrology, Dialysis and Transplantation* (*NDT*), between 1993 and 1999, following the tenure of his friend A.M. Davison from the UK. Although citation tools had already started to influence the whole publication process, Eberhard resisted their dominance. He was not aiming for a high citation index, but rather for a journal that was highly useful to its readers. At the same time, he recognized the need for a publication platform for an expanding European kidney research community. Eberhard saw his role as an Editor-in-Chief as not only to select the best publications, but also to be a scout, continuously watching the field and not infrequently inviting colleagues to submit position statements, reviews, or case reports. When Tilman Drueke followed Eberhard as the next Editor-in-Chief of *NDT*, he faced the challenge of maintaining the popularity of the journal while reducing its size, which had significantly increased.

Eberhard also served professional societies in other capacities, which he always considered opportunities to improve education, as well as diagnostic and therapeutic standards. He was a council member of the Gesellschaft für Nephrologie and the European Renal Association (ERA), chairman of the Eastern Europe Committee of the Commission for the Global Advancement of Nephrology (COMGAN) of the ISN and Congress President of the unique World Congress of Nephrology 2003, organized jointly by ERA, ISN, two German societies, the European Kidney Research Association (EKRA), and the European Society of Pediatric Nephrology (ESPN). Between 2007 and 2009, he was president of the ISN.

Reflecting a high level of international recognition, Eberhard Ritz was an honorary member of not only the German Nephrological Society, but also 9 additional renal societies on 3 continents. Moreover, the Slesian Academy of Medicine (Katowice), the Pomerian Medical Academy (Szszecin), the Semmelweis University Budapest (Hungary), and the Gr. Z. Poppa University of Medicine and Pharmacy in Iasi (Romania) each awarded him with an honorary doctorate. The most outstanding recognitions among his many prestigious awards are the John P. Peters Award of the American Society of Nephrology (ASN), given in 2003, as well as the lifetime award of the ERA, and the Jean-Hamburger Award of the ISN, both of which he received in 2011.

Along with his multiple talents, drivers of Eberhard's success include his enormous diligence, self-discipline, and a deep humanitarian conviction that he applied similarly to the care of individual patients in Heidelberg and his activities in the ISN. He was self-confident and humble at the same time. Despite all the recognition he received at the center of his field, he was concerned about the future of nephrology; he deplored the fact that it lagged behind other medical disciplines with respect to the molecular understanding of disease processes and targeted interventions. Unfortunately, he was not able to witness the very recent innovative developments in nephrology that hopefully indicate a turning point in this regard. He would have analyzed them with intellectual joy and embraced them with enthusiasm, two of his outstanding qualities for which we will always remember him.

Eberhard is survived by his loving wife Christina, and their 4 children and 5 grandchildren, whose warm and continuous support has been a very important source of strength for him in his personal and professional life.

ACKNOWLEDGMENTS
The authors thank Martin Zeier and Johannes Mann for their assistance in the preparation of this obituary.

REFERENCES
1. Lewis EJ, Hunsicker LG, Clarke WR, et al. *N Engl J Med*. 2001;345:851–860.
2. Wanner C, Krane V, März W, et al. Atrovastatin in patients with type 2 diabetes mellitus undergoing hemodialysis. *N Engl J Med*. 2005;353:238–248.
3. Amann K, Wiest G, Zimmer G, et al. Reduced capillary density in the myocardium of uremic rats. *Kidney Int*. 1992;42:1079–1085.
4. Keller G, Zimmer G, Mall G, et al. Nephron number in patients with primary hypertension. *N Engl J Med*. 2003;348:101–108.
5. Eberhard Ritz: Pioneers of European Nephrology. Accessed December 13, 2023. https://www.youtube.com/watch?v=e8sSiNxk720

A tribute to Edmund J Lewis, MD

Kidney International (2024) 105, 403–405; https://doi.org/10.1016/j.kint.2024.01.003

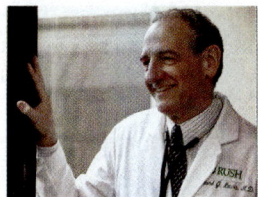

Ed Lewis circa 1990.

Stephen M. Korbet[1]

[1]Division of Nephrology, Department of Internal Medicine, Rush University Medical Center, Chicago, Illinois, USA

Correspondence: Stephen M. Korbet, Division of Nephrology, Department of Internal Medicine, Rush University Medical Center, 1426 W. Washington Blvd., Chicago, Illinois 60607, USA. E-mail: stephen_m_korbet@rush.edu

On November 12, 2023, the world lost an amazingly talented and brilliant individual. I personally lost a mentor, colleague, collaborator, and friend.

Edmund Jean Lewis was born on November 10, 1936, into a working-class Jewish family in New York City. His father was a high steel welder, and his mother was an accountant. He had a younger sister who died at the age of 12 from kernicterus, an event that had an effect on him for the rest of his life. Although he made his career as a physician working in hospitals, he absolutely hated being a patient, and I think it was in no small part a result of the experience that he had watching his sister suffer.

Ed graduated college cum laude in 1958 with a BS degree from McGill University in Montreal. He was also on the varsity swim team. He attended medical school at the University of British Columbia in Vancouver, was elected into Alpha Omega Alpha, and graduated in 1962. He told me that he trained in Canada because at that time there were limits to admission for Jews in many universities in the United States and it was not uncommon to leave the country to matriculate.

He completed his residency in internal medicine at Johns Hopkins Hospital and was a research fellow at the Robert Breck Brigham Hospital, Harvard Medical School in Boston under the guidance of John Merrill, MD. In 1969, he became the Chief of the renal division at the Thorndike Memorial Laboratory of Harvard Medical Unit in Boston City Hospital where his research career really began.

Ed's primary research interest was in the immunology of glomerulonephritis. Even at an early stage of his career, it was clear that he was a visionary, publishing an article in the *New England Journal of Medicine*, which supported the concept that glomerulonephritis could in part be a result of cellular hypersensitivity to glomerular basement membrane antigens.[1] This theory came under great criticism at a time when it was felt that glomerular injury was due to autoantibodies and immune complexes. Several decades later, Ed was vindicated when the proof of this mechanism was provided first by his former fellow Kline Bolton at the University of Virginia and later by several other laboratories.

Dr. Lewis' work in the area of immunologic mechanisms of renal disease caught the attention of 2 aspiring nephrologists, William (Bill) Couser and Kline Bolton, who were completing their internal medicine residency at the Harvard Medical Unit at the Boston City Hospital. They were so intrigued by Ed's research that they elected to work with him at the Thorndike Medical Laboratory. In 1971, Ed was recruited to be the head of the Section of Nephrology at the University of Chicago, Pritzker School of Medicine, and Bill and Kline followed him as his first nephrology fellows.

After completing their fellowship, Dr. Couser, first at Boston University and later as Scribner Professor and Head of the Division of Nephrology at the University of Washington, continued studying immunologic mechanisms of glomerulonephritis, and his first fellow, David Salant, continued research in the field leading to the discovery of the PLA2R antigen in membranous glomerulonephritis. Kline Bolton became Chief of the Nephrology Division at the University of Virginia, where his laboratory was the first to confirm Ed's hypothesis that T cells could mediate several forms of glomerulonephritis.

In 1973, Ed was recruited to be Director of the Section of Nephrology at Rush Presbyterian St. Luke's Medical Center (now Rush University Medical Center) by Dr. Robert Kark. Dr. Kark felt that Ed's interest in immunologic mechanisms of renal disease made him a perfect candidate to carry on the legacy that Drs. Kark, Muehrcke, Pollack, and Pirani had established in defining lupus nephritis. Ed became the Muehrcke Family Professor of Nephrology at Rush and held this position for over 40 years.

After arriving at Rush, he recruited a young nephropathologist, Dr. Melvin M. Schwartz, whom he had met at Boston City Hospital. In the early days at Rush, Ed and Mel along with their colleagues, Jimmy Roberts and Zev Sharon, continued to pursue basic research in the area of immunologic renal disease. And, as part of the Nephrology Fellowship Training Program, Ed and Mel instituted the renal biopsy conference, which was held every Thursday afternoon and attracted nephrologists from other local institutions. This conference continues to this day but is now live virtually with an international audience.

I first met Ed in 1976 as a second-year medical student at Rush when he was leading the renal pathophysiology course. It was the best course I had experienced, consisting of 12 lectures and 8 three-hour workshops that were "case-based." The case-based method may not seem novel today, but it was completely revolutionary at the time. I later met Ed as a second-year resident during my rotation on the nephrology service. I was struck by his charisma and how knowledgeable he was. And, I found him to be an exceptional clinician. At that point, I was hooked on nephrology.

Through the years, medical students and residents from outside institutions would rotate on the Nephrology Service at Rush to experience the genius of Ed Lewis. In 1982, when Ed was the attending and I was the fellow, a fourth-year medical student from the University of Illinois, Brad Rovin, made a point to rotate on the nephrology service at Rush in order to be with Ed. Dr. Rovin's subsequent success in the field of glomerulonephritis is well known.

In 1979, Ed directed his focus from bench research to conducting clinical trials. He along with Marc Pohl (Cleveland Clinic Foundation), Lee Hebert (Ohio State University), and Larry Hunsicker (University of Iowa) organized the Lupus Nephritis Collaborative Study Group (later to become the Collaborative Study Group [CSG]). Ed believed that studies should be "investigator-directed," which meant the CSG would exclusively be responsible for developing the protocols, managing the data, and writing the final manuscripts, not "industry." There was no compromise on this, and as the CSG's principal investigator, he subsequently passed up many opportunities for major clinical trials in which he felt that the CSG did not have the ultimate control.

The CSG's initial study (National Institutes of Health–funded) sought to address whether the addition of plasmapheresis to standard immunosuppressive therapy would be beneficial in the treatment of severe lupus nephritis. Plasmapheresis was becoming a popular therapy for severe lupus nephritis despite the lack of controlled data to support its use. And while the study, published in the *New England Journal of Medicine* in 1992,[2] reported that plasmapheresis offered no significant advantage in the treatment of severe lupus nephritis, the clinical pathologic information gained from this study was instrumental in the revised lupus nephritis classification published in 2004 by the International Society of Nephrology/Renal Pathology Society. There were at least 20 more publications that arose from the data generated from the "plasmapheresis" trial. In addition, Ed edited a book entitled *Lupus Nephritis* with editions in 1999 and 2011.

The CSG turned their efforts to evaluating the effect of angiotensin-converting enzyme inhibitors and angiotensin receptor blockers on type I and type II diabetic nephropathy, respectively. The results of the industry-sponsored "Captopril Trial"[3] and the Irbesartan in Diabetes nephropathy trial[4] took the laboratory work of Barry Brenner of the effect of renin-angiotensin-aldosterone system inhibition on the progression of renal disease in animal models to humans. These were landmark trials that changed the trajectory of progressive kidney disease in patients with diabetic as well as nondiabetic renal disease. It is arguable that fewer things in nephrology have had a larger impact on the lives of patients with kidney disease than renoprotection afforded by renin-angiotensin-aldosterone system inhibition. Over these impactful clinical trials, the CSG grew from investigators at 12 institutions in the United States to over 250 investigators in 25 countries internationally.

Ed ran the section of nephrology at Rush for over 40 years and, during that time, fostered the careers of over 100 fellows. Ed loved tradition. Every Friday afternoon in the nephrology conference room, a bottle of wine would be served during the "sign-out" of the clinical service to the attending, fellow, and residents who would be covering for the weekend. At Christmas time, he and the chief research technician, Richard Rohde, would make "renal punch." This was a concoction that consisted of grain alcohol, champagne, and peach brandy, and orange juice was added to give it the appearance of urine. Ed would proudly serve this potent brew up using a urinal. Although these events are clearly a thing of the past, they were legendary during their time. Whenever an attending was promoted or some honor was bestowed to one of the faculty, Ed would take the entire faculty to an exclusive private French restaurant that he was a member at.

Ed was truly a renaissance man. He loved the opera and the symphony and had season tickets to both. He was a world traveler, but his favorite destination was Hawaii, where he and his family

obituary

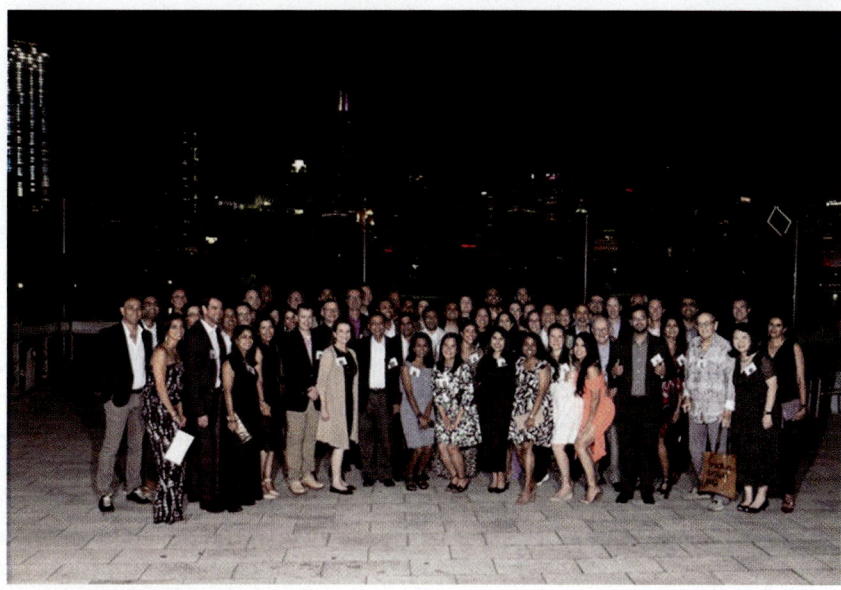

Figure 1 | September 2023 fellow reunion. Ed is in the front row, second from the right.

would go once or twice a year. One of his greatest loves, however, was Asian art. Just as he excelled in medicine, he approached Asian art the same way. He amassed an amazing collection that on 2 occasions was the subject of exhibits at prestigious museums. He wrote numerous academic articles about Asian art and published 2 books. Ed had 2 separate lives, one in the world of art and the other in the world of medicine. I will never forget when he and the love of his life, Julia, were married in 1997; I met a number of his friends from the art world, and all were amazed to find out that Ed was actually a physician. He had never talked about it with them, and thus, they had no idea.

I am grateful that I had 40 years with this amazing individual. My experiences and collaboration with him and Mel were truly some of the best times in my life. I cannot imagine my professional trajectory without him. When Ed turned 80, Julie had a birthday party for him at Brown's Hotel in London, which was attended by his family and 40 of his closest friends in the Asian art world and medicine. I was fortunate that at that occasion, I was able to formally tell him how much I appreciated him and how much he had changed my life.

About a month before his passing, our colleague and fellowship program director, Roger Rodby, organized a reunion of fellows who had trained at Rush over the past 50 years. Over 70 fellows attended the reunion as did Ed (Figure 1) and Mel Schwartz. One after another of his former trainees used this opportunity to thank him for the role he played in their career. Giants like Edmund Jean Lewis do not leave this earth without a huge impact.

ACKNOWLEDGMENTS

The author would like to thank Dr. Roger Rodby for his much-appreciated assistance in editing this tribute. And, I greatly appreciate Drs. William Couser, Kline Bolton, Marc Pohl, and Julia Lewis for their valuable input.

REFERENCES

1. Rocklin RE, Lewis EJ, David JR. In vitro evidence for cellular hypersensitivity to glomerular-basement-membrane antigens in human glomerulonephritis. *N Engl J Med*. 1970;283:497–501.
2. Lewis EJ, Hunsicker LG, Lan SP, et al. A controlled trial of plasmapheresis therapy in severe lupus nephritis. The Lupus Nephritis Collaborative Study Group. *N Engl J Med*. 1992;326:1373–1379.
3. Lewis EJ, Hunsicker LG, Bain RP, Rohde RD. The effect of angiotensin-converting-enzyme inhibition on diabetic nephropathy. The Collaborative Study Group. *N Engl J Med*. 1993;329:1456–1462.
4. Lewis EJ, Hunsicker LG, Clarke WR, et al. Renoprotective effect of the angiotensin-receptor antagonist irbesartan in patients with nephropathy due to type 2 diabetes. *N Engl J Med*. 2001;345:851–860.

editorial: special report

Mind the gap in kidney care: translating what we know into what we do

Valerie A. Luyckx[1,2,3,18], Katherine R. Tuttle[4,5,18], Dina Abdellatif[6], Ricardo Correa-Rotter[7], Winston W.S. Fung[8], Agnès Haris[9], Li-Li Hsiao[2], Makram Khalife[10,19], Latha A. Kumaraswami[11], Fiona Loud[10,19], Vasundhara Raghavan[10,19], Stefanos Roumeliotis[12], Marianella Sierra[10,19], Ifeoma Ulasi[13], Bill Wang[10,19], Siu-Fai Lui[14], Vassilios Liakopoulos[15] and Alessandro Balducci[16]; for the World Kidney Day Joint Steering Committee[17]

[1]Department of Public and Global Health, Epidemiology, Biostatistics and Prevention Institute, University of Zurich, Zurich, Switzerland; [2]Renal Division, Department of Medicine, Brigham and Women's Hospital, Harvard Medical School, Boston, Massachusetts, USA; [3]Department of Paediatrics and Child Health, University of Cape Town, Cape Town, South Africa; [4]Providence Medical Research Center, Providence Inland Northwest Health, Spokane, Washington, USA; [5]Nephrology Division, Department of Medicine, University of Washington, Seattle, Washington, USA; [6]Department of Nephrology, Cairo University Hospital, Cairo, Egypt; [7]Department of Nephrology and Mineral Metabolism, National Medical Science and Nutrition Institute Salvador Zubiran, Mexico City, Mexico; [8]Department of Medicine and Therapeutics, Prince of Wales Hospital, The Chinese University of Hong Kong, Shatin, Hong Kong, China; [9]Nephrology Department, Péterfy Hospital, Budapest, Hungary; [10]ISN Patient Liaison Advisory Group; [11]Tamilnad Kidney Research (TANKER) Foundation, Chennai, India; [12]2nd Department of Nephrology, AHEPA University Hospital Medical School, Aristotle University of Thessaloniki, Thessaloniki, Greece; [13]Department of Medicine, College of Medicine, University of Nigeria, Ituku-Ozalla, Enugu, Nigeria; [14]Division of Health System, Policy and Management, Jockey Club School of Public Health and Primary Care, The Chinese University of Hong Kong, Hong Kong; [15]2nd Department of Nephrology, AHEPA University Hospital Medical School, Aristotle University of Thessaloniki, Thessaloniki, Greece; and [16]Italian Kidney Foundation, Rome, Italy

Historically, it takes an average of 17 years to move new treatments from clinical evidence to daily practice. Given the highly effective treatments now available to prevent or delay kidney disease onset and progression, this is far too long. The time is now to narrow the gap between what we know and what we do. Clear guidelines exist for the prevention and management of common risk factors for kidney disease, such as hypertension and diabetes, but only a fraction of people with these conditions worldwide are diagnosed, and even fewer are treated to target. Similarly, the vast majority of people living with kidney disease are unaware of their condition, because in the early stages it is often silent. Even among patients who have been diagnosed, many do not receive appropriate treatment for kidney disease. Considering the serious consequences of kidney disease progression, kidney failure, or death, it is imperative that treatments are initiated early and appropriately. Opportunities to diagnose and treat kidney disease early must be maximized beginning at the primary care level. Many systematic barriers exist, ranging from patient to clinician to health systems to societal factors. To preserve and improve kidney health for everyone everywhere, each of these barriers must be acknowledged so that sustainable solutions are developed and implemented without further delay.

Kidney International (2024) **105**, 406–417; https://doi.org/10.1016/j.kint.2023.12.003
KEYWORDS: chronic kidney disease; equity; kidney care; public health; World Kidney Day
Copyright © 2024 World Kidney Day Steering Committee. Published by Elsevier Inc., on behalf of the International Society of Nephrology. This is an open access article under the CC BY-NC-ND license (http://creativecommons.org/licenses/by-nc-nd/4.0/).

At least 1 in 10 people worldwide is living with kidney disease.[1] According to the Global Burden of Disease study, in 2019, >3.1 million deaths were attributed to kidney dysfunction, making it the seventh leading risk factor for death worldwide (Figure 1 and Supplementary Figure S1).[2] However, global mortality from all kidney diseases may actually range between 5 and 11 million per year if the estimated lives lost, especially in lower-resource settings, from acute kidney injury and from lack of access to kidney replacement therapy for kidney failure (KF) are also counted.[3] These high global death rates reflect disparities in prevention, early detection, diagnosis, and treatment of chronic kidney disease (CKD).[4] Death rates from CKD are especially prominent in some regions, and particularly high in Central Latin America and Oceania (islands of the South Pacific Ocean), indicating the need for urgent action.[5]

CKD also poses a significant global economic burden, with costs increasing exponentially as CKD progresses, not only because of the costs of dialysis and transplantation, but also because of the multiple comorbidities and complications that accumulate over time.[6,7] In the United States, Medicare fee-for-service spending for all beneficiaries with CKD was $86.1 billion in 2021 (22.6% of the total expenditure).[8] Data from many lower-resource settings are absent, where most costs are paid for out of pocket. A recent study from Vietnam reported that the cost of CKD per patient was higher than the gross

editorial: special report

This article is being published in *Kidney International* and is being reprinted in several journals. The articles cover identical concepts and wording, but vary in minor stylistic and spelling changes, detail, and length of manuscript in keeping with each journal's style. Any of these versions may be used in citing this article.

Correspondence: *Winston Fung, Department of Medicine and Therapeutics, Prince of Wales Hospital, The Chinese University of Hong Kong, Ninth Floor, Lui Che Woo Clinical Science Bldg, 32 Ngan Shing St, Shatin, Hong Kong. E-mail: fws898@ha.org.hk; or Valerie A. Luyckx, Department of Public and Global Health, Epidemiology, Biostatistics and Prevention Institute, University of Zurich, Hirschengraben 84, Zurich 8001, Switzerland. E-mail: valerie.luyckx@uzh.ch; or Katherine R. Tuttle, Providence Medical Research Center, Providence Inland Northwest Health, 105 W 8th Avenue, Suite 250 E, Spokane, Washington 99204, USA. E-mail: katherine.tuttle@providence.org*

domestic product per capita.[7] In Australia, it has been estimated that early diagnosis and prevention of CKD could save the health system $10.2 billion over 20 years.[9]

Although there is regional variation in the causes of CKD, the risk factors with the highest population-attributable factors for age-standardized CKD-related disease-adjusted life years were as follows: high blood pressure (51.4%), high fasting plasma glucose level (30.9%), and high body mass index (26.5%).[10] These risk factors are also global leading risk factors for death (Figure 1). Only 40% and 60% of those with hypertension and diabetes, respectively, are aware of their diagnosis, and far smaller proportions are receiving treatment and at target goals.[11,12] Moreover, at least 1 in 5 people with hypertension and 1 in 3 people with diabetes also have CKD.[13]

A large proportion of CKD can be prevented through healthy lifestyles, prevention and control of risk factors, avoidance of acute kidney injury, optimization of maternal and child health, mitigation of climate change, and addressing social and structural determinants of health.[3] Nevertheless, the benefits of some of these measures may only be seen in generations to come. In the meantime, early diagnosis and risk stratification create opportunities to institute therapies to slow, halt, or even reverse CKD.[14] Concerningly, CKD awareness was strikingly low among individuals with kidney dysfunction, with ≈80% to 95% of patients being unaware of their diagnosis across world regions (Figure 2).[15–20] People are dying because of missed opportunities to detect CKD early and deliver optimal care!

More important, CKD is a major risk factor for cardiovascular disease, and as kidney disease progresses, cardiovascular death and KF become competing risks.[21] Indeed, the Global Burden of Disease study data from 2019 showed that more people died of cardiovascular disease attributed to kidney dysfunction (1.7 million people) than from CKD itself (1.4 million people).[2] Therefore, cardiovascular disease care must also be a priority for people with CKD.

GAPS BETWEEN KNOWLEDGE AND IMPLEMENTATION IN KIDNEY CARE

Strategies to prevent and treat CKD have been built on a strong evidence base over the past 3 decades (Figure 3).[19,22] Clinical practice guidelines for CKD are clear; however, adherence to these guidelines is suboptimal (Figure 2).[15,19,20]

Regardless of the cause, control of major risk factors, particularly diabetes and hypertension, forms the foundation of optimal care for CKD.[19,23] Beyond lifestyle changes and risk factor control, the initial pharmacologic classes of agents proven to provide kidney protection

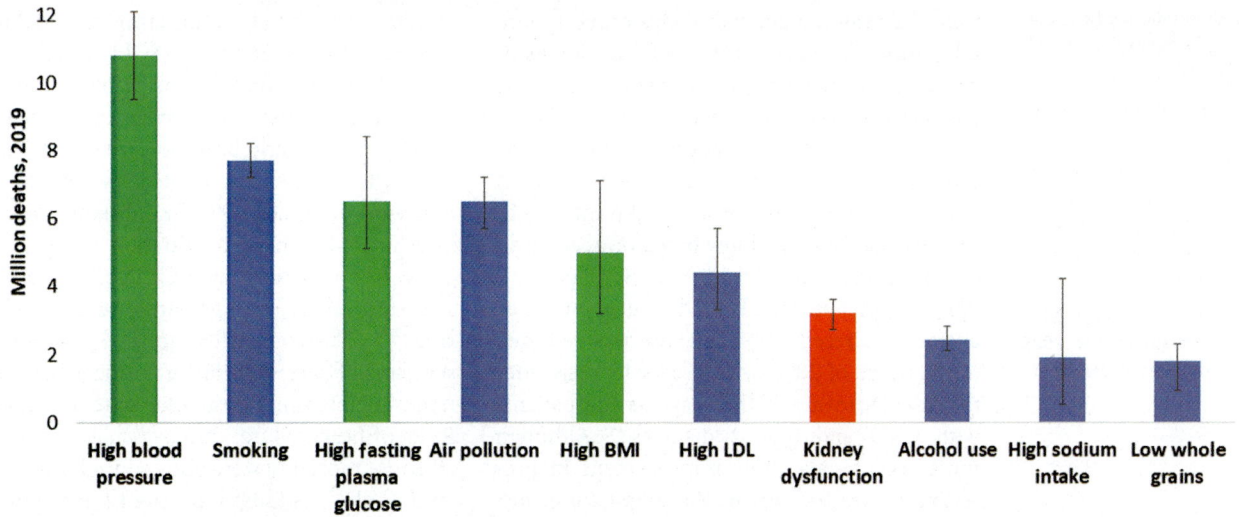

Figure 1 | All ages, top 10 global risk factors for death, 2019. Kidney dysfunction (defined as estimated glomerular filtration rate <60 ml/min per 1.73 m^2 or albumin-to-creatinine ratio ≥30 mg/g) was the seventh leading global level 3 risk factor for death in 2019. The 3 leading global risk factors for kidney disease, including hypertension, diabetes, and overweight/obesity, are also leading global risk factors for death; therefore, holistic strategies are required to address all risk factors simultaneously. Ranking is depicted by millions if deaths are attributed to the risk factors. Error bars depict the confidence range. Global ranking of kidney dysfunction stratified by World Bank income category and gender is shown in Supplementary Figure S1. Data obtained from the Global Burden of Disease Study.[2] BMI, body mass index; LDL, low-density lipoprotein.

editorial: special report

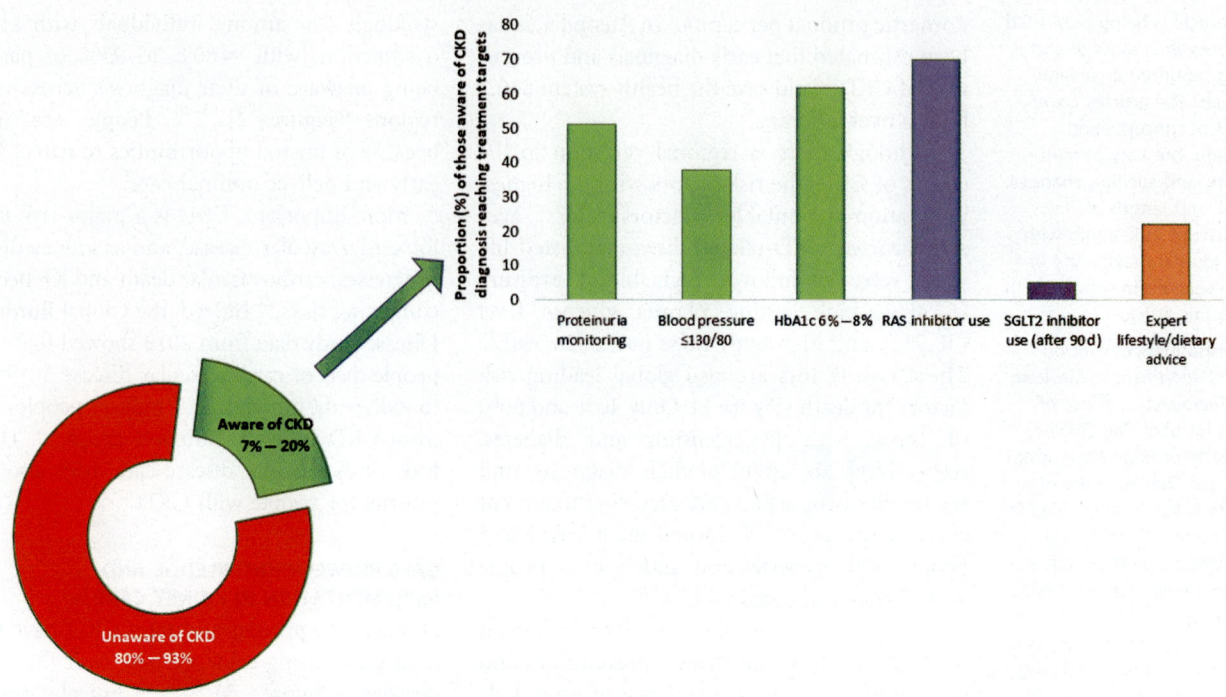

Figure 2 | Proportion of people with chronic kidney disease (CKD) who are aware of their diagnosis and are receiving appropriate guideline-recommended care. The proportion of people with CKD who are aware of their diagnosis varies globally, with rates ranging from 7% to 20%. As CKD stage worsens, knowledge of CKD increases. Among those with a diagnosis of CKD, the average proportion of patients receiving appropriate medication to delay CKD progression (renin-angiotensin-aldosterone system [RAS] inhibitors and sodium-glucose cotransporter 2 [SGLT2] inhibitors) is suboptimal as are those reaching target blood pressure, diabetes control, and nutrition advice. The treatment targets depicted in the figure follow the Kidney Disease: Improving Global Outcomes (KDIGO) 2012 guidelines.[15] Most data come from higher-resource settings; these proportions are likely lower in lower-resource settings. Data are shown for proportions of patients reaching blood pressure of <130/80 mm Hg. Data compiled from previous studies.[15–20] HbA1c, hemoglobin A1c.

[17]The World Kidney Day Joint Steering Committee is listed in the Appendix.

[18]VAL and KRT are joint first authors.

[19]MK, FL, VR, MS, and BW are patient representatives of the Patient Liaison Advisory Group of the International Society of Nephrology.

Received 25 October 2023; revised 18 November 2023; accepted 1 December 2023

were the renin-angiotensin-aldosterone system inhibitors in the form of angiotensin-converting enzyme inhibitors (ACEIs) and the angiotensin receptor blockers.[14,19] However, despite decades of knowledge that these medications have important protective effects on kidney and heart function in people with CKD, their use has remained low based on real-world data from electronic health records (Figure 2). For example, in the United States, ACEI or angiotensin receptor blocker use was reported in the range of 20% to 40% at ≥15 years after the last approvals of these agents for patients with CKD and type 2 diabetes.[24] Although more recent data show improvement in prescribing rates to 70% in this population, just 40% persist on an ACEI or angiotensin receptor blocker for at least 90 days.[20] These data illustrate gaps in both prescribing kidney protective medication and continuity of care over time, potentially related to cost, lack of patient education, polypharmacy, and adverse effects.[25]

Although initial enthusiasm for sodium-glucose cotransporter 2 (SGLT2) inhibitors focused on their benefits for diabetes and cardiovascular disease, unprecedented therapeutic benefits have clearly been observed for CKD as well. The relative risk reductions with SGLT2 inhibitors approach 40% for substantial decline in estimated glomerular filtration rate, KF, and death in populations with CKD of several causes, heart failure, or high cardiovascular disease risk.[26,27] These benefits accrued on top of standard-of-care risk factor management and renin-angiotensin-aldosterone system inhibitor. Risks of heart failure, cardiovascular death, and all-cause mortality were also reduced in patients with CKD.[26] Addition of SGLT2 inhibitor to renin-angiotensin-aldosterone system inhibitors could delay the need for kidney replacement therapy by several years, depending on when they are started.[28] Moreover, for every 1000 patients with CKD treated with an SGLT2 inhibitor on top of standard therapy, 83 deaths, 19

editorial: special report

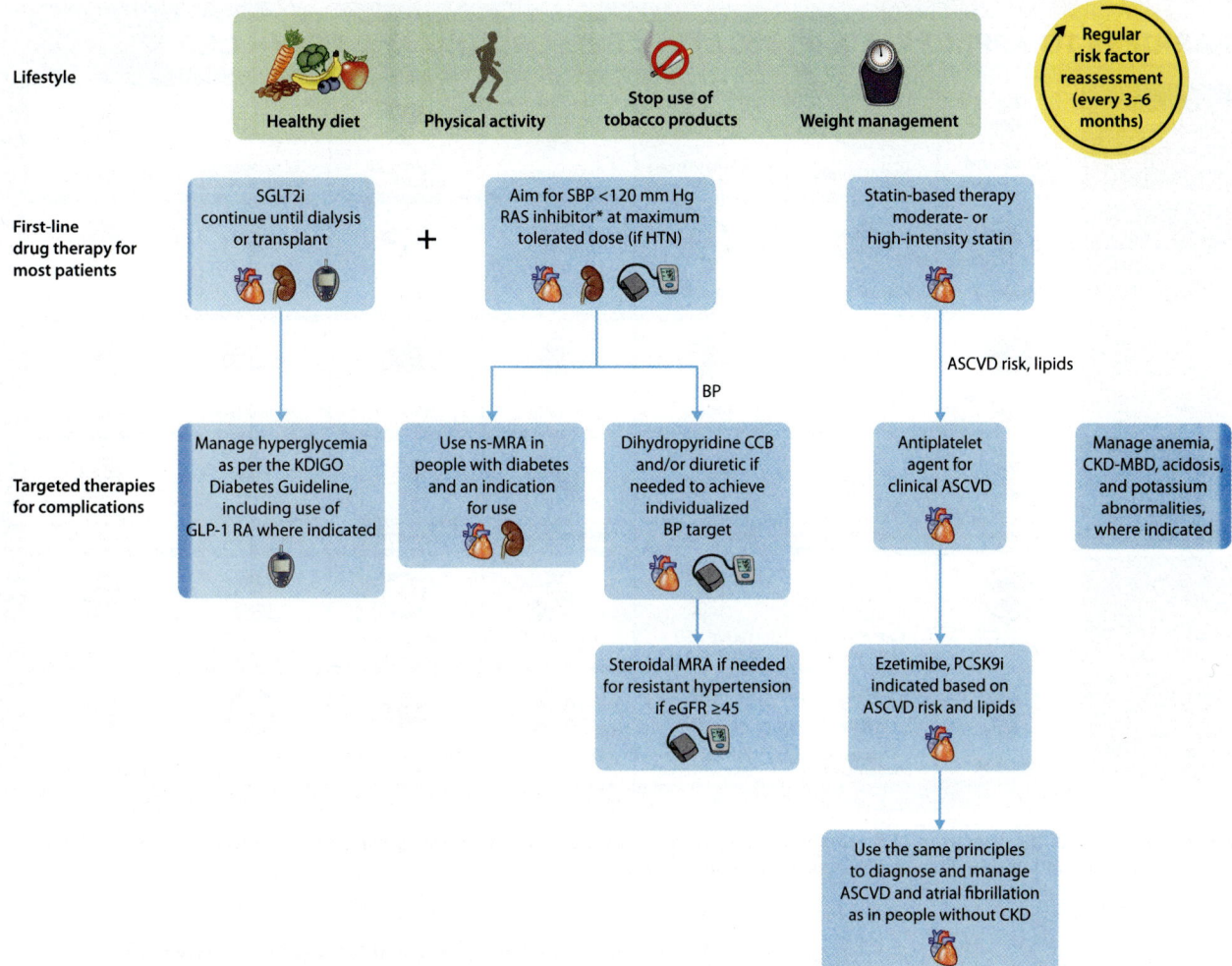

Figure 3 | Recommended optimal lifestyle and therapeutic management for chronic kidney disease (CKD) in diabetes. Illustration of a comprehensive and holistic approach to optimizing kidney health in people with CKD. In addition to the cornerstone lifestyle adjustments, attention to diabetes, blood pressure (BP), and cardiovascular risk factor control is intergral to kidney care. *Angiotensin-converting enzyme inhibitor or angiotensin II receptor blocker should be first-line therapy for BP control when albuminuria is present; otherwise dihydropyridine calcium channel blocker (CCB) or diuretic can also be considered. Figure reproduced from Kidney Disease: Improving Global Outcomes (KDIGO) CKD Work Group. KDIGO 2024 Clinical Practice Guideline for the Evaluation and Management of Chronic Kidney Disease. *Kidney Int*. https://doi.org/10.1016/j.kint.2023.10.018.[22] Copyright © 2023, Kidney Disease: Improving Global Outcomes (KDIGO). Published by Elsevier Inc. on behalf of the International Society of Nephrology under the CC BY-NC-ND license (http://creativecommons.org/licenses/by-nc-nd/4.0/). ASCVD, atherosclerotic cardiovascular disease; CKD-MBD, chronic kidney disease-mineral and bone disorder; eGFR, estimated glomerular filtration rate; GLP-1 RA, glucagon-like peptide-1 receptor agonist; HTN, hypertension; MRA, mineralocorticoid receptor antagonist; ns-MRA, nonsteroidal mineralocorticoid receptor antagonist; PCSK9i, proprotein convertase subtilisin/kexin type 9 inhibitor; RAS, renin-angiotensin-aldosterone system; SBP, systolic blood pressure; SGLT2i, sodium-glucose cotransporter 2 inhibitor.

heart failure hospitalizations, 51 dialysis initiations, and 39 episodes of acute kidney function worsening can be prevented.[29]

Concerningly, marked underuse of these and other guideline-recommended therapies, including SGLT2 inhibitors, persists (Figure 2).[20,24] In the CURE-CKD registry, only 5% and 6.3% of eligible patients with CKD and diabetes, respectively, continued on SGLT2 inhibitor and glucagon-like peptide-1 receptor agonist at 90 days.[18] Notably, lack of commercial health insurance and treatment in community-based versus academic institutions were associated with lower likelihoods of SGLT2 inhibitor, ACEI, or angiotensin receptor blocker prescriptions among patients with diabetes and CKD.[20] In low- or middle-income countries (LMICs), the gap between evidence and implementation is even wider given the high cost and inconsistent availability of these medications, despite availability of generics.[30] Such gaps in delivering optimal treatment for CKD are unacceptable.

In addition to the SGLT2 inhibitors, nonsteroidal mineralocorticoid receptor antagonists have been demonstrated to reduce the

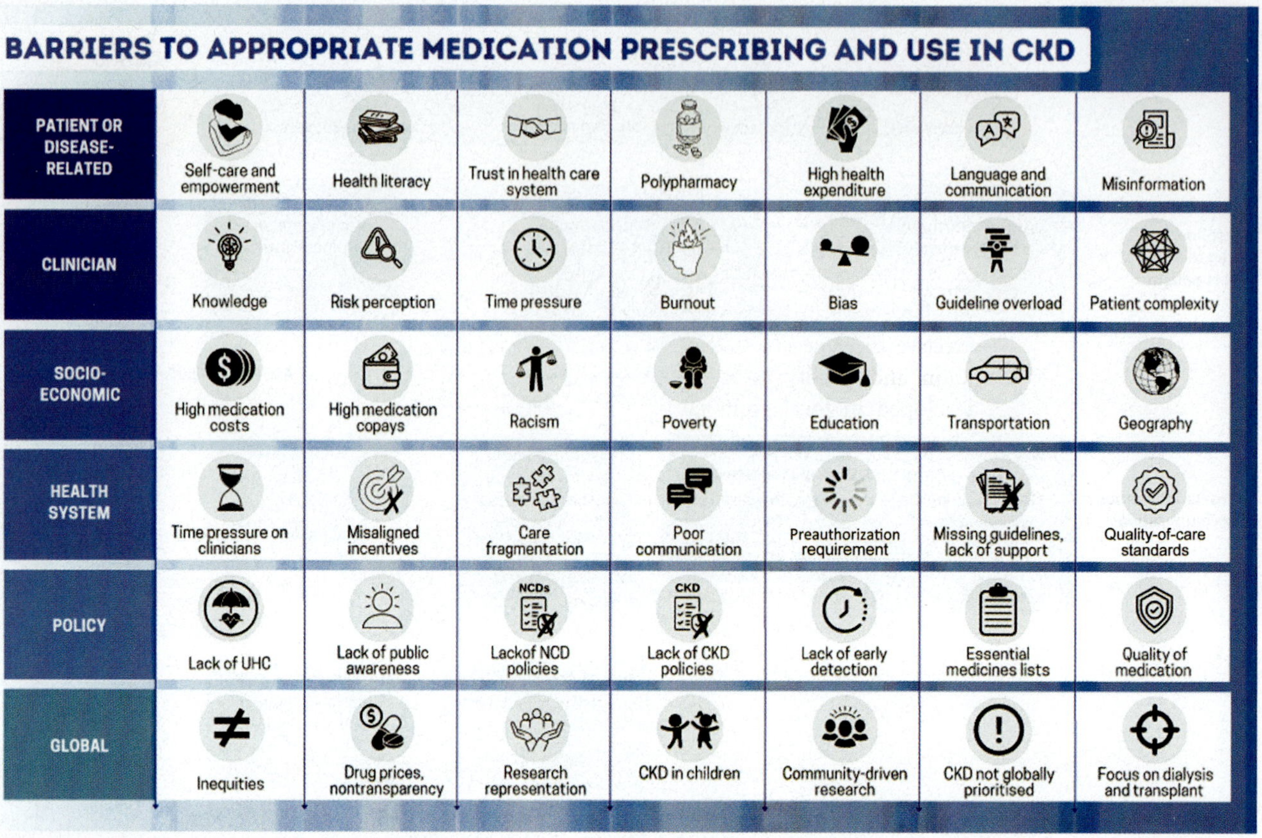

Figure 4 | Depiction of the spectrum of factors impacting implementation of timely and quality kidney care. CKD, chronic kidney disease; NCD, noncommunicable disease; UHC, universal health coverage.

risks of CKD progression, KF, cardiovascular events, and deaths, on top of the standard of care with renin-angiotensin-aldosterone system inhibitors, in type 2 diabetes.[31] A growing portfolio of promising therapeutic options is on the horizon with glucagon-like peptide-1 receptor agonists (NCT03819153, NCT04865770), aldosterone synthase inhibitors (NCT05182840), and dual-to-triple incretins (Supplementary Table S1).[26,32] Furthermore, the evidence is already clear that in patients with CKD and diabetes, glucagon-like peptide-1 receptor agonists reduce cardiovascular events, are safe and effective glucose-lowering therapies, and aid with weight loss.[32]

Historically, it has taken an average of 17 years to move new treatments from clinical evidence to daily practice.[33] With millions of people with CKD dying each year, this is far too long to wait.

CLOSING THE "Gap" BETWEEN WHAT WE KNOW AND WHAT WE DO
Lack of policies, global inequities

Health policy. Since the launch of the World Health Organization Action Plan for Non-Communicable Diseases (NCDs) in 2013, there has been global progress in the proportion of countries with a national NCD action plan and dedicated NCD units.[34] However, CKD is only incorporated into NCD strategies in approximately one-half of countries.[4] Policies are required to integrate kidney care within essential health packages under universal health coverage (Figure 4).[30] Multisectoral policies must also address the social determinants of health, which are major amplifiers of CKD risk and severity, limiting people's opportunities to improve their health.[3] Lack of investment in kidney health promotion, along with primary and secondary prevention of kidney disease, hinders progress.[14]

Health systems. Two major goals of universal health coverage are to achieve coverage of essential health services and reduce financial hardship imposed by health care. However, universal health coverage alone is insufficient to ensure adequate access to kidney care.[3] Health systems must be strengthened and quality of care must also be prioritized, as poor quality care contributes to more deaths than lack of access in low-resource settings.[35] Quality care requires a well-trained health care workforce, sustainable availability of accurate diagnostics, reliable infrastructure, and medication supplies and should be monitored in an ongoing process of quality improvement (Figure 4). The quality of medications, especially in LMICs, may be an additional barrier to successful management of CKD.[36] Regulation and monitoring of drug manufacturing and quality standards are important to ensure safe and effective therapies. Strategies to support regulation and quality assurance will need to be developed in local contexts and guidance, as outlined elsewhere.[37]

Establishing a credible case for CKD detection and management based on risks, interventions and outcomes, and costs, based on real-world data, will help to translate theoretical cost-effectiveness (currently established primarily in high-income countries with minimal data from elsewhere) into economic reality.[30,38] Screening should include evaluation of risk factors for CKD, eliciting a family history, recognizing potential symptoms (usually advanced—fatigue, poor appetite, edema, itching etc.), and measuring blood pressure, serum creatinine, urinalysis, and urine albumin/protein to creatinine ratios, as outlined in established guidelines.[19,39] Addressing CKD upstream beginning in primary care should lower costs over time by reducing CKD complications and KF. Medications required for kidney care are already included in the World Health Organization Essential Medication List (Table 1). These must be provided at national levels under universal health coverage.[40] Pharmaceutical companies should provide these at affordable prices.

Challenges in primary care, clinical inertia

Health care professionals. A shortage of primary care professionals is compounded by inconsistent access to specialists and allied health professionals in both high-income countries and LMICs. Defining roles and responsibilities for kidney care is essential. Solutions may include multidisciplinary team care (primary care physicians, pharmacists, advanced practitioners, nurses, therapists, educators, nutritionists, and mental health professionals) with well-established mechanisms of collaboration of all elements and promptly

Table 1 | Essential medicines for patients with kidney disease

Medication/technology	Example	Reason	On WHO model list of essential medicines
ACE inhibitor	Enalapril, lisinopril	Delays CKD progression, benefits cardiovascular disease and stroke	Yes
Angiotensin receptor blocker	Losartan, telmisartan	Delays CKD progression, cardiovascular disease, and stroke	Yes
Calcium channel blocker	Amlodipine, verapamil	Blood pressure control	Yes
Loop diuretics	Furosemide, torsemide	Good when GFR is low, good for heart failure	Yes
Thiazide diuretics	Hydrochlorothiazide, metolazone, indapamide	Good for BP, especially in the Black population	Yes
SGLT2 inhibitor	Empagliflozin, canagliflozin, dapagliflozin	Diabetes control, delays CKD progression, cardiovascular disease, and death	Yes
GLP1 agonist	Semaglutide	Diabetes control, weight loss	No
Mineralocorticoid inhibitor	Spironolactone, finerenone	Delays CKD progression, reduces heart failure risk. Caution: risk of hyperkalemia in patients with kidney disease	Yes/no
β-Blocker	Bisoprolol	Prevention and treatment of ischemic heart disease	Yes
Statins	Simvastatin	Prevention of CAD in patients with CKD, transplant	Yes
Aspirin		Secondary prevention of MI in patients with CKD, transplant	Yes
Fixed-dose combinations (polypill)[a]	Aspirin + atorvastatin + ramipril	Simultaneous management of CKD and cardiovascular disease and risk factors where indicated[a]	Yes
	Aspirin + simvastatin + ramipril + atenolol + hydrochlorthiazide		Yes
	Aspirin + perindopril + amlodipine		Yes
Oral hypoglycemic medication	Gliclazide, metformin, SGLT2 inhibitors	DM management. Caution with dosing and glomerular filtration rate	Yes
Insulin	Long and short acting	DM management	Yes

ACE, angiotensin-converting enzyme; BP, blood pressure; CAD, coronary artery disease; CKD, chronic kidney disease; DM, diabetes mellitus; GFR, glomerular filtration rate; GLP1, glucagon-like peptide-1; MI, myocardial infarction; SGLT2, sodium-glucose cotransporter 2; WHO, World Health Organization.
[a]Polypills containing aspirin may not be appropriate for patients with early CKD without other cardiovascular indications.

available communication technologies within health systems and between professionals to support care and decision-making.[41,42] Brain drain in low-resource settings is complex and must be tackled.

Mobilization of community health workers yields cost savings in infectious disease programs in LMICs, and may facilitate early detection, diagnosis, and management of NCDs.[43] Protocolized CKD management, possibly supported by electronic decision-support systems, lends itself well to interventions at the community level, with integration of primary care physicians and backup from nephrology and other professionals.[44,45] In some environments, pharmacists, for example, could identify people with diabetes or hypertension, at risk of CKD, based on their prescriptions, and could offer testing on site and reference if needed.[46] Pharmacists can also provide medication reconciliation and medication advice for safety, effectiveness, and adherence. Social workers and pharmacists can help patients with medications access programs.[46]

Challenges for clinical inertia. Clinical "inertia," commonly blamed for low prescribing rates, has many facets (Figure 4).[47] Many knowledge gaps regarding CKD exist among primary care clinicians.[48] Such gaps are remediable with focused public and professional education. Additional factors include fear of medication adverse effects, misaligned incentives within the health system, excessive workload, formulary restrictions, and clinician burnout.[47] Furthermore, discrepancies in guideline recommendations from different professional organizations may add to confusion. A major impediment to optimal care is the time constraints imposed on individual clinicians. The average primary care practitioner in the United States would require ≈26.7 hours per day to implement guideline-recommended care for a 2500 patient panel.[49] Innovation is required to support guideline implementation, especially for primary care practitioners who must implement many different guidelines to meet the needs of various patients. Electronic health records, reminders, team-based nudges, and decision support tools offer a promising support for quality kidney care in busy clinical practices.[50] The extra time and effort spent negotiating preauthorizations or completing medication assistance program requests, along with need for frequent monitoring of multiple medications, however, also hinder appropriate prescribing.[25] Many primary care practitioners have only a few minutes allocated per patient because of institutional pressure or patient volume. "Inertia" can hardly be applied to clinicians working at this pace. The number of health professionals must increase globally.

Visits for patients with CKD are complex as multimorbidity is high. Patients are often managed by multiple specialists, leading to fragmentation of care, lack of holistic oversight, and diffusion of responsibility for treatment. Multidisciplinary care improved transition to kidney replacement therapy and lowered mortality in single and combined outcomes analyses.[51] Novel models of "combined clinics" with on-site collaboration and coparticipation (nephrologist-cardiologist-endocrinologist) may prove to be of substantial benefit for patients, in terms of reduced fragmentation of care, logistics, and cost saving.

Patient centeredness

Health literacy. Self-care is the most important aspect of kidney care. A patient's ability to understand his/her health needs, make healthy choices, and feel safe and respected in the health system, and psychosocial support are important to promote health decision-making (Figure 4). Communication should start from good communication that requires quality information and importantly confirmation of "understanding" on the side of the patient and often family. Electronic apps and reminders may become useful tools to support patients by improving disease knowledge, promoting patient empowerment, and improving self-efficacy, although it is unlikely that one size will fit all.[52] Insufficient patient health information, poor communication, and mistrust, among other elements, are important barriers, especially in marginalized and minoritized communities, where CKD is common.[30] Patients may also be confused by contradictory recommendations for care between health care professionals, as well as conflicting messaging in lay media. Innovative platforms to improve communication between patients and clinicians about CKD are promising and may promote optimal prescribing and adherence.[53,54]

To overcome barriers and promote equity, patient perspectives are essential to designing and testing better health strategies. Collaborative

Box 1 | Barriers impacting medication use as expressed by people living with kidney disease

> "I have to pay for my medications so I either settle for less expensive options or ration the regular dose."
> "I am seeing doctors of different specialties each of whom prescribe separate regimens which makes me concerned about drug interactions."
> "As an experienced patient, I sometimes stop, or modify the dose of the prescribed medications without referring to my doctors. If they do ask, I would tell them that I am in full compliance."
> "Over time, the dose and varieties of my medication keep increasing. I am not sure whether it's because of condition worsening or medications becoming less effectiveness."
> "My knowledge of medication mostly comes from a peer patient who appears to be very knowledgeable about this stuff."

care models must include patients, families, community groups, diverse health care professionals, health systems, government agencies, and payers.[38] Advocacy organizations and local community groups and peer navigators, having trusted voices and relationships, can be conduits for education and may provide input for development of patient tools and outreach programs.[55] Most important, patients must be at the center of their care.

Cost and availability of medication. In high-income countries, people without health insurance and those with high copays paradoxically pay the most for even essential medications.[38] Across LMICs, kidney disease is the leading cause of catastrophic health expenditure because of reliance on out-of-pocket payments.[56] Across 18 countries, 4 cardiovascular disease medications (statins, ACEIs, aspirin, and β-blockers), all often indicated in CKD, were more available in private than in public settings, mostly unavailable in rural communities, and unaffordable for 25% of people in upper middle-income countries and 60% of people in low-income countries.[57] Newer therapies may be prohibitively expensive worldwide, especially where generics may not yet be available. In the United States, the retail price for a 1-month supply of an SGLT2 inhibitor or finerenone is ≈$500 to $700; and for glucagon-like peptide-1 receptor agonists, ≈$800 to $1200 per month.[38] Reliance on out-of-pocket payment for vital, lifesaving basic medications is unacceptable (Figure 4).

Special considerations

Not all kidney diseases are the same. Much of what has been discussed here relates to the most common forms of CKD (e.g., diabetes and hypertension). Some forms of CKD not yet completely understood have different risk profiles, including environmental exposures, genetic predisposition, and autoimmune or other systemic disorders. Highly specialized therapies may be required. Pharmaceutical companies should be accountable to ensure that research studies include disease-representative participants with appropriate race, ethnicity, and sex and gender representation, that effective drugs are made available after studies, and that the balance between profit and prices is fair and transparent. Many novel therapies are offering new hope for diverse kidney diseases; and once approved, there must be no delay in extending the benefits to all affected patients (Supplementary Table S1).

An important group often overlooked is children with kidney diseases. This group is especially vulnerable in LMICs, where nephrology services and resources are limited, and families must often make the choice to pay for treatment for 1 child or support the rest of their family.[58] Children with CKD are also at high risk of cardiovascular disease, even in high-income settings, and more attention is required to control risk factors and achieve treatment targets.[59]

Fostering innovation

Implementation science and knowledge translation. Given that we know how to treat CKD based on a rigorous evidence base, we must now optimize implementation.[60] Implementation research aims to identify effective solutions by understanding how evidence-based practices, often developed in high-income countries, can be integrated into care pathways in lower-resource settings. The management of CKD lends itself to implementation research: optimal therapeutic strategies are known, outcomes are easily measurable, and essential diagnostics and medications should already be in place. Eliciting local patient preferences and understanding challenges are crucial components of such research. Ministries of health should commit to overcoming identified barriers and scaling up successful and sustainable programs.

Table 2 | Examples of strategies to improve implementation of appropriate CKD care

Domain	Potential solutions
Health policy	Include NCD and CKD as health care priorities; ensure sustainable financing; monitor disease burdens and outcomes; registries; multisectoral action; promote kidney health through public health measures; achieve SDGs
Health systems	Integrate CKD care into primary care under UHC; establish quality standards; include necessary diagnostics and medications in national essential medication/diagnostic lists; monitoring and evaluation; reduce brain drain; monitor equity; simplify and streamline guidelines
Quality assurance	Regulation and monitoring of medication quality, especially of generics. Monitoring of health outcomes and care processes to permit iterative improvement
Health care professionals	Reduce time pressure; improve knowledge; broaden scope of practice (e.g., pharmacists); engage community health workers
Patient empowerment	Health literacy; education; community engagement; involvement in research design and conduct
Medication cost	Quality generics; reduce prices; UHC for essential medications
Implementation research	Identify barriers within local contexts; test solutions to overcome barriers
Polypills	Reduce cost; lower pill burden
Digital technologies	Electronic pill boxes, bags, bottles; blister pack technology; ingestible sensors; electronic medication management systems; patient self-report technology; video-based technology; motion sensor technology; telemedicine; smartphone apps; electronic health records

CKD, chronic kidney disease; NCD, noncommunicable disease; SDG, sustainable development goal; UHC, universal health coverage.

Polypills as an example of simple innovation. Polypills are attractive on multiple levels: fixed doses of several guideline-recommended medications are present within 1 tablet (Table 1); lower price; reduced pill burden; and simplicity of the regimen.[61] Polypills have been shown to prevent cardiovascular disease, and to be cost-effective for patients with CKD.[62] More studies are needed, but given the alternatives of costly kidney replacement therapy or early death, it is likely that polypills will prove cost-effective to reduce CKD progression.

Harnessing digital technologies. Integration of telehealth and other types of remotely delivered care can improve efficiency and reduce costs.[63] Electronic health records and registries can support monitoring of quality of care and identify gaps to guide implementation and improve outcomes within learning health care systems. Artificial intelligence may also be harnessed to risk stratify and personalize medication prescribing and adherence.[64] The use of telenephrology for communication between primary care and subspecialists may also prove of use and benefit for patient treatment.[65]

Patient perspectives

Multiple methods support elicitation of patient preferences for CKD care, including interviews, focus groups, surveys, discrete choice experiments, structured tools, and simple conversations.[66,67] At present, many of these are in research stages. Translation into the clinic will require contextualization and determination of local and individual acceptability.

The journey of each person living with CKD is unique; however, challenges and barriers exist in common. As examples of lived experiences, comments solicited from patients about their medications and care are outlined in Box 1 and Supplementary Table S2. These voices must be heard and headed to close gaps and improve quality of kidney care everywhere.

Call to action

A stalemate in kidney care has been tolerated far too long. The new therapeutic advances offer real hope that many people with CKD can survive without developing KF. The evidence of clinical benefit is overwhelming and unequivocal. We cannot wait another 17 years for this evidence to trickle into clinical practice.[33] The time is now to ensure that all who are eligible to receive CKD treatment equitably receive this care.

Known barriers and global disparities in access to diagnosis and treatment must be urgently addressed (Figure 4). To achieve health equity for people with and at risk of kidney diseases, we must raise awareness from policy makers to patients and the general population, harness innovative strategies to support all cadres of health care workers, and balance profits with reasonable prices (Table 2). If we narrow the gap between what we know and what we do, kidney health will become a reality worldwide.

APPENDIX
Members of the World Kidney Day Joint Steering Committee

Alessandro Balducci, Vassilios Liakopoulos, Li-Li Hsiao, Ricardo Correa-Rotter, Ifeoma Ulasi, Latha Kumaraswami, Siu Fai Lui, Dina Abdellatif, and Ágnes Haris.

DISCLOSURE

VL is chair of the Advocacy Working Group, International Society of Nephrology, no financial disclosures. KRT has received research grants from the National Institutes of Health (National Institute of Diabetes and Digestive and Kidney Diseases, National Heart, Lung, and Blood Institute, National Center for Advancing Translational Sciences, National Institute on Minority Health and Health Disparities, director's office), the US Centers for Disease Control and Prevention, and Travere Therapeutics; and consultancy fees from AstraZeneca, Bayer, Boehringer Ingelheim, Eli Lilly, and Novo Nordisk. She is chair of the Diabetic Kidney Disease Collaborative for the American Society of Nephrology. RC-R is a member of the Steering Committee of World Kidney Day, a member of the Diabetes Committee of the Latin-American Society of Nephrology and Hypertension (SLANH), and a member of the Latin American Regional Board, International Society of Nephrology. He is a member of the Steering Committee of the Dapagliflozin and Prevention of Adverse Outcomes in Chronic Kidney Disease (DAPA-CKD) trial (AstraZeneca), the Study of Diabetic Nephropathy with Atrasentan (SONAR) (Abbvie), A Non-interventional Study Providing Insights Into the Use of Finerenone in a Routine Clinical Setting (FINE-REAL) (Bayer), and CKD-ASI (Boehringer). He has received research grants from AstraZeneca, GlaxoSmithKline, Roche, Boehringer, and Novo Nordisk; and has received honoraria as a speaker from AstraZeneca, Bayer, Boehringer Ingelheim, and Amgen. All the other authors declared no competing interests.

ACKNOWLEDGMENTS

The authors are grateful for the thoughtful input provided by members of the Advocacy Working Group and the Patient Liaison Advisory Group of the International Society of Nephrology: Elliot Tannor, Marcello Tonelli, Boris Bikbov, Maria Carlota Gonzalez, Vivekanand Jha, and Viviane Calice-Silva.

SUPPLEMENTARY MATERIAL

Supplementary File (Word)
Supplementary Figure S1. Ranking of kidney dysfunction as a cause of death stratified by world-income category and gender by level 2 risk factors for death.
Supplementary Table S1. Approved and emerging novel therapeutic agents for various kidney diseases.
Supplementary Table S2. Patient comments on accessibility, affordability, knowledge, facilitators and barriers to optimal kidney care.

REFERENCES

1. Jager KJ, Kovesdy C, Langham R, et al. A single number for advocacy and communication-worldwide more than 850 million individuals have kidney diseases. *Kidney Int.* 2019;96:1048–1050.
2. Institute for Health Metrics and Evaluation (IHME). GBD compare data visualization. Accessed November 18, 2023. http://vizhub.healthdata.org/gbd-compare
3. Luyckx VA, Tonelli M, Stanifer JW. The global burden of kidney disease and the sustainable development goals. *Bull World Health Organ.* 2018;96:414–422D.
4. International Society of Nephrology. ISN Global Kidney Health Atlas. 3rd ed. Accessed November 18, 2023. https://www.theisn.org/initiatives/global-kidney-health-atlas/
5. GBD Chronic Kidney Disease Collaboration. Global, regional, and national burden of chronic kidney disease, 1990-2017: a systematic analysis for the Global Burden of Disease Study 2017. *Lancet.* 2020;395:709–733.
6. Vanholder R, Annemans L, Brown E, et al. Reducing the costs of chronic kidney disease while delivering quality health care: a call to action. *Nat Rev Nephrol.* 2017;13:393–409.
7. Nguyen-Thi HY, Le-Phuoc TN, Tri Phat N, et al. The economic burden of chronic kidney disease in Vietnam. *Health Serv Insights.* 2021;14:11786329211036011.
8. US Renal Data System. Healthcare expenditures for persons with CKD. Accessed November 18, 2023. https://usrds-adr.niddk.nih.gov/2023/chronic-kidney-disease/6-healthcare-expenditures-for-persons-with-ckd
9. Kidney Health Australia. Transforming Australia's kidney health: a call to action for early detection and treatment of chronic kidney disease. Accessed January 16, 2024. https://kidney.org.au/uploads/resources/Changing-the-CKD-landscape-Economic-benefits-of-early-detection-and-treatment.pdf
10. Ke C, Liang J, Liu M, et al. Burden of chronic kidney disease and its risk-attributable burden in 137 low-and middle-income countries, 1990-2019: results from the global burden of disease study 2019. *BMC Nephrol.* 2022;23:17.
11. Gregg EW, Buckley J, Ali MK, et al. Improving health outcomes of people with diabetes: target setting for the WHO Global Diabetes Compact. *Lancet.* 2023;401:1302–1312.
12. Geldsetzer P, Manne-Goehler J, Marcus ME, et al. The state of hypertension care in 44 low-income and middle-income countries: a cross-sectional study of nationally representative individual-level data from 1.1 million adults. *Lancet.* 2019;394:652–662.
13. Chu L, Bhogal SK, Lin P, et al. AWAREness of Diagnosis and Treatment of Chronic Kidney Disease in Adults With Type 2 Diabetes (AWARE-CKD in T2D). *Can J Diabetes.* 2022;46:464–472.
14. Levin A, Tonelli M, Bonventre J, et al. Global kidney health 2017 and beyond: a roadmap for closing gaps in care, research, and policy. *Lancet.* 2017;390:1888–1917.
15. Stengel B, Muenz D, Tu C, et al. Adherence to the Kidney Disease: Improving Global Outcomes CKD guideline in nephrology practice across countries. *Kidney Int Rep.* 2021;6:437–448.
16. Chu CD, Chen MH, McCulloch CE, et al. Patient awareness of CKD: a systematic review and meta-analysis of patient-oriented questions and study setting. *Kidney Med.* 2021;3:576–585.e1.
17. Ene-Iordache B, Perico N, Bikbov B, et al. Chronic kidney disease and cardiovascular risk in six regions of the world (ISN-KDDC): a cross-sectional study. *Lancet Global Health.* 2016;4:e307–e319.
18. Gummidi B, John O, Ghosh A, et al. A systematic study of the prevalence and risk factors of CKD in Uddanam, India. *Kidney Int Rep.* 2020;5:2246–2255.

19. Kidney Disease: Improving Global Outcomes (KDIGO) Diabetes Work Group. KDIGO 2022 Clinical Practice Guideline for Diabetes Management in Chronic Kidney Disease. *Kidney Int*. 2022;102(5S):S1–S127.
20. Nicholas SB, Daratha KB, Alicic RZ, et al. Prescription of guideline-directed medical therapies in patients with diabetes and chronic kidney disease from the CURE-CKD Registry, 2019-2020. *Diabetes Obes Metab*. 2023;25:2970–2979.
21. Grams ME, Yang W, Rebholz CM, et al. Risks of adverse events in advanced CKD: the Chronic Renal Insufficiency Cohort (CRIC) study. *Am J Kidney Dis*. 2017;70:337–346.
22. Kidney Disease: Improving Global Outcomes (KDIGO) CKD Work Group. KDIGO 2024 Clinical Practice Guideline for the Evaluation and Management of Chronic Kidney Disease. *Kidney Int*. https://doi.org/10.1016/j.kint.2023.10.018
23. Kidney Disease: Improving Global Outcomes (KDIGO) Blood Pressure Work Group. KDIGO 2021 clinical practice guideline for the management of blood pressure in chronic kidney disease. *Kidney Int*. 2021;99(3S):S1–S87.
24. Tuttle KR, Alicic RZ, Duru OK, et al. Clinical characteristics of and risk factors for chronic kidney disease among adults and children: an analysis of the CURE-CKD registry. *JAMA Netw Open*. 2019;2:e1918169.
25. Ismail WW, Witry MJ, Urmie JM. The association between cost sharing, prior authorization, and specialty drug utilization: a systematic review. *J Manag Care Spec Pharm*. 2023;29:449–463.
26. Heerspink HJL, Vart P, Jongs N, et al. Estimated lifetime benefit of novel pharmacological therapies in patients with type 2 diabetes and chronic kidney disease: a joint analysis of randomized controlled clinical trials. *Diabetes Obes Metab*. 2023;25:3327–3336.
27. Nuffield Department of Population Health Renal Studies Group. SGLT2 Inhibitor Meta-Analysis Cardio-Renal Trialists' Consortium. Impact of diabetes on the effects of sodium glucose co-transporter-2 inhibitors on kidney outcomes: collaborative meta-analysis of large placebo-controlled trials. *Lancet*. 2022;400:1788–1801.
28. Fernández-Fernandez B, Sarafidis P, Soler MJ, et al. EMPA-KIDNEY: expanding the range of kidney protection by SGLT2 inhibitors. *Clin Kidney J*. 2023;16:1187–1198.
29. McEwan P, Boyce R, Sanchez JJG, et al. Extrapolated longer-term effects of the DAPA-CKD trial: a modelling analysis. *Nephrol Dial Transplant*. 2023;38:1260–1270.
30. Vanholder R, Annemans L, Braks M, et al. Inequities in kidney health and kidney care. *Nat Rev Nephrol*. 2023;19:694–708.
31. Agarwal R, Filippatos G, Pitt B, et al. Cardiovascular and kidney outcomes with finerenone in patients with type 2 diabetes and chronic kidney disease: the FIDELITY pooled analysis. *Eur Heart J*. 2022;43:474–484.
32. Tuttle KR, Bosch-Traberg H, Cherney DZI, et al. Post hoc analysis of SUSTAIN 6 and PIONEER 6 trials suggests that people with type 2 diabetes at high cardiovascular risk treated with semaglutide experience more stable kidney function compared with placebo. *Kidney Int*. 2023;103:772–781.
33. Rubin R. It takes an average of 17 years for evidence to change practice-the burgeoning field of implementation science seeks to speed things up. *JAMA*. 2023;329:1333–1336.
34. World Health Organisation. Mid-point evaluation of the implementation of the WHO global action plan for the prevention and control of noncommunicable diseases 2013–2020 (NCD-GAP). Accessed November 18, 2023. https://cdn.who.int/media/docs/default-source/documents/about-us/evaluation/ncd-gap-final-report.pdf?sfvrsn=55b22b89_5&download=true
35. Kruk ME, Gage AD, Joseph NT, et al. Mortality due to low-quality health systems in the universal health coverage era: a systematic analysis of amenable deaths in 137 countries. *Lancet*. 2018;392:2203–2212.
36. Kingori P, Peeters Grietens K, Abimbola S, et al. Uncertainties about the quality of medical products globally: lessons from multidisciplinary research. *BMJ Glob Health*. 2023;6:e012902.
37. Pan American Health Organization Quality control of medicines. Accessed November 18, 2023. https://www.paho.org/en/topics/quality-control-medicines
38. Tuttle KR, Wong L, St Peter W, et al. Moving from evidence to implementation of breakthrough therapies for diabetic kidney disease. *Clin J Am Soc Nephrol*. 2022;17:1092–1103.
39. Kalyesubula R, Conroy AL, Calice-Silva V, et al. Screening for kidney disease in low- and middle-income countries. *Semin Nephrol*. 2022;42:151315.
40. Francis A, Abdul Hafidz MI, Ekrikpo UE, et al. Barriers to accessing essential medicines for kidney disease in low- and lower middle-income countries. *Kidney Int*. 2022;102:969–973.
41. Rangaswami J, Tuttle K, Vaduganathan M. Cardio-renal-metabolic care models: toward achieving effective interdisciplinary care. *Circ Cardiovasc Qual Outcomes*. 2020;13:e007264.
42. Neumiller JJ, Alicic RZ, Tuttle KR. Overcoming barriers to implementing new therapies for diabetic kidney disease: lessons learned. *Adv Chronic Kidney Dis*. 2021;28:318–327.
43. Mishra SR, Neupane D, Preen D, et al. Mitigation of non-communicable diseases in developing countries with community health workers. *Global Health*. 2015;11:43.
44. Joshi R, John O, Jha V. The potential impact of public health interventions in preventing kidney disease. *Semin Nephrol*. 2017;37:234–244.
45. Patel A, Praveen D, Maharani A, et al. Association of multifaceted mobile technology-enabled primary care intervention with cardiovascular disease risk management in rural Indonesia. *JAMA Cardiol*. 2019;4:978–986.
46. Ardavani A, Curtis F, Khunti K, et al. The effect of pharmacist-led interventions on the management and outcomes in chronic kidney disease (CKD): a systematic review and meta-analysis protocol. *Health Sci Rep*. 2023;6:e1064.
47. Sherrod CF, Farr SL, Sauer AJ. Overcoming treatment inertia for patients with heart failure: how do we build systems that move us from rest to motion? *Eur Heart J*. 2023;44:1970–1972.
48. Ramakrishnan C, Tan NC, Yoon S, et al. Healthcare professionals' perspectives on facilitators of and barriers to CKD management in primary care: a qualitative study in Singapore clinics. *BMC Health Services Res*. 2022;22:560.
49. Porter J, Boyd C, Skandari MR, et al. Revisiting the time needed to provide adult primary care. *J Gen Intern Med*. 2023;38:147–155.
50. Peralta CA, Livaudais-Toman J, Stebbins M, et al. Electronic decision support for management of CKD in primary care: a pragmatic randomized trial. *Am J Kidney Dis*. 2020;76:636–644.
51. Rios P, Sola L, Ferreiro A, et al. Adherence to multidisciplinary care in a prospective chronic kidney disease cohort is associated with better outcomes. *PLoS One*. 2022;17:e0266617.
52. Stevenson JK, Campbell ZC, Webster AC, et al. eHealth interventions for people with chronic kidney disease. *Cochrane Database Syst Rev*. 2019;8:Cd012379.
53. Tuot DS, Crowley ST, Katz LA, et al. Usability testing of the kidney score platform to enhance communication about kidney disease in primary care settings:

qualitative think-aloud study. *JMIR Form Res.* 2022;6: e40001.
54. Verberne WR, Stiggelbout AM, Bos WJW, et al. Asking the right questions: towards a person-centered conception of shared decision-making regarding treatment of advanced chronic kidney disease in older patients. *BMC Med Ethics.* 2022;23:47.
55. Taha A, Iman Y, Hingwala J, et al. Patient navigators for CKD and kidney failure: a systematic review. *Kidney Med.* 2022;4:100540.
56. Essue BM, Laba M, Knaul F, et al. Economic burden of chronic ill health and injuries for households in low- and middle-income countries. In: Jamison DT, Gelband H, Horton S, et al., eds. *Disease Control Priorities: Improving Health and Reducing Poverty, 3rd ed.* The International Bank for Reconstruction and Development/The World Bank; 2017. https://doi.org/10.1596/978-1-4648-0527-1_ch6
57. Khatib R, McKee M, Shannon H, et al. Availability and affordability of cardiovascular disease medicines and their effect on use in high-income, middle-income, and low-income countries: an analysis of the PURE study data. *Lancet.* 2016;387:61–69.
58. Kamath N, Iyengar AA. Chronic kidney disease (CKD): an observational study of etiology, severity and burden of comorbidities. *Indian J Pediatr.* 2017;84: 822–825.
59. Cirillo L, Ravaglia F, Errichiello C, et al. Expectations in children with glomerular diseases from SGLT2 inhibitors. *Pediatr Nephrol.* 2022;37:2997–3008.
60. Donohue JF, Elborn JS, Lansberg P, et al. Bridging the "know-do" gaps in five non-communicable diseases using a common framework driven by implementation science. *J Healthc Leadersh.* 2023;15: 103–119.
61. Population Health Research Institute. Polypills added to WHO essential medicines list. Accessed November 18, 2023. https://www.phri.ca/eml/
62. Sepanlou SG, Mann JFE, Joseph P, et al. Fixed-dose combination therapy for prevention of cardiovascular diseases in CKD: an individual participant data meta-analysis. *Clin J Am Soc Nephrol.* 2023;18:1408–1415.
63. Dev V, Mittal A, Joshi V, et al. Cost analysis of telemedicine use in paediatric nephrology-the LMIC perspective. *Pediatr Nephrol.* 2024;39:193–201.
64. Musacchio N, Zilich R, Ponzani P, et al. Transparent machine learning suggests a key driver in the decision to start insulin therapy in individuals with type 2 diabetes. *J Diabetes.* 2023;15:224–236.
65. Zuniga C, Riquelme C, Muller H, et al. Using telenephrology to improve access to nephrologist and global kidney management of CKD primary care patients. *Kidney Int Rep.* 2020;5:920–923.
66. van der Horst DEM, Hofstra N, van Uden-Kraan CF, et al. Shared decision making in health care visits for CKD: patients' decisional role preferences and experiences. *Am J Kidney Dis.* 2023;82:677–686.
67. Hole B, Scanlon M, Tomson C. Shared decision making: a personal view from two kidney doctors and a patient. *Clin Kidney J.* 2023;16:i12–i19.

journal club

Sparsentan versus irbesartan in focal segmental glomerulosclerosis

Rheault *et al.* (N Engl J Med. 2023;389:2436–2445.)

Focal segmental glomerulosclerosis (FSGS) is a term used both for a lesion of segmental glomerular scarring that may be caused by any injury and for a disease caused by specific podocyte injury linked to as yet unidentified circulating factor(s). Previous treatment strategies have relied on immunosuppression, but with limited effectiveness. Studies in experimental animal models have shown that inhibiting angiotensin or endothelin decreased proteinuria and sclerosis. The DUPLEX phase 3 trial of 108-week duration compared sparsentan, a novel antagonist selective for both endothelin A receptor and angiotensin II type 1 receptor, with irbesartan, an angiotensin receptor blocker. Patients had biopsy-proven FSGS or a pathogenic variant in a podocyte protein known to be linked with FSGS, with significant proteinuria (urine protein:creatinine ratio ≥ 1.5) and estimated glomerular filtration rate (eGFR) >30 ml/min per 1.73 m^2. A total of 371 patients were randomized equally to the 2 treatment groups. Patients in the 2 groups were on average 41.7 versus 41.5 years of age, ranging from 9 to 75 years, and mostly White. The authors stated that those with "FSGS resulting from another cause were excluded," but total 27 patients with *COL4A3-5* variants were included (12 sparsentan and 15 irbesartan group). These patients should be considered as having Alport with secondary FSGS lesions. In addition, 9 patients in the sparsentan group but only 5 in the irbesartan group had high-risk *APOL1* variants, which are associated with increased risk for kidney disease. Partial remission of proteinuria was achieved in significantly more patients treated with sparsentan versus irbesartan

(42.0% vs. 26.0%). Complete remission was also more frequent with sparsentan (Figure 1). As expected, because of hemodynamic effects, eGFR decreased over the first 6 weeks, but to a greater degree with sparsentan versus irbesartan. However, eGFR slopes did not differ at the end of the study. Of note, the lack of a superior effect of sparsentan on eGFR slope may reflect the inclusion of patients with podocyte-specific genetic causes of FSGS, those with Alport-related secondary FSGS, and those with *APOL1* high-risk variants, who may have different mechanisms underlying podocyte injury and scarring. The promising effects to significantly decrease proteinuria may yet translate into GFR preservation over longer term, particularly in those patients without genetic contribution to their FSGS lesions.
—Agnes B. Fogo

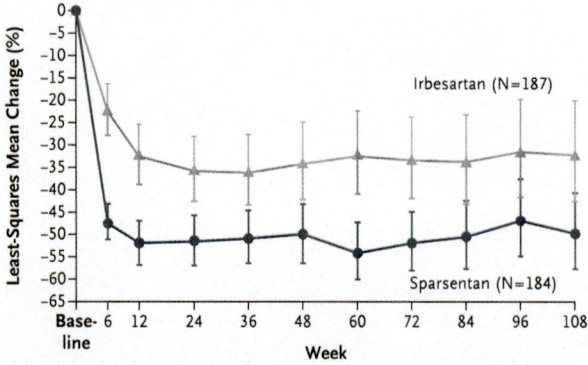

Figure 1 | Changes over time in the urine protein:creatinine ratio shown as percent change from baseline with bars indicating 95% confidence intervals. From *New England Journal of Medicine*, Rheault MN, Alpers CE, Barratt J, et al.; DUPRO Steering Committee and DUPLEX Investigators. Sparsentan versus irbesartan in focal segmental glomerulosclerosis, volume 389, pages 2436–2445, Copyright © (2023) Massachusetts Medical Society. Reprinted with permission from Massachusetts Medical Society.

Effect of a novel multicomponent intervention to improve patient access to kidney transplant and living kidney donation: the EnAKT LKD cluster-randomized clinical trial

Garg *et al.* (JAMA Intern Med. 2023;183:1366–1375.)

Globally, there are significant barriers to access to kidney transplantation services. Not all patients who are eligible for transplantation will have the opportunity to receive one during their lifetime. There are many initiatives to improve equity in access to both deceased and living donor kidney transplantation, but the gaps remain persistent and excessive, particularly for those living in rural/remote areas and patients from lower socioeconomic backgrounds. In the Enhance Access to Kidney Transplantation and Living Kidney Donation (EnAKT LKD) trial, the investigators aimed to assess the effectiveness of a multicomponent intervention to improve access to kidney transplantation in Canada.

The EnAKT LKD trial is a pragmatic, 2-arm, parallel-group, registry-based, clustered randomized controlled trial. A total of 26 chronic kidney disease (CKD) programs in Ontario, Canada, were enrolled into the study and randomly assigned (1:1) to receive the intervention or standard of care. The intervention involved a multicomponent strategy that consisted of 4 main components: administrative support to facilitate local quality improvement, transplant educational resources, patient engagement, and program-level performance evaluation and oversight by administrative leaders. The primary outcome was the rate of steps completed toward receiving a kidney transplant. The maximum number of steps that each individual participant could complete was 4. These steps included: (i) referral to a transplanting center for evaluation, (ii) had a potential living donor contact a transplant center for evaluation, (iii) enlisted on the deceased donor waitlist, and (iv) received a living or deceased donor kidney transplant. During the 4.2-year trial period, 9780 patients from 13 CKD programs received the intervention, and 10,595 patients from another 13 CKD programs received standard care. Participants were followed for a median (interquartile range) period of 2.1 (1.0–3.6) years. There were no differences in the rate of the primary outcome between the intervention and standard of care arm (5334 vs. 5638 steps; 24.8 vs. 24.1 steps per 100 patient-years; adjusted hazard ratio 1.00 [95% confidence interval {CI}, 0.87–1.15]). Despite adequate intervention uptake, there were substantial challenges related to the delivery of the intervention as the trial was conducted during the peak of the COVID-19 pandemic. Rates of living and deceased donor kidney transplantation were reduced considerably, and clinical staff was retrained and redeployed to work in COVID-19 wards and emergency services. Although the null results are disappointing, this trial highlights the barriers and hurdles to conducting and delivering a complex intervention trial during an unexpected global health crisis.

—Germaine Wong

Effect of thiazides in kidney stone disease?

Triozzi et al. (Mendelian randomization analysis of genetic proxies of thiazide diuretics and the reduction of kidney stone risk. *JAMA Netw Open.* 2023;6:e2343290.)

Thiazides are commonly used to reduce urine calcium excretion and hence the recurrence of calcium-containing kidney stones. The authors of the randomized, placebo-controlled NOSTONE study recently reported that the administration of hydrochlorothiazide was of no apparent benefit in patients with recurrent kidney stones.[1] This study had several strengths but also some limitations. Triozzi et al. set out to determine whether there is an association between genetic proxies of thiazide diuretics and the risk of developing kidney stones using Mendelian randomization analysis. Mendelian randomization allows investigating potential causal relationships between exposures and disease outcomes. The genetic proxies of thiazide diuretics were derived from naturally occurring genetic variation in the thiazide-sensitive sodium chloride cotransporter gene, based on data of the International Consortium for Blood Pressure. Genetic proxies of β-blockers and systolic blood pressure served as negative controls. Kidney stone outcomes were derived from 3 biobanks. The main outcome was the odds of kidney stones. Secondary outcomes were serum laboratory values relevant to the treatment of kidney stones. The main analysis included more than 1 million individuals, with more than 50,000 kidney stone cases and more than 1 million controls. In a meta-analysis of all cohorts, genetic proxies of thiazide diuretics were associated with a lower odds of kidney stones (odds ratio, 0.85; 95% CI, 0.81–0.89; $P < .001$). Figure 2 demonstrates this association. Genetic proxies of β-blockers and systolic blood pressure were not associated with kidney stones. Furthermore, genetic proxies of thiazide diuretics were associated with higher serum calcium and total cholesterol levels, but lower serum potassium levels. The association of genetic proxies of thiazide diuretics with reduced kidney stone risk reflects a drug effect over the course of a lifetime, unconstrained by the limited follow-up period of clinical trials. This finding is in favor of a beneficial role of thiazide diuretics in the prevention of kidney stones.

—Tilman B. Drüeke

[1]Dhayat NA, Bonny O, Roth B, et al. Hydrochlorothiazide and prevention of kidney-stone recurrence. *N Engl J Med.* 2023;388:781–791.

Exposure	OR (95% CI)
Thiazide diuretics	
MVP[31]	0.84 (0.80-0.89)
UKB[56]	0.90 (0.79-1.04)
FinnGen[57]	0.83 (0.73-0.95)
Total	0.85 (0.81-0.89)
Heterogeneity: $\chi_2^2 = 0.92$ ($P = .63$); $I^2 = 0\%$	
β Blockers	
MVP[31]	1.03 (1.02-1.05)
UKB[56]	0.96 (0.92-0.99)
FinnGen[57]	1.06 (1.01-1.10)
Total	1.02 (0.96-1.07)
Heterogeneity: $\chi_2^2 = 15.53$ ($P < .001$); $I^2 = 87\%$	
Systolic blood pressure	
MVP[31]	1.00 (1.00-1.01)
UKB[56]	1.00 (0.99-1.01)
FinnGen[57]	1.00 (0.99-1.01)
Total	1.00 (1.00-1.01)
Heterogeneity: $\chi_2^2 = 0.59$ ($P = .74$); $I^2 = 0\%$	

Figure 2 | Association of genetic proxies of thiazide diuretics, β-blockers, and systolic blood pressure with risk of kidney stones. From Triozzi JL, Hsi RS, Wang G, et al. Mendelian randomization analysis of genetic proxies of thiazide diuretics and the reduction of kidney stone risk. *JAMA Netw Open.* 2023;6:e2343290. This is an open access article distributed under the terms of the CC-BY License. © 2023 Triozzi JL et al. JAMA Network Open.

journal club

Cumulative incidence of thiazide-induced hyponatremia: a population-based cohort study

Andersson et al. (Ann Intern Med. Published online December 19, 2023.)
https://doi.org/10.7326/M23-1989

For nephrologists who frequently incur cases of thiazide-induced hyponatremia, it can be surprising to learn that most thiazide drug labels report a risk of hyponatremia that is unknown or uncommon. A Danish linked registries study published in the *Annals of Internal Medicine* emulated 2 pragmatic target trials of the cumulative incidence of hyponatremia after the new use of thiazide diuretics compared with the new use of alternative first-intention antihypertensive drugs, such as calcium channel blockers (CCBs) and renin-angiotensin system inhibitors (RASis).

Danish residents (outside the Central Denmark Region) aged 40 years or older between January 1, 2014, and October 31, 2018, with no prescriptions for antihypertensive medication within the previous year were included in the study. To isolate participants with general practice–initiated treatments of uncomplicated hypertension, the researchers excluded those with secondary hypertension and an indication for one medication over another. Treatment assignment, defined as filling a first prescription for the drug, could not be modified after baseline, regardless of the actual use, switching, or addition of another antihypertensive medication, consistent with an emulated intention-to-treat design. The study's primary outcome was hyponatremia, defined as sodium level <130 mmol/l.

The comparison of bendroflumethiazide versus a CCB included 82,749 participants, and combined hydrochlorothiazide and RASi versus RASi alone included 97,727 participants. Standardized differences for baseline characteristics, including but not limited to age, sex, comorbidities, income, and education level, across groups were below 10% after inverse probability of treatment weighting. Timing, frequency, and proportion of participants with blood sodium level ascertainment were similar among thiazide and non-thiazide users.

The 2-year cumulative incidence of hyponatremia among bendroflumethiazide first-time users was 3.83%, with an estimated 2-year risk difference of 1.35% (95% CI, 1.04%–1.66%) compared with first-time CCB users. Hydrochlorothiazide + RASi users had a 2-year cumulative incidence of hyponatremia of 3.51% and an estimated risk difference of 1.38% (95% CI, 1.01%–1.75%) compared with RASi alone. The risk of hyponatremia was highest during the first months after treatment initiation and increased with older age and comorbidity burden. Severe hyponatremia (<125 mmol/l) and hospitalization with hyponatremia were also more common among the thiazide users.

In this large-scale real-world registry data study, the 2-year cumulative incidence of sodium levels <130 mmol/l with initiation of thiazide diuretics was between 3.5% and 3.8%. Considering the selection of a general practice population and the lack of consideration for the actual intake as well as antihypertensive medications added after baseline, this is likely to be a conservative estimate of the risk of thiazide-induced hyponatremia.

—Amélie Bernier-Jean

translational science

Secrets and myths between tubules—new insights on erythropoietin production from single-cell technology

Kai-Uwe Eckardt[1] and Armin Kurtz[2]

Refers to: Kragesteen BK, Giladi A, David E, et al. The transcriptional and regulatory identity of erythropoietin producing cells. *Nat Med.* 2023;29:1191–1200.

Kidney International (2024) **105,** 421–423; https://doi.org/10.1016/j.kint.2023.09.007

KEYWORDS: anemia; cell signaling; erythropoietin; fibroblast; hypoxia; nephrology

Copyright © 2023, International Society of Nephrology. Published by Elsevier Inc. All rights reserved.

[1]Department of Nephrology and Medical Intensive Care, Charité-Universitätsmedizin Berlin, Berlin, Germany; and [2]Insititute of Physiology, University of Regensburg, Regensburg, Germany

Correspondence: Kai-Uwe Eckardt, Department of Nephrology and Medical Intensive Care, Charité-Universitätsmedizin Berlin, Augustenburger Platz 1, Berlin 13353, Germany. E-mail: kai-uwe.eckardt@charite.de

Where within the kidney erythropoietin (EPO) is produced and how its production is adjusted to renal oxygen supply, thereby establishing a negative feedback-loop, have been longstanding questions. Given the prevailing nephron-centric view focused on glomerular and tubular epithelial cells, it came as a surprise when *in situ* hybridization for EPO pointed to cells located in the cortical interstitium.[1] Although first presumed to be capillary endothelial cells, these cells were subsequently identified as peritubular fibroblast-like cells. Little was known about these peritubular cells before that observation; they were primarily considered to be of structural relevance by producing extracellular matrix and filling the niches between adjacent tubules. Subsequently, investigators used different surface markers and genetic labeling strategies in mice to characterize these cells. Not all observations are consistent, but most data indicate that the vast majority of the EPO-producing cells are of mesenchymal origin, are located in cortex and outer medulla, and share properties and surface markers with fibroblasts. However, subpopulations sharing pericyte and neuronal cell markers may also contribute to EPO production.[2,3] To distinguish the cells producing EPO from the larger population of cells located in the interstitium, the term renal EPO-producing (REP) cells came into use.

Parallel studies on EPO regulation led to the discovery of hypoxia-inducible transcription factors (HIFs), core elements of a widespread oxygen-sensing mechanism that activates more than a hundred target genes in response to reduced oxygen availability.[4] HIFs are heterodimers formed by 1 of 3 oxygen-regulated α-subunits and a constitutive β-subunit (HIF1, HIF2, and HIF3). Several lines of evidence indicate that EPO is regulated by the HIF2 isoform. Consistent with this concept, hypoxia leads to HIF2 accumulation in peritubular kidney cells. The oxygen dependence of prolyl hydroxylase domain enzymes, which target HIFα-subunits for proteasomal degradation, serves as the oxygen-sensing mechanism.[4]

Although these findings define the main elements of the control of EPO production in the kidney, at least 2 levels of unresolved complexity remain. First, the increase in EPO production with decreasing oxygen availability is to a large extent mediated by an increase in the number of peritubular cells that activate the EPO gene. However, even under conditions of severe hypoxia, less than 20% of cells carrying REP cell markers produce EPO.[5] Whether these cells represent a distinct subpopulation and how they are gradually recruited remains unclear. Second, whether the impaired ability to increase EPO production appropriately in response to falling hemoglobin concentrations in chronic kidney disease (CKD) is less clear than frequently assumed. Although it is plausible that interstitial fibrosis interferes with the sophisticated function of REP cells, prolyl hydroxylase inhibitors that stabilize HIF in the presence of oxygen, thereby mimicking cellular hypoxia, are able to (re)activate an EPO response even in people with kidney failure.[6] Recent work by Kragesteen *et al.*[7] published in *Nature Medicine* provides interesting novel insight into EPO production by the kidneys by applying cutting-edge single-cell technologies.

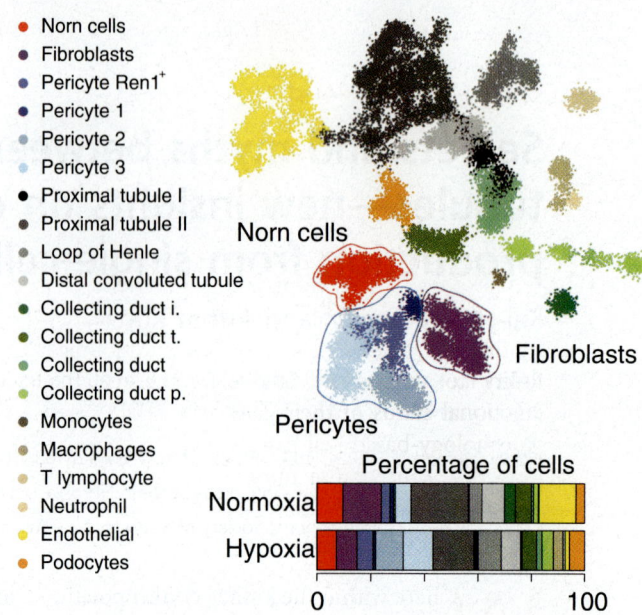

Figure 1 | Two-dimensional projection of 35,834 renal cells combined from normoxic and hypoxic mice. Hypoxia was induced by exposure to 0.1% carbon monoxide for 4 hours. Cells were grouped into 385 metacells, based on the MetaCell algorithm. The dots represent single cells and colors denote cell-type annotation. Cells differentiated from other cells on the basis of their ability to express erythropoietin gene transcripts are labeled as "Norn cells." The stack bar shows the percentage of renal cell types obtained from mice under hypoxic and normoxic conditions. Cells were pooled from 52 mice. Adapted from Kragesteen BK, Giladi A, David E, et al. The transcriptional and regulatory identity of erythropoietin producing cells. *Nat Med.* 2023;29:1191–1200.[7] https://doi.org/10.1038/s41591-023-02314-7, reproduced with permission from Springer Nature.

What did the study show?

The investigators used an elegant mouse model, previously developed by Wenger's group, in which cells actively producing EPO are permanently labeled.[8] As a first step, they developed a sophisticated enrichment strategy for REP cells, which then allowed further molecular analysis using single-cell RNA sequencing (scRNA-seq). Grouping cells according to their transcriptome in conjunction with a scRNA-seq atlas distinguished many kidney cell types, including different types of fibroblasts and pericytes, plus an additional group of cells with EPO transcripts (Figure 1). Although these cells express some fibroblast and pericyte markers, the authors concluded that they are a distinct cell population, as they exhibit hundreds of differentially expressed genes. The investigators then isolated cells with these characteristics from normoxic and hypoxic wild-type mice. Although EPO transcripts were confined to these cells, only 11% of those harvested from hypoxic mice contained EPO mRNA, consistent with previous observations. Comparison between normoxic and hypoxic conditions revealed 134 differentially expressed genes, of which more than a third were restricted to this population of cells.

In subsequent analyses, the investigators determined transposase-accessible chromatin regions to identify thousands of candidate enhancer regions that are likely to play a role in cell identity and function. These regions include 5 open chromatin regions upstream and downstream of the EPO gene and were enriched in motifs of several transcription factors, which could potentially act in concert with HIF to drive the hypoxia response. Importantly, the authors also provided several lines of evidence indicating that the described EPO-producing kidney cells, characterized by the combination of multiple markers, are conserved from mice to humans.

Why is it important?

This work represents a major advance by providing the most detailed and comprehensive characterization of REP cells achieved so far. At the same time, the analysis sheds further light on the functional heterogeneity of cells in the kidney interstitium, a still understudied territory. The ability to respond to changes in oxygen may be important for processes beyond EPO production, including inflammation and matrix production, as some of the marker genes suggest. Future identification of the full regulatory region of the EPO gene *in vivo* may lead to novel approaches to activate this gene. Although current prolyl hydroxylase inhibitors effectively ameliorate anemia in CKD, safety signals were observed in large phase 3 trials, which are potentially due to off-target effects, and may limit the use of the agents.[9] More specific targeting of EPO gene expression could therefore be advantageous.

The work by Kragesteen *et al.* highlights another important issue. With the exploding ability to categorize cells according to the functional status of their genome, our current morphology-based cell categorization must be expanded. One of the important questions is how to distinguish a "cell type" from a "functional status" of a given cell type. This question is not constrained to the kidney, but of special relevance to kidney researchers given the large number of kidney cell types and states that have already been identified. Related to this are questions about terminology. Kragesteen *et al.* propose the term "Norn" cells for the cells that they describe, inspired by Norse mythology.[10] Whether this proper name will be helpful for disclosing the secrets of EPO production remains to be shown. Novel findings, such as those presented by Kragesteen *et al.*, rather than myths are likely to expand our understanding of the important functions of REP cells and their alterations during the course of CKD.

DISCLOSURE
All the authors declared no competing interests.

REFERENCES
1. Lacombe C, Da Silva JL, Bruneval P, et al. Peritubular cells are the site of erythropoietin synthesis in the murine hypoxic kidney. *J Clin Invest*. 1988;81:620–623.
2. Broeker KAE, Fuchs MAA, Schrankl J, et al. Different subpopulations of kidney interstitial cells produce erythropoietin and factors supporting tissue oxygenation in response to hypoxia in vivo. *Kidney Int*. 2020;98:918–931.
3. Dahl SL, Bapst AM, Khodo SN, et al. Fount, features, and function of renal erythropoietin-producing cells. *Pflügers Arch*. 2022;474:783–797.
4. Schödel J, Ratcliffe PJ. Mechanisms of hypoxia signalling: new implications for nephrology. *Nat Rev Nephrol*. 2019;10:641–659.
5. Yamazaki S, Souma T, Hirano I, et al. A mouse model of adult-onset anaemia due to erythropoietin deficiency. *Nat Commun*. 2013;4:1950.
6. Bernhard WM, Wiesener MS, Scigalla P, et al. Inhibition of prolyl hydroxylases increases erythropoietin production in ESRD. *J Am Soc Nephrol*. 2010;12:2151–2156.
7. Kragesteen BK, Giladi A, David E, et al. The transcriptional and regulatory identity of erythropoietin producing cells. *Nat Med*. 2023;29:1191–1200.
8. Imeri F, Nolan KA, Bapst AM, et al. Generation of renal Epo-producing cell lines by conditional gene tagging reveals rapid HIF-2 driven Epo kinetics, cell autonomous feedback regulation, and telocyte phenotype. *Kidney Int*. 2019;95:375–387.
9. Ku E, Del Vecchio L, Eckardt K-U, et al. for Conference Participants. Novel anemia therapies in chronic kidney disease: conclusions from a Kidney Disease: Improving Global Outcomes (KDIGO) controversies conference. *Kidney Int*. 2023;104:655–680.
10. Norse mythology. Accessed June 24, 2023. https://en.wikipedia.org/wiki/Norse_mythology

---

translational science

Reconstructing the interface between the human intestine and immune system: potential to advance mechanistic studies in IgA nephropathy

Huamin Wang[1,3], James Zuiani[2,3], P. Toby Coates AO[2] and Yun Xia[1]

[1]Lee Kong Chian School of Medicine, Nanyang Technological University Singapore, Singapore; and [2]Central Northern Adelaide Renal and Transplantation Service, Royal Adelaide Hospital, Adelaide, South Australia, Australia

Correspondence: *P. Toby Coates AO, Royal Adelaide Hospital, 1 Port Road, Adelaide, South Australia 5000, Australia. E-mail: Toby.coates@sa.gov.au; or Yun Xia, Lee Kong Chian School of Medicine, Nanyang Technological University Singapore, 11 Mandalay Road, Singapore 308232. E-mail: yunxia@ntu.edu.sg*

[3]HW and JZ contributed equally.

Refers to: Bouffi C, Wikenheiser-Brokamp KA, Chaturvedi P, et al. In vivo development of immune tissue in human intestinal organoids transplanted into humanized mice. *Nat Biotechnol*. 2023;41:824–831.

Kidney International (2024) **105,** 423–426; https://doi.org/10.1016/j.kint.2023.07.027

KEYWORDS: human intestinal organoid (HIO); humanized mouse; immune cell; intestinal epithelial cell; lymphoid follicle

Copyright © 2023, International Society of Nephrology. Published by Elsevier Inc. All rights reserved.

Organoids are 3-dimensional cell clusters, derived from pluripotent or adult stem cells, that self-organize into tissue- or organ-like structures enriched for cell types of the cognate tissue/organ. Although current organoids represent a valuable tool for understanding human development and disease, the lack of a native tissue microenvironment has limited their usefulness in recapitulating pathophysiological processes that involve "generic" cell types, such as vascular endothelial cells and immune cells. The internal boundaries of the human body, such as the intestinal epithelium, possess the highest concentration of immune cells, constituting the first line of defense against infection. Because of the inherent differences between mouse and human immune systems, murine models do not faithfully reproduce crosstalk between intestinal epithelial cells and immune cells that is essential for tissue homeostasis, defense against pathogens, and immunologic tolerance to dietary antigens and commensal bacteria.

Human intestinal organoids (HIOs) harbor intestinal stem cells (ISCs) and their progenies, which adopt a 3-dimensional architecture reminiscent of human intestinal epithelium.[1,2] Coculture of HIOs and immune cells has been established to study immune-epithelial interaction in disease pathogenesis. However, such in vitro coculture does not precisely emulate the physiological communication between intestinal epithelial cells and immune cells. Recently, Bouffi et al.[3] developed an in vivo human intestinal organoid model, which successfully re-establishes the interface between human intestinal epithelial cells and immune system for the first time. This new model may provide new opportunities to study the pathogenesis of diseases driven by mucosal immunity, including inflammatory bowel diseases (IBD) and IgA nephropathy (IgAN).

What did the study show?
In this study, the authors used cord blood cells to humanize immunodeficient mice (NSGS, NOD/SCID/Il2rg$^{-/-}$ mice with transgenic expression of stem cell factor, granulocyte-macrophage colony-stimulating factor, and interleukin 3), providing the mice with a full array of human immune cells.[3] Fourteen days later, human pluripotent stem cell–derived intestinal organoids were transplanted underneath the kidney capsule of the humanized mice and harvested at different time points for analysis (Figure 1). The HIOs transplanted in humanized mice demonstrated all major intestinal cell lineages, as well as growing to a similar size as organoids in nonhumanized mice. Human CD45+ cells, derived from the injected cord blood, migrated to the mucosal layer and populated the lamina propria of the HIOs.[3] In both the transplanted HIOs and small intestine of humanized mice, mass cytometry and unsupervised analysis of tissue samples revealed a similar composition of 12 immune cell types including T cells, B cells, and innate lymphoid cells, largely recapitulating the immune landscape of human intestine (Figure 1).[3] Notably, B cells and CD4+ T cells were present in higher numbers in HIOs compared with the small intestine, which may reflect the lack of interleukin 2 receptor γ and associated lymphoid follicles and Peyer's patches in the immunodeficient mice.[3] Aggregation and zonation of T and B cells was observed in the transplanted HIOs, suggesting that HIOs promote the formation of lymphoid follicular structures (Figure 1).[3]

Infiltration, aggregation, and zonation of T and B cells followed a similar program to human fetal intestine development, occurring 11 to 19 weeks after conception. At 16 and 20 weeks posttransplantation, T-cell zones of HIOs showed a high proportion of CD4+ and a low proportion of CD8+ T cells, reminiscent of human fetal intestine 19 weeks after conception.[3] Plasma cells and neutrophils were observed in both 16- and 20-week HIOs, indicating the acquisition of cellular complexity over time.[3] The authors also evaluated the presence and function of specialized intestinal epithelial cells known as microfold (M) cells, which uptake antigens at the luminal side and deliver the antigens to mononuclear phagocytes via transcytosis.[3] Although the M-cell marker glycoprotein 2 (GP2) was not expressed in HIOs transplanted in humanized mice, GP2 expression was induced in enteroids derived from the transplanted HIOs.[3] Bacterial challenge at 16 weeks after transplantation resulted in increased levels of M cells in HIOs, represented by the acquisition of GP2 expression.[3] Subsequently, translocation of luminal antigens by M cells leads to the production of IgA antibodies, indicating that immune cells within these lymphoid-like structures can mount an appropriate immune response.

Why is this study important?
Mice and humans exhibit distinct developmental programs of gut-associated lymphoid tissue (GALT). Although B cells colonize Peyer's patches in postnatal mouse intestine,[4] zonation of T and B cells is already present in the lymphoid follicles of human intestine by post-conception week 19.[5] This and various other interspecies differences both during and after intestinal development preclude the use of mouse models to investigate gastrointestinal diseases caused by defective programming of GALT. This study successfully incorporated allogenic immune cells into HIOs, representing a feasible model of the

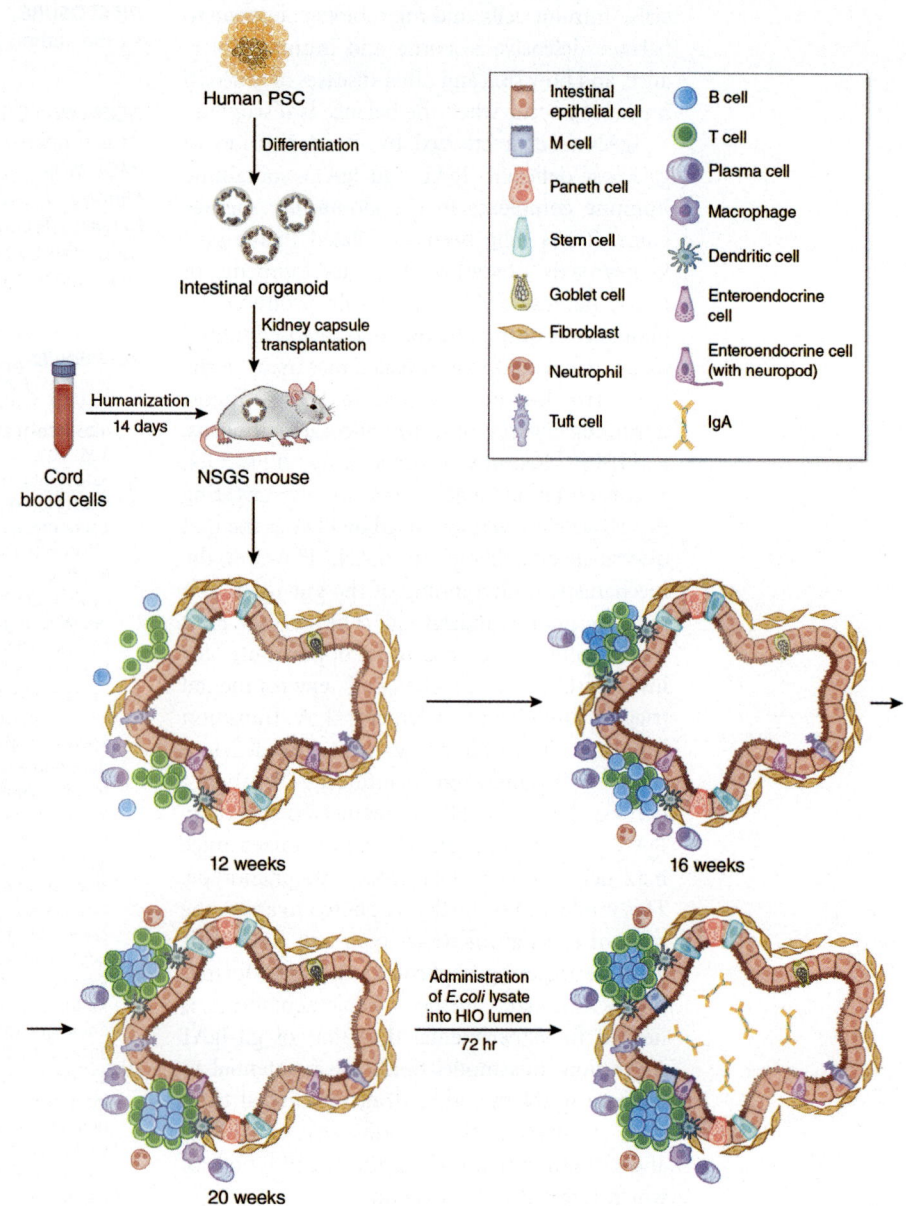

Figure 1 | Diagram of the experimental workflow. Human pluripotent stem cells (PSCs) were differentiated into intestinal organoids (HIOs) and transplanted into immunodeficient mice (NSGS mice, NOD/SCID/Il2rg$^{-/-}$ mice with transgenic expression of stem cell factor [SCF], granulocyte-macrophage colony-stimulating factor [GM-CSF], and interleukin 3 [IL-3]) that were humanized with cord blood cells 14 days in advance. The transplanted HIOs were collected for analysis in the absence or presence of luminal administration of *Escherichia coli* lysates.

developing human gut and associated diseases, such as necrotizing enterocolitis, which is commonly observed in premature infants.

Human GALT are broadly categorized into programmed (Peyer's patches) and induced (isolated lymphoid follicles). While Peyer's patches are formed during fetal gut development, isolated lymphoid follicles develop after birth and mature alongside colonization of the intestine by commensal bacteria.[6] In the current study, HIOs were engrafted under the kidney capsule of humanized mice. Although this conformation is highly effective in establishing the interface between intestinal epithelial cells and immune cells, it does not accommodate the introduction of microbiota. Orthotopic transplantation of HIOs in humanized mice will enable the colonization of microbiota to fully reconstruct the cognate intestinal immune microenvironment. The establishment of this more complex intestinal organoid model will allow us to understand how intestinal epithelial cells, immune cells, and microbiota cooperate to balance defensive response and immune tolerance, and how IBD and other diseases of mucosal immunity occur when the balance is disrupted.

IgAN is characterized by the deposition of galactose-deficient IgA1 (gd-IgA1)–containing immune complexes in the glomerular mesangium. It has long been speculated that a gut-kidney axis underlies the development of IgAN, because IgA1 is primarily produced by plasma cells of the mucosa-associated lymphoid tissues. Genetic studies revealed that many of the IgAN risk loci are involved in IgA synthesis, immunogenic response to mucosal pathogens, and IBD.[7,8] Recently, the novel drug NEFECON, a corticosteroid that works locally targeting Peyer's patches, was approved by FDA as the first disease-specific therapy for IgAN.[9] However, the mechanistic underpinning of the gut-IgAN axis remains poorly understood. The *in vivo* HIO model offers unprecedented opportunity for investigating the genetic and environmental triggers underlying polymeric IgA transition from O-glycosylation to galactose-deficient state. For instance, transplanting IgAN patient–derived HIOs or HIOs engineered to carry IgAN predisposing genes into humanized mice may help correlate genotype with phenotype. This model can be further exploited to assess the roles of specific microbial type and food antigens in triggering nephrotoxic gd-IgA1 formation. Although further implementation is needed for experimental detection of gd-IgA1 deposition, this model holds great potential to evaluate IgAN candidate drugs in clinical trials such as BION-1301 (antibody against APRIL) and Blisbimod (antibody against BAFF), both of which target B-cell activation.

DISCLOSURE
All the authors declared no competing interest.

ACKNOWLEDGMENTS
YX is supported by Ministry of Education Singapore (MOE-MOET32020-0004, MOE-T2EP30220-0008), Ministry of Healthy Singapore (MOH-001214), and Nanyang Technological University Singapore. HW is supported by Ministry of Education Singapore (MOE-MOET32020-0004).

REFERENCES
1. Spence JR, Mayhew CN, Rankin SA, et al. Directed differentiation of human pluripotent stem cells into intestinal tissue in vitro. *Nature*. 2011;470:105–109.
2. Sato T, Stange DE, Ferrante M, et al. Long-term expansion of epithelial organoids from human colon, adenoma, adenocarcinoma, and Barrett's epithelium. *Gastroenterology*. 2011;141:1762–1772.
3. Bouffi C, Wikenheiser-Brokamp KA, Chaturvedi P, et al. In vivo development of immune tissue in human intestinal organoids transplanted into humanized mice. *Nat Biotechnol*. 2023;41:824–831.
4. Hashi H, Yoshida H, Honda K, et al. Compartmentalization of Peyer's patch anlagen before lymphocyte entry. *J Immunol*. 2001;166:3702–3709.
5. Spencer J, MacDonald TT, Finn T, et al. The development of gut associated lymphoid tissue in the terminal ileum of fetal human intestine. *Clin Exp Immunol*. 1986;64:536–543.
6. Eberl G, Lochner M. The development of intestinal lymphoid tissues at the interface of self and microbiota. *Mucosal Immunol*. 2009;2:478–485.
7. Gharavi AG, Kiryluk K, Choi M, et al. Genome-wide association study identifies susceptibility loci for IgA nephropathy. *Nat Genet*. 2011;43:321–327.
8. Kiryluk K, Li Y, Scolari F, et al. Discovery of new risk loci for IgA nephropathy implicates genes involved in immunity against intestinal pathogens. *Nat Genet*. 2014;46:1187–1196.
9. Barratt J, Lafayette R, Kristensen J, et al. Results from part A of the multi-center, double-blind, randomized, placebo-controlled NefIgArd trial, which evaluated targeted-release formulation of budesonide for the treatment of primary immunoglobulin A nephropathy. *Kidney Int*. 2023;103:391–402.

Mining the amyloid-plaque proteome to uncover disease mechanisms in renal amyloidoses

Mario Nuvolone[1,2] and Giampaolo Merlini[1,2]

Beyond typing amyloid deposits and discovering new forms of amyloidosis, laser microdissection and mass spectrometry enable the analysis of the amyloid-plaque proteome constituents—amyloid fibrillar proteins, matrix and cellular components, and absorbed blood-borne proteins. Charalampous *et al.* analyzed the amyloid-plaque proteomes of the 7 most common renal amyloidoses to gain preliminary mechanistic insights on cellular and molecular perturbations elicited during gradual amyloid deposition and potential tissue repair or damage mechanisms. Clinical correlations identified a prognostic pattern.

Kidney International (2024) 105, 427–429; https://doi.org/10.1016/j.kint.2023.12.013

Copyright © 2023, International Society of Nephrology. Published by Elsevier Inc. All rights reserved.

see basic research on page 484

Amyloidosis is caused by misfolded proteins that aggregate and form insoluble beta-sheet fibrils that deposit in tissues, causing progressive organ damage and failure.[1] The kidney and heart are the 2 most common targets in systemic amyloidosis. Heart involvement determines survival, particularly during the first 6 months from diagnosis, and kidney involvement, leading to kidney failure, contributes significantly to morbidity. In most types of amyloidosis, amyloid is deposited in the glomeruli, interstitium, and/or arteries, whereas the medulla is preferentially involved in amyloidosis caused by the deposition of apolipoprotein A-I and A-IV. Although the mechanisms of heart damage have been investigated extensively, the pathogenesis of amyloid renal damage is less defined. Progressive organ dysfunction derives from aberrant interactions between prefibrillar oligomers and fibrils with cellular components, and physical disruption caused by large amounts of amyloid deposits. Misfolded proteins and their aggregates trigger local inflammatory changes involving the complement system. Inflammation produces oxidative stress, which in turn promotes protein misfolding and aggregation, establishing a vicious cycle that underlies progressive organ injury. The contribution of each of these basic mechanisms to organ damage varies in the different types of amyloidosis. Early clinical observations, in both amyloidosis caused by monoclonal immunoglobulin light chains (AL amyloidosis) and amyloidosis caused by serum amyloid A protein (AA amyloidosis), indicate that the nephrotic syndrome caused by amyloid renal damage can promptly regress upon etiologic therapy leading to a profound reduction of the amyloidogenic precursor, despite the amyloid deposits being almost unchanged, as assessed through renal biopsy.[2,3] These observations indicate that in certain types of renal amyloidosis, the interactions of the amyloid proteins with cellular constituents result in cytotoxicity that contributes substantially to kidney failure. Furthermore, in AL amyloidosis, the interaction between amyloid light chains and glomerular mesangial cells has been reported to play a crucial role in amyloid fibril formation.[4]

In this issue, Charalampous and coworkers explored the largest database of amyloid plaque proteomes from diagnostic mass spectrometry–based typing analyses on renal biopsies available worldwide, to build a proteomic atlas of renal amyloidosis[5] that contains a mine of information on amyloid-related kidney pathology. Proteomic data were obtained through laser microdissection of amyloid deposits, coupled with tandem mass spectrometry from 2650 cases of 7 different types of renal amyloidosis (AL, AA, and amyloidosis formed by immunoglobulin heavy chains [AH], leukocyte chemotactic factor 2 [ALECT2], variants fibrinogen alpha chain [AFib], apolipoprotein A-IV [AApoAIV], and apolipoprotein C-II variants [AApoCII]) and 14 nondisease tissue controls (membranous nephropathies or day-zero renal transplants). Analyses were aimed at identifying differences between amyloid plaques and control tissues, as well as commonalities and individual specificities of the different types of renal amyloidosis. As reported by the authors, the main limitation of this work is that the analysis was confined to the amyloid plaques that contain only remnant proteins of dying renal cells that adhere to amyloid plaques, limiting the investigation of the interactions between renal cells and amyloid species. However, this study provides several valuable insights into the complex pathophysiology of the most common forms of renal amyloidoses. The detailed analysis of this large set of data would require an extensive dissertation; here, we discuss aspects related to pathogenic mechanisms and clinical implications.

The most distinctive proteomes were identified in both types of hereditary renal amyloidosis included in the analysis (AFib and AApoCII), as well as in AA amyloidosis, with the remaining types clustering closer to one another.

---

[1]Department of Molecular Medicine, University of Pavia, Pavia, Italy; and [2]Amyloidosis Research and Treatment Center, Fondazione IRCCS Policlinico San Matteo, Pavia, Italy

Correspondence: *Giampaolo Merlini, Department of Molecular Medicine, University of Pavia, V.le Forlanini, 6, Pavia 27100, Italy. E-mail: gmerlini@unipv.it*

Of note, ALECT2 and AL amyloidosis showed the highest intragroup amyloid plaque heterogeneity, which in the latter case was explained only partly through differences between AL kappa and lambda cases. The extent to which these observations are influenced by basic demographics (age, sex, ethnicity), underlying predisposing conditions, and other factors is presently unknown. An unexpected finding is the clusterization of ALECT2 amyloidosis with AL and AH amyloidosis, implying some proteomic overlap and possibly common pathogenic mechanisms, despite their having different clinical presentations. ALECT2 amyloidosis, of which the pathogenesis is still undefined, is a relatively benign type of renal amyloidosis associated with a slow glomerular filtration rate decline and rare full nephrotic syndrome. Conversely, AL amyloidosis is characterized by a rapid decline of kidney function associated with full nephrotic proteinuria, suggesting a substantial proteotoxicity of the amyloid light chains, as also indicated by the presence in the AL amyloid plaque of proteins implicated in kidney damage (A1AT, HSPB1). This finding stimulates further investigation of the molecular mechanisms of ALECT2 amyloidosis.

Another compelling observation is that, besides the main amyloidogenic fibrillar protein and the ubiquitous amyloid signature proteins, the amyloid proteome consisted of only a few hundred proteins, likely representing proteins from residual cellular debris entrapped in amyloid deposits, and blood-borne proteins adsorbed to the amyloid deposits. Such proteins can provide valuable information on cellular and molecular perturbations elicited by exposure to amyloidogenic species, the gradual formation of amyloid deposits within the kidney, and potential tissue repair or damage mechanisms. In this context, several interesting observations were made. Ubiquitins and heat shock proteins were underrepresented within amyloid plaques of most amyloid types, compared to controls. Considering that ubiquitins play a central role in intracellular protein catabolism through the ubiquitin–proteasome system and that heat shock proteins are well established anti-amyloid chaperones, these changes reflect a reduction in proteostatic capacities as an important determinant of amyloid organ damage. Also, complement components were ubiquitously present, and their relative abundance was the strongest determinant of proteomic heterogeneity across different amyloid types. The source of complement components accumulating within amyloid deposits, particularly their derivation from blood or their local production as an atypical response to a danger signal represented by toxic species, remains to be determined. The complement components also could play a role in the pathogenesis of renal damage, as several complement proteins are proteases that are themselves activated by proteolytic cleavage. As a major component of the inflammatory response, they may contribute to sustaining local inflammation and the consequent progression of kidney damage. Several collagen proteins were increased in AL and AH. Recent cryogenic electron microscopy data provided the first structural evidence of interactions between AL amyloidosis fibrils and collagen VI.[6] Collagen has been recently reported to inhibit the phagocytosis of amyloid fibrils, hindering the clearance of amyloid deposits, thus representing a possible therapeutic target.

Charalampous et al. also observed that the most indolent, non-AL types of amyloid plaques had a higher proteomic content, considering proteins other than the main plaque constituents. A highly intriguing finding is that, when the focus was on AL cases with available clinical information, patients with earlier stages of amyloid kidney involvement (renal stages I and II)[7] displayed higher proteomic content and lower intra-plaque light-chain levels than did patients with the most advanced disease (stage III). This finding may reflect that in earlier stages of renal amyloid deposition, the amyloid fibril density is lower (lower light-chain content), and amyloid fibrils might be intermingled with trapped renal cells (higher proteomic content). Conversely, in more advanced disease stages, when most of the cells have succumbed to the amyloid-induced cytotoxicity, the amyloid fibrils are more densely packed (higher light-chain content), whereas only remnants of cells are attached to the amyloid plaque (lower proteomic content). Indeed, a specific proteomic profile (cluster 1) was prognostic in this series, being significantly associated with a lower renal stage and prolonged kidney survival. Notably, proteins associated with the protection from oxidative stress were increased in the early stages, indicating that oxidative stress plays a key role in renal toxicity, as already reported in the case of light chain–induced cardiotoxicity. By contrast, proteins related to matrix fibrosis had a greater presence in the proteome of cases with a higher renal stage and adverse outcome, likely denoting irreversible tissue-remodeling changes associated with kidney function deterioration (Figure 1).

The proteomic database generated within this study is openly available and will provide an unprecedented opportunity for the scientific community to mine protein changes across high numbers of patients with the most common forms of renal amyloidosis. Following a similar analytical approach, the same group previously reported on the amyloid plaque proteomes within the heart.[8] Comparison of the 2 studies will offer the possibility to deepen our current understanding of molecular mechanisms of organ toxicity by examining generalized and organ-specific amyloid plaque proteomic changes and possibly identifying potential targets amenable to therapeutic interventions.

Clinical and experimental evidence, including data stemming from this study, converges to indicate that the aberrant interactions between the amyloidogenic precursors and tissue-resident cells play an important role in the disease. Once more, achieving a deep and rapid reduction, or possibly the elimination, of the amyloidogenic precursor

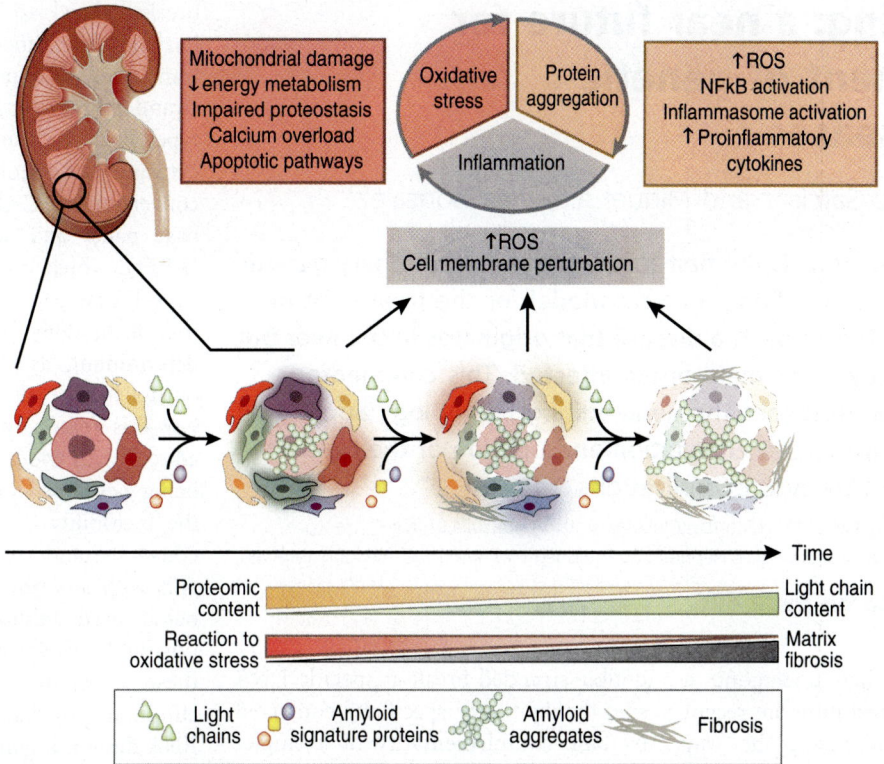

Figure 1 | **Amyloid-plaque proteome sheds light on pathogenic mechanisms of renal amyloidosis caused by monoclonal immunoglobulin light chains (AL amyloidosis).** Schematic representation of pathogenic mechanisms underlying renal AL amyloidosis and associated changes identified in the amyloid-plaque proteome. Amyloidogenic light chains misfold, aggregate, and deposit in the extracellular space in the form of amyloid fibrils, along with amyloid signature proteins. Amyloid fibrils cause cytotoxicity through aberrant interactions with cell membranes and oxidative stress. Misfolded light chains and/or their aggregates can enter resident cells. Intracellular aggregates generate oxidative stress and sequester ubiquitin and chaperones, unbalancing protein homeostasis, impairing mitochondrial function, reducing adenosine triphosphate (ATP) production, altering calcium influx, and releasing cytochrome C, leading to proteostatic collapse and apoptotic cell death. Protein aggregates can trigger local inflammatory changes and oxidative stress, establishing a vicious cycle that sustains disease progression. Over time, fibril density increases, amyloid deposits progressively replace the normal tissue, and matrix fibrosis ensues. These pathogenic events are reflected by temporal changes in the amyloid-plaque proteome, the analysis of which provides important hints on disease pathophysiology and harbors prognostic information. ↑: increase; ↓: decrease; ROS: reactive oxygen species.

is vital. Our group reported that prompt treatment at the early stages of kidney involvement in AL amyloidosis can abrogate the risk of kidney failure and dialysis and reduce morbidity and mortality.[7] New therapies that include amyloid protein stabilizers, gene silencers, gene-editing, and monoclonal antibodies to enhance the clearance of amyloid deposits[9] are available or are under development in AL and transthyretin amyloidosis (ATTR). They also offer hope to patients with other types of systemic amyloidosis.

DISCLOSURE

MN reports receiving research funding from Gate Bioscience and being a member of its Advisory Board; receiving honoraria and research funding from Pfizer; receiving honoraria from Jannsen-Cilag; and receiving research funding from Oncopeptides. The other author declared no competing interests.

REFERENCES

1. Merlini G, Bellotti V. Molecular mechanisms of amyloidosis. *N Engl J Med*. 2003;349:583–596.
2. Kyle RA, Wagoner RD, Holley KE. Primary systemic amyloidosis: resolution of the nephrotic syndrome with melphalan and prednisone. *Arch Intern Med*. 1982;142:1445–1447.
3. Lee YH, Kim EY, Jeong DW, et al. Complete remission of nephrotic syndrome without resolution of amyloid deposit after anti-tumor necrosis factor alpha therapy in a patient with ankylosing spondylitis. *J Clin Rheumatol*. 2016;22:86–88.
4. Herrera GA. Renal amyloidosis: pathogenesis. *Ultrastruct Pathol*. 2021;45:267–275.
5. Charalampous C, Dasari S, McPhail E, et al. A proteomic atlas of kidney amyloidosis provides insights into disease pathogenesis. *Kidney Int*. 2024;105:484–495.
6. Schulte T, Chaves-Sanjuan A, Speranzini V, et al. Helical superstructures between amyloid and collagen VI in heart-derived fibrils from a patient with light chain amyloidosis. Preprint. Research Square. Posted online November 21, 2023. https://doi.org/10.21203/rs.3.rs-3625869/v1
7. Palladini G, Hegenbart U, Milani P, et al. A staging system for renal outcome and early markers of renal response to chemotherapy in AL amyloidosis. *Blood*. 2014;124:2325–2332.
8. Kourelis TV, Dasari SS, Dispenzieri A, et al. A proteomic atlas of cardiac amyloid plaques. *JACC CardioOncol*. 2020;2:632–643.
9. Nuvolone M, Nevone A, Merlini G. Targeting amyloid fibrils by passive immunotherapy in systemic amyloidosis. *BioDrugs*. 2022;36:591–608.

commentary

Gene editing: a near future for the treatment of genetic kidney diseases

Fernando Gómez-García[1,2] and Miguel A. Garcia-Gonzalez[1]

The study by Chen et al. is the first to apply the revolutionary genetic engineering tool, base editing, in a rat model for the treatment of primary hyperoxaluria type 1, a disease that originates in the liver but in which the kidney is the main organ affected. This commentary contextualizes and describes the gene-editing technology applied by the authors, provides an interpretation and opinion of their results, and indicates possible future applications.

Kidney International (2024) **105**, 430–433; https://doi.org/10.1016/j.kint.2024.01.004

Copyright © 2024, International Society of Nephrology. Published by Elsevier Inc. All rights reserved.

see basic research on page 496

Gene editing has undergone a fascinating evolution in recent years, revolutionizing the way we understand and manipulate genes. From its beginnings to the latest emerging technologies, the field has gone through several key stages that have led to important scientific and technological breakthroughs, but one deserves special attention.

CRISPR-Cas9: a new starting point

In 2012, the scientific community witnessed a revolutionary moment when the researchers Jennifer Doudna and Emmanuelle Charpentier successfully used the CRISPR-Cas9 (Clustered Regularly Interspaced Short Palindromic Repeats-CRISPR associated protein 9) system as a gene-editing tool. The Cas9 endonuclease generates a double-stranded break at specific DNA site, thanks to the specificity conferred by base complementarity of a single-guide RNA, and a nucleotide sequence called protospacer adjacent motif (PAM).[1] The double-stranded break triggers subsequent endogenous cellular repair through the nonhomologous end-joining pathway or the homology-directed repair pathway. The nonhomologous end-joining pathway often leads to the insertion or deletion of nucleotides and can be used to introduce frameshifts into the coding sequence of a gene causing premature truncation of the protein (knock out). On the other hand, the homology-directed repair pathway can be applied to insert or correct a specific mutation at the target loci thanks to a donor DNA template (knock in).[1] A technical limitation is the relatively low efficiency of exogenous DNA integration by CRISPR/Cas9-directed homology-directed repair. This limitation has forced researchers to continue searching for new systems that allow greater efficiency.

Base editing: a small change makes a big difference

In 2016, David Liu's group described an innovative CRISPR-Cas9-based tool called base editing. This system contains a Cas9 nickase (produces single-strand breaks) fused to a DNA deaminase enzyme that can generate nucleotide transitions without the need for double-stranded breaks or DNA templates. Two types of base editors are distinguished: cytosine base editors, which catalyze the conversion of C-G base pairs to T-A base pairs, and adenine base editors (ABEs), which catalyze the conversion of A-T base pairs to G-C base pairs. In this technology, PAM is particularly determinant, as effective editing only occurs in a small nucleotide window.[1] For this reason, new variants of base editors with wider editing windows are being developed (although it increases the possibility of unwanted secondary edits—bystander edits), and Cas9 variants with less restrictive PAMs are also being used (although it widens the possibility of off-targets).[1] Interestingly, these problems can be reduced or eliminated by methodical single-guide RNA design, highlighting the great potential of this tool for the treatment of human disease.

Base editing has already been successfully applied in humans to treat acute lymphoblastic leukemia, not by rectifying a point mutation in a single gene but by inducing a nonsense mutation in 3 genes. The assay involved transducing T cells from healthy volunteer donors using a lentivirus to express a chimeric antigen receptor (CAR) with specificity for CD7 (CAR7), a protein expressed in T-cell acute lymphoblastic leukemia. Base editing was used to inactivate the CD52, CD7, and TRB genes to prevent lymphodepleting serum therapy, CAR7 T-cell fratricide, and graft-versus-host disease, respectively.[2]

Undoubtedly, this is a clear demonstration of the great potential of base editing, which corroborates the statement by Chen et al.[3] on the application of this tool for the development of personalized and precision medicine.

Base editing against primary hyperoxaluria type 1

In this issue, Chen et al.[3] applied base editing technology to correct both *in vitro* and *in vivo* a mutation in the

---

[1]Group of Genetics and Developmental Biology of Renal Diseases, Health Research Institute of Santiago de Compostela, Santiago de Compostela, Spain; and [2]Group of Genomic Medicine, University of Santiago de Compostela Center for Research in Molecular Medicine and Chronic Diseases, Santiago de Compostela, Spain

Correspondence: Miguel Garcia-Gonzalez, Complexo Hospitalario Universitario de Santiago (CHUS), Fundación IDIS—Laboratorio No. 11 (Genética y Biología del desarrollo de las enfermedades renales (NEFROCHUS), Edificio de Consultas Planta-2, Travesía da Choupana, 15706 Santiago de Compostela, Spain. E-mail: miguel.garcia.gonzalez@sergas.es

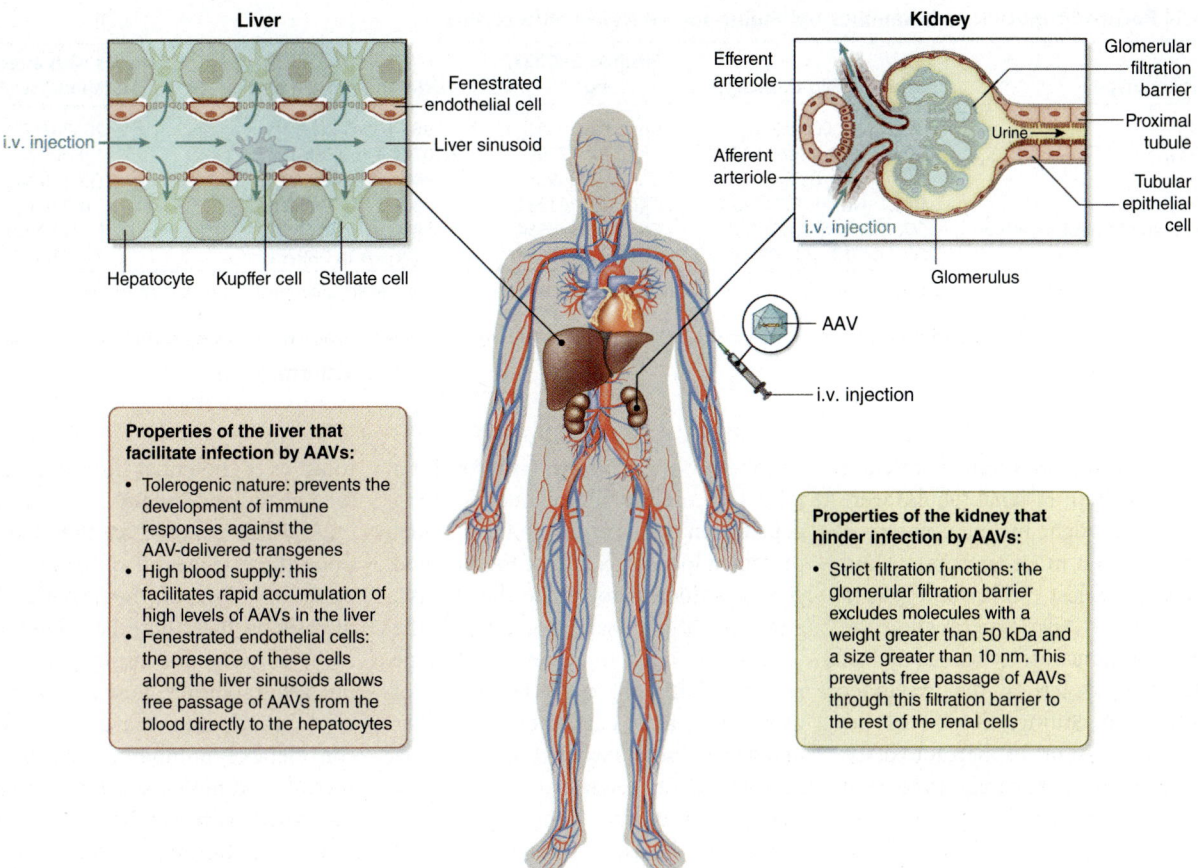

Figure 1 | Liver and kidney infection after i.v. injection of adeno-associated virus (AAV). AAV would mainly infect the liver due to the accessibility and tropism of these vectors for liver cells. On the other hand, the kidney would be minimally infected, infecting mainly glomerular cells, due to the difficulty of these cells to cross the glomerular filtration barrier. The infection is represented by the cells shaded in blue.

alanine glyoxylate aminotransferase ($Agxt^{Q84X}$) gene. For the *in vitro* assay, they used 2 different types of base editors: (i) ABE8e, characterized by a wider window of action, and (ii) ABEmax, with a narrower window. In addition, each type of editor was also composed of different Cas9 variants, which recognize different PAMs. The use of 2 different editors to correct the same mutation highlighted the differences between them in terms of desired editing efficiency and generation of bystander edits. The editing efficiency of target adenine (A_6) with ABE8e-VQR (SpCas9-VQR variant that recognizes PAM-NGA) was a staggering 95.3%. However, it also performed bystander editing 5 nucleotides away from the target nucleotide—adenine (A_{11})—generating the $Agxt^{I82T}$ mutation with an efficiency of 13.1%. On the other hand, using ABEmax-VQR, the authors achieved a lower editing efficiency (81.3%) in A_6, but the percentage of bystander editing was also considerably lower (3.1%), providing some advantage over ABE8e-VQR. Despite this, the authors decided to apply ABE8e-VQR editing technology for the *in vivo* assay, stating that the perfect correction efficiency (only the A_6>G modification) was higher in ABE8e-VQR (82.2%) compared with ABEmax-VQR (78.2%) although with no statistically significant difference.

For *in vivo* experiments, one of the main limitations is to deliver the gene editing tool to the target organ. Viral vectors, and more specifically adeno-associated virus (AAV), have become the most widely used vectors for gene delivery. This is because they can infect different organs in multiple vertebrate species (including humans) with relatively low immunogenicity. However, it has been observed that infection is not equal in all organs. For example, the liver is an organ that is easily infected by AAVs compared with other organs such as the kidney (Figure 1).[4] Although both organs receive a high blood flow, being even 4 to 5 times higher in the kidney in relation to the weight of the organ, the liver presents particular qualities such as its tolerogenic nature, which prevents the development of immune responses against AAV-delivered transgenes, or its anatomic properties, which allow AAV particles present in the blood to directly access hepatocytes, making it an ideal organ for AAV-based gene therapies.[5] Taking advantage of this, Chen *et al.*[3] used AAV serotype 8 to deliver the ABE8e-VQR to the liver, achieving an A_6 correction efficiency of 13.3%. Despite this editing percentage, a reduction in endogenous oxalate synthesis, a decrease in kidney

Table 1 | Recurrent mutations in families belonging to the NefroCHUS cohort

OMIM phenotype	Gene (RefSeq transcript)	Position GRCh37, hg19	cDNA and protein change	Families with a recurrent mutation,[a] % (n/N)
ADPKD type 2	PKD2 (NM_000297.4)	Chr4: 88929481	c.595+1G>C	20 (34/171)
ARPKD type 1	PKHD1 (NM_138694.4)	Chr6: 51947999	c.107C>T (p.T36M)	9 (5/57)
ADTKD type 1	UMOD (NM_003361.4)	Chr16: 20359859	c.764G>A (p.C255Y)	35 (12/34)
ADTKD type 2	MUC1 (NM_001371720.1)	Chr1: 155161732	c.428dup (p.A144SfsTer288)	100 (6/6)
Collagen type IV nephropathies	COL4A3 (NM_000091.5)	Chr2: 228176554	c.4981C>T (p.R1661C)	10 (11/113)
	COL4A4 (NM_000092.5)	Chr2: 227920687	c.2690G>A (p.G897E)	21 (21/102)

ADPKD, autosomal dominant polycystic kidney disease; ADTKD, autosomal dominant tubulointerstitial disease; ARPKD, autosomal recessive PKD; OMIM, Online Mendelian Inheritance in Man.
[a]The number of Galician families from the NefroCHUS cohort with the mentioned mutation versus the total number of families with some type of mutation in that gene is indicated in parentheses.

damage, and a diminution in calcium oxalate deposition in renal tubules were achieved. Although, in our opinion, it would have been more appropriate and rigorous to select ABEmax-VQR to perform the *in vivo* experiments, the authors demonstrate the safety of ABE8e-VQR by testing the bystander and off-target editing, as well as the possible generation of hepatotoxicity. These results further highlight the great potential of treating this disease with this gene editing tool.

Another important and noteworthy observation by Chen et al.[3] was the *in vitro* verification of the possible applicability of the base editing technology for the correction of 39 transitional mutations observed in patients with primary hyperoxaluria type 1. In this way, the authors achieved the perfect correction of 32.4% of the mutations observed in patients. Undoubtedly, these results support this technology as a promising and effective therapy for primary hyperoxaluria type 1. Although there are effective therapies to treat this disease, such as those based on RNAi,[6] their administration to patients lasts a lifetime and this may affect to a greater or lesser extent their quality of life. Therefore, it is worth investing in the search for alternative therapies that contribute to improving the well-being of patients for the rest of their lives.

Gene editing: a promising future in genetic kidney disease treatment

Several reasons could lead us to think that gene editing will be an invaluable technology for genetic kidney disorders. As demonstrated by Chen et al.[3] in the treatment of primary hyperoxaluria type 1, a disease whose manifestation depends on the dose effect of functional protein, a low correction of the mutated gene is sufficient to rescue the disease, and it is not necessary to correct all the cells of the organ to achieve phenotype recovery. This raises the possibility of using the genetic editing tools in other hereditary diseases where the dose effect also influences disease evolution, for example, autosomal dominant polycystic kidney disease (ADPKD), the most common genetic cause of kidney failure worldwide. Interestingly, ADPKD is autosomal dominant in inheritance but is recessive at the cellular level in both PKD and polycystic liver disease, and cystogenesis is initiated after a somatic mutation occurs in the unaffected allele, increasing the functional loss of the causative gene from 50% to 100%.[7] Furthermore, mutational analyses in human patients suggest that ADPKD is also dose dependent and that alleles with incomplete penetrance determine disease development and progression.[8] More importantly for a potential therapeutic approach, recent studies have demonstrated renal plasticity that fully restores kidney structure and function after the recovery of gene expression.[9] However, new strategies need to be developed to deliver gene-editing technologies to hard-to-reach organs, such as the kidney.[4] Moreover, many cystic disorders present both kidney and liver cysts at the same time, which opens the possibility of easily addressing both PKD and polycystic liver disease with a single treatment. Taken together, all these concepts position gene-editing tools as a potential future treatment for hepatic and kidney cystic disorders.

Another possible feature that positions the application of these technologies in many of the genetic kidney diseases is that there is a high recurrence of mutations in many of them. In our geographically closed cohort (Galicia, Spain), we have identified a considerable number of families with several common recurrent mutations associated with ADPKD type 2 (PKD2 gene), autosomal recessive PKD (PKHD1 gene), autosomal dominant tubulointerstitial disease (UMOD and MUC1 genes), and collagen IV nephropathies (COL4A3 and COL4A4 genes) (NefroCHUS cohort; Table 1). The development of specific single-guide RNAs with proven safety and efficacy for mutations associated with well-characterized familial cohorts or recurrent mutations in different families would position gene editing as a promising hope for treating these diseases. Moreover, given the speed at which gene editing is advancing, it is to be expected that its application will eventually be extended to rare or ultrarare kidney diseases, which would take the term "personalized medicine" to its maximum expression.

In conclusion, the study by Chen et al. adds to the growing preclinical research demonstrating the great potential of CRISPR tools for the treatment of genetic diseases. However, it should be noted that many challenges remain, such as addressing long-term safety issues, ensuring equitable access to gene therapies, public acceptance of gene editing, and the possibility of nontherapeutic uses.

Although there is still a considerable journey ahead, the first steps have already been taken, and the prospect of using these tools to treat diseases is starting to become a reality. If technological progress finally allows it, what better treatment for a genetic disease than to correct the mutation that causes it?

DISCLOSURE
All the authors declared no competing interests.

REFERENCES
1. Anzalone AV, Koblan LW, Liu DR. Genome editing with CRISPR-Cas nucleases, base editors, transposases and prime editors. *Nat Biotechnol.* 2020;38:824–844.
2. Chiesa R, Georgiadis C, Syed F, et al. Base-edited CAR7 T cells for relapsed T-cell acute lymphoblastic leukemia. *N Engl J Med.* 2023;389:899–910.
3. Chen Z, Zhang D, Zheng R, et al. *In vivo* base editing rescues primary hyperoxaluria type 1 in rats. *Kidney Int.* 2024;105:496–507.
4. Gómez-García F, Martínez-Pulleiro R, Carrera N, et al. Genetic kidney diseases (GKDs) modeling using genome editing technologies. *Cells.* 2022;11:1571.
5. Kattenhorn LM, Tipper CH, Stoica L, et al. Adeno-associated virus gene therapy for liver disease. *Hum Gene Ther.* 2016;27:947–961.
6. Groothoff JW, Metry E, Deesker L, et al. Clinical practice recommendations for primary hyperoxaluria: an expert consensus statement from ERKNet and OxalEurope. *Nat Rev Nephrol.* 2023;19:194–211.
7. Chebib FT, Torres VE. Autosomal dominant polycystic kidney disease: core curriculum 2016. *Am J Kidney Dis.* 2016;67:792–810.
8. Hopp K, Ward CJ, Hommerding CJ, et al. Functional polycystin-1 dosage governs autosomal dominant polycystic kidney disease severity. *J Clin Invest.* 2012;122:4257–4273.
9. Dong K, Zhang C, Tian X, et al. Renal plasticity revealed through reversal of polycystic kidney disease in mice. *Nat Genet.* 2021;53:1649–1663.

Advancing parathyroid anatomy understanding through single-cell RNA sequencing in uremic secondary hyperparathyroidism

Iddo Z. Ben-Dov[1]

This commentary explores the recent application of single-cell RNA sequencing in the study of uremic secondary hyperparathyroidism, shedding light on the cellular dynamics within parathyroid glands. The use of single-cell RNA sequencing reveals new insights into the differentiation processes of chief and oxyphil cells, challenging traditional views and highlighting the potential of this technology in advancing our understanding of parathyroid anatomy.

Kidney International (2024) **105,** 433–435; https://doi.org/10.1016/j.kint.2023.12.005
Copyright © 2023, International Society of Nephrology. Published by Elsevier Inc. All rights reserved.

see clinical investigation on page 562

For over a century, investigations into parathyroid anatomy have played a crucial role in expanding our understanding of both normal and pathologic states. Techniques ranging from histologic and ultrastructural analyses to more recent single-cell cytological[1] approaches have contributed to this knowledge base. However, in comparison to the rapid progress in cellular[2] and molecular[3] biology, advancements in parathyroid anatomy, particularly in the context of chronic kidney disease, have been relatively modest.

Enter single-cell RNA sequencing (scRNA-seq), a revolutionary technology that enables the examination of gene expression profiles at the single-cell level.[4] This method holds immense promise in elevating our understanding of parathyroid anatomy, offering a higher-resolution view of cellular heterogeneity compared with conventional methods. The ability to analyze individual cells provides an unprecedented opportunity to validate and refine our existing knowledge of tissue anatomy and, crucially, to uncover novel subpopulations of cells. The method can also be used to investigate gene expression shifts in various cell types during diseases and can map developmental trajectories and differentiation pathways, illuminating relationships between cell types.

In the context of human parathyroid glands, 2 distinct cell populations, chief cells and oxyphil cells, have long been recognized. Chief cells, predominant in abundance, exhibit a basophilic appearance with lighter eosin staining. These cells play a central role in parathyroid hormone (PTH) production, sensing blood calcium levels and secreting PTH in response to low calcium. On the other hand, oxyphil cells, less abundant and located predominantly in the periphery of the gland, display an eosinophilic appearance because of their high mitochondrial content.[5] Traditionally considered aged chief cells, recent research challenges this notion, suggesting that oxyphil cells may have distinct functions and origins. Ritter *et al.* have documented a 5-fold increase in the proportion of oxyphil cells in the parathyroid glands of uremic patients compared with normal individuals.[6] This suggests that oxyphil cells are sensitive to the stimulatory environment associated with uremia, such as high phosphate levels and low calcium levels. The increase in oxyphil cell number generally parallels the increase in total parathyroid gland weight in uremic patients, further supporting their stimulated state. In addition, Ritter *et al.* suggest that different treatment regimens associate with the oxyphil/chief cell ratio in uremic hyperparathyroidism. Cinacalcet is linked with a

---

[1]Internal Medicine B, Department of Nephrology and Hypertension and Laboratory of Medical Transcriptomics, Hadassah–Hebrew University Medical Center, Jerusalem, Israel

Correspondence: *Iddo Z. Ben-Dov, Internal Medicine B, Hadassah University Medical Center, Kiryat Hadassah 1, Jerusalem, 9112001 Israel. E-mail: iddo@hadassah.org.il*

commentary

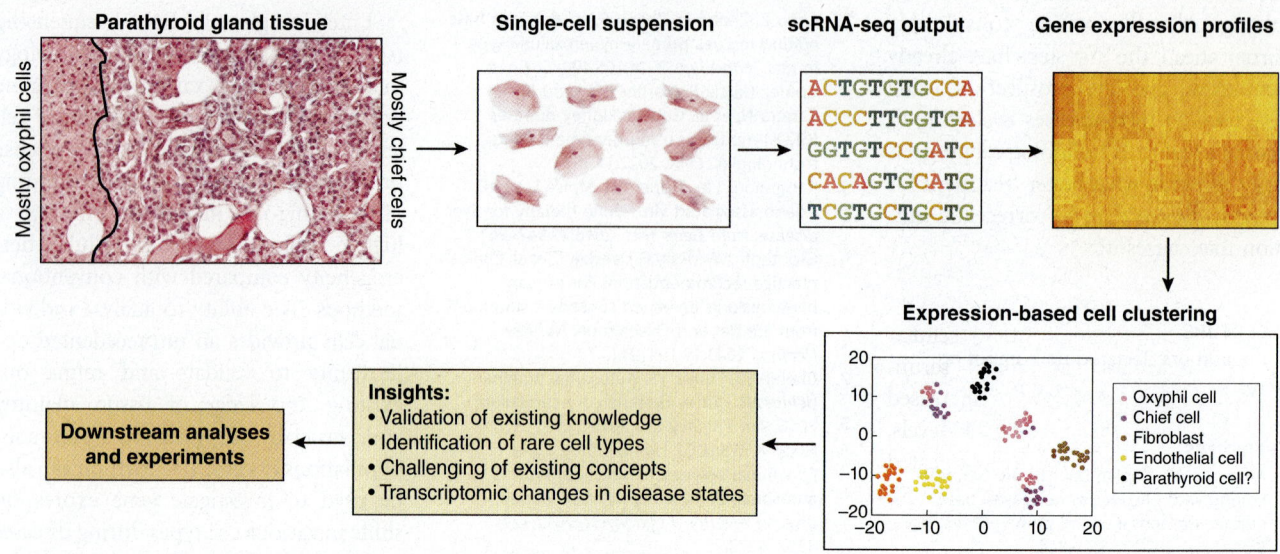

Figure 1 | An illustration describing a possible workflow using single-cell RNA sequencing (scRNA-seq) to generate new knowledge and hypotheses to be tested in follow-up investigations.

further increase in the proportion of oxyphil cells, whereas paricalcitol is not.

In this issue of the journal, Mao et al. delve into the molecular intricacies of uremic secondary hyperparathyroidism, employing scRNA-seq to delineate cell diversity in parathyroid tissues from affected patients.[7] This investigation, involving 20 uremic patients with secondary hyperparathyroidism, presents a fascinating exploration into the pathologic types observed—chief cell nodules, oxyphil cell nodules, and mixed nodules. (According to biochemical parameters, many participants must have had tertiary hyperparathyroidism, a condition in which the glands function autonomously, continuing to produce excess PTH independently of the original triggering factor.)

Surgical parathyroidectomy led to a significant decrease in serum PTH, calcium, and phosphorus levels. Parathyroid tissues exhibited 3 pathologic types: chief cell nodules, oxyphil cell nodules, and mixed nodules. scRNA-seq of parathyroid tissues from 3 uremic secondary hyperparathyroidism patients with mixed nodules revealed 16 distinct cell clusters. Clusters were identified using specific markers, and parathyroid-specific factors, like *PTH* and *GCM2* (a parathyroid-specific transcription factor, required for gland development), were highly expressed in certain clusters.

Trajectory analysis suggested a differentiation relationship between chief and oxyphil cells, with oxyphil cells showing gradual mitochondrial enrichment. (Trajectory analysis in scRNA-seq is a computational approach that examines gene expression patterns across individual cells to infer developmental paths and cell fate decisions. Using dedicated tools, this method orders cells along trajectories, identifies branching points, and visualizes high-dimensional data with t-distributed stochastic neighbor embedding plots. Pseudotime represents the progression of cells, whereas RNA velocity analysis validates trajectory findings, collectively offering insights into the dynamics of cellular development and differentiation in heterogeneous cell populations.) *NRF1* (nuclear factor erythroid 2–related factor 1) and *PPARGC1A* (peroxisome proliferator-activated receptor γ coactivator 1α, also known as PGC1α, a coactivator interacting with *NRF1* and other transcription factors) regulate mitochondrial biogenesis, stimulating expression of genes involved in mitochondrial DNA replication, transcription, and translation. Also, genes involved in mitochondrial fusion, such as *MFN1* and *MFN2*, which promote the formation of interconnected mitochondrial networks, may be upregulated in the differentiation process.

Involvement of the mammalian target of rapamycin pathway, which regulates cellular growth and metabolism,[8] may also influence mitochondrial function. Using their current data and previous findings, Mao et al. identified specific transcription factors involved in transdifferentiation, including *PPARGC1A*. Increased expression of *PPARGC1A* in oxyphil cells suggests its role in their enhanced mitochondrial content. Notably, *PPARGC1A* also regulates energy metabolism in other tissues.

Further investigations by Mao et al. revealed differences in mitochondrial quality control and metabolic function between chief and oxyphil cells. Kyoto Encyclopedia of Genes and Genomes (KEGG) pathway enrichment analysis highlighted pathways related to immunity and inflammation, lipid and energy metabolism, mineral metabolism disorder, endocrine metabolic disorder, kinase signal transduction, cell growth, development and death, and cell adhesion and junction. (KEGG pathway enrichment analysis is a computational method to interpret large-scale biological data, typically gene expression profiles, in the context of known biological pathways documented in KEGG. It identifies whether specific biological pathways are overrepresented or underrepresented in a set of genes of interest compared with what would be expected by chance. It provides insights into the functional relevance of the genes and helps uncover the underlying biological processes at play.) These findings are postulated to reflect the impact of the uremic milieu on mitochondrial biogenesis in parathyroid cells.

Transplantation experiments, involving the implantation of hyperplastic nodules into nude mice, provided insights into the systemic effects of these cellular changes. Changes in host serum biochemical indexes, including increased serum calcium and (human) PTH levels, were observed. Further analyses indicated a reduced proliferation ability of both chief and oxyphil cells posttransplantation, with specific changes in mitochondrial biogenesis in oxyphil cell nodules. Bulk RNA sequencing confirmed the amelioration of the oxyphil cell phenotype after transplantation into nonuremic nude mice.

Although the study by Mao *et al.* significantly contributes to our understanding of uremic secondary hyperparathyroidism, it also prompts critical reflections. The commentary suggests a need for a nuanced reevaluation of the chief cell–oxyphil cell dichotomy, especially given the intricate clustering map observed (Figure 1). The potential reclassification of parathyroid cells based on this state-of-the-art phenotyping modality could offer additional insights, challenging existing perspectives.

In conclusion, the study by Mao *et al.* exemplifies the power of scRNA-seq in unraveling the cellular intricacies of parathyroid glands, particularly in the context of uremic secondary hyperparathyroidism. The comprehensive analysis provides a foundation for future investigations, urging the scientific community to explore shared data for further insights. (Fortunately, using the authors' shared data, one can reanalyze to obtain additional insights from different viewpoints [with a reservation that at the time of writing this commentary the accession the authors provided to the deposited data exists, but data are not yet available].) As we continue to unravel the mysteries of parathyroid anatomy, scRNA-seq stands out as a transformative tool, offering unprecedented insights into cellular dynamics and differentiation processes.

DISCLOSURE
The author declared no competing interests.

REFERENCES
1. Lever J. Cytological appearances in the normal and activated parathyroid of the rat: a combined study by electron and light microscopy with certain quantitative assessments. *J Endocrinol.* 1958;17:210–217.
2. Drüeke T. Cell biology of parathyroid gland hyperplasia in chronic renal failure. *J Am Soc Nephrol.* 2000;11:1141–1152.
3. Hassan AK, Kilav-Levin N, Nechama R, et al. Molecular mechanisms of parathyroid disorders in chronic kidney disease. *Metabolites.* 2022;12:111.
4. Jovic D, Liang X, Zeng H, et al. Single-cell RNA sequencing technologies and applications: a brief overview. *Clin Transl Med.* 2022;12:e694.
5. Ritter C, Haughey B, Miller B, Brown A. Differential gene expression by oxyphil and chief cells of human parathyroid glands. *J Clin Endocrinol Metab.* 2012;97:E1499–E1505.
6. Ritter C, Miller B, Coyne D, et al. Paricalcitol and cinacalcet have disparate actions on parathyroid oxyphil cell content in patients with chronic kidney disease. *Kidney Int.* 2017;92:1217–1222.
7. Mao J, You H, Wang M, et al. Single-cell RNA sequencing reveals transdifferentiation of parathyroid chief cells into oxyphil cells in patients with uremic secondary hyperparathyroidsism. *Kidney Int.* 2024;105: 562–581.
8. Saxton RA, Sabatini DM. mTOR signaling in growth, metabolism and disease. *Cell.* 2017;169:361–371.

Refining GFR estimation: a quest for the unobservable truth?

Tariq Shafi[1]

Assessing glomerular filtration rate (GFR), which is central to evaluating kidney health, remains challenging. Measured GFR is not widely available and lacks standardization. Estimated GFR can be highly inaccurate for some patients and has limited applicability to many patient populations, such as those who are acutely ill. Recent metabolomic advances show promise for identifying new filtration markers that might enhance GFR estimation. Improving GFR assessment will require refinement in both GFR measurement and estimation methods.

Kidney International (2024) **105**, 435–437; https://doi.org/10.1016/j.kint.2023.12.004

Copyright © 2023, International Society of Nephrology. Published by Elsevier Inc. All rights reserved.

see clinical investigation on page 582

Glomerular filtration rate (GFR) is widely regarded as the best available index of overall kidney health.[1] The GFR of individual nephrons is a dynamic physiological process that is currently immeasurable in humans.

[1]*Division of Nephrology, Department of Medicine, Houston Methodist Hospital and Houston Methodist Research Institute, Houston, Texas, USA*

Correspondence: *Tariq Shafi, Houston Methodist Hospital and Houston Methodist Research Institute, 6550 Fannin Ave, Houston, Texas 77030, USA. E-mail: tshafi@houtonmethodist.org*

Measured GFR (mGFR) reflects the time-averaged GFR of all the functioning nephrons during the measurement period. Clinically, GFR is typically estimated from the serum levels of endogenous filtration markers, such as creatinine, and can be approximated to mGFR by equations. Estimated GFR (eGFR), the predicted average mGFR of the people in the equation derivation cohorts, converts serum creatinine from a biochemical mg/dl scale to a more clinically intuitive ml/min per 1.73 m^2 scale. Advances in GFR estimation have allowed advances in kidney disease epidemiology and standardized disease definitions, aided large-scale clinical trials, and simplified communication of the severity of the kidney disease among clinicians and with patients.

Yet, eGFR's limitations are often underrecognized. First, eGFR's applicability is limited to the patient populations similar to those used in its development. Thus, eGFR is unreliable in acutely ill and hospitalized patients and in those with heart failure, cirrhosis, acute kidney failure, extremes of muscle mass, and advanced chronic kidney disease, among others. Second, statistical metrics reported for equation models have appropriately focused on minimizing the population-level difference between mGFR and eGFR (bias), but clinicians commonly misunderstand the negligible bias to mean that the eGFR is highly accurate for individual patients. Thus, the universal reporting of eGFR with each serum creatinine as a single number without its prediction interval has led clinicians to consider the reported eGFR "measurement" the same as inulin mGFR that they learned about in medical school physiology. We recently documented that at an individual level, eGFR was highly inaccurate in assessing mGFR; at an eGFR creatinine of 60 ml/min per 1.73 m^2, 50% of the mGFR values were either >67 ml/min per 1.73 m^2 or <52 ml/min per 1.73 m^2.[2] Thus, new GFR assessment methods are needed in clinical scenarios where current eGFR equations are not applicable and in situations where a more exact value of GFR may be used, such as anticancer drug eligibility and dosing, nephrectomy for kidney donors, and kidney transplant referral and listing eligibility.

The inaccuracies in the current methods to estimate GFR result from the characteristics of the endogenous filtration markers and the variability in mGFR. An ideal endogenous filtration marker would be produced at a steady rate in the human body, independent of diet or gut microbiota, freely filtered at the glomerulus, neither secreted nor reabsorbed, and not have any nonrenal elimination. The factors besides GFR influencing the plasma concentration of filtration markers are referred to as the non-GFR determinants. It has been hypothesized that combining multiple endogenous filtration markers might cancel out the errors from the non-GFR determinants.[3] The addition of cystatin C to serum creatinine reduces the inaccuracy (giving a higher P30, i.e., the percentage of eGFR values within 30% of mGFR) with further improvements using a panel of metabolites.[4] The variability in mGFR also contributes to the error in GFR estimation. The variability in mGFR could be due to the normal physiological variability of GFR or measurement error due to the pharmacokinetic properties of external filtration markers, errors in the GFR measurement procedure, and the accuracy of the markers' assays. The technique of GFR measurement can also influence the results. For example, plasma clearance methods using bolus injection are unreliable in the presence of edema, ascites, or third spacing due to the unpredictable diffusion of the external filtration marker in those fluid compartments. Thus, plasma clearance methods should not be used to assess GFR in patients with decompensated heart failure, cirrhosis, or acute kidney failure. Enhancing the accuracy of eGFR will need to overcome these sources of inaccuracy, and different methods may be more useful in different circumstances. The ideal study design would recruit participants from the specific populations of interest; obtain detailed information on medical and dietary history; perform deep physical and physiological phenotyping; use standardized and reproducible GFR measurement protocols that are calibrated to inulin clearance; obtain, process, and store plasma and urine samples under optimal conditions; and repeat the measurements to quantify intraindividual sources of variability in GFR and metabolites.

In this issue of *Kidney International*, Fino *et al.* present the results of a study designed to identify potential endogenous filtration markers that could be included in a multimarker panel eGFR.[5] The goal of this panel eGFR would be to improve eGFR accuracy and eliminate the need for demographic variables for GFR estimation. They used data from 7 research studies with untargeted metabolomic profiling performed on a single commercial metabolomics platform at different periods. GFR was measured using plasma clearance of iohexol in 3 studies, plasma clearance of nonradiolabeled iothalamate in 1 study, urinary clearance of radiolabeled iothalamate in 2 studies, and plasma clearance of ^{51}chromium ethylenediamine tetraacetic acid in 1 study. Of the 2851 participants included in the study, 29% (n = 816) were not previously included in the equation development data sets, with the vast majority (n = 613) from the Chronic Kidney Disease in Children Study. Samples used for metabolite profiling were collected simultaneously as mGFR, except in the Chronic Kidney Disease in Children Study, where there is a 6-month gap between mGFR and samples for metabolomics. The investigators considered metabolites as candidates for further evaluation if their average Pearson correlation with mGFR across studies was less than –0.5. Using a rigorous iterative modeling approach that prioritized accuracy of estimation and independence from demographic factors, they identified 12 potential endogenous filtration markers. The accuracy metric used in selecting the candidate markers was the root mean square error. The root mean square error calculates how far off a model's predictions (eGFR) are from the actual observed values (mGFR). The smallest root mean square error value possible is the most desirable. The study's strengths include using existing data sets and a rigorous modeling approach. The limitations include a limited evaluation of patients with cancer (cohort n = 100), cirrhosis (cohort n = 103), and advanced chronic kidney disease, groups in which improvement in estimation is desirable. Notably, the cirrhosis cohort used plasma iothalamate clearance following a bolus injection to measure GFR. As discussed above, this method can be erroneous in individuals with ascites or edema. The investigators acknowledge other limitations, including the cross-sectional design and lack of repeated measurements.

The investigators describe their next steps in developing an improved panel eGFR: understanding the markers' biological properties, developing a targeted mass spectrometry multiplex panel, and then developing and validating this panel. It is unclear what methods will be used to understand the markers' biological properties. Furthermore, it is also unclear if the data from the existing cohorts will be sufficient to validate a panel eGFR that could be used when a precise GFR number is needed for clinical decisions.

As we maintain GFR as the paramount indicator of kidney function, refining its estimation is as important as efforts to improve and standardize mGFR methods. Initiatives like those by the European Kidney Function Consortium to develop consensus on plasma iohexol clearance methods mark significant strides in this direction. However, the journey does not end here. We need similar endeavors to refine urinary clearance methods and align both plasma and urinary clearance techniques to a universal standard. Beyond these technical advancements, assessing the real-world impact of these improvements is critical. Key questions remain: Will refining GFR estimation for the general population significantly enhance our ability to estimate GFR in individual patients with a level of accuracy beyond what is provided by current clinical data? How do we define a desired level of accuracy and who makes this decision? How will the proposed scientific advancements translate into concrete benefits for patients? How do we measure the clinical utility of additional testing at increased cost? In answering these questions, we must not overlook the importance of engaging a broader spectrum of stakeholders: patients, health care providers, and payers alike. Their perspectives are pivotal in shaping a patient-centric approach that aligns scientific progress with practical health care needs.

DISCLOSURE

TS is both a scientific and site principal investigator for numares Health on the AGENTA Study, which is evaluating the reliability of a panel estimated glomerular filtration rate in patients with heart failure. All payments are made to the institution.

REFERENCES

1. Levey AS, Coresh J, Tighiouart H, et al. Measured and estimated glomerular filtration rate: current status and future directions. *Nat Rev Nephrol*. 2020;16:51–64.
2. Shafi T, Zhu X, Lirette ST, et al. Quantifying individual-level inaccuracy in glomerular filtration rate estimation. *Ann Intern Med*. 2022;175:1073–1082.
3. Inker LA, Levey AS, Coresh J. Estimated glomerular filtration rate from a panel of filtration markers—hope for increased accuracy beyond measured glomerular filtration rate? *Adv Chronic Kidney Dis*. 2018;25:67–75.
4. Coresh J, Inker LA, Sang Y, et al. Metabolomic profiling to improve glomerular filtration rate estimation: a proof-of-concept study. *Nephrol Dial Transplant*. 2019;34:825–833.
5. Fino NF, Adingwupu OM, Coresh J, et al. Evaluation of novel candidate filtration markers from a global metabolomics discovery for glomerular filtration rate estimation. *Kidney Int*. 2024;105:582–592.

APOL1-mediated and Mendelian forms of "heretofore" idiopathic collapsing glomerulopathy: lessons from Brazil

Nicholette D. Palmer[1] and Barry I. Freedman[2]

APOL1-mediated kidney diseases have forever changed nephrology and kidney transplantation. Neves *et al.* extend this field with analyses in admixed Brazilians with the most severe type of *APOL1*-mediated kidney disease, idiopathic collapsing glomerulopathy. Causative gene variants were detected in 58.6% of patients; 80.5% had *APOL1* high-risk genotypes, and 19.5% had causative Mendelian variants. Their work identifies the cause of previous idiopathic collapsing glomerulopathy and provides opportunities to identify novel modifiers in severe *APOL1*-mediated kidney diseases that are relevant beyond Brazil.

Kidney International (2024) **105,** 437–439; https://doi.org/10.1016/j.kint.2023.12.014

Copyright © 2024, International Society of Nephrology. Published by Elsevier Inc. All rights reserved.

see clinical investigation on page 593

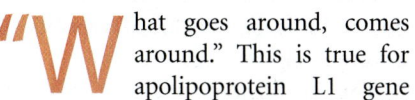hat goes around, comes around." This is true for apolipoprotein L1 gene

[1]Department of Biochemistry, Wake Forest University School of Medicine, Winston-Salem, North Carolina, USA; and [2]Department of Internal Medicine, Section on Nephrology, Wake Forest University School of Medicine, Winston-Salem, North Carolina, USA

Correspondence: *Barry I. Freedman, Section on Nephrology, Wake Forest University School of Medicine, Medical Center Boulevard, Winston-Salem, North Carolina 27157-1053, USA. E-mail: bfreedma@wakehealth.edu*

(*APOL1*)–mediated kidney disease (AMKD). In the early 1990s, 36.1% of African Americans (AAs) initiating renal replacement therapy (RRT) in North Carolina reported close relatives with end-stage kidney disease; surprisingly, disparate causes of chronic kidney disease (CKD) were common in families.[1] This led to the hypothesis that variation in a single gene underlies multiple forms of CKD in AAs.[2] The 2010 discovery of *APOL1* as the cause of nondiabetic CKD closed the loop.[3] AMKD explains most of the excess

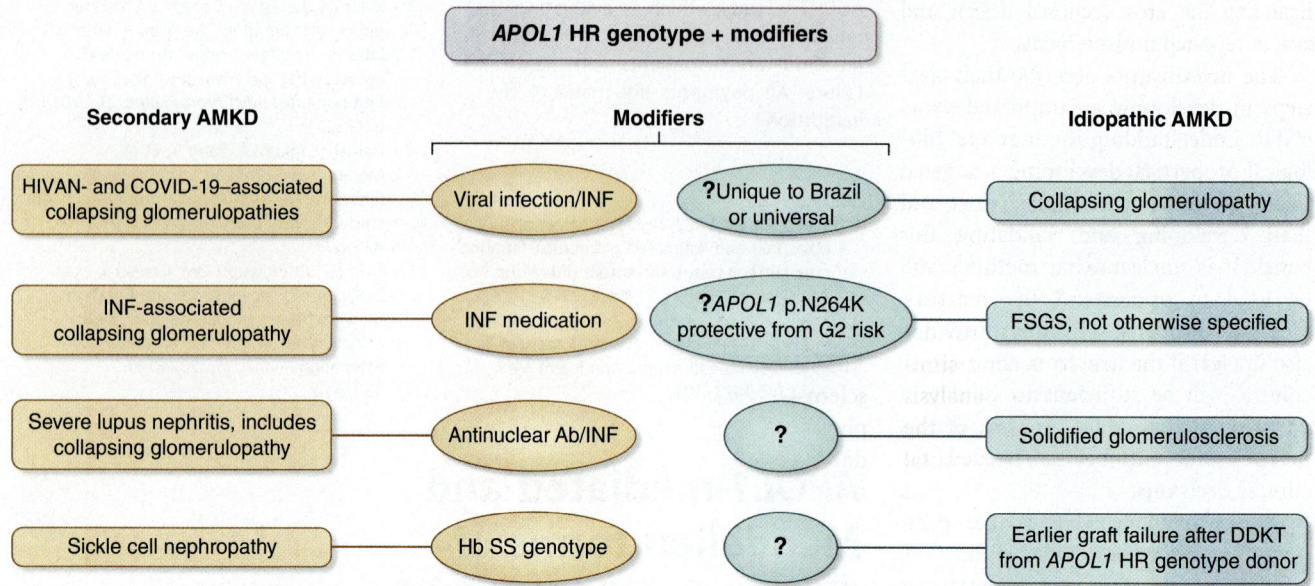

Figure 1 | Idiopathic and secondary forms of *APOL1*-mediated kidney disease (AMKD). Ab, antibodies; COVID-19, coronavirus disease 2019; DDKT, deceased donor kidney transplant; FSGS, focal segmental glomerular sclerosis; Hb, hemoglobin; HIVAN, HIV-associated nephropathy; HR, high risk; INF, interferon.

risk for end-stage kidney disease in AAs versus Europeans, solidified glomerulosclerosis with low-level/absent proteinuria causes the disorder long misattributed to essential hypertension, and the broad spectrum of diseases caused by *APOL1* has been defined (Figure 1).[4]

Fast forward to 2023 and results of a study of idiopathic collapsing glomerulopathy (iCG) in the highly admixed Brazilian population.[5] The frequency of recent African ancestry is considerably lower in Brazilians than AAs. Nonetheless, 36.4% of patients with iCG reported a family history of CKD, and these relatives had poorly described renal phenotypes (unknown, proteinuria, and focal segmental glomerular sclerosis [FSGS]). Despite being a continent away from North Carolina, 58.6% had an inherited cause of iCG, and >80% of those were due to *APOL1*. As in the United States, patients with *APOL1*-mediated iCG had earlier onset (9 to 44 years), as opposed to a wider age distribution in those with *APOL1* low-risk genotypes. These idiopathic cases predated the coronavirus disease 2019 (COVID-19) pandemic, and secondary collapsing glomerulopathy (CG) cases related to COVID-19 vaccination, HIV, schistosomiasis, and lymphoma were excluded.

These investigators analyzed DNA from a carefully phenotyped cohort of adult and pediatric patients with biopsy-proven iCG. Toward variant discovery, they applied targeted gene-based panels or whole-exome sequencing. Assessment of variant pathogenicity included population-specific databases with resequencing to confirm potential causative variants identified in accordance with American College of Medical Genetic and Genomics criteria and included variants of uncertain significance.

The investigators chose 2 complementary approaches for selection and implementation of a sequencing strategy to discover causative gene variants: targeted gene resequencing and whole-exome sequencing. Both methods achieve efficiency in overall cost, particularly with low sample quantity, but they can limit the discovery of novel causative variants. Targeted resequencing strategies often lack uniform coverage because of genomic content that is related to biased enrichment methods (e.g., repeated sequences, base composition). As a result, there will be differential representation of the genomic regions, despite a relatively high mean coverage. Secondarily, the *a priori* selection of genes to sequence significantly limits genetic inquiry as the lack of contributory findings does not confirm the complete lack of genetic contribution. Although whole-exome sequencing may provide a broader view of the genome, it remains limited by our simplistic view of functionally important regions and may fail to provide insight into more complex genomic variations and regulatory contributions.

As a component of their integrated analysis, the investigators considered genetic ancestry data in this highly genetically admixed cohort. In this study, individual genetic ancestry was ascertained through high-density single-nucleotide polymorphism array data anchored on samples of African, European, East-Asian, and Native American ancestry. Although anchoring from preselected populations can inform genetic similarity, it can bias the results toward those populations when other genetic backgrounds may be present. In addition, *a priori* selection of anchoring samples combined with array selection can limit the number of informative markers, acknowledging that there have to be significant allele frequency differences to be informative. More broadly, this approach provides only a global picture of genetic similarity. In contrast, admixture analysis targeted toward specific regions of the genome, potentially harboring causal variants, may provide a better view of the local ancestry and suggest a more homogeneous genetic ancestry.

Among the 70 study patients classified with iCG, the median age of disease onset was 23 (range, 17–31) years, with most patients reporting White ethnicity (64.3%), fewer reporting a family history of kidney disease (22.9%), and half (51.4%) progressing to CKD-RRT by 36 months following diagnosis and represented by a larger proportion of younger patients. Forty-one patients possessed an *APOL1* high-risk genotype (defined as *G1G1*, *G2G2*, or *G1G2*) or a causative Mendelian variant (MV). Among the 33 patients with an *APOL1* high-risk genotype, generally higher proportions of African ancestry were detected. The 8 patients with an MV included more adults, all of whom progressed to CKD-RRT. Among the pathogenic MV, 2 novel variants in the collagen type IV α 5 chain gene (*COL4A5*), a major structural component of basement membranes, were identified. Mutations in *COL4A5* have been associated with X-linked Alport syndrome and FSGS. These mutations included a coding variant resulting in a frameshift and a variant in an exon/intron boundary that could impact splicing. Regarding demographic characteristics, older age and remission of any type (i.e., partial or complete) were protective for CKD-RRT; however, possessing an MV increased the risk of progressive CKD.

Several aspects of this novel study could shed light on modifying factors underlying severe AMKD. We believe the range of histologic findings in AMKD (from solidified glomerulosclerosis, FSGS, CG, sickle cell nephropathy, and lupus nephritis, to donor allograft failure) likely result from exposure to different second hits or mediators (Figure 1). High interferon states (infection with HIV or COVID-19, medical interferon administration, and lupus nephritis) induce *APOL1*-mediated CG.[6,7] These carefully phenotyped cases from Brazil reveal that 47.2% of idiopathic CG cases were *APOL1* mediated. Second hits initiating iCG are not yet known; but novel viral, parasitic, or environmental causes may be detectable in Brazil. These factors may also be relevant to AMKD in patients from Africa, the Caribbean, and the United States. Blocking or treating second hits could prevent or slow progression of nephropathy. A role for the protective *APOL1* p.n264K variant on *G2*-mediated disease in FSGS can also be studied in iCG to determine whether it modifies risk.[8] Finally, these data reveal that the proportion of CG cases deemed "idiopathic" is dwindling as its genetic underpinnings are identified. It has become apparent that a large percentage of iCG cases in Brazil, and likely elsewhere, can be reclassified as due to AMKD. This finding provides exciting hope for the treatment of Brazilians using novel therapies directed specifically against *APOL1* to prevent or slow the inexorable progression of iCG to end-stage kidney disease.[9]

DISCLOSURE

Wake Forest University Health Sciences and BIF have rights to a US patent related to *APOL1* gene testing (https://www.apol1genetest.com). BIF is a consultant for and receives research support from AstraZeneca and Renalytix. The other author declared no competing interests.

REFERENCES

1. Freedman BI, Spray BJ, Tuttle AB, Buckalew VM Jr. The familial risk of end-stage renal disease in African Americans. *Am J Kidney Dis*. 1993;21:387–393.
2. Freedman BI, Iskandar SS, Appel RG. The link between hypertension and nephrosclerosis. *Am J Kidney Dis*. 1995;25:207–221.
3. Genovese G, Friedman DJ, Ross MD, et al. Association of trypanolytic ApoL1 variants with kidney disease in African Americans. *Science*. 2010;329:841–845.
4. Freedman BI, Limou S, Ma L, Kopp JB. APOL1-associated nephropathy: a key contributor to racial disparities in CKD. *Am J Kidney Dis*. 2018;72:S8–S16.
5. Neves PD, Watanabe A, Watanabe EH, et al. Idiopathic collapsing glomerulopathy is associated with *APOL1* high-risk genotypes or Mendelian variants in most affected individuals in a highly admixed population. *Kidney Int*. 2024;105:593–607.
6. Nichols B, Jog P, Lee JH, et al. Innate immunity pathways regulate the nephropathy gene apolipoprotein L1. *Kidney Int*. 2015;87:332–342.
7. Velez JCQ, Caza T, Larsen CP. COVAN is the new HIVAN: the re-emergence of collapsing glomerulopathy with COVID-19. *Nat Rev Nephrol*. 2020;16:565–567.
8. Gupta Y, Friedman DJ, McNulty MT, et al. Strong protective effect of the APOL1 p.N264K variant against G2-associated focal segmental glomerulosclerosis and kidney disease. *Nat Commun*. 2023;14:7836.
9. Egbuna O, Zimmerman B, Manos G, et al. Inaxaplin for proteinuric kidney disease in persons with two APOL1 variants. *N Engl J Med*. 2023;388:969–979.

commentary

Anti-nephrin antibodies in recurrence of focal segmental glomerulosclerosis: closer to discovering the Holy Grail?

Marina Vivarelli[1] and Manuela Colucci[1]

Recurrent forms of primary focal segmental glomerulosclerosis (FSGS) pose an unmet challenge to nephrologists, both in terms of understanding the underlying pathophysiology and in terms of identifying an effective management strategy of this disease, which frequently leads to kidney graft loss. In the past few decades, experimental observations both in patients and in animal models have led to the hypothesis of the existence of circulating factors driving the loss of integrity of the glomerular filtration barrier in FSGS. Although different circulating factor candidates have been postulated, none has been unequivocally shown to be pathogenic. In the current study, Shirai et al. propose a new candidate for this role by identifying circulating anti-nephrin autoantibodies in a cohort of patients with post-transplant recurrence of primary FSGS. Recent evidence by Watts et al. has also identified anti-nephrin autoantibodies in the circulation and in the kidney biopsies of patients with minimal change disease. If confirmed, the identification of these autoantibodies would both contribute to identifying the elusive circulating factor in FSGS and increase our understanding of the spectrum of proteinuric glomerular lesions, spanning from minimal change disease to FSGS. The quest for the Holy Grail is perhaps closer to completion.

Kidney International (2024) 105, 440–442; https://doi.org/10.1016/j.kint.2023.12.015
Copyright © 2024, International Society of Nephrology. Published by Elsevier Inc. All rights reserved.

see clinical investigation on page 608

[1]Laboratory of Nephrology, IRCCS Ospedale Pediatrico Bambino Gesù, Rome, Italy

Correspondence: Marina Vivarelli, UO Nefrologia e Dialisi, IRCCS Ospedale Pediatrico Bambino Gesù, Piazza S. Onofrio 4, Rome 00165, Italy. E-mail: marina.vivarelli@opbg.net

The pathogenic role of a circulating glomerular permeability factor inducing podocyte foot process effacement followed by the intense proteinuria typical of nongenetic idiopathic nephrotic syndrome was hypothesized more than 50 years ago. A very recent review reports all the scientific evidence of the existence of this extrarenal permeability factor, which could mediate the podocyte damage in both minimal change disease (MCD) and primary and recurrent focal segmental glomerulosclerosis (FSGS), which are the 2 most frequent pathologic findings when kidney biopsy is performed in patients with idiopathic nephrotic syndrome.[1] Some proofs supporting the concept of a pathogenic circulating permeability factor derive from indirect evidence of an early recurrence in approximately 30% of patients with FSGS after kidney transplantation and of the ability of plasma exchange to reduce the risk of FSGS recurrence.[1] However, the most direct evidence stems from the study of Gallon et al.,[2] who demonstrated in 2012 that a kidney removed from a post-transplant early recurrent FSGS patient could be efficiently retransplanted into a different non-FSGS recipient with a complete recovery of the glomerular filtration function. Several potential candidates have been described over the years, but the most convincing seemed to be cardiotrophin-like cytokine factor 1, purified from plasma samples of patients with recurrent FSGS by Savin et al.[3] and showing the same ability of plasma samples of patients with recurrent FSGS to induce glomerular permeabilization in injected rats and in rat-perfused glomeruli. Despite these interesting results, several discrepancies between experimental observations and FSGS patient unresponsiveness to galactose treatment targeting cardiotrophin-like cytokine factor 1 suggest that further mechanisms could be at play.[1] Therefore, whereas its immune origin is largely supported by the therapeutic efficacy of immunosuppressive drugs and of immunoadsorption in inducing remission after FSGS recurrence, the circulating permeability factor remained elusive for several years.[1]

In 2022, Watts et al.[4] described for the first time the presence of a punctate positivity to IgG colocalizing with nephrin in the glomerulus of approximately 30% pediatric and adult nongenetic MCD patients. The authors also aimed to measure the presence of circulating anti-nephrin autoantibodies by setting up an enzyme-linked immunosorbent assay and an immunoprecipitation method by testing the reactivity against a manufactured recombinant extracellular domain of the nephrin and found a direct association between autoantibody positivity and activity of the disease.[4] They also identified a pretransplant positivity of anti-nephrin antibodies in an adult patient who experienced a rapid recurrence of proteinuria after kidney transplantation.[4] In the current issue of Kidney International, Shirai et al.[5] expanded their first observation in a single pediatric case report investigating the role of anti-nephrin antibodies in mediating post-transplant FSGS recurrence in a Japanese pediatric multicentric cohort. Twenty-two pediatric

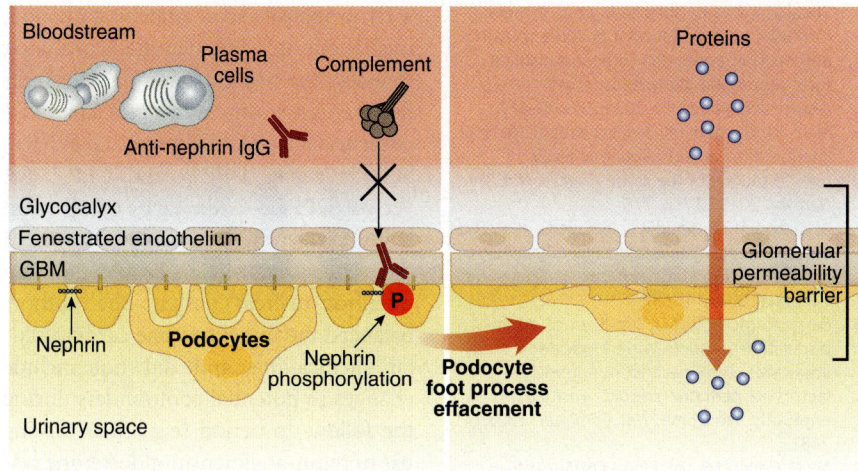

Figure 1 | Anti-nephrin antibodies directly mediate post-transplant focal segmental glomerulosclerosis (FSGS) recurrence. Anti-nephrin IgG secreted by antibody-producing plasma cells binds podocyte nephrin and induces nephrin tyrosine phosphorylation, causing podocyte foot process effacement and intense proteinuria typical of post-transplant FSGS recurrence. These effects seem to be complement-independent because no colocalization with complement factors is found in graft biopsies. GBM, glomerular basement membrane.

patients with FSGS receiving kidney transplantation with available plasma samples and graft biopsy specimens were enrolled; among them, 8 patients resulted in disease-causing variants secondary to genetic mutations, and 11 of 14 nongenetic patients experienced FSGS recurrence.[5] Plasma samples from a total of 30 healthy or disease (membranous nephropathy or lupus nephritis) controls as well as from 13 patients with MCD were also assessed. Graft biopsies were evaluated for the presence of punctate IgG colocalizing with nephrin and for the nephrin tyrosine phosphorylation, whereas circulating anti-nephrin antibody levels were determined by the same enzyme-linked immunosorbent assay method but performed with a commercially available recombinant human nephrin.[5] Shirai et al. found that 100% of patients with recurrent FSGS had autoantibodies against nephrin in both graft biopsies and plasma samples, in contrast to none of the patients with genetic or nonrecurrent FSGS or the healthy or disease controls. Circulating anti-nephrin antibody positivity was also found in 5 of 13 patients with MCD during active disease and was significantly reduced during remission, as previously reported.[4] Biopsies resulting positive for anti-nephrin autoantibody staining also showed nephrin tyrosine phosphorylation, altered nephrin distribution, and intense foot process effacement. In addition, these alterations, as well as the presence of anti-nephrin autoantibodies, decreased or disappeared in 9 of 11 patients with recurrent FSGS who achieved remission after plasma exchange, rituximab, or no treatment, whereas anti-nephrin antibody levels before plasma exchange were similar among patients who responded compared with those who failed to reach remission after treatment.[5] Of note, no colocalization with complement deposition was found in graft biopsies of recurrent FSGS.[5] Altogether, the reported results strongly support a direct pathogenic role of anti-nephrin autoantibodies in mediating post-transplant FSGS recurrence and podocyte foot process effacement by inducing nephrin tyrosine phosphorylation in a complement-independent manner and suggest their role as a new circulating factor causing FSGS (Figure 1).

Of note, the presence of autoantibodies against nephrin in both MCD and primary FSGS strongly suggests a common pathogenic origin of these 2 different clinical and histologic entities, as previously hypothesized.[6] The pathogenic role of anti-nephrin autoantibodies is also supported by 2 important observations in pediatric forms of steroid-sensitive nephrotic syndrome (SSNS), which constitutes the vast majority of children with MCD. One is a very recent study aimed at characterizing the peripheral blood B-cell repertoire by single-cell RNA-sequencing analysis in children with SSNS. This study reports an altered transcriptional profile in extrafollicular and antibody-producing B-cell subsets.[7] Although the mechanisms underlying the expansion of these specific B-cell subsets are still unknown, this study strongly implicates pathogenic antibody production in the underlying disease pathophysiology. The second is the recent observation that genetic variants at the NPHS1 locus can predispose to a higher risk of developing primary SSNS in East Asians but not in patients of other ethnicities.[8] However, both Watts et al.[4] and Shirai et al.,[5] albeit in very small numbers of children with SSNS, found a comparable prevalence of anti-nephrin antibodies in patients with MCD of different ethnic backgrounds.

In parallel with the dissection of the precise mechanism(s) underlying the induction of anti-nephrin autoantibodies and their role in disease pathogenesis, a major effort must be made to set up a reproducible, standardized laboratory method to correctly evaluate the presence and the amount of circulating anti-nephrin autoantibodies. Several issues are emerging on the published assays aimed at measuring anti-nephrin IgG, and the sensitivity and the specificity required by a validated diagnostic method are still far, as recently reported as an Abstract at the "American Society of Nephrology Kidney Week 2023."[9]

Taken altogether, the identification of anti-nephrin autoantibodies, if confirmed in larger, well-characterized, and multiethnic cohorts, will provide a true breakthrough in our understanding of the glomerular spectrum, as it is delineating itself, of MCD and primary FSGS, allowing early and noninvasive identification of patients with an autoantibody-mediated glomerular disease responsive to immunosuppressive treatment.

commentary

DISCLOSURE
All the authors declared no competing interests.

REFERENCES

1. Salfi G, Casiraghi F, Remuzzi G. Current understanding of the molecular mechanisms of circulating permeability factor in focal segmental glomerulosclerosis. *Front Immunol.* 2023;14:1247606.
2. Gallon L, Leventhal J, Skaro A, et al. Resolution of recurrent focal segmental glomerulosclerosis after retransplantation. *N Engl J Med.* 2012;366:1648–1649.
3. Savin VJ, Sharma M, Zhou J, et al. Renal and hematological effects of CLCF-1, a B-cell-stimulating cytokine of the IL-6 family. *J Immunol Res.* 2015;2015:714964.
4. Watts AJB, Keller KH, Lerner G, et al. Discovery of autoantibodies targeting nephrin in minimal change disease supports a novel autoimmune etiology. *J Am Soc Nephrol.* 2022;33:238–252.
5. Shirai Y, Miura K, Ishizuka K, et al. A multi-institutional study found a possible role of anti-nephrin antibodies in post-transplant focal segmental glomerulosclerosis recurrence. *Kidney Int.* 2024;105:608–617.
6. Maas RJ, Deegens JK, Smeets B, et al. Minimal change disease and idiopathic FSGS: manifestations of the same disease. *Nat Rev Nephrol.* 2016;12:768–776.
7. Al-Aubodah TA, Aoudjit L, Pascale G, et al. The extrafollicular B cell response is a hallmark of childhood idiopathic nephrotic syndrome. *Nat Commun.* 2023;14:7682.
8. Barry A, McNulty MT, Jia X, et al. Multi-population genome-wide association study implicates immune and non-immune factors in pediatric steroid-sensitive nephrotic syndrome. *Nat Commun.* 2023;14:2481.
9. Liu P, Gallon LG, Jin J. SA-PO971—anti-nephrin autoantibodies broadly detected in the general population and in non-kidney disease patients. *J Am Soc Nephrol.* 2023;34:100–101.

Exploring nontraditional cardiorenal advantages of SGLT-2 inhibitors and GLP-1 receptor agonists

Jia-Jin Chen[1], Tao-Han Lee[2] and Huang-Yu Yang[1,3]

This commentary provides an analysis of the study by Fu *et al.* in *Kidney International*, which employs 3 administrative databases to investigate the hyperkalemia protective effects of sodium-glucose cotransporter-2 inhibitors, glucagon-like peptide-1 receptor agonists, and dipeptidyl peptidase-4 inhibitors. It emphasizes the methodological approach, notably the use of a fixed-effect model to aggregate pairwise comparisons from 3 data sets. In addition, we explored the broader cardiorenal and potential nonrenal benefits of these drug classes, underscoring the imperative for continued research in this domain.

Kidney International (2024) **105**, 442–444; https://doi.org/10.1016/j.kint.2024.01.002

Copyright © 2024, International Society of Nephrology. Published by Elsevier Inc. All rights reserved.

see clinical investigation on page 618

---

[1]Kidney Research Center, Nephrology Department, Linkou Chang Gung Memorial Hospital, Taoyuan City, Taiwan; [2]Department of Nephrology, Chansn Hospital, Taoyuan City, Taiwan; and [3]Department of Health Policy and Management, Johns Hopkins Bloomberg School of Public Health, Baltimore, Maryland, USA

Correspondence: Huang-Yu Yang, Department of Nephrology, Chang Gung Memorial Hospital, No. 5, Fusing Street, Gueishan District, Taoyuan City 333, Taiwan. E-mail: hyyang01@gmail.com

In the latest issue of *Kidney International*, Fu *et al.* present a study using 3 administrative claims databases to compare the hyperkalemia protective effects of sodium-glucose cotransporter-2 inhibitors (SGLT2i), glucagon-like peptide-1 receptor agonists (GLP-1 RA), and dipeptidyl peptidase-4 inhibitors (DPP4i). The study's design and statistical methods were noteworthy. They use a 1:1 propensity score matching method, incorporating >140 identified covariates, to assess the hyperkalemia protective effects. This assessment involves 3 pairwise comparisons—SGLT2i versus GLP-1 RA, SGLT2i versus DPP4i, and GLP-1 RA versus DPP4i—with each comparison being exclusively analyzed in 1 of the 3 different databases. Employing an intention-to-treat design, the authors balanced the initial baseline cardiovascular medications and did not include changes in potential confounders during the follow-up period (e.g., time-varying use of renin-angiotensin-aldosterone system inhibitors) in this study. For the follow-up period, an "as-treated" approach was applied. Patients were followed up until the development of the outcome, death, or drug discontinuation (defined by a 30-day period)/switch. Additional sensitivity analyses using a 60-day period for drug discontinuation definition and an intention-to-treat follow-up approach yielded results consistent with the primary analysis.

Fu *et al.* illustrate that, compared with DPP4i, both SGLT2i and GLP-1 RA are linked with a lower hazard ratio for hyperkalemia. In addition, they performed a fixed-effect meta-analysis to pool hyperkalemia incidence data from various databases. Despite some baseline characteristic variations, the authors report comparable propensity score–matched hazard ratios for GLP-1 RA versus DPP4i across 3 databases (not provided in the main text). A similar trend was observed for SGLT2i versus DPP4i across 3 databases. Consequently, Fu *et al.* suggest that employing a fixed-effect model is appropriate. The result of this study might be the first real-world evidence of GLP-1 RA's hyperkalemia protective effect.[1]

Fu *et al.* discuss several mechanisms potentially underlying this effect, including the following: (i) increased sodium excretion in the proximal tubule, enhancing potassium excretion in the distal nephron; (ii) changes in dietary habits (although this was not directly analyzed, as acknowledged in their limitations); and (iii) reduced albuminuria, leading to better kidney

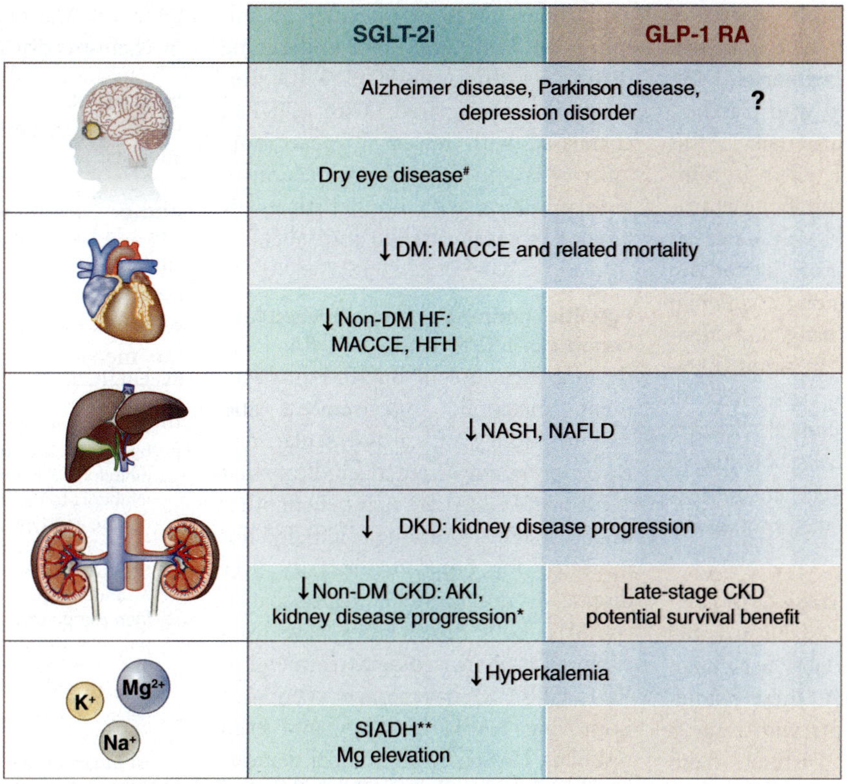

Figure 1 | Potential clinical application and cardio-renal benefit of glucagon-like peptide-1 receptor agonists (GLP-1 RA) and sodium-glucose cotransporter-2 inhibitors (SGLT-2i). Although the roles of SGLT2i in neuroprotection and anti-inflammation have been explored, robust clinical effectiveness remains unproven because of the lack of randomized controlled trials (RCTs). Similarly, although GLP-1 RA have been studied in RCTs and cohort studies for Parkinson disease, Alzheimer disease, and depression, their benefits remain uncertain based on the current evidence. In the context of populations with late-stage chronic kidney disease (CKD) and kidney failure on dialysis, a cohort study noted that prescribing GLP-1 RA, as opposed to dipeptidyl peptidase-4 inhibitors, was linked with a reduced hazard ratio for all-cause mortality. #SGLT2i were associated with lower hazard for dry eye disease development in comparison with GLP-1 RA from a cohort study. *SGLT2i in non–diabetes mellitus (DM) CKD were examined with more preserved renal function until recently. Specific population-like autosomal dominant or autosomal recessive polycystic kidney disease and lupus nephritis were not included in RCTs. **Empagliflozin was examined in 2 RCTs for treatment of syndrome of inappropriate secretion of antidiuretic hormone (SIADH). AKI, acute kidney injury; DKD, diabetic kidney disease; HF, heart failure; HFH, heart failure hospitalization; MACCE, major adverse cardiac and cerebrovascular event; NAFLD, nonalcoholic fatty liver disease; NASH, nonalcoholic steatohepatitis.

function preservation and further less risk for hyperkalemia, which is a common complication with kidney function decline. They also address previous contradictory findings of increased kidney potassium excretion effect from randomized controlled trials (RCTs) comparing GLP-1 RA with DPP4i.[1] In our view, it remains to be confirmed whether this hyperkalemia protection effect results from enhanced renal potassium excretion or from unmeasured confounding factors, like kidney protection or dietary changes. Prospective trials are needed for this confirmation.

In summary, the large-scale, multi-cohort study of Fu et al. highlights that, in stage 3 to 5 chronic kidney disease (CKD) populations, both SGLT2i and GLP-1 RA are associated with a protective effect against hyperkalemia.[1] Further research is needed to ascertain if this benefit extends to patients with diabetic kidney disease with better-preserved kidney function or to non-CKD, diabetes mellitus patients who are at low risk for hyperkalemia.

In addition to this newly identified hyperkalemia preventive effect of GLP-1 RA, we would like to discuss a range of recently recognized nontraditional cardiorenal benefits associated with GLP-1 RA and SGLT2i. These benefits have emerged from both RCTs and observational studies in real-world settings.

SGLT2i in SIADH management and magnesium elevation effect

Refardt et al. demonstrated through 2 randomized controlled trials that empagliflozin, by increasing electrolyte-free water excretion and urine volume, can be effective in treating the syndrome of inappropriate secretion of antidiuretic hormone (SIADH), both in acute inpatient[2] and chronic outpatient settings.[3] In acute SIADH-associated hyponatremia, a 4-day course of 25 mg daily empagliflozin resulted in a significantly greater increase in serum sodium levels (10 vs. 7 mmol/L) compared with standard care.[2] Furthermore, a small-scale trial in chronic outpatient SIADH patients showed that 25 mg daily empagliflozin over 4 weeks led to an estimated serum sodium increase of 4.09 mmol/L (95% confidence interval, 1.68–6.49 mmol/L) compared with placebo.[3] However, it remains uncertain if this hyponatremic treatment effect is common to all SGLT2i or specific to empagliflozin, as network meta-analysis suggests a slight variation in sodium elevation effects among different SGLT2i.[4] In addition, Zhang et al. identified a slight elevation in serum magnesium as a potential class effect of SGLT2i.[4] However, the clinical relevance of this subtle effect and its potential to induce hypermagnesemia in patients with CKD has yet to be determined.[4]

GLP-1 RA in advanced stage CKD

Although RCTs have established the cardiovascular and mortality benefits of SGLT2i and GLP-1 RA, these studies largely excluded patients with stage 5 CKD and dialysis. Distinct from SGLT2i, whose use in late-stage CKD has only recently become a topic of discussion, GLP-1 RA, such as dulaglutide and albiglutide, are already approved for use in advanced stages of CKD. The clinical benefit of GLP-1 RA in this late-stage CKD population remained unclear until recent observational cohorts based on real-world evidence filled this gap. Using a nationwide claims database, our study showed that for patients with stage 5 CKD and kidney failure on dialysis, GLP-1 RA prescriptions, in comparison to DDP4i, were associated with lower hazard ratios (HRs) for all-cause mortality (HR, 0.79; 95% confidence interval, 0.63–0.98) and infection-related mortality (HR, 0.61; 95% confidence interval, 0.40–0.91).[5] No significant difference in cardiovascular-related mortality was found between the 2 groups,[5] possibly reflecting differing cardiovascular death pathogeneses in patients with late-stage CKD and kidney failure on dialysis compared with the general population. A similar outcome was observed in another multicenter cohort study,[6] which included patients with estimated glomerular filtration rate of <30 ml/min per 1.73 m^2 and those undergoing dialysis. In this study, GLP-1 RA prescriptions, compared with DDP4i, correlated with lower all-cause mortality HRs and delayed progression to kidney failure, with no statistical difference in cardiovascular mortality.[6]

Potential nonrenal, noncardiovascular benefits of SGLT2i and GLP-1 RA

Beyond their use in diabetes management, metabolic improvement, and various kidney or cardiovascular diseases, recent advancements indicate that SGLT2i and GLP-1 RA may benefit other organ systems. Although initially not indicated for nonalcoholic fatty liver disease or nonalcoholic steatohepatitis (NASH), both drug classes have been explored as pharmacologic treatments in RCTs. GLP-1 RA have shown potential in improving NASH histology and even resolving NASH,[7] with SGLT2i demonstrating similar effects.[7] GLP-1 RA were also studied in patients with depression, Alzheimer disease, and Parkinson disease,[8] hypothesized to offer neuroprotection by activating GLP-1 receptors in the central nervous system to reduce inflammation, oxidative stress, and apoptosis, and activate dopaminergic neurons, potentially countering Parkinson disease.[8] However, recent RCTs have not yet confirmed significant effectiveness in these neurodegenerative diseases.[8] In addition, SGLT2i, because of their potential ocular anti-inflammatory effects, were associated with a lower HR for the development of dry eye disease.[9]

In conclusion, this innovative study by Fu et al.,[1] along with prior research, reveals significant potential for SGLT2i and GLP-1 RA in nontraditional cardiorenal benefit areas. This expanding body of evidence not only reinforces their recognized cardiorenal advantages but also their promising role in complex conditions, like SIADH, hyperkalemia, and beyond, including nonalcoholic fatty liver disease/NASH and neurodegenerative diseases (Figure 1). Further prospective trials and retrospective observational studies are essential to deepen our understanding of these benefits and the mechanisms driving them.

DISCLOSURE
All the authors declared no competing interests.

Author Contributions
J-JC and T-HL drafted the manuscript. T-HL created the figure. H-YY supervised. All authors have read and approved the final version of the manuscript.

REFERENCES

1. Fu EL, Mastrorilli J, Bykov K, et al. A population-based cohort defined risk of hyperkalemia after initiating SGLT-2 inhibitors, GLP-1 receptor agonists or DPP-4 inhibitors to patients with chronic kidney disease and type 2 diabetes. *Kidney Int*. 2024;105:618–628.
2. Refardt J, Imber C, Sailer CO, et al. A randomized trial of empagliflozin to increase plasma sodium levels in patients with the syndrome of inappropriate antidiuresis. *J Am Soc Nephrol*. 2020;31:615–624.
3. Refardt J, Imber C, Nobbenhuis R, et al. Treatment effect of the SGLT2 inhibitor empagliflozin on chronic syndrome of inappropriate antidiuresis: results of a randomized, double-blind, placebo-controlled, crossover trial. *J Am Soc Nephrol*. 2023;34:322–332.
4. Zhang J, Huan Y, Leibensperger M, et al. Comparative effects of sodium-glucose cotransporter 2 inhibitors on serum electrolyte levels in patients with type 2 diabetes: a pairwise and network meta-analysis of randomized controlled trials. *Kidney360*. 2022;3:477–487.
5. Chen JJ, Wu CY, Jenq CC, et al. Association of glucagon-like peptide-1 receptor agonist vs dipeptidyl peptidase-4 inhibitor use with mortality among patients with type 2 diabetes and advanced chronic kidney disease. *JAMA Netw Open*. 2022;5:e221169.
6. Lin Y, Wang TH, Tsai ML, et al. The cardiovascular and renal effects of glucagon-like peptide 1 receptor agonists in patients with advanced diabetic kidney disease. *Cardiovasc Diabetol*. 2023;22:60.
7. Mantovani A, Byrne CD, Targher G. Efficacy of peroxisome proliferator-activated receptor agonists, glucagon-like peptide-1 receptor agonists, or sodium-glucose cotransporter-2 inhibitors for treatment of non-alcoholic fatty liver disease: a systematic review. *Lancet Gastroenterol Hepatol*. 2022;7:367–378.
8. Laurindo LF, Barbalho SM, Guiguer EL, et al. GLP-1a: going beyond traditional use. *Int J Mol Sci*. 2022;23:739.
9. Su YC, Hung JH, Chang KC, et al. Comparison of sodium-glucose cotransporter 2 inhibitors vs glucagonlike peptide-1 receptor agonists and incidence of dry eye disease in patients with type 2 diabetes in Taiwan. *JAMA Netw Open*. 2022;5:e2232584.

commentary

Alternative creatinine-based GFR estimates in United States populations—similar performance, same gaps—is it time to move on?

June Fabian[1,2]

This study evaluated performance of the European Kidney Function Consortium (EKFC) equation in a US cohort, comparing population-specific (EKFCPS) with race-free (EKFCRF) Q values (median normal creatinine). Both EKFCPS and EKFCRF equations showed less bias than the Chronic Kidney Disease Epidemiology Collaboration (CKD-EPI) 2021 equation. The percentage of estimated glomerular filtration rate (GFR) within 30% of measured GFR was similar for CKD-EPI 2021 (79.2% [range, 78.5%–79.9%]) and EKFCRF (80.1% [range, 79.4%–80.7%]) equations but improved with the EKFCPS equation (81.1% [range, 80.5%–81.8%]), confirming utility of the EKFC equation in US populations.

Kidney International (2024) **105**, 445–446; https://doi.org/10.1016/j.kint.2024.01.001

Copyright © 2024, International Society of Nephrology. Published by Elsevier Inc. All rights reserved.

see clinical investigation on page 629

Across the globe, evaluating kidney function is a critical component of everyday clinical and laboratory practice, informing diagnoses of kidney disease, specialist nephrology referrals, and dosing regimens for nephrotoxic drugs. Although measured glomerular filtration rate (GFR) is considered the reference, it is invasive, time-consuming, and more expensive relative to creatinine-based estimates of GFR (eGFR).[1] Currently, all the available eGFR equations have been developed and validated in predominantly European and North American White populations, with surprisingly little validation in continental Africa, the American and European African diaspora, Latin America, India, and Asia. The era of race-based adjustments of eGFR was introduced in 1999 with the Modification of Diet in Renal Disease equation and further perpetuated in the modeling of the first Chronic Kidney Disease Epidemiology Collaboration (CKD-EPI) equation in 2009.[2,3] It is noteworthy that such adjustments were based on a relatively small proportion of Black US study participants with established CKD, with most observed population-based differences in men rather than women.

Recently, race-based adjustments of GFR estimates have come under the spotlight, heavily criticized in Black Lives Matter for perpetuating inequalities in the US health system, especially in the provision of nephrology services. Such services include timeous specialist referral, initiation of directed treatment for prevention of CKD progression, and, for those with end-stage kidney disease, access to chronic dialysis and listing for transplantation. Overestimating GFR as an artefactual consequence of race-based adjustments especially impacts women, younger people, and those with better-preserved kidney function, with similar findings replicated in non-US populations.[4] Despite the ensuing debate that polarized the nephrology community, there was a collective sigh of relief when the National Kidney Foundation–American Society of Nephrology Task Force called for a reappraisal of race coefficients in GFR equations, resulting in the modeling of a race-free CKD-EPI equation that only includes age and sex as variables.[5] Likewise, in the United Kingdom, we took another step forward when the revised National Institute for Health and Care guidelines were published, recommending the omission of race-based GFR estimates from clinical practice.[6]

In this edition of *Kidney International*, acknowledging the utility of the new creatinine-based European Kidney Function Consortium (EKFC) equation remained confined to mainly European populations, Delanaye *et al.* elegantly demonstrate its equivalent performance to that of the race-free CKD-EPI equation in a large pooled US cohort.[7] The EKFC equation is based on rescaling creatinine using the Q value, which is defined as the median normal creatinine for a given population. Two options for the EKFC are subsequently proposed: the first is defined as population specific (which is race based), and the second is race free. Overall, for both forms of the EKFC equation, their respective bias, accuracy, and precision have such small differences they can be considered comparable with each other, and with the race-free CKD-EPI equation. The strength of the study lies in the large number of participants sourced from multiple US-based studies with a broad range of GFR; however, the representation of those who were self-identified as Black remained relatively small (21%).

We could argue that the missed opportunities lie in the absence of an

---

[1]*Division of Internal Medicine, University of the Witwatersrand Faculty of Health Sciences–Wits Donald Gordon Medical Centre, School of Clinical Medicine, Johannesburg, South Africa; and* [2]*Medical Research Council/Wits University Rural Public Health and Health Transitions Research Unit (Agincourt), School of Public Health, Faculty of Health Sciences, University of the Witwatersrand, Johannesburg, South Africa*

Correspondence: *June Fabian, University of the Witwatersrand Faculty of Health Sciences–Wits Donald Gordon Medical Centre, School of Clinical Medicine, 27 Eton Rd, Parktown, Johannesburg, Gauteng 2193, South Africa. E-mail: june.fabian@mweb.co.za*

evaluation of EKFC in children and adolescents, as we know a focus on improving the detection of kidney disease in this group would be of immense value because of their burgeoning risk of CKD. Also, the absence of an evaluation of cystatin C as a biomarker for eGFR, either in combination with creatinine, or as cystatin C alone, is disappointing. We know that cystatin C improves the accuracy of eGFR equations and is a prognostic indicator of outcome; thus, the more evidence we have accumulated in multiple studies, the more informed our approaches can be to defining its role in eGFR testing going forward.

A few aspects of this study provide opportunity for reflection, especially if we want to practice nephrology that is truly global. As there was little difference between the population-specific and race-free versions of the new EKFC equation, we could ask ourselves why we continue to perform race-based analyses in GFR estimates. Although one could justify there is some heritability relating to creatinine and that self-reported race may be a proxy for heritability, which varies considerably in African American populations, the data presented do not justify this differentiation. Furthermore, the European-American comparison in this work reflects the dominant narrative in nephrology, which remains that of the Global North. Thus, this study contributes relevant information to an already well-studied population. Although this is not a phenomenon specific to nephrology, as most research is done in well-resourced environments, mostly from high-income countries, the (unintentional) fallout is obvious. The voices of many populations from low- and middle-income countries in the Global South remain silent or are silenced.

Finally, the authors state in their discussion that the ambition of the EKFC equation is for it to be applicable to different populations. There have been numerous ongoing debates about which GFR estimating equation is better, and in the case of creatinine-based performance—most accept there are limitations that no amount of modeling will overcome, and alternative biomarkers must be sought. The notion of a "one-size fits all" equation for global use is an oversimplification with the potential to compromise individual-level care and population-based policy for the management of kidney disease. Incorrectly estimating GFR (as seen in Africa and Asia)—mostly overestimating true GFR—has devastating consequences in resource-limited settings with restricted access to kidney replacement therapy. The missed diagnosis of early-stage CKD is a death sentence.

DISCLOSURE

The author declared no competing interests.

REFERENCES

1. Delanaye P, Ebert N, Melsom T, et al. Iohexol plasma clearance for measuring glomerular filtration rate in clinical practice and research: a review. Part 1: how to measure glomerular filtration rate with iohexol? *Clin Kidney J*. 2016;9:682–699.
2. Levey AS, Bosch JP, Lewis JB, et al. Modification of Diet in Renal Disease Study Group. A more accurate method to estimate glomerular filtration rate from serum creatinine: a new prediction equation. *Ann Intern Med*. 1999;130:461–470.
3. Levey AS, Stevens LA, Schmid CH, et al; CKD-EPI (Chronic Kidney Disease Epidemiology Collaboration). A new equation to estimate glomerular filtration rate. *Ann Intern Med*. 2009;150:604–612.
4. Chu CD, Powe NR, Crews DC, Tuot DS. CKD Progression from the time of estimated GFR-based waitlist eligibility and racial disparities in transplant access. *Am J Kidney Dis*. 2022;79:841–848.e1.
5. Delgado C, Baweja M, Crews DC, et al. A unifying approach for GFR estimation: recommendations of the NKF-ASN task force on reassessing the inclusion of race in diagnosing kidney disease. *Am J Kidney Dis*. 2022;79:268–288.e1.
6. Martinez YV, Benett I, Lewington AJP, Wierzbicki AS, Guideline Committee. Chronic kidney disease: summary of updated NICE guidance. *BMJ*. 2021;374:n1992.
7. Delanaye P, Rule AD, Schaeffner E, et al. Performance of the European Kidney Function Consortium (EKFC) creatinine-based equation in United States cohorts. *Kidney Int*. 2024;105:629–637.

www.kidney-international.org

KDIGO executive conclusions

Executive summary of the KDIGO 2024 Clinical Practice Guideline for the Management of ANCA–Associated Vasculitis

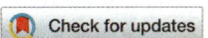

OPEN

Jürgen Floege[1], David R.W. Jayne[2], Jan-Stephan F. Sanders[3], Vladimír Tesar[4], Ethan M. Balk[5], Craig E. Gordon[6], Gaelen Adam[5], Marcello A. Tonelli[7], Michael Cheung[8], Amy Earley[8] and Brad H. Rovin[9]

[1]Division of Nephrology, University Hospital, Rheinisch-Westfälische Technische Hochschule (RWTH) Aachen, Aachen, Germany; [2]Division of Experimental Medicine & Immunotherapeutics, School of Clinical Medicine, University of Cambridge, Cambridge, UK; [3]Division of Nephrology, Department of Internal Medicine, University of Groningen, Groningen, The Netherlands; [4]Department of Nephrology, 1st Faculty of Medicine and General University Hospital, Charles University, Prague, Czech Republic; [5]Center for Evidence Synthesis in Health, Brown University School of Public Health, Providence, Rhode Island, USA; [6]Division of Nephrology, Tufts Medical Center, Boston, Massachusetts, USA; [7]Department of Medicine, Cumming School of Medicine, University of Calgary, Calgary, Alberta, Canada; [8]KDIGO, Brussels, Belgium; and [9]Department of Internal Medicine, The Ohio State University College of Medicine, Columbus, Ohio, USA

In 2021, the Kidney Disease: Improving Global Outcomes (KDIGO) Guideline for the Management of Glomerular Diseases was published. KDIGO is committed to providing the nephrology community with periodic updates, based on new developments for each disease. For patients with anti-neutrophil cytoplasmic antibody (ANCA)–associated vasculitis (AAV), avacopan received regulatory approval in late 2021, leading to this KDIGO guideline update. In addition, the evidence supporting a lower-dose glucocorticoid induction regimen or even complete replacement of glucocorticoids has become stronger. Herein, an executive summary of the most important guideline changes from the AAV chapter is provided as a quick reference.

Kidney International (2024) **105**, 447–449; https://doi.org/10.1016/j.kint.2023.10.009

KEYWORDS: ANCA-associated vasculitis; glomerular diseases; glomerulonephritis; guideline; KDIGO; systematic review

Copyright © 2023, Kidney Disease: Improving Global Outcomes (KDIGO). Published by Elsevier Inc. on behalf of the International Society of Nephrology. This is an open access article under the CC BY-NC-ND license (http://creativecommons.org/licenses/by-nc-nd/4.0/).

Correspondence: *Jürgen Floege, Division of Nephrology, RWTH Aachen University Hospital, Pauwelsstrasse 30, Aachen 52074, Germany. E-mail: jfloege@ukaachen.de*

The complete KDIGO 2024 Clinical Practice Guideline for the Management of Antineutrophil Cytoplasmic Antibody (ANCA)–Associated Vasculitis is published in *Kidney International*, volume 105, issue 3S, 2024, which is available online at www.kidney-international.org.

Received 11 September 2023; revised 20 October 2023; accepted 20 October 2023

In 2021, a major revision of the Kidney Disease: Improving Global Outcomes (KDIGO) Clinical Practice Guideline for the Management of Glomerular Diseases was published.[1] Since publication, important data concerning anti-neutrophil cytoplasmic antibody (ANCA)–associated vasculitis (AAV) have become available, prompting this guideline update. Probably the most significant development has been the approval of the C5a receptor inhibitor avacopan by the United States Food and Drug Administration (FDA) and the European Medicines Agency (EMA) as add-on therapy to standard-of-care for the treatment of AAV.[2,3] This development directly relates to the second major emerging novel approach to the treatment of AAV, namely, a reduction of systemic glucocorticoid exposure. Although the latter is obviously desirable, given the short- and long-term complications of glucocorticoids, it is less clear which patients need avacopan in order to allow for lower glucocorticoid dosages. At the same time, this new therapy adds significant cost to treatment, and long-term safety data are currently lacking.

This Executive Summary provides a brief snapshot of the updated guideline, but readers are encouraged to view the full chapter for detailed discussion and useful practice points (Supplementary Table S1; https://kdigo.org/guidelines/gd/).

No major changes have been made in sections related to diagnosis and assessment of prognosis of AAV (https://kdigo.org/guidelines/gd/). The most important update in the ANCA guideline relates to induction therapy. Recommendation 9.3.1.1, "**We recommend that glucocorticoids in combination with cyclophosphamide or rituximab be used as initial treatment of new-onset AAV (1B),**" did not change, but the discussion now places stronger emphasis on a more rapid reduction of glucocorticoid dose, based on the recent Low-Dose Glucocorticoid Vasculitis Induction Study (LoVAS), among others.[4] The study randomized patients with AAV to receive reduced-dose prednisolone (0.5 mg/kg/d) or high-dose prednisolone (1 mg/kg/d) plus 4 doses of 375 mg/m^2/wk rituximab. Reduced-dose glucocorticoids led to a similar remission rate, but the frequency of severe infections was

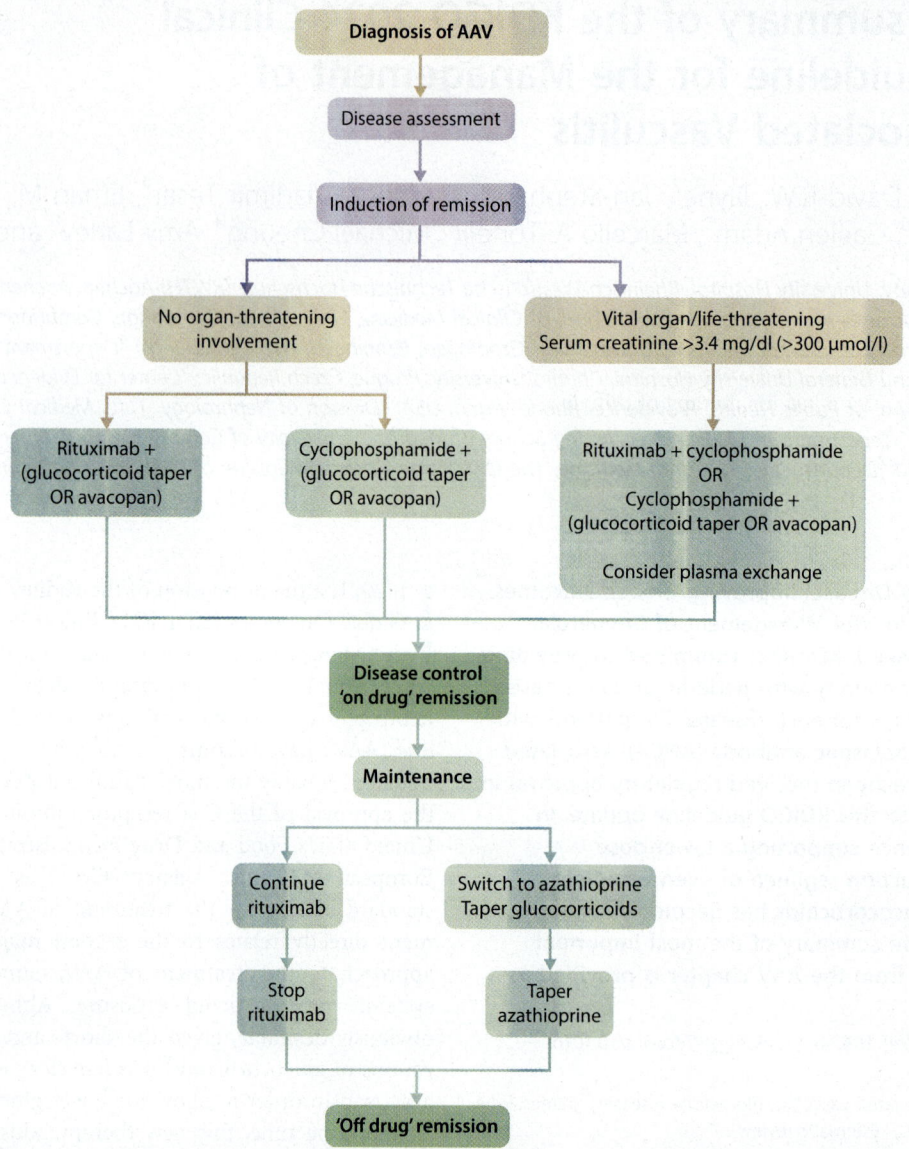

Figure 1 | Practical treatment regimen for antineutrophil cytoplasmic antibody–associated vasculitis (AAV).

reduced. A limitation of the study is that it included only Japanese patients with predominantly myeloperoxidase (MPO)-ANCA-associated vasculitis. Nonetheless, these data support the "reduced-glucocorticoid dose" as used in the Plasma Exchange and Glucocorticoids for the Treatment of ANCA-Associated Vasculitis (PEXIVAS) trial.[5]

The most important change in AAV induction therapy is the availability of avacopan for AAV (Figure 1; **Practice Point 9.3.1.1 and Practice Point 9.3.1.7 in guideline**). Two placebo-controlled randomized controlled trials (RCTs) studied avacopan in AAV; one of the RCTs (A Phase 3 Clinical Trial of CCX168 [Avacopan] in Patients with ANCA-Associated Vasculitis [ADVOCATE]) had no serious methodological concerns,[6] but the other RCT (Clinical ANCA Vasculitis Safety and Efficacy Study of Inhibitor of C5aR [CLASSIC]) had a high dropout rate and changed the *a priori* primary outcome.[7] The certainty of the evidence for sustained remission and severe adverse events was graded as moderate, but the certainty of evidence for infections and discontinuation due to adverse events were graded as low. The Work Group considered the results of both randomized controlled trials (RCTs) when deciding to make avacopan a practice point rather than a recommendation. Patients with an increased risk of glucocorticoid toxicity are likely to benefit most from avacopan. Furthermore, a *post hoc* analysis of patients with low glomerular filtration rate (GFR) (<30 ml/min per 1.73 m^2) suggested greater GFR recovery with avacopan as compared to glucocorticoid therapy.[8]

Controversy still surrounds the value of plasma exchange in AAV patients with a severe clinical course. From the Public Review, approval for Practice Point 9.3.1.9. was relatively low, at 75%: "Consider plasma exchange for patients with serum creatinine (SCr) >3.4 mg/dl (>300 μmol/l), patients requiring dialysis or with rapidly increasing SCr, and patients with diffuse alveolar hemorrhage who have hypoxemia." However, a 2022 meta-analysis concluded that there is a reduction of kidney failure at 12 months with plasma exchange, with no evidence of subgroup effects, but it comes at the cost of an increased risk of serious infections.[9] At present, the routine use of plasma exchange is not recommended for patients presenting with a GFR <50 ml/min per 1.73 m^2, but it can be considered in patients with more severe presentations (SCr >3.4 mg/dl [>300 μmol/l], especially if oliguric) or those with alveolar hemorrhage and hypoxemia, in whom early mortality is high. Plasma exchange should be used in patients with concomitant anti-glomerular basement membrane (GBM) disease. Conversely, plasma exchange is not required for therapy of diffuse alveolar hemorrhage in the absence of hypoxemia.

Maintenance therapy has not changed in the 2024 guideline update, and Recommendation 9.3.2.1 still states "**We recommend maintenance therapy with either rituximab, or azathioprine and low-dose glucocorticoids after induction of remission (1C).**" For both azathioprine and rituximab, the updated guideline now mentions an optimal duration of therapy of between 18 months and 4 years after the induction of remission. As a maintenance drug, rituximab can be dosed on a fixed schedule or upon reappearance of CD19+ B cells and/or ANCA, but dosing based on B cell counts led to fewer infusions and thus lower cost.[10,11]

Even in patients on kidney replacement therapy, extrarenal AAV can and does relapse, and a remission should be consolidated with maintenance therapy. In patients with kidney failure, anti-MPO positivity, and no extrarenal symptoms, long-term maintenance may not be necessary. In this situation, the need for (and length of) maintenance treatment should be assessed at an individual level.

There is no new information to guide clinical approaches to AAV in patients with relapsing or refractory disease, or after kidney transplantation; thus, the content of the 2021 guideline did not change. Finally, research recommendations from this 2024 guideline still call for RCTs that incorporate patient-reported outcomes, more prolonged long-term outcome studies, studies aimed at defining the role of rituximab in severe AAV, and studies conducted in ethnically diverse populations. Another area in which there is a large unmet need is the identification of biomarkers to better guide treatment. Hopefully, these future trials, if successful, will lead to yet another update of the KDIGO AAV guideline in the near-term.

DISCLOSURE

The development and publication of this guideline were supported by Kidney Disease: Improving Global Outcomes (KDIGO). The opinions or views expressed in this summary are those of the authors and do not necessarily reflect the opinions or recommendations of the International Society of Nephrology or Elsevier. Dosages, indications, and methods of use for products that are referred to in the supplement by the authors may reflect their clinical experience or may be derived from the professional literature or other clinical sources. Because of the differences between *in vitro* and *in vivo* systems and between laboratory animal models and clinical data in humans, *in vitro* and animal data do not necessarily correlate with clinical results.

JF reports receiving consultancy fees and/or speaker honoraria from AstraZeneca, Bayer, Calliditas, Chinook, GlaxoSmithKline, Novartis, Omeros, Otsuka, Stadapharm, and Travere; and serving on data safety monitoring boards for Novo Nordisk and Visterra. DRWJ reports receiving consultancy fees from AstraZeneca, GlaxoSmithKline, Novartis, Takeda, and Vifor; grant/research support from GlaxoSmithKline*, Roche*, and Vifor*; funding for lectures, presentations, speakers' bureaus, manuscript writing or educational events from Otsuka and Vifor; serving on a Data Safety Monitoring Board or Advisory Board for Chinook and GlaxoSmithKline; receiving funding support for a leadership or fiduciary role at Aurinia; and receiving stock or stock options from Aurinia. VT reports receiving funding for a leadership or fiduciary role at Calliditas, Novartis, Omeros, Otsuka, and Travere. CEG reports receiving consultancy fees from Alexion; serving on the speaker bureau for Alexion; and receiving funding for travel and/or accommodation from Alexion. MAT reports receiving payment for expert testimony from Gilead Sciences (not related to the guideline topic). BHR reports receiving consultancy fees from Alexion, AstraZeneca, Aurinia, Bristol Myers Squibb, Exagen, Genentech, GlaxoSmithKline, Kezar Life Sciences, Kyverna, Novartis, and Otsuka; and grant/research support from Biogen*. All the other authors declared no competing interests. *Monies paid to institution.

SUPPLEMENTARY MATERIAL

Supplementary File (PDF)

Supplementary Table S1. Comparison of the 2021 and 2024 KDIGO Clinical Practice Guideline for the Management of Antineutrophil Cytoplasmic Antibody (ANCA)–Associated Vasculitis.

REFERENCES

1. Kidney Disease: Improving Global Outcomes (KDIGO) Glomerular Diseases Work Group. KDIGO 2021 clinical practice guideline for the management of glomerular diseases. *Kidney Int*. 2021;100(4S):S1–S276.
2. European Medicines Agency. First-in-class medicine recommended for treatment of rare blood vessel inflammation. Accessed September 11, 2023. https://www.ema.europa.eu/en/news/first-class-medicine-recommended-treatment-rare-blood-vessel-inflammation
3. US Food and Drug Administration. FDA approves add-on drug for adults with rare form of blood vessel inflammation. Accessed September 11, 2023. https://www.fda.gov/drugs/news-events-human-drugs/fda-approves-add-drug-adults-rare-form-blood-vessel-inflammation
4. Furuta S, Nakagomi D, Kobayashi Y, et al. Effect of reduced-dose vs high-dose glucocorticoids added to rituximab on remission induction in ANCA-associated vasculitis: a randomized clinical trial. *JAMA*. 2021;325: 2178–2187.
5. Walsh M, Merkel PA, Peh CA, et al. Plasma exchange and glucocorticoids in severe ANCA-associated vasculitis. *N Engl J Med*. 2020;382:622–631.
6. Jayne DRW, Merkel PA, Schall TJ, et al. Avacopan for the treatment of ANCA-associated vasculitis. *N Engl J Med*. 2021;384:599–609.
7. Merkel PA, Niles J, Jimenez R, et al. Adjunctive treatment with avacopan, an oral C5a receptor inhibitor, in patients with antineutrophil cytoplasmic antibody-associated vasculitis. *ACR Open Rheumatol*. 2020;2:662–671.
8. Cortazar FB, Niles JL, Jayne DRW, et al. Renal recovery for patients with ANCA-associated vasculitis and low eGFR in the ADVOCATE trial of avacopan. *Kidney Int Rep*. 2023;8:860–870.
9. Walsh M, Collister D, Zeng L, et al. The effects of plasma exchange in patients with ANCA-associated vasculitis: an updated systematic review and meta-analysis. *BMJ*. 2022;376:e064604.
10. Charles P, Terrier B, Perrodeau E, et al. Comparison of individually tailored versus fixed-schedule rituximab regimen to maintain ANCA-associated vasculitis remission: results of a multicentre, randomised controlled, phase III trial (MAINRITSAN2). *Ann Rheum Dis*. 2018;77: 1143–1149.
11. Walters GD, Willis NS, Cooper TE, et al. Interventions for renal vasculitis in adults. *Cochrane Database Syst Rev*. 2020;1:CD003232.

meeting report

Post-transplant recurrence of focal segmental glomerular sclerosis: consensus statements

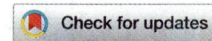

Rupesh Raina[1,2,31], Swathi Jothi[1,31], Dieter Haffner[3], Michael Somers[4], Guido Filler[5,6,7], Prabhav Vasistha[1], Ronith Chakraborty[1,2], Ron Shapiro[8], Parmjeet S. Randhawa[9], Rulan Parekh[10], Christopher Licht[11], Timothy Bunchman[12], Sidharth Sethi[13], Guneive Mangat[1], Joshua Zaritsky[14], Franz Schaefer[15], Bradley Warady[16], Sharon Bartosh[17], Mignon McCulloch[18], Khalid Alhasan[19,20], Agnieszka Swiatecka-Urban[21], William E. Smoyer[22], Anil Chandraker[23], Hui Kim Yap[24,25], Vivekanand Jha[26,27,28], Arvind Bagga[29] and Jai Radhakrishnan[30]

[1]Department of Nephrology, Akron Nephrology Associates/Cleveland Clinic Akron General Medical Center, Akron, Ohio, USA; [2]Department of Nephrology, Akron Children's Hospital, Akron, Ohio, USA; [3]Department of Pediatric Kidney, Liver and Metabolic Diseases, Hannover Medical School, Hannover, Germany; [4]Division of Nephrology, Department of Medicine, Boston Children's Hospital, Harvard Medical School, Boston, Massachusetts, USA; [5]Department of Pediatrics, Schulich School of Medicine and Dentistry, University of Western Ontario, London, Ontario, Canada; [6]Department of Medicine, Schulich School of Medicine and Dentistry, University of Western Ontario, London, Ontario, Canada; [7]Department of Pathology and Laboratory Medicine, Schulich School of Medicine and Dentistry, University of Western Ontario, London, Ontario, Canada; [8]Recanati/Miller Transplantation Institute, The Mount Sinai Medical Center, New York, New York, USA; [9]Department of Pathology, Thomas E Starzl Transplant Institute, University of Pittsburgh School of Medicine, Pittsburgh, Pennsylvania, USA; [10]Department of Medicine, School of Medicine, Johns Hopkins University, Baltimore, Maryland, USA; [11]Division of Pediatric Nephrology, The Hospital for Sick Children, University of Toronto, Toronto, Ontario, Canada; [12]Pediatric Nephrology and Transplantation, Children's Hospital of Richmond at Virginia Commonwealth University (VCU), Richmond, Virginia, USA; [13]Pediatric Nephrology, Kidney Institute, Medanta, The Medicity Hospital, Gurgaon, Haryana, India; [14]Division of Pediatric Nephrology, Nemours, A.I. duPont Hospital for Children, Wilmington, Delaware, USA; [15]Department of Pediatric Nephrology, University Children's Hospital Heidelberg, Heidelberg, Germany; [16]Division of Nephrology, University of Missouri–Kansas City School of Medicine, Children's Mercy, Kansas City, Missouri, USA; [17]Department of Pediatrics, University of Wisconsin Medical School, Madison, Wisconsin, USA; [18]Red Cross War Memorial Children's Hospital, University of Cape Town, Cape Town, South Africa; [19]Nephrology Unit, Pediatrics Department, College of Medicine, King Saud University, Riyadh, Saudi Arabia; [20]Pediatric Kidney Transplant Division, Organ Transplant Center, King Faisal Specialist Hospital and Research Center, Riyadh, Saudi Arabia; [21]University of Virginia Children's Hospital, University of Virginia School of Medicine, Charlottesville, Virginia, USA; [22]Center for Clinical and Translational Research and Division of Nephrology, Nationwide Children's Hospital, The Ohio State University College of Medicine, Columbus, Ohio, USA; [23]Transplantation Research Center, Kidney and Pancreas Transplantation, Brigham and Women's Hospital, Harvard Medical School, Boston, Massachusetts, USA; [24]Department of Pediatrics, Yong Loo Lin School of Medicine, National University of Singapore, Singapore, Singapore; [25]Khoo Teck Puat-National University Children's Medical Institute, National University Hospital, Singapore, Singapore; [26]George Institute for Global Health, University of New South Wales (UNSW), New Delhi, India; [27]School of Public Health, Imperial College, London, UK; [28]Prasanna School of Public Health, Manipal Academy of Higher Education, Manipal, India; [29]Division of Pediatric Nephrology, All India Institute of Medical Sciences, New Delhi, India; and [30]Department of Medicine (Nephrology), Columbia University Medical Center, New York, New York, USA

Focal segmental glomerular sclerosis (FSGS) is 1 of the primary causes of nephrotic syndrome in both pediatric and adult patients, which can lead to end-stage kidney disease. Recurrence of FSGS after kidney transplantation significantly increases allograft loss, leading to morbidity and mortality. Currently, there are no consensus guidelines for identifying those patients who are at risk for recurrence or for the management of recurrent FSGS. Our work group performed a literature search on PubMed/Medline, Embase, and Cochrane, and recommendations were proposed and graded for strength of evidence. Of the 614 initially identified studies, 221 were found suitable to formulate consensus guidelines for recurrent FSGS. These guidelines focus on the definition, epidemiology, risk factors, pathogenesis, and management of recurrent FSGS. We conclude that additional studies are required to strengthen the recommendations proposed in this review.

Kidney International (2024) **105**, 450–463; https://doi.org/10.1016/j.kint.2023.10.017

KEYWORDS: focal segmental glomerular sclerosis; plasmapheresis; post-transplant

Copyright © 2023, International Society of Nephrology. Published by Elsevier Inc. All rights reserved.

Correspondence: *Jai Radhakrishnan, Division of Nephrology, Department of Medicine, Columbia University, 622 W 168th Street, PH4124, New York, New York 10032, USA. E-mail: jr55@cumc.columbia.edu*

[31]RR and SJ are joint first authors.

Received 22 December 2021; revised 3 October 2023; accepted 17 October 2023; published online 22 December 2023

SUMMARY OF RECOMMENDATIONS
Diagnosis recommendations
- We recommend that the diagnosis of recurrent focal segmental glomerular sclerosis (FSGS) in the transplanted

kidney be made in patients with history of primary FSGS in native kidneys, both children and adults, who show:
  - Nephrotic-range proteinuria > 3.5 g/24 h or protein-to-creatinine ratio > 3g/g (>300 mg/mmol) in adults, and first morning or 24-hour protein-to-creatinine ratio >2 g/g (>200 mg/mmol) or > 3+ on urine dipstick in children, AND hypoalbuminemia (serum albumin <3.0 g/dl) (1A). (Supplementary Table S1 explains the grading system for the recommendations.)
  - Allograft biopsy showing FSGS pattern of injury and widespread podocyte effacement (1A).
- We recommend that all patients with FSGS undergoing kidney transplantation be monitored for recurrent FSGS. Patients may be monitored for proteinuria and serum creatinine daily for 1 week, twice weekly in week 2, weekly for 4 weeks, monthly for the first year, and every 3 months thereafter; preferably with use of a first morning void urine sample (1B).

Risk assessment
- We recommend that if the recipient is known to possess a causal pathogenic variant associated with FSGS, potential living-related donors should undergo genetic testing before being accepted as kidney donors, to preclude the donor from a risk of chronic kidney disease, and although uncommon, to assess the risk of development of FSGS in transplanted kidney (1A).
- We recommend kidney transplantation in patients with primary FSGS after the risk of recurrence is discussed with the recipient (2C).
- Recurrent FSGS leading to loss of a prior allograft is associated with a high risk of recurrence in a subsequent allograft. In such a situation, candidacy for a subsequent kidney transplant (especially a living-donor transplant) should be carefully considered.

Treatment recommendations
- We recommend prompt initial therapy of recurrent FSGS with plasmapheresis (2A).
- We recommend not providing prophylactic plasmapheresis or rituximab before the kidney transplant (2C).

SECTION 1: INTRODUCTION

Focal segmental glomerular sclerosis (FSGS) is a leading cause of corticosteroid-resistant nephrotic syndrome in children and adults. FSGS is a term that was coined to reflect the histopathologic findings where the glomeruli show hyalinosis, sclerosis, and scarring and can result from several underlying pathophysiological mechanisms. The condition may progress to end-stage kidney disease (ESKD), especially in patients who are treatment resistant.[1]

FSGS may recur in the kidney allograft and is a notable cause of post-transplant morbidity and mortality. Recurrent FSGS (rFSGS) refers to the development of primary FSGS (pFSGS) in the transplanted kidney of patients who had ESKD secondary to pFSGS in their native kidney. Rarely, recurrence of proteinuria may be seen with certain types of genetic FSGS.

The incidence of post-transplant rFSGS ranges from 6% to 57%,[1–3] and various predisposing factors have been identified. There is a large variability in the incidence rate; this can be attributed to the fact that rFSGS is rare and most incidence rates come from studies with a small sample size and limited power. rFSGS is typically diagnosed when transplant recipients manifest nephrotic-range proteinuria with hypoalbuminemia and with or without edema. If rFSGS is suspected, allograft biopsy is necessary to confirm the diagnosis and rule out other causes of allograft injury. Studies have reported varying success with various treatment regimens for rFSGS, including the use of plasmapheresis, immunoadsorption, and immunosuppression.[4]

Familial FSGS has a low risk of recurrence.[5,6] It is hypothesized that a circulating factor, possibly of immune origin, may be responsible for other nongenetic forms of FSGS through podocyte injury.[7,8] Studies have attempted to isolate this circulating factor, and some of the potential candidates include interleukins, tumor necrosis factor, cardiotrophin-like cytokine-1, and soluble urokinase receptor.[9–15] However, none of these contenders has been consistently shown to be the permeability factor in rFSGS.

In this systematic review, we performed a literature search for data pertaining to risk factors, pathogenesis, and management of rFSGS to formulate graded recommendations for management of rFSGS in adult and pediatric patients.

1.1 METHODS
Data searches and sources

This study was registered in the International Prospective Register for Systematic Reviews (2019). To find potential studies, a database search using PubMed/Medline, Embase, and Cochrane was performed to include publications on rFSGS in the adults and children from January 1974 to October 2019. Medical subject headings used in the creation of the search strategy included focal glomerulosclerosis, recurrence, *kidney transplantation, post renal transplant, postoperative complications, graft rejection, and delayed graft function. An asterisk (*) was used to denote when a term was "exploded" to search for all related terms on the familial hierarchy. The search strategy was limited to the English language. Two reviewers (PV and SJ) assessed each title, abstract, and the full-text article. Case reports, case-control studies, and retrospective observational studies, performed among the pediatric and adult population, pertaining to rFSGS were assessed. A third reviewer (RR) reconciled incongruent reviews and assessed for similar data. A population, intervention, comparator, outcome, and study design table was constructed to illustrate the inclusion and exclusion criteria. Our search yielded 614 studies, of which 159 duplicates (studies published in >1 database) were deleted. Next, systematic reviews, meta-analyses, and abstracts were excluded; 221 eligible studies were chosen, and their methods and quality were analyzed. A Preferred Reporting Items for Systematic Reviews and Meta-Analyses flow diagram of the complete selection process is depicted in Supplementary Figure S1. The methods, search strategy, and population, intervention, comparator, outcome, and study design/Delphi methods[16] are summarized in Supplementary Appendix S1 and Supplementary Figure S2.

Data extraction and statistical analysis

The following data were extracted from transplant recipients: age, sex, ethnicity of patient, type of donor, number of acute rejection episodes, and 5-year graft survival rates. Outcomes (with 95% confidence interval [CI]) were the incidence of rFSGS, episodes of acute rejection, and 5-year graft survival. A meta-analysis of these outcomes was conducted. The degree of between-study heterogeneity was assessed using the I^2 test; $I^2 \geq 50\%$ indicated high heterogeneity. Pooled estimate was calculated with random-effects model for high heterogeneity and fixed-effects model for low heterogeneity. Forest plot was used to visualize outcomes in each study, with estimate of combined outcomes. Publication bias was assessed graphically using funnel plots; $P \leq 0.05$ was considered statistically significant. Statistical analyses were performed with R software, version 3.1.0.

Data were extracted to evaluate the efficacy of rituximab in therapy of rFSGS. Data on 58 patients across 23 studies were collected as follows: age and sex of patient, concurrent treatment, and use of rituximab within 2 weeks of onset of rFSGS. Continuous variables were compared using Mann-Whitney U test, whereas association of categorical variables with remission was analyzed by χ^2 or Fisher exact test.

FSGS is a pattern of histologic glomerular injury where "focal segments" of glomeruli are subject to hyalinosis, sclerosis, and scarring. pFSGS is diagnosed when all other causes of the biopsy-proven FSGS have been ruled out. rFSGS was diagnosed when transplant recipients experienced recurrence of massive proteinuria (>40 mg/m^2 per day in children and >1g/L in adults), hypoalbuminemia (<2.5 g/dl) following transplantation,[8] and biopsy showing FSGS pattern of injury in the allograft.

Supplementary Appendix S2 provides a comprehensive overview on the diagnosis and classifications of FSGS. Supplementary Appendix S3 shows a practice algorithm for diagnosis and treatment. A recent study of the Australian and New Zealand Dialysis and Transplant Registry defined recurrence as histologically proven rFSGS and defined date of onset of recurrent disease as either clinically by the onset of nephrotic-range proteinuria with a decrease in serum albumin or as the date of histologic confirmation on tissue biopsy. With this strict definition, they revealed that only 10.3% patients (51 adults and 25 children) showed signs of recurrence occurring within the first 2 years of transplantation.[17]

SECTION 2: DIAGNOSIS AND CLINICAL PRESENTATION

- We recommend that the diagnosis of rFSGS in the transplanted kidney be made in patients with a history of pFSGS in native kidneys, both children and adults, who show:
  - Nephrotic-range proteinuria > 3.5 g/24 h or protein-to-creatinine ratio > 3 g/g (>300 mg/mmol) in adults, and first morning or 24-hour protein-to-creatinine ratio >2 g/g (>200 mg/mmol) or $> 3+$ on urine dipstick in children, AND hypoalbuminemia (serum albumin <3.0 g/dl) (1A).
  - Allograft biopsy showing FSGS pattern of injury and widespread podocyte effacement (1A).
- We recommend that all patients with FSGS undergoing kidney transplantation be monitored for rFSGS. Patients may be monitored for proteinuria and serum creatinine daily for 1 week, twice weekly in week 2, weekly for 4 weeks, monthly for the first year, and every 3 months thereafter, preferably with use of a first-morning void urine sample (1B).

rFSGS is suspected when a patient with biopsy-proven FSGS in the native kidney develops significant proteinuria (albuminuria $\geq 3+$) following transplantation. The diagnosis may be confirmed by an allograft biopsy, which may be normal by light microscopy in the initial stages, with only electron microscopy showing extensive fusion of podocyte foot processes. The treatment of recurrent nephrotic syndrome in patients with pFSGS should not be delayed in such circumstance because the typical focal segmental sclerosis lesions recognizable by routine[18,19] microscopy can take several weeks to develop. The term "focal" is a misnomer because ultrastructural examination shows a diffuse distribution of podocyte injury in all glomeruli. Furthermore, FSGS lesions are more prevalent in deeper (i.e., juxtamedullary) sections rather than the superficial cortex and may not always be sampled by needle biopsy.[20]

The timing of FSGS recurrence may vary: early recurrence (within 48 hours; typically seen in children); infrequent and insidious late recurrence (≥ 1 month); or intermediate recurrence (2 days to 1 month).[4] Clinical and laboratory changes precede the histologic change by 10 days to 2 months. Three histologic stages are visualized: normal appearing glomeruli; early segmental lesions with foam cell change, endocapillary cellularity, or podocyte hyperplasia; and late focal sclerosing lesions characteristic of late-onset disease defined by some as occurring after 3 months.[21,22] In patients with either acute tubular necrosis or delayed graft function, proteinuria may be missed because of the initial oliguria/anuria.

Late recurrence takes an indolent course, with proteinuria typically appearing at least 3 months after transplantation.[23] Some authors suggest that an adequate biopsy sample should comprise ≥ 8 glomeruli and examination of 12 to 15 serial sections.[20] However, this issue is best viewed as a statistical problem of estimating a probability. It has been calculated that >25 glomeruli need to be present in a biopsy if one is to confidently detect a lesion that affects 10% of glomeruli.[24] The number of glomeruli required would be larger if a smaller proportion of the glomeruli were diseased or if it is desired that a specific subtype of FSGS be reliably identified.

An important issue is to distinguish between recurrence of pFSGS and *de novo* occurrence of secondary forms of the disease. The latter include chronic T-cell or antibody-mediated rejection, calcineurin inhibitor toxicity with arteriolar hyalinosis, recurrent glomerulonephritis, renal artery stenosis, atheroembolism, thrombotic microangiopathy, reflux nephropathy, viral infections (HIV, parvovirus, cytomegalovirus, or coronavirus disease 2019 [COVID-19]), drug-induced injury (interferon, lithium, or pamidronate), and light chain podocytopathies.[25]

Adaptive FSGS is a unique cause of FSGS that results from excessive nephron stress brought on by a lowered nephron capacity, an increase in body mass, or isolated glomerular

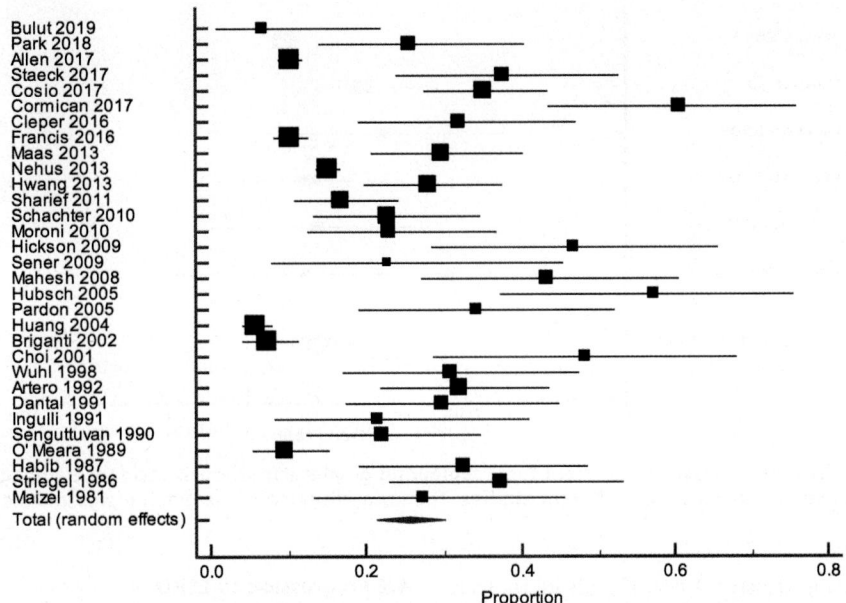

Figure 1 | Forest plot of the meta-analysis of recurrent focal segmental glomerular sclerosis incidence among kidney transplant recipients. The lower diamond in the graph represents the pooled estimate.[S1–S31]

hyperfiltration linked to particular disorders. It is distinguished by a more gradual onset of proteinuria, the lack of hypoalbuminemia, and a less severe fusion of the foot processes of the podocyte.[26] In seeking to distinguish primary from adaptive FSGS by electron microscopy, examination should focus on nonsclerotic glomeruli that do not show ischemic changes. Clinical correlation is of paramount importance because some forms of secondary disease, such as HIV-associated collapsing glomerulopathy and drug-induced injury, can result in extensive podocyte injury. Another caveat is that biopsies taken in the resolving phase of disease, possibly after therapy has been started, may show only mild changes.

SECTION 3: EPIDEMIOLOGY
3.1 Incidence
Determining the precise incidence of rFSGS and its contribution to graft failure is challenging. Thus, it may be difficult to differentiate between donor transmitted, *de novo*, secondary, and recurrent disease.[27,28] Proteinuria occurring early in the post-transplant course is usually indicative of rFSGS. Lesions of FSGS may be incidentally present in transplanted kidneys with good function, even in the absence of proteinuria, and may not always progress to allograft failure.[29,30] Chronic allograft nephropathy and nephrotoxicity due to calcineurin inhibitors may be associated with FSGS lesions in allograft recipients.

The systematic review showed that the pooled incidence of rFSGS in adults was 16.6% (95% CI, 7.5%–28.3%; Supplementary Table S8).[26,31–34] The reported pooled incidence of rFSGS in our systematic review among children was 39.6% (95% CI, 7.5%–49.9%).[26,31–34] Overall, an odds ratio (OR) for rFSGS in children compared with adults was 4.52 (95% CI, 1.82-11.28; Figure 1 and Supplementary Table S9), with younger age (6–10 years) of onset being an important determinant of rFSGS (Supplementary Table S10).[35–37] The pooled incidence of subgroup analysis based on sample size and study design was observed to be within the 95% CI of the OR, indicating that the results of this meta-analysis are robust enough. Also, no publication bias was observed on the basis of the Egger test ($P = 0.98$). We hypothesize that the variability in the reported incidence in individual studies may be attributable to confounding factors, such as cause of FSGS, patients' race, and donor graft characteristics.

3.2 Race
Although pFSGS is more common in African Americans,[38–43] our review shows that rFSGS is more common in patients of European descent (27.98% [range, 17.27%–40.14%]) than non-European patients (14.0% [range, 12.2%–15.9%]), with total fixed-effect OR of Caucasian to non-Caucasian incidence of 1.48 (95% CI, 2.29-1.84; Figure 2 and Supplementary Table S11).[1,31,33,36,37,44] The pooled incidence of subgroup analysis based on sample size and study design was observed to be within the 95% CI of the OR, indicating that the results of this meta-analysis are robust enough. Also, no publication bias was observed on the basis of the Egger test ($P = 0.10$).

3.3 Survival of allografts with rFSGS recurrence
According to an analysis of the European Renal Association–European Dialysis and Transplant Association database, recurrent glomerular disease accounts for 3% of primary graft loss and 48% of secondary graft losses.[45] In the United

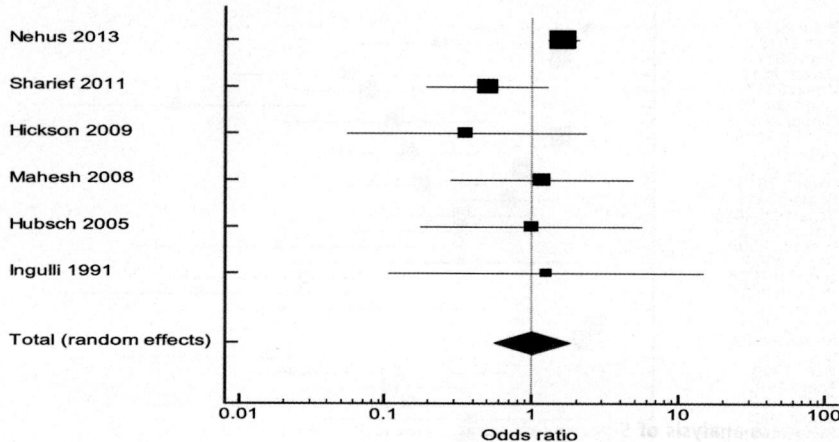

Figure 2 | Forest plot of the meta-analysis of recurrent focal segmental glomerular sclerosis incidence among Caucasian and non-Caucasian kidney transplant recipients across different studies. The lower diamond in the graph represents the pooled estimate.[S11,S14,S16,S17,S25,S30]

Network of Organ Sharing registry, 1.8% of graft losses were attributed to recurrent glomerular disease.[46] Of the various glomerular diseases, rFSGS poses the highest risk of graft failure, with a relative risk of 2.25.[25,47,48] The highest risk of recurrence and graft loss is during the first 2 years after transplantation.

Among all causes of graft loss in patients with rFSGS, recurrence is implicated in the failure of >6% of primary transplant and 12% of secondary transplant.[42,49] In adult patients with rFSGS in our systematic review, recurrence confers a 5-year graft survival rate of 52.59% (95% CI, 50.09%–62.00%; n = 116) compared with a rate of 82.77% (95% CI, 79.76%–85.30%; n = 749) without recurrence (Supplementary Table S12). The pooled odds of 5-year graft survival were significantly higher among those without rFSGS versus those with rFSGS (OR, 4.24; 95% CI, 2.77–6.48; $P < 0.001$), as shown in Figure 3. There was no evidence of publication bias on the basis of the Egger test ($P = 0.11$). In a retrospective study in the pediatric population, graft survival in patients with rFSGS was 68% after a minimum follow-up of 4 years, whereas a 93% graft survival was observed in patients with other causes of ESKD.[17] Supplementary Table S13 summarizes the outcomes of kidney transplantation in patients with rFSGS included in our systematic review.

SECTION 4: RISK FACTORS
4.1 Histology
Patients with the mesangial proliferation subtype have been shown to have a higher risk of post-transplant recurrence.[50] However, the Columbia University histologic classification of FSGS does not recognize a mesangioproliferative form of the disease, although it recognizes a cellular variant with endocapillary hypercellularity. Two studies using the Columbia classification did not show a higher risk of recurrence with any subtype,[51,52] but additional studies are needed to address the recurrence rate of the relatively uncommon cellular and collapsing variants.

4.2 Progression to ESKD
A progression to ESKD in pFSGS (within 3 years from FSGS diagnosis)[32,53,54] or rFSGS in a prior kidney allograft increases the risk for rFSGS after subsequent transplantation.[6] Sex, duration of dialysis, and choice of post-transplant therapy did not influence the recurrence of FSGS.[4,55,56] Supplementary Table S14 highlights the various risk factors for rFSGS.

4.3 Genetic factors
- We recommend that if the recipient is known to possess a causal pathogenic variant associated with FSGS, potential living-related donors should undergo genetic testing before being accepted as kidney donors, to preclude the donor from a risk of chronic kidney disease, and in the recipient, to assess the risk of development of FSGS in transplanted kidney (1A).

A study evaluated steroid-resistant nephrotic syndrome in 101 pediatric patients followed up for a median of 58.5 months with age >9 years and at least 1 human leukocyte antigen-AB match and found that there were independent risk factors for disease recurrence. Notably, the patients with genetic steroid-resistant nephrotic syndrome experienced no recurrence.[57]

There are also various syndromic and nonsyndromic forms of genetic FSGS that have been described. Syndromic forms include Alport, Fabry, Frasier, Leigh, Nail-Patella, and Renal-Coloboma-Oligomeganephronia syndromes. Nonsyndromic forms of FSGS are associated with pathogenic variants in podocyte genes, such as *NPHS1*, *NPHS2*, *WT1*, α-actin-4, *CDAP*, *TRP6*, *ACTN4*, *PLCE1*, and *INF2*, which have been associated with FSGS.[58] Inheritance patterns include autosomal recessive (e.g., *NPHS1*, *NPHS2*) or autosomal dominant (e.g., *ACTN4*). Morphologically, patients with genetic forms of FSGS are indistinguishable from those with nongenetic FSGS. Mitochondrial genetic variants may also be associated with FSGS with dysmorphic mitochondria on electron microscopy.[59] The risk of recurrent proteinuria in genetic forms of FSGS is generally low. However, some

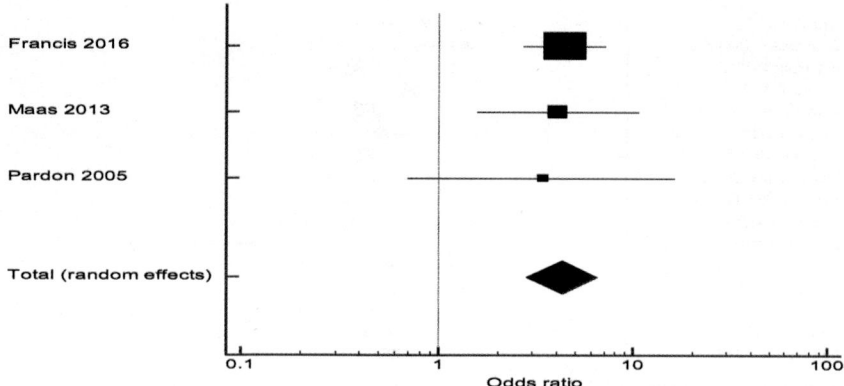

Figure 3 | Forest plot of the meta-analysis of 5-year graft survival among recurrent and nonrecurrent focal segmental glomerular sclerosis kidney transplant recipients across different studies. The lower diamond in the graph represents the pooled estimate.[57,S8,S18]

patients with NPHS1 pathogenic variants (especially with a homozygous truncating variant, leading to total absence of nephrin) may develop anti-nephrin antibodies, resulting in nephrotic-range proteinuria.[60,61] In the kidney biopsy, the immunofluorescence staining for nephrin in podocytes occurs in an irregular pattern along the glomerular basement membranes.[62] Plasma exchange in combination with cyclophosphamide or anti–CD-20 antibody treatment is generally successful in treating these episodes. Although rFSGS has been reported in association with *NPHS2* gene variants, the response to immunosuppression/plasmapheresis in these patients occurred at rates comparable to pFSGS. This suggests that the pathomechanism of rFSGS was similar to that of pFSGS.[63] It is important to screen prospective family donors of recipients, who should be excluded if they exhibit similar risk genotype as the recipient.

Bertelli *et al.* observed that the recurrence of FSGS associated with the *NPHS2* gene variants is unlikely to recur in the kidney allograft, thus demonstrating that genetic forms of FSGS have a lower risk of recurrence.[64]

Morello *et al.* conducted a meta-analysis to investigate the role of genetic factors and corticosteroid sensitivity in post-transplant recurrence FSGS. The children with a genetic mutation experienced an exclusion of recurrence compared with recurrence seen in 61% of patients with no genetic mutations. Sensitivity to initial corticosteroid therapy in children was associated with significantly higher rates of recurrence after transplant. In a total of 7 studies included with a total cohort of 135 genetic patients, there was no recurrence reported. On the contrary, 129 children (negative genetic test) from 6 studies showed 61% recurrence rate with no heterogeneity.[65] In Supplementary Appendix S4 and Supplementary Table S15, some biomarkers associated with rFSGS have been discussed.

4.4 Impact of kidney donor type on rFSGS

- We recommend kidney transplantation in patients with primary FSGS after the risk of recurrence is discussed with the recipient (2C).

- Recurrent FSGS leading to loss of a prior allograft is associated with a high risk of recurrence in a subsequent allograft. In such a situation, candidacy for a subsequent kidney transplant (especially a living donor transplant) should be carefully considered (2A).

- We suggest that the choice between deceased donor (DD) and living donor (LD) kidney transplantation should be based on availability of grafts from DDs and complications from ongoing chronic dialysis therapy. We suggest the use of LD grafts in individuals with low risk for rFSGS because this confers potential benefits of shorter waiting times (2C).

The recommendation for LD versus DD transplantation grafts in patients with FSGS is controversial. In other forms of ESKD, LD grafts are typically associated with improved graft outcomes compared with DD kidneys. In recessive forms of FSGS (e.g., NPHS2-associated FSGS), allografts from LDs who are heterozygous were observed to have a better graft survival compared with those from DDs.[58] Physicians have avoided using LD grafts in patients with primary FSGS because of the risk of disease recurrence and lack of adequate treatment options.[66]

Data from the North American Pediatric Renal Trials and Collaborative Studies showed that, in the setting of rFSGS, the expected advantage in graft survival for kidneys arising from living donation was lost.[49,53] Along these lines, a review of the US Renal Data System database suggested that rFSGS accounted for more graft losses in the LD group with rFSGS than the DD group with rFSGS (18.7% vs. 7.8%).[67] By contrast, studies from the United Network of Organ Sharing and the Renal Allograft Disease Registries did not show a difference in frequency of disease recurrence between LD and DD recipients after correcting for confounding factors.[26,36,67] Conversely, analysis of the Australian and New Zealand Dialysis and Transplant registry revealed better 5-year LD graft survival (85% vs. 76% in adults; 80% vs. 46% in children), with a median graft survival advantage of 2.7 years.[17]

In our analysis, the pooled incidence of rFSGS was 22.9% (range, 17.6%–28.6%) in LD recipients and 21.8% (range, 15.3%–29.3%; n = 2492) in DD recipients (Supplementary

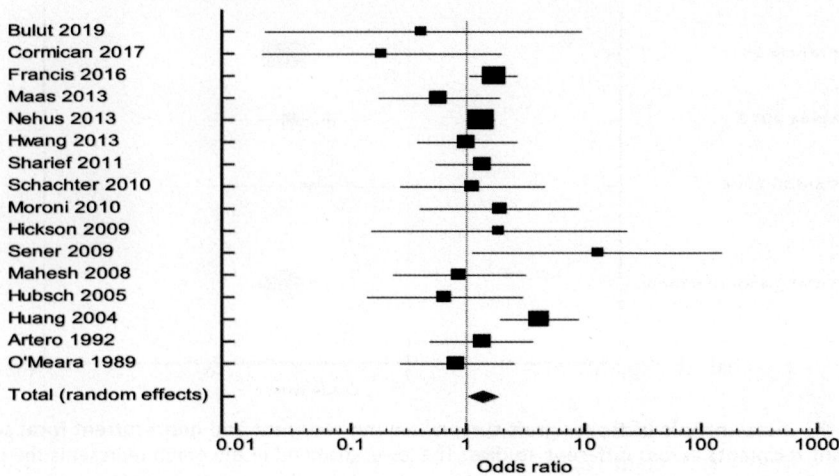

Figure 4 | Forest plot of the meta-analysis of recurrent focal segmental glomerular sclerosis among living and deceased donor kidney transplant recipients across different studies. The lower diamond in the graph represents the pooled estimate.[S1,S5,S7,S8,S10–S17,S19,S23,S30,S31]

Table S16).[1,17,31–34,36,44,66,68–73] Our analysis found that DDs may have lower risk of rFSGS than LDs. We propose that genetic testing should be done for donors whose family members have genetic FSGS, presuming that genetic studies should have been done pretransplant in all children with FSGS.

The pooled odds of rFSGS were significantly higher among LDs when compared with DDs (OR, 1.39; 95% CI, 1.17–1.66; $P < 0.001$), as shown in Figure 4. The pooled incidence of subgroup analysis based on sample size, study design, and setting (single center/multicenter) was observed to be within the 95% CI of the OR, indicating that the results of this meta-analysis are robust enough. Also, no publication bias was observed on the basis of the Egger test ($P = 0.57$). However, the data are not adjusted for recipient race, recipient age, and genetic basis of FSGS in the native kidneys. After lengthy discussions, there still is insufficient data to make a definitive recommendation on whether DD offers a lower risk of rFSGS compared with LD.

4.5 Effect of induction therapy on rFSGS

Data on the effects of induction therapy are derived from observation studies with a wide variation in reported incidence of rFSGS (Supplementary Table S17). Raafat et al. were the first to analyze the effect of induction therapy on rFSGS.[74] Induction with antilymphocyte globulin and antithymocyte globulin was compared with controls with no induction. The antithymocyte globulin group had 88% recurrence as opposed to 43% recurrence in the antilymphocyte globulin group. In contrast, Pascual et al. demonstrated that there were no major differences in the incidence of recurrence following induction therapy with alemtuzumab, interleukin 2 receptor antagonists, or antithymocyte globulin group. At this time, it is unclear if specific induction therapy has an effect on rFSGS.[74–76]

4.6 Effect of nephrectomy

A survey done on the current practice regarding FSGS recurrence after pediatric kidney transplantation found that 37% of patients underwent unilateral or bilateral nephrectomy before transplant.[77] The literature search did not reveal any evidence for or against native kidney nephrectomy. Thus, bilateral native kidney nephrectomy before kidney transplantation as a preventive measure of recurrence cannot be recommended.

4.7 The role of autoantibodies

The role of anti-nephrin antibodies in nongenetic recurrent FSGS is being actively investigated. Circulating anti-actin and anti-ATP synthase antibodies were reported in 8 of 60 children with nongenetic idiopathic nephrotic syndrome.[78] In a single case of rFSGS, anti-angiotensin-1 receptor antibody was found, with improvement of symptoms with plasmapheresis, i.v. Ign therapy, and losartan therapy.[79] A panel of seven Abs (CD40, PTPRO, CGB5, FAS, P2RY11, SNRPB2, and APOL2) were found to predict post-transplant FSGS recurrence with 92% accuracy.[80] Anti-nephrin antibodies were first implicated in minimal change disease.[81] Pretransplant anti-nephrin antibody was reported in 1 patient who presented with early post-transplant recurrence of FSGS.[82] In a recent study of 22 Japanese pediatric kidney transplant recipients with nongenetic FSGS, 11 experienced post-transplant recurrence. Elevated levels of anti-nephrin antibodies were noted in these patients, with punctate IgG deposition observed in graft biopsies. Biopsies after remission showed no IgG staining and a normal nephrin expression pattern. Anti-nephrin antibody levels decreased after remission. In contrast, patients with genetic FSGS and those with nongenetic FSGS without recurrence showed comparable anti-nephrin antibody levels to control individuals, with normal graft biopsy results. The role of autoantibodies needs to be further validated in larger cohorts.

SECTION 5: TREATMENT OF RECURRENT FSGS
5.1 Overview of treatment of rFSGS

Because of the paucity of well-designed randomized trials, the management of rFSGS has not been standardized. Multiple treatments have been prescribed, making it difficult to analyze the specific outcomes associated with any 1 particular therapy. Current treatment options include plasmapheresis or immunoadsorption therapy, immunosuppressive therapy with a calcineurin inhibitor and use of anti-CD20 monoclonal antibodies for B-cell depletion, and management of concomitant modifiable risk factors (Supplementary Appendix S5). Supplementary Appendix S6 highlights the current ongoing trials. Pulse methylprednisolone therapy has been shown to be effective in a few studies but warrants more investigation.[22,83]

- We recommend prompt initial therapy of rFSGS with intensive plasmapheresis (1C).
- We recommend not providing prophylactic plasmapheresis or rituximab before the kidney transplant (2C).

5.1A Plasmapheresis

Therapeutic plasma exchange (TPE), or plasmapheresis, has been considered as a treatment for rFSGS because of the underlying putative pathogenic role of a circulating factor.[57,84] This was demonstrated with resolution of urinary albumin excretion in rats following plasmapheresis.[85] Subsequent clinical use and efficacy of intermittent TPE in the post-transplant period has been evaluated and shows promising results (Supplementary Table S18).

The probability of achieving remission is dependent on the time of initiation of TPE.[86] Early initiation of TPE for patients with rFSGS is associated with higher remission rates.[87] One commonly used regimen includes 1.5 times plasma volume exchanges for 3 consecutive days, followed by every other day for a total of 2 weeks.[88] The regimen is combined with standard anti-rejection medications, including cyclosporine, mycophenolate mofetil, and corticosteroids.[89] In a study by Restropo et al., of 17 patients with rFSGS, 12 achieved remission after treatment with plasmapheresis while on corticosteroid-based immunosuppression.[90] Demir et al. also demonstrated remission in patients with rFSGS after the administration of plasma exchange and i.v. cyclosporine.[91] A case study by Ino et al. followed the case of a 29-year-old female patient with rFSGS who achieved remission after plasmapheresis along with maintenance therapy with rituximab.[92] Hansrivijit et al. conducted a meta-analysis that showed combination therapy of plasmapheresis and rituximab achieved remission in 72.7% of patients (n = 85), thus indicating its success in treating patients with rFSGS.[92]

The use of preemptive TPE in the perioperative period has also been considered in high-risk patients (those who had rapid progression to ESKD or had rFSGS in their first transplant) for prophylaxis against rFSGS. In 1 study, high-risk patients were perioperatively treated with 8 sessions of TPE. None of the patients experienced recurrence, and 50% of patients with rFSGS in their first transplant experienced recurrence following their second transplant.[89] However the beneficial effect of prophylactic plasmapheresis was not corroborated by subsequent studies.[33] Vallianou et al. conducted a study with 26 patients. Sixteen of these patients underwent plasmapheresis, thereby achieving remission in all of those patients.[93]

Clinical practice guidelines

- We suggest that treatment be initiated promptly in a patient with a clinical diagnosis of rFSGS while kidney biopsy confirmation is awaited.
- The suggested regimen for plasmapheresis in rFSGS includes daily plasmapheresis for 3 days and then 3 times a week for 2 weeks. Exchanges of 1 to 1.5 plasma volumes, using citrate or heparin anticoagulation, with replacement by human albumin or hemofiltration solution should be targeted; fresh frozen plasma should be used as replacement fluid if plasma fibrinogen is low. Plasmapheresis may be terminated after reduction of proteinuria (<1 g/d).

5.1B Immunoadsorption

In our systematic review, 5 case series (n = 23) considered the efficacy of immunoadsorption (IA) in the treatment of rFSGS, reporting that ≈91% achieved complete or partial remission (Supplementary Table S13). Allard et al. observed 12 patients between the ages of 2 and 13 years who were started on IA.[94] They received a median of 4.2 IA sessions during the first week and 2.5 sessions during the second week. Two of the 12 patients (17%) achieved complete remission, and 8 of the 12 patients (66%) had partial remission, with no graft losses reported. In addition, various studies have also assessed the use of IA in combination with plasmapheresis[86,95] (Supplementary Table S19). Because of the absence of randomized trials with this combination therapy, we recommend against combined therapy (immunoadsorption and plasmapheresis) and believe the therapeutic choice between plasmapheresis or IA should depend on local availability, cost, and experience.[86,96]

IA is a selective procedure that mitigates some of the potential adverse effects observed with TPE, such as postoperative bleeding due to loss of coagulation factors.[97] Nonetheless, IA poses its own set of adverse effects. Citrate toxicity has been reported because of the use of citrate as a systemic or regional anticoagulant in the plasma circuit. Depression of humoral immunity can cause acute bacterial infections (urinary tract infections, pneumonia, and bronchitis), fungal infections, or viral infections. Reactivation of hepatitis B virus has also been reported. When the indications for Ig supplementation are met, they should be meticulously followed to avoid the risk of life-threatening anaphylaxis and transmission of blood-borne viruses.[98] In highly dependent patients, the frequency of IA sessions can potentially impact the quality of life.[94] In a study by Neciri et al., treatment with immunoadsorption showed remission in 5 of 7 patients. Of these patients, 4 had LD transplant, whereas 3 had DD transplant.[99]

Clinical practice guidelines

- Immunoadsorption should initially be conducted with 2.5 to 3 plasma volumes and should be performed every day for

1 week, followed by alternate-day treatments for 2 more weeks, and then twice weekly for another 2 weeks.
- We suggest that either plasmapheresis or immunoadsorption be reinstituted in patients who successfully respond to initial sessions of plasmapheresis but later relapse (2C).

5.1C Calcineurin inhibitors and corticosteroids

In our systematic review, 3 case series (n = 21) evaluated the efficacy of cyclosporine A (CsA) in patients with rFSGS and showed that ≈81% (17 of 21) of patients achieved complete or partial remission. All the patients were treated with CsA in these case series. Canaud et al. described 10 patients with rFSGS who received high-dose oral corticosteroids (1 mg/kg per day, tapered to 10 mg/d over 8–12 weeks), i.v. CsA (for 14 days, to achieve 2-hour CsA levels of 1200–1400 ng/ml), and prolonged plasmapheresis (6–9 months) supplemented with angiotensin pathway blockers once remission was achieved. All patients achieved complete remission, with 90% able to maintain a sustained remission compared with only 27% achieving long-term remission in controls.[88] There are limited data on high-dose tacrolimus in children or adults with rFSGS. Given the widespread use of tacrolimus, and its potential early benefit in transplant recipients, most centers prefer to continue tacrolimus instead of switching to CsA. The aim is to target tacrolimus levels around the higher recommended limit.[100,101] Shishido et al. demonstrated that a course of i.v. pulse methylprednisone infusions combined with high-dose oral CsA therapy can lead to complete remission in up to 70% of pediatric patients within 18 months of beginning treatment.[83] The participants received infusions of methylprednisolone on 3 consecutive days during weeks 1, 3, and 5, then monthly until 6 months after transplant. At this point, if they were in complete or partial remission, pulse therapy was continued for an additional 18 months. CsA dose was titrated on the basis of area under the curve of 0 to 4 (Supplementary Table S20).

Clinical practice guidelines

- We suggest consideration of the use of calcineurin inhibitors with concomitant high-dose corticosteroids and apheresis in selected patients with rFSGS (2B).

5.1D Low-density lipoprotein apheresis

Low-density lipoprotein apheresis, which removes potential nephrotoxic lipids, may prevent kidney injury and improve nephrotic symptoms.[102–106] A 47-year-old man with rFSGS resistant to therapy with methylprednisolone and TPE experienced partial remission with low-density lipoprotein apheresis, resulting in a decrease in proteinuria from 9.6 to 2.0 g/d.[107] A case series conducted among pediatric patients showed that 9 weeks of low-density lipoprotein apheresis therapy combined with pulse methylprednisolone produced either complete or partial remission of rFSGS proteinuria in all 7 participants.[108] Low-density lipoprotein apheresis may be considered in patients who are resistant to TPE and IA; however, more studies are warranted in evaluating the efficacy of this procedure and its use.

Clinical practice guideline

- Low-density lipid apheresis may be considered in patients who are refractory to plasmapheresis and immunoadsorption.

5.1E Rituximab

Several case reports have been published detailing the efficacy of rituximab in treating rFSGS, with variable conclusions.[109–118]

We conducted a meta-analysis of 58 patients across 23 studies and found a total remission rate of 63.8%, a complete remission rate of 48.3%, and a partial remission rate of 15.5%. On performing a subgroup analysis, we noted that age ($P = 0.24$) and rituximab ($P = 0.70$) were not significantly associated with remission. The various doses used in these 23 studies are illustrated in Supplementary Table S21. We analyzed the OR for sex (the term *sex* is used as the biological classification of individuals as males, females, or intersex) (1.66; 95% CI, 0.39–7.07; $P = 0.73$) and for starting rituximab within 2 weeks of recurrence (2.44; 95% CI, 0.80–7.50; $P = 0.11$) and noted that these 2 factors were not significantly associated with remission. The various studies on the efficacy of rituximab are shown in Supplementary Table S21. Our analysis is concurrent with a previously conducted systematic review by Araya et al., who also showed similar remission rates.[119] They noted that fewer rituximab infusions and normal serum albumin at the time of recurrence were associated with higher response. Contrary to our analysis, on multivariate analysis, they found that male sex and shorter initiation time of rituximab following relapse was associated with response.

Rituximab has demonstrated a 50% remission rate in patients who did not respond to plasma exchange and i.v. cyclosporine.[120] A large group study done in kidney transplant recipients showed that rituximab can be recommended as a rescue treatment in cases refractory to initial therapy or in those who failed weaning from plasmapheresis.[118] Bharati et al. observed 6 patients who were treated with TPE (3 sessions per week for a total of 7–10 sessions) and single-dose rituximab (375 mg/m^2) after completion of TPE.[121] Of the 6 patients, 5 (83.3%) achieved remission in proteinuria, with the other patient requiring ongoing plasma exchange. On the other hand, El Khashab et al. observed 8 patients (aged 17–36 years) who were treated with a single dose of rituximab (375 mg/m^2) post-transplant, with no patients having graft loss and 1 patient developing proteinuria after 4 months.[122] Koutroutsos et al. conducted a study and demonstrated that combination of rituximab and plasmapheresis helped achieved remission in 9 of 10 patients with rFSGS.[123]

Rituximab as preemptive therapy. Case reports and small case series have reported on the role of rituximab for patients with a history of rFSGS post-transplant for recurrence prophylaxis in a subsequent kidney transplant (Supplementary

Table S22). A study by Boonpheng et al. assessed the risk of FSGS recurrence by the use of rituximab with or without plasmapheresis in patients after kidney transplantation.[124] As per this analysis, there was no difference in recurrence in patients receiving rituximab, with a pooled risk ratio of 0.82. There is no strong evidence to suggest the preemptive role of rituximab in prevention of FSGS recurrence.

Clinical practice guidelines
- Therapy with rituximab should be considered in patients with rFSGS who have contraindications to plasmapheresis, or who fail to improve despite treatment with plasmapheresis or immunoadsorption. Rituximab doses ranged from 75 to 3375 mg (median dose, 1500 mg/m^2) (2B).
- Plasmapheresis/immunoadsorption should be withheld for 48 hours following any rituximab infusion to prevent immediate drug removal.

5.1F Abatacept and belatacept
Few studies have investigated the efficacy of abatacept or belatacept (Supplementary Table S23). Yu et al. described resolution of proteinuria in 4 patients with rituximab-resistant rFSGS and 1 patient with primary FSGS who received abatacept at 250 or 500 mg per day.[125] Similar encouraging results were reported by Sprenger-Mähr et al. and Shah et al.[125–127]

Of concern, combination therapy with plasmapheresis and abatacept has been associated with severe sepsis.[125] Delville et al. prospectively treated 9 patients with rFSGS using either abatacept or belatacept but failed to induce remission or detect B7-1 in the patient biopsies.[128]

5.1G Cyclophosphamide
Cyclophosphamide has been reported to be associated with varying response rates in the treatment of rFSGS. Used as induction therapy, Kershaw et al. reported a complete remission in 2 of 3 patients and partial remission in 1 of 3 patients.[129] Two studies used cyclophosphamide as a substitute for an antimetabolite medication post-transplant concurrently with TPE and pulse corticosteroids, and this led to sustained rFSGS remission in all 3 patients in 1 study but only 33% of 16 children in the other study.[129,130] In another report, cyclophosphamide and TPE alone produced a sustained remission in 7 of 11 patients.[4]

5.1H Renin-angiotensin system blockade
Increased expression of nuclear factor-κB and the angiotensinogen gene has been observed in patients with rFSGS.[131] This is consistent with mouse models, where it was hypothesized that angiotensin II may contribute to rFSGS by causing preferential constriction of the afferent arteriole and associated increased intraglomerular pressure.[132]

Recently, various case series have reported the antiproteinuric efficacy of renin-angiotensin system blockers in rFSGS.[121,133,134] A study by Abuzeineh et al. found an association of angiotensin II type 1 receptors and rFSGS, leading to worse allograft outcome.[133]

Clinical practice guidelines
- We suggest therapy with angiotensin-converting enzyme inhibitors or angiotensin receptor blockers in patients with persistent proteinuria in the absence of contraindications, with close monitoring of kidney function (2C).

5.1I Newer therapies
Novel anti-CD20 antibodies. Ofatumumab has been used in rFSGS. Data are limited to case reports and small case series, and responses include complete or partial remission or no effect on proteinuria or kidney function. The positive results with the combination of obinutuzumab and the anti-CD38 (plasma cell) antibody daratumumab in patients with multidrug-resistant minimal change disease offers a future consideration for the treatment of rFSGS.[135–140]

Anti–tumor necrosis factor-α. Leroy et al. reported the successful treatment of a case of biopsy-proven rFSGS with only prior partial response to plasma exchange using bimonthly infliximab at a dose of 3 mg/kg along with high-dose corticosteroids (60 mg/1.73 m^2 per day).[141] During several periods when treatment was discontinued, relapses ensued that were not controlled by high-dose corticosteroids (3 methylprednisolone pulses, followed by 60 mg/1.73 m^2 per day) or etanercept (25 mg biweekly) provided alone, suggesting a synergistic action of dual concomitant therapy. In fact, when the relapses were treated with a combination of therapies again, remission was achieved.

Mesenchymal stem cell. Belingheri et al. proposed an innovative treatment with mesenchymal stem cells (MSCs) in a 13-year-old boy with rFSGS dependent on chronic plasma exchange. MSCs were administered in 6 doses, divided into 3 cycles of 2 infusions (1×10^6 cells/kg per dose). After the first MSC cycle, the patient did not need plasma exchange for 50 days. In view of worsening proteinuria, the patient was treated with a second and a third MSC dose at 3 and 7 months, respectively. Notably, after MSC dosing, there was a sustained decrease in the number of circulating inflammatory factors (CD40L, EN-RAGE, eotaxin-3, interleukin 16, migration inhibitory factor, myeloperoxidase [MPO], N-terminal pro–B-type natriuretic peptide [NT-proBNP], plasminogen activator inhibit [PAI-1], and thrombospondin-1). Epidermal growth factor receptor ligands (amphiregulin, epidermal growth factor, heparin-binding epidermal growth factor, and transforming growth factor-α), which are upregulated in experimental models of FSGS and in mesangial cell proliferation, were also found at significantly lower levels following MSC treatment in this patient. MSCs could potentially exert a paracrine effect, modulating the microenvironment or stimulating native kidney stem cells.[142]

RECENT STUDIES
A total of 7 studies reported the data on remission among subjects with recurrent FSGS on treatment.[18,90,91,93,99,123,133] The total sample size among these studies was 134, with the median age of the subjects ranging from 3.2 to 51 years (male, 56%; female, 44%; LD, 63%; DD, 37%; Hispanic, 16.8%; Caucasian, 42.6%; Black, 14.9%; Asian, 18.8%; others, 6.9%).

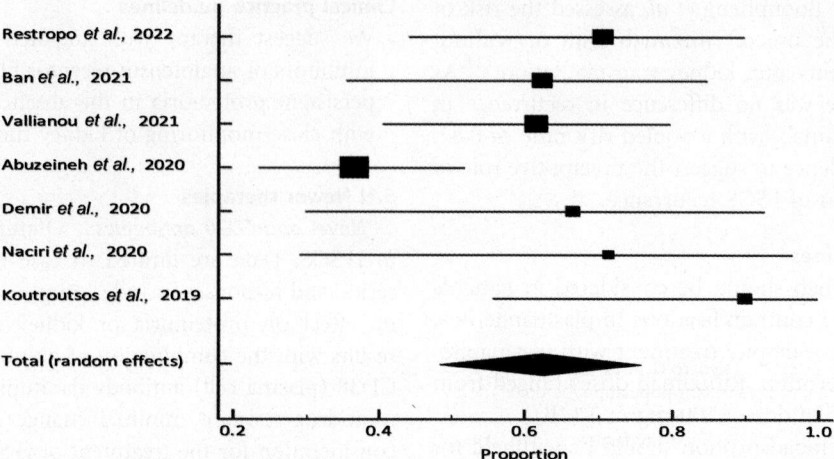

Figure 5 | Forest plot of the meta-analysis of remission among subjects with recurrent focal segmental glomerular sclerosis on treatment. The lower diamond in the graph represents the pooled estimate.[S115–S121]

The different treatments included plasmapheresis, thymoglobulin, angiotensin receptor blockers/angiotensin-converting enzyme inhibitors, cyclophosphamide, immunoadsorption, and rituximab. The pooled proportion of remission among subjects with recurrent FSGS on these treatments was 62.51% (95% CI, 48.38%–75.61%) (I^2 = 61.57%; range, 12.28%–83.16%; P = 0.016; df = 6; random effects; 7 studies; Supplementary Table S24; Figure 5). A publication bias was observed on the basis of the Egger test (P = 0.0174).

DISCLOSURE
All the authors declared no competing interests.

SUPPLEMENTARY MATERIAL
Supplementary File (Word)
Supplementary Appendix S1. Methods.
Supplementary Appendix S2. Diagnosis, clinical presentation, and classifications of focal segmental glomerular sclerosis (FSGS).
Supplementary Appendix S3. Practice algorithms.
Supplementary Appendix S4. Biomarkers.
Supplementary Appendix S5. Current treatment options for recurrent focal segmental glomerular sclerosis (rFSGS).
Supplementary Appendix S6. Ongoing trials on recurrent focal segmental glomerular sclerosis (rFSGS).
Supplementary Figure S1. PRISMA chart of included and excluded studies.
Supplementary Figure S2. Delphi method.
Supplementary Table S1. Grading the quality of evidence and strength of the recommendation.
Supplementary Table S2. Complete search strategy.
Supplementary Table S3. Population, intervention, comparator, outcome, and study design (PICOS) table.
Supplementary Table S4. The Joanna Briggs risk-of-bias tool.
Supplementary Table S5. Time line of guideline creation.
Supplementary Table S6. Delphi round results for guideline and practice points.
Supplementary Table S7. AMSTAR checklist.
Supplementary Table S8. Meta-analysis of recurrent focal segmental glomerular sclerosis (FSGS) incidence among kidney transplant recipients across different studies.
Supplementary Table S9. Meta-analysis of recurrent focal segmental glomerular sclerosis (FSGS) incidence among pediatric and adult kidney transplant recipients across different studies.
Supplementary Table S10. Incidence of recurrent focal segmental glomerular sclerosis (FSGS) among pediatric kidney transplant recipients stratified by age groups across different studies.
Supplementary Table S11. Recurrent focal segmental glomerular sclerosis (FSGS) incidence among Caucasian and non-Caucasian kidney transplant recipients.
Supplementary Table S12. Meta-analysis of 5-year graft survival among recurrent and nonrecurrent focal segmental glomerular sclerosis (FSGS) kidney transplant recipients across different studies.
Supplementary Table S13. Studies on efficacy of immunoadsorption in the treatment of recurrent focal segmental glomerular sclerosis (rFSGS).
Supplementary Table S14. Factors affecting the risk of recurrent focal segmental glomerular sclerosis (rFSGS).
Supplementary Table S15. Biomarker candidates for recurrent focal segmental glomerular sclerosis (rFSGS).
Supplementary Table S16. Meta-analysis of recurrent focal segmental glomerular sclerosis (FSGS) among living and deceased donor kidney transplant recipients across different studies.
Supplementary Table S17. The effects of induction therapy on focal segmental glomerular sclerosis (FSGS) recurrence.
Supplementary Table S18. The use of prophylactic plasmapheresis to prevent recurrent focal segmental glomerular sclerosis (rFSGS).
Supplementary Table S19. Studies on efficacy of the combined use of immunoadsorption with plasmapheresis and other modalities in the treatment of recurrent focal segmental glomerular sclerosis (rFSGS).
Supplementary Table S20. Studies on efficacy of cyclosporine in the treatment of recurrent focal segmental glomerular sclerosis (rFSGS).
Supplementary Table S21. Studies on efficacy of rituximab in the treatment of recurrent focal segmental glomerular sclerosis (rFSGS).
Supplementary Table S22. Studies on efficacy of prophylactic rituximab in recurrent focal segmental glomerular sclerosis (rFSGS).
Supplementary Table S23. Studies on efficacy of abatacept/belatacept in the treatment of recurrent focal segmental glomerular sclerosis (rFSGS).
Supplementary Table S24. Data of remission among subjects with recurrent focal segmental glomerular sclerosis (FSGS) on treatment across different studies from year 2020 to 2022.
Supplementary References.

REFERENCES

1. Hubsch H, Montané B, Abitbol C, et al. Recurrent focal glomerulosclerosis in pediatric renal allografts: the Miami experience. *Pediatr Nephrol.* 2005;20:210–216.
2. Hoyer JR, Raij L, Vernier RL, et al. Recurrence of idiopathic nephrotic syndrome after renal transplantation. *Lancet.* 1972;300:343–348.
3. Uffing A, Pérez-Sáez MJ, Mazzali M, et al. Recurrence of FSGS after kidney transplantation in adults. *Clin J Am Soc Nephrol.* 2020;15:247–256.
4. Dall'Amico R, Ghiggeri G, Carraro M, et al. Prediction and treatment of recurrent focal segmental glomerulosclerosis after renal transplantation in children. *Am J Kidney Dis.* 1999;34:1048–1055.
5. Winn MP, Conlon PJ, Lynn KL, et al. Medicine: a mutation in the TRPC6 cation channel causes familial focal segmental glomerulosclerosis. *Science.* 2005;308:1801–1804.
6. Felldin M, Nordén G, Svalander C, Nyberg G. Focal segmental glomerulosclerosis in a kidney transplant population: hereditary and sporadic forms. *Transplant Int.* 1998;11:16–21.
7. Maas RJ, Deegens JK, Wetzels JF. Permeability factors in idiopathic nephrotic syndrome: historical perspectives and lessons for the future. *Nephrol Dial Transplant.* 2014;29:2207–2216.
8. Maas RJH, Wetzels JFM, Deegens JKJ. Serum-soluble urokinase receptor concentration in primary FSGS. *Kidney Int.* 2012;81:1043–1044.
9. Hamie L, Daoud G, Nemer G, et al. SuPAR, an emerging biomarker in kidney and inflammatory diseases. *Postgrad Med J.* 2018;94:517–524.
10. Alachkar N, Li J, Matar D, et al. Monitoring suPAR levels in post-kidney transplant focal segmental glomerulosclerosis treated with therapeutic plasma exchange and rituximab. *BMC Nephrol.* 2018;19:361.
11. Wei C, Trachtman H, Li J, et al. Circulating suPAR in two cohorts of primary FSGS. *J Am Soc Nephrol.* 2012;23:2051–2059.
12. Savin VJ. Cardiotrophin-like cytokine 1, a candidate molecule for the FSGS factor. Accessed June 1, 2023. http://grantome.com/grant/NIH/R21-DK081148-01A1
13. Bitzan M, Babayeva S, Vasudevan A, et al. TNF α pathway blockade ameliorates toxic effects of FSGS plasma on podocyte cytoskeleton and β3 integrin activation. *Pediatr Nephrol.* 2012;27:2217–2226.
14. Chung CF, Kitzler T, Kachurina N, et al. Intrinsic tumor necrosis factor-α pathway is activated in a subset of patients with focal segmental glomerulosclerosis. *PLoS One.* 2019;14:e0216426.
15. Kacprzyk F, Chrzanowski W. Czynnik martwicy nowotworu (TNF) i interleukina-6 (IL-6) w k??ebuszkowych zapaleniach nerek. *Pol Arch Med Wewn.* 1996;96:224–233.
16. Guyatt GH, Oxman AD, Vist GE, et al. GRADE: an emerging consensus on rating quality of evidence and strength of recommendations. *BMJ.* 2008;336:924–926.
17. Francis A, Trnka P, McTaggart SJ. Long-term outcome of kidney transplantation in recipients with focal segmental glomerulosclerosis. *Clin J Am Soc Nephrol.* 2016;11:2041–2046.
18. Ban H, Miura K, Kaneko N, et al. Amount and selectivity of proteinuria may predict the treatment response in post-transplant recurrence of focal segmental glomerulosclerosis: a single-center retrospective study. *Pediatr Nephrol.* 2021;36:2433–2442.
19. Pardon A, Audard V, Caillard S, et al. Risk factors and outcome of focal and segmental glomerulosclerosis recurrence in adult renal transplant recipients. *Nephrol Dial Transplant.* 2006;21:1053–1059.
20. Fuiano G, Comi N, Magri P, et al. Serial morphometric analysis of sclerotic lesions in primary "focal" segmental glomerulosclerosis. *J Am Soc Nephrol.* 1996;7:49–55.
21. Verani RR, Hawkins EP. Recurrent focal segmental glomerulosclerosis: a pathological study of the early lesion. *Am J Nephrol.* 1986;6:263–270.
22. Cheong H, Han HW, Park HW, et al. Early recurrent nephrotic syndrome after renal transplantation in children with focal segmental glomerulosclerosis. *Nephrol Dial Transplant.* 2000;15:78–81.
23. Swaminathan S, Lager DJ, Qian X, et al. Collapsing and non-collapsing focal segmental glomerulosclerosis in kidney transplants. *Nephrol Dial Transplant.* 2006;21:2607–2614.
24. Shi J, Hu Y, Shao G, et al. Quantifying podocyte number in a small sample size of glomeruli with CUBIC to evaluate podocyte depletion of db/db mice. *J Diabetes Res.* 2023;2023:1901105.
25. Hariharan S, Peddi VR, Savin VJ, et al. Recurrent and de novo renal diseases after renal transplantation: a report from the renal allograft disease registry. *Am J Kidney Dis.* 1998;31:928–931.
26. Cravedi P, Kopp JB, Remuzzi G. Recent progress in the pathophysiology and treatment of FSGS recurrence. *Am J Transplant.* 2013;13:266–274.
27. Cosio FG, Cattran DC. Recent advances in our understanding of recurrent primary glomerulonephritis after kidney transplantation. *Kidney Int.* 2017;91:304–314.
28. Radha S, Afroz T, Prasad CR, et al. Focal segmental glomerulosclerosis in renal allografts: is it possible to diagnose the etiology? *Indian J Nephrol.* 2015;25:82–85.
29. Choy BY, Chan TM, Lai KN. Recurrent glomerulonephritis after kidney transplantation. *Am J Transplant.* 2006;6:2535–2542.
30. Chadban SJ. Glomerulonephritis recurrence in the renal graft. *J Am Soc Nephrol.* 2001;12:394–402.
31. Sharief S, Mahesh S, Del Rio M, et al. Recurrent focal segmental glomerulosclerosis in renal allograft recipients: role of human leukocyte antigen mismatching and other clinical variables. *Int J Nephrol.* 2011;2011:506805.
32. Hwang JH, Han SS, Huh W, et al. Outcome of kidney allograft in patients with adulthood-onset focal segmental glomerulosclerosis: comparison with childhood-onset FSGS. *Nephrol Dial Transplant.* 2012;27:2559–2565.
33. Hickson LJ, Gera M, Amer H, et al. Kidney transplantation for primary focal segmental glomerulosclerosis: outcomes and response to therapy for recurrence. *Transplantation.* 2009;87:1232–1239.
34. Artero M, Biava C, Amend W, et al. Recurrent focal glomerulosclerosis: natural history and response to therapy. *Am J Med.* 1992;92:375–383.
35. Huang K, Ferris ME, Andreoni KA, Gipson DS. The differential effect of race among pediatric kidney transplant recipients with focal segmental glomerulosclerosis. *Am J Kidney Dis.* 2004;43:1082–1090.
36. Nehus EJ, Goebel JW, Succop PS, Abraham EC. Focal segmental glomerulosclerosis in children: multivariate analysis indicates that donor type does not alter recurrence risk. *Transplantation.* 2013;96:550–554.
37. Ingulli E, Tejani A. Incidence, treatment, and outcome of recurrent focal segmental glomerulosclerosis posttransplantation in 42 allografts in children — a single-center experience. *Transplantation.* 1991;51:401–405.
38. Braden GL, Mulhern JG, O'Shea MH, et al. Changing incidence of glomerular diseases in adults. *Am J Kidney Dis.* 2000;35:878–883.
39. Pontier PJ, Patel TG. Racial differences in the prevalence and presentation of glomerular disease in adults. *Clin Nephrol.* 1994;42:79–84.
40. Korbet SM, Genchi RM, Borok RZ, Schwartz MM. The racial prevalence of glomerular lesions in nephrotic adults. *Am J Kidney Dis.* 1996;27:647–651.
41. Ingulli E, Tejani A. Racial differences in the incidence and renal outcome of idiopathic focal segmental glomerulosclerosis in children. *Pediatr Nephrol.* 1991;5:393–397.
42. Bakir AA, Bazilinski NG, Rhee HL, et al. Focal segmental glomerulosclerosis: a common entity in nephrotic black adults. *Arch Intern Med.* 1989;149:1802–1804.
43. Sorof JM, Hawkins EP, Brewer ED, et al. Age and ethnicity affect the risk and outcome of focal segmental glomerulosclerosis. *Pediatr Nephrol.* 1998;12:764–768.
44. Mahesh S, Del Rio M, Feuerstein D, et al. Demographics and response to therapeutic plasma exchange in pediatric renal transplantation for focal glomerulosclerosis: a single center experience. *Pediatr Transplant.* 2008;12:682–688.
45. Kramer A, Pippias M, Noordzij M, et al. The European Renal Association - European Dialysis and Transplant Association (ERA-EDTA) registry annual report 2016: a summary. *Clin Kidney J.* 2019;12:702–720.
46. Cecka JM, Terasaki PI. The UNOS scientific renal transplant registry: United Network for Organ Sharing. *Clin Transpl.* 1995;1–18.
47. Briganti EM, Russ GR, McNeil JJ, et al. Risk of renal allograft loss from recurrent glomerulonephritis. *N Engl J Med.* 2002;347:103–109.
48. Koh LJ, Martz K, Blydt-Hansen TD. Risk factors associated with allograft failure in pediatric kidney transplant recipients with focal segmental glomerulosclerosis. *Pediatr Transplant.* 2019;23:e13469.
49. Baum MA, Stablein DM, Panzarino VM, et al. Loss of living donor renal allograft survival advantage in children with focal segmental glomerulosclerosis. *Kidney Int.* 2001;59:328–333.
50. Durkan AM, Robinson LA. Chapter 60 - acute allograft dysfunction. In: Geary DF, Schaefer F, eds. *Comprehensive Pediatric Nephrology.* Mosby; 2008:931–945.
51. D'Agati V. Pathologic classification of focal segmental glomerulosclerosis. *Semin Nephrol.* 2003;23:117–134.
52. Ijpelaar DHT, Farris AB, Goemaere N, et al. Fidelity and evolution of recurrent FSGS in renal allografts. *J Am Soc Nephrol.* 2008;19:2219–2224.

53. Tejani A, Stablein DH. Recurrence of focal segmental glomerulosclerosis posttransplantation: a special report of the North American pediatric renal transplant cooperative study. *J Am Soc Nephrol*. 1992;2(suppl): S258–S263.
54. Pinto J, Lacerda G, Cameron JS, et al. Recurrence of focal segmental glomerulosclerosis in renal allografts. *Transplantation*. 1981;32:83–89.
55. Schachter AD, Strehlau J, Zurakowski D, et al. Increased nuclear factor-κB and angiotensinogen gene expression in posttransplant recurrent focal segmental glomerulosclerosis. *Transplantation*. 2000;70:1107–1110.
56. Ponticelli C. Recurrence of focal segmental glomerular sclerosis (FSGS) after renal transplantation. *Nephrol Dial Transplant*. 2010;25:25–31.
57. Morello W, Puvinathan S, Puccio G, et al. Post-transplant recurrence of steroid resistant nephrotic syndrome in children: the Italian experience. *J Nephrol*. 2020;33:849–857.
58. Weber S, Tönshoff B. Recurrence of focal-segmental glomerulosclerosis in children after renal transplantation: clinical and genetic aspects. *Transplantation*. 2005;80(suppl):S128–S134.
59. Govers LP, Toka HR, Hariri A, et al. Mitochondrial DNA mutations in renal disease: an overview. *Pediatr Nephrol*. 2021;36:9–17.
60. Holmberg C, Jalanko H. Congenital nephrotic syndrome and recurrence of proteinuria after renal transplantation. *Pediatr Nephrol*. 2014;29: 2309–2317.
61. Becker-Cohen R, Bruschi M, Rinat C, et al. Recurrent nephrotic syndrome in homozygous truncating NPHS2 mutation is not due to anti-podocin antibodies. *Am J Transplant*. 2007;7:256–260.
62. Patrakka J, Kestilä M, Wartiovaara J, et al. Congenital nephrotic syndrome (NPHS1): features resulting from different mutations in Finnish patients. *Kidney Int*. 2000;58:972–980.
63. Carraro M, Caridi G, Bruschi M, et al. Serum glomerular permeability activity in patients with podocin mutations (NPHS2) and steroid-resistant nephrotic syndrome. *J Am Soc Nephrol*. 2002;13:1946–1952.
64. Bertelli R, Ginevri F, Caridi G, et al. Recurrence of focal segmental glomerulosclerosis after renal transplantation in patients with mutations of podocin. *Am J Kidney Dis*. 2003;41:1314–1321.
65. Morello W, Proverbio E, Puccio G, Montini G. A systematic review and meta-analysis of the rate and risk factors for post-transplant disease recurrence in children with steroid resistant nephrotic syndrome. *Kidney Int Rep*. 2023;8:254–264.
66. Schachter ME, Monahan M, Radhakrishnan J, et al. Recurrent focal segmental glomerulosclerosis in the renal allograft: single center experience in the era of modern immunosuppression. *Clin Nephrol*. 2010;74:173–181.
67. Abbott KC, Sawyers ES, Oliver JD, et al. Graft loss due to recurrent focal segmental glomerulosclerosis in renal transplant recipients in the United States. *Am J Kidney Dis*. 2001;37:366–373.
68. Bulut IK, Taner S, Keskinoglu A, et al. Long-term follow-up results of renal transplantation in pediatric patients with focal segmental glomerulosclerosis: a single-center experience. *Transplant Proc*. 2019;51: 1064–1069.
69. Maas RJH, Deegens JKJ, Van Den Brand JAJG, et al. A retrospective study of focal segmental glomerulosclerosis: clinical criteria can identify patients at high risk for recurrent disease after first renal transplantation. *BMC Nephrol*. 2013;14:47.
70. Moroni G, Gallelli B, Quaglini S, et al. Long-term outcome of renal transplantation in adults with focal segmental glomerulosclerosis. *Transplant Int*. 2010;23:208–216.
71. Sener A, Bella AJ, Nguan C, et al. Focal segmental glomerular sclerosis in renal transplant recipients: predicting early disease recurrence may prolong allograft function. *Clin Transplant*. 2009;23:96–100.
72. O'Meara Y, Green A, Carmody M, et al. Recurrent glomerulonephritis in renal transplants: fourteen years' experience. *Nephrol Dial Transplant*. 1989;4:730–734.
73. Cormican S, Kennedy C, O'Kelly P, et al. Renal transplant outcomes in primary FSGS compared with other recipients and risk factors for recurrence: a national review of the Irish Transplant Registry. *Clin Transplant*. 2018;32:e13152.
74. Raafat R, Travis LB, Kalia A, Diven S. Role of transplant induction therapy on recurrence rate of focal segmental glomerulosclerosis. *Pediatr Nephrol*. 2000;14:189–194.
75. Pascual J, Mezrich JD, Djamali A, et al. Alemtuzumab induction and recurrence of glomerular disease after kidney transplantation. *Transplantation*. 2007;83:1429–1434.
76. Kirk AD. Induction immunosuppression. *Transplantation*. 2006;82:593–602.
77. Bouts A, Veltkamp F, Tönshoff B, Vivarelli M. European Society of Pediatric Nephrology survey on current practice regarding recurrent focal segmental glomerulosclerosis after pediatric kidney transplantation. *Pediatr Transplant*. 2019;23:e13385.
78. Musante L, Candiano G, Bruschi M, et al. Circulating anti-actin and anti-ATP synthase antibodies identify a sub-set of patients with idiopathic nephrotic syndrome. *Clin Exp Immunol*. 2005;141:491–499.
79. Alachkar N, Gupta G, Montgomery RA. Angiotensin antibodies and focal segmental glomerulosclerosis. *N Engl J Med*. 2013;368:971–973.
80. Delville M, Sigdel TK, Wei C, et al. A circulating antibody panel for pretransplant prediction of FSGS recurrence after kidney transplantation. *Sci Transl Med*. 2014;6:256ra136.
81. Watts AJB, Keller KH, Lerner G. Discovery of autoantibodies targeting nephrin in minimal change disease supports a novel autoimmune etiology. *J Am Soc Nephrol*. 2022;33:238–252.
82. Hattori M, Shirai Y, Kanda S, et al. Circulating nephrin autoantibodies and post-transplant recurrence of primary focal segmental glomerulosclerosis. *Am J Transplant*. 2022;22:2478–2480.
83. Shishido S, Satou H, Muramatsu M, et al. Combination of pulse methylprednisolone infusions with cyclosporine-based immunosuppression is safe and effective to treat recurrent focal segmental glomerulosclerosis after pediatric kidney transplantation. *Clin Transplant*. 2013;27:E143–E150.
84. Sharma M, Sharma R, McCarthy ET, Savin VJ. The focal segmental glomerulosclerosis permeability factor: biochemical characteristics and biological effects. *Exp Biol Med*. 2004;229:85–98.
85. Zimmerman SW. Plasmapheresis and dipyridamole for recurrent focal glomerular sclerosis. *Nephron*. 1985;40:241–245.
86. Fencl F, Simková E, Vondrák K, et al. Recurrence of nephrotic proteinuria in children with focal segmental glomerulosclerosis after renal transplantation treated with plasmapheresis and immunoadsorption: case reports. *Transplant Proc*. 2007;39:3488–3490.
87. Cleper R, Krause I, Bar Nathan N, et al. Focal segmental glomerulosclerosis in pediatric kidney transplantation: 30 years' experience. *Clin Transplant*. 2016;30:1324–1331.
88. Canaud G, Zuber J, Sberro R, et al. Intensive and prolonged treatment of focal and segmental glomerulosclerosis recurrence in adult kidney transplant recipients: a pilot study. *Am J Transplant*. 2009;9:1081–1086.
89. Gohh RY, Yango AF, Morrissey PE, et al. Preemptive plasmapheresis and recurrence of FSGS in high-risk renal transplant recipients. *Am J Transplant*. 2005;5:2907–2912.
90. Restrepo JM, Torres-Canchala L, Londoño H, et al. Treatment of post-transplant recurrent FSGS in children using plasmapheresis and augmentation of immunosuppression. *BMC Nephrol*. 2022;23:131.
91. Demir ME, Uyar M, Merhametsiz O. Combination of high-dose intravenous cyclosporine and plasma exchange treatment is effective in post-transplant recurrent focal segmental glomerulosclerosis: results of case series. *Transplant Proc*. 2020;52:843–849.
92. Hansrivijit P, Ghahramani N. Combined rituximab and plasmapheresis or plasma exchange for focal segmental glomerulosclerosis in adult kidney transplant recipients: a meta-analysis. *Int Urol Nephrol*. 2020;52: 1377–1387.
93. Vallianou K, Marinaki S, Skalioti C, et al. Therapeutic options for recurrence of primary focal segmental glomerulonephritis (FSGS) in the renal allograft: single-center experience. *J Clin Med*. 2021;10: 373.
94. Allard L, Kwon T, Krid S, et al. Treatment by immunoadsorption for recurrent focal segmental glomerulosclerosis after paediatric kidney transplantation: a multicentre French cohort. *Nephrol Dial Transplant*. 2018;33:954–963.
95. Belson A, Yorgin PD, Al-Uzri AY, et al. Long-term plasmapheresis and protein A column treatment of recurrent FSGS. *Pediatr Nephrol*. 2001;16: 985–989.
96. Fencl F, Vondrák K, Rosík T, et al. Recurrence of nephrotic proteinuria in children with focal segmental glomerulosclerosis: early treatment with plasmapheresis and immunoadsorption should be associated with better prognosis. *Minerva Pediatr*. 2016;68:348–354.
97. Dantal J, Baatard R, Hourmant M, et al. Recurrent nephrotic syndrome following renal transplantation in patients with focal glomerulosclerosis: a one-center study of plasma exchange effects. *Transplantation*. 1991;52:827–831.

98. Ponikvar R, Ponikvar JB. Side effects of protein A immunoadsorption and plasma exchange in renal allograft recipients. *Transplant Proc.* 2002;34:2910–2913.
99. Naciri Bennani H, Bonzi JY, Noble J, et al. Immunoadsorption for recurrent primary focal segmental glomerulosclerosis on kidney allografts: a single-center experience and literature review. *Blood Purif.* 2020;49:322–333.
100. Salomon R, Gagnadoux MF, Niaudet P. Intravenous cyclosporine therapy in recurrent nephrotic syndrome after renal transplantation in children. *Transplantation.* 2003;75:810–814.
101. Sannomiya A, Murakami T, Koyama I, et al. Preoperative low-density lipoprotein apheresis for preventing recurrence of focal segmental glomerulosclerosis after kidney transplantation. *J Transplant.* 2018;2018:8926786.
102. Muso E. Beneficial effect of LDL-apheresis in refractory nephrotic syndrome. *Clin Exp Nephrol.* 2014;18:286–290.
103. Muso E, Yashiro M, Sasayama S, et al. Does LDL-apheresis in steroid-resistant nephrotic syndrome affect prognosis? *Nephrol Dial Transplant.* 1994;9:257–264.
104. Muso E, Mune M, Yorioka N, et al. Beneficial effect of low-density lipoprotein apheresis (LDL-A) on refractory nephrotic syndrome (NS) due to focal glomerulosclerosis (FGS). *Clin Nephrol.* 2007;67:341–344.
105. Muso E, Mune M, Fujii Y, et al. Significantly rapid relief from steroid-resistant nephrotic syndrome by LDL apheresis compared with steroid monotherapy. *Nephron.* 2001;89:408–415.
106. Raina R, Krishnappa V. An update on LDL apheresis for nephrotic syndrome. *Pediatr Nephrol.* 2019;34:1655–1669.
107. Masutani K, Katafuchi R, Ikeda H, et al. Recurrent nephrotic syndrome after living-related renal transplantation resistant to plasma exchange: report of two cases. *Clin Transplant Suppl.* 2005;19(suppl 14):59–64.
108. Shah L, Hooper DK, Okamura D, et al. LDL-apheresis-induced remission of focal segmental glomerulosclerosis recurrence in pediatric renal transplant recipients. *Pediatr Nephrol.* 2019;34:2343–2350.
109. Nozu K, Iijima K, Fujisawa M, et al. Rituximab treatment for posttransplant lymphoproliferative disorder (PTLD) induces complete remission of recurrent nephrotic syndrome. *Pediatr Nephrol.* 2005;20:1660–1663.
110. Pescovitz MD, Book BK, Sidner RA. Resolution of recurrent focal segmental glomerulosclerosis proteinuria after rituximab treatment. *N Engl J Med.* 2006;354:1961–1963.
111. Yabu JM, Ho B, Scandling JD, Vincenti F. Rituximab failed to improve nephrotic syndrome in renal transplant patients with recurrent focal segmental glomerulosclerosis. *Am J Transplant.* 2008;8:222–227.
112. Dello Strologo L, Guzzo I, Laurenzi C, et al. Use of rituximab in focal glomerulosclerosis relapses after renal transplantation. *Transplantation.* 2009;88:417–420.
113. Bayrakci US, Baskin E, Sakalli H, et al. Rituximab for post-transplant recurrences of FSGS. *Pediatr Transplant.* 2009;13:240–243.
114. Damodar A, Mustafa R, Bhatnagar J, et al. Use of anti-CD20 antibody in the treatment of post-transplant glomerulonephritis. *Clin Transplant.* 2011;25:375–379.
115. Stewart ZA, Shetty R, Nair R, et al. Case report: successful treatment of recurrent focal segmental glomerulosclerosis with a novel rituximab regimen. *Transplant Proc.* 2011;43:3994–3996.
116. Grenda R, Jarmużek W, Piątosa B, Rubik J. Long-term effect of rituximab in maintaining remission of recurrent and plasmapheresis-dependent nephrotic syndrome post-renal transplantation - case report. *Pediatr Transplant.* 2011;15:E121–E125.
117. Spinner ML, Bowman LJ, Horwedel TA, et al. Single-dose rituximab for recurrent glomerulonephritis post-renal transplant. *Am J Nephrol.* 2015;41:37–47.
118. Garrouste C, Canaud G, Büchler M, et al. Rituximab for recurrence of primary focal segmental glomerulosclerosis after kidney transplantation: clinical outcomes. *Transplantation.* 2017;101:649–656.
119. Araya CE, Dharnidharka VR. The factors that may predict response to rituximab therapy in recurrent focal segmental glomerulosclerosis: a systematic review. *J Transplant.* 2011;2011:1–7.
120. Basu B, Mahapatra TKS, Mondal N. Mycophenolate mofetil following rituximab in children with steroid-resistant nephrotic syndrome. *Pediatrics.* 2015;136:e132–e139.
121. Bharati J, Gupta KL, Kenwar DB, et al. Recurrent focal segmental glomerulosclerosis after kidney transplant in adults: a report on various treatment regimens. *Indian J Transplant.* 2018;12:193–198.
122. El Khashab S, El Khashab O, El Ghoneimy M, AbdelRassoul MA. Rituximab as a preemptive treatment to prevent recurrence of primary focal segmental glomerulosclerosis: a novel approach. *Exp Clin Transplant.* 2019;17:326–329.
123. Koutroutsos K, Charif R, Moran L, et al. Successful management of post-transplant focal segmental glomerulosclerosis with therapeutic plasma exchange and rituximab. *Clin Exp Nephrol.* 2019;23:700–709.
124. Boonpheng B, Hansrivijit P, Thongprayoon C, et al. Rituximab or plasmapheresis for prevention of recurrent focal segmental glomerulosclerosis after kidney transplantation: a systematic review and meta-analysis. *World J Transplant.* 2021;11:303–319.
125. Yu CC, Fornoni A, Weins A, et al. Abatacept in B7-1-positive proteinuric kidney disease. *N Engl J Med.* 2013;369:2416–2423.
126. Shah Y, Almeshari K, Aleid H, et al. Successful treatment with abatacept in recurrent focal segmental glomerulosclerosis after kidney transplant. *Exp Clin Transplant.* 2019;17:178–180.
127. Sprenger-Mähr H, Zitt E, Soleiman A, Lhotta K. Successful treatment of focal segmental glomerulosclerosis after kidney transplantation with plasma exchange and abatacept in a patient with juvenile rheumatoid arthritis. *Case Rep Transplant.* 2016;2016:7137584.
128. Delville M, Baye E, Durrbach A, et al. B7-1 blockade does not improve post-transplant nephrotic syndrome caused by recurrent FSGS. *J Am Soc Nephrol.* 2016;27:2520–2527.
129. Kershaw DB, Sedman AB, Kelsch RC, Bunchman TE. Recurrent focal segmental glomerulosclerosis in pediatric renal transplant recipients: successful treatment with oral cyclophosphamide. *Clin Transplant.* 1994;8:546–549.
130. Cochat P, Kassir A, Colon S, et al. Recurrent nephrotic syndrome after transplantation: early treatment with plasmaphaeresis and cyclophosphamide. *Pediatr Nephrol.* 1993;7:50–54.
131. Requião-Moura LR, Moscoso-Solorzano GT, Franco MF, et al. Prognostic factors associated with poor graft outcomes in renal recipients with post-transplant glomerulonephritis. *Clin Transplant.* 2007;21:363–370.
132. Arai M, Wada A, Isaka Y, et al. *In vivo* transfection of genes for renin and angiotensinogen into the glomerular cells induced phenotypic change of the mesangial cells and glomerular sclerosis. *Biochem Biophys Res Commun.* 1995;206:525–532.
133. Abuzeineh M, Aala A, Alasfar S, Alachkar N. Angiotensin II receptor 1 antibodies associate with post-transplant focal segmental glomerulosclerosis and proteinuria. *BMC Nephrol.* 2020;21:253.
134. Freiberger V, Amann K, Heemann U, Frank H. Effect of a triple blockade of the renin-angiotensin-system in recurrent focal segmental glomerulosclerosis after kidney transplantation. *Transplant Int.* 2009;22:1110–1113.
135. Zhang B. Ofatumumab. *MAbs.* 2009;1:326–331.
136. Basu B. Ofatumumab for rituximab-resistant nephrotic syndrome. *N Engl J Med.* 2014;370:1268–1270.
137. Wang CS, Liverman RS, Garro R, et al. Ofatumumab for the treatment of childhood nephrotic syndrome. *Pediatr Nephrol.* 2017;32:835–841.
138. Bonanni A, Rossi R, Murtas C, Ghiggeri GM. Low-dose ofatumumab for rituximab-resistant nephrotic syndrome. *BMJ Case Rep.* 2015;2015:bcr2015210208.
139. Solomon S, Zolotnitskaya A, Del Rio M. Ofatumumab in post-transplantation recurrence of focal segmental glomerulosclerosis in a child. *Pediatr Transplant.* 2019;23:e13413.
140. Reynolds BC, Lamb A, Jones CA, et al. UK experience of ofatumumab in recurrence of focal segmental glomerulosclerosis post-kidney transplant. *Pediatr Nephrol.* 2022;37:199–207.
141. Leroy S, Guigonis V, Bruckner D, et al. Successful anti-TNFα treatment in a child with posttransplant recurrent focal segmental glomerulosclerosis. *Am J Transplant.* 2009;9:858–861.
142. Belingheri M, Lazzari L, Parazzi V, et al. Allogeneic mesenchymal stem cell infusion for the stabilization of focal segmental glomerulosclerosis. *Biologicals.* 2013;41:439–445.

policy forum

Kidney biopsies among persons living in hotspots of CKDu: a position statement from the International Society of Nephrology's Consortium of Collaborators on CKDu

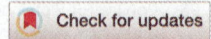

Eranga Wijewickrama[1], Suman Behera[2,3], Pablo Garcia[4], Carmen Avila-Casado[5], Ben Caplin[6,7], Vicente Sanchez Paolo[8], Karen Courville[9,10], David Friedman[11], Magdalena Madero[12], Vivekanand Jha[13,14,15], Neeraja Kambham[16], Adeera Levin[17] and Shuchi Anand[18]; on behalf of the International Society of Nephrology's International Consortium of Collaborators on CKDu[19]

[1]Department of Clinical Medicine, Faculty of Medicine, University of Colombo, Colombo, Sri Lanka; [2]Division of Nephrology, McMaster University, Hamilton, Ontario, Canada; [3]Division of Nephrology, William Osler Health System, Brampton, Ontario, Canada; [4]Department of Medicine (Nephrology), University of New Mexico, Albuquerque, New Mexico, USA; [5]Department of Laboratory Medicine & Pathology, University Health Network, University of Toronto, Toronto, Ontario, Canada; [6]Department of Renal Medicine, University College London, London, UK; [7]Department of Nephrology, Royal Free London NHS Foundation Trust, London, UK; [8]Nephrology and Kidney Transplant Division, Social Security Guatemalan Institute, Concepción, Guatemala; [9]Section of Nephrology, Department of Medicine, Hospital Dr. Gustavo Nelson Collado, Chitré, Herrera, Panama; [10]Instituto de Ciencias Médicas and Sistema Nacional de Investigación, Las Tablas, Los Santos, Panamá; [11]Division of Nephrology, Beth Israel Deaconess Medical Center, Harvard Medical School, Boston, Massachusetts, USA; [12]Division of Nephrology, Instituto Nacional de Cardiologia Ignacio Chávez, Mexico City, Mexico; [13]George Institute for Global Health, UNSW, New Delhi, India; [14]School of Public Health, Imperial College, London, UK; [15]Prasanna School of Public Health, Manipal Academy of Medical Education, Manipal, India; [16]Department of Pathology, Stanford University School of Medicine, Palo Alto, California, USA; [17]Division of Nephrology, Department of Medicine, University of British Columbia, Vancouver, British Columbia, Canada; and [18]Division of Nephrology, Stanford University School of Medicine, Palo Alto, California, USA

Kidney International (2024) 105, 464–469; https://doi.org/10.1016/j.kint.2023.12.012

Copyright © 2023, International Society of Nephrology. Published by Elsevier Inc. All rights reserved.

Correspondence: *Eranga Wijewickrama, Department of Clinical Medicine, Faculty of Medicine, University of Colombo, 25 Kynsey Road, Colombo 00800, Sri Lanka. E-mail: erangasw@clinmed.cmb.ac.lk*

[19]Members of the International Society of Nephrology's International Consortium of Collaborators on CKDu are listed in the Appendix.

Received 3 September 2023; revised 2 November 2023; accepted 1 December 2023; published online 30 December 2023

Chronic kidney disease of unknown etiology (CKDu) is a progressive primary tubulointerstitial kidney disease affecting persons in rural, agricultural communities worldwide. Some of the other terms used to identify this disease include Mesoamerican nephropathy (MeN) in Central America, Uddanam nephropathy in India, and chronic interstitial nephritis in agricultural communities (CINAC). Well-described hotspots exist in Central America, Sri Lanka, and India, with investigations to assess epidemiology and cause(s) ongoing in many regions of the world.[1,2] Although the disease is suggested in a person living in a CKDu endemic area and presenting with declining kidney function without alternative explanations (e.g., diabetes, heavy proteinuria or hematuria indicative of glomerulonephritis, or structural kidney disease), definitive diagnosis requires findings of chronic tubulointerstitial disease on kidney biopsy.

However, clinicians may not be enthusiastic about performing kidney biopsies among patients suspected to have CKDu, for several reasons. These reasons include the following: (i) undefined thresholds of kidney function decline at which to pursue biopsy; (ii) the experiential evidence that a clinical diagnosis of CKDu is predictive of biopsy diagnosis; (iii) the lack of a specific treatment for CKDu at present; and (iv) concerns about safety and risk and cost to the patient. Kidney biopsies offer definitive diagnosis, provide prognostic information, and advance our knowledge about the spectrum of disease putatively to enable the institution of preventive and/or therapeutic strategies. The tension among limited resources, patient burden, and quest for accuracy in disease diagnostics leads to the following question: Are kidney biopsies clinically indicated among persons suspected of having CKDu in regions known to be CKDu hotspots?

In 2022 and 2023, the International Society of Nephrology's (ISN) i3C (International Consortium CKDu Collaborators) Working Group and the ISN Renal Pathology Working Group held 3 consensus-building meetings to explore the pros and cons of pursuing kidney biopsies in CKDu hotspots. In addition, a survey was circulated to ISN members through 3 ISN regional boards (Latin America, South Asia, and Oceania and South East Asia) to assess biopsy practices in nonproteinuric kidney diseases. Acknowledging that a group of research-intensive, internationally engaged nephrologists and associated research scientists participated in this endeavor, we summarize the key considerations and describe the group's consensus. The contents of this article were reviewed by the chairpersons of the 3 ISN Regional Boards.

We note that, ideally, a rigorous, research-based approach to biopsies will be pursued in many CKDu hotspots, but the reality on the ground, including the lack of resources to apply advanced tissue-processing techniques, means that such studies may not have a broad or immediate reach, and in the meantime, clinicians are faced with counseling patients with CKDu. Thus, our aim is to provide practicing clinicians with a framework around which to anchor personalized discussions with patients, and to maximize the clinical and scientific output of clinically indicated biopsies in CKDu hotspots.

Clinical utility of kidney biopsy in a person suspected to have CKDu

Traditional indications for kidney biopsy emphasize proteinuria (with or without hematuria), or unexplained acute kidney injury. Persons with CKDu may not fall under any of these categories, as they may experience variable and insidious loss of kidney function without an active urinary sediment. We implemented a simple survey posing several scenarios of nonproteinuric kidney disease presentation at young and middle age and in patients of male and female sex (Figure 1). A total of 68 nephrologists responded, a majority from affected regions (32% and 36% from South Asia and Latin America). A total of 40% of the responding nephrologists would opt to recommend a kidney biopsy on a 36-year-old male or female, with an estimated glomerular filtration rate (eGFR) of 80 ml/min per 1.73 m^2, and evidence of kidney function decline by an eGFR change > 5 ml/min per 1.73 m^2 over a short time frame; fewer (∼25%) would pursue a biopsy if the patient were a 60-year-old male. A similar pattern of responses held if eGFR were < 60 ml/min per 1.73 m^2 and no clear evidence of eGFR decline over a short time frame. More than 70% would pursue biopsy in patients with an eGFR of 58 ml/min per 1.73 m^2, and evidence of eGFR decline, independent of age or sex.

A biopsy in any of these 3 scenarios, with CKDu being suspected, could address diagnostic uncertainty, and even in the case of pathologically confirmed tubulointerstitial nephritis, could potentially point to known etiologies other

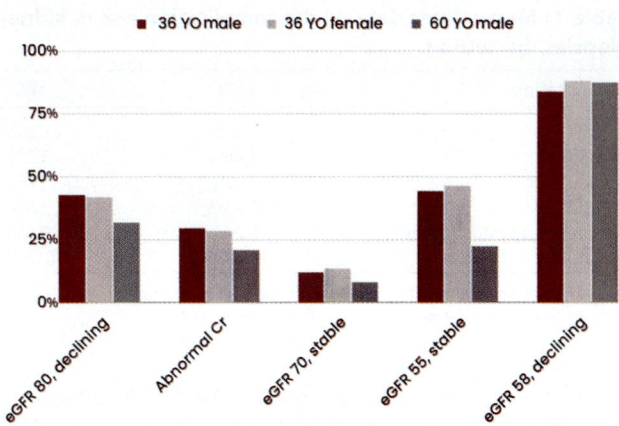

Figure 1 | Survey results on kidney biopsy in nonproteinuric kidney diseases. Proportions indicate % of survey respondents indicating that a biopsy is indicated for these scenarios: estimated glomerular filtration rate (eGFR) 80, declining—eGFR 80 ml/min per 1.73 m^2, and a >5 ml/min decline between 2 time points; abnormal Cr—serum creatinine level higher than laboratory range, at 2 time points; eGFR 70, stable—eGFR 70 ml/min per 1.73 m^2, stable at 2 time points; eGFR 55, stable—eGFR 55 ml/min per 1.73 m^2, stable at 2 time points; eGFR 58 declining—eGFR 58 ml/min per 1.73 m^2 and a >5 ml/min decline between 2 time points. The 2 time points were specified to be least 3 months apart. YO, year old.

than CKDu (e.g., nephrocalciniosis, oxalate nephropathy, granulomatous inflammation indicating tuberculosis or sarcoid, or plasma-rich infiltrate indicating IgG4 disease). In addition, kidney biopsy can provide valuable information for prognostication by quantifying the extent of tubular atrophy, interstitial fibrosis, and secondary glomerulosclerosis, which is essential for developing a treatment plan. Conceivably, clinical trials targeting either tubular inflammation or fibrosis may be offered in the near future, and a kidney biopsy could facilitate patient enrollment.

The uncertainty that exists in the utility of kidney biopsy was acknowledged by ISN i3C Working Group discussants, especially in the context of socioeconomic constraints on the patients, many of whom may need to travel or miss work to undergo the procedure. Some clinically important questions—such as, does biopsy alter outcomes—remain unanswered, and in fact, they can be answered only with systematic approaches to biopsy. Furthermore, the ISN i3C Working Group consists largely of academically focused nephrologists who aim to investigate CKDu in depth, and thus, they have an inherent bias toward gaining more information when doing so is feasible.

Ultimately, the decision to pursue biopsy in clinical encounters is reliant on physician-facilitated personalized discussion of risks and benefits, with patient autonomy at the center of these discussions.

Considering the safety of kidney biopsies in low-resource settings in general, and specifically for CKDu

The best-described CKDu hotspots exist in low- and middle-income countries.[3] A recent review of 39 studies described safety data from 19,500 kidney biopsies performed

Table 1 | Metanalyses data on the complication risk in kidney biopsies, by setting

Complication	LMIC	HIC
Biopsy, n	19,500	118,064
Hematuria	1.48%	3.5%
Hematomas	2.4%	11%
Transfusion	0.24%	1.6%
Nephrectomy/intervention	0.04%	0.3%
Death	0.01%	0.06%

HIC, high-income countries; LMIC, low- and middle-income countries.
Data are from Kajawo et al.[4] (LMIC) and Poggio et al.[5] (HIC).

Table 2 | ISN i3C recommendations for kidney biopsy in CKDu endemic regions

Recommendation	Rationale
Kidney biopsies for clinical indication should be considered routinely in cases of suspected CKDu	Diagnostic uncertainty without biopsy; Prognostic data; Phenotype of potentially affected patients has low risk for complications
Standard of care for kidney biopsy safety must exist when offering kidney biopsies: ultrasound guidance, biopsy gun, trained nephrologist or radiologist, biochemical and bleeding risk profile review	Decreases risk for complications when these conditions are met, regardless of resource setting
Standard clinical data inclusive of occupational history and residence, biopsy processing protocol, and pathology review output should be gathered among all persons undergoing biopsy for any reason in CKDu-endemic region	Standard minimal dataset and pathology scoring approach will enable optimal use of available clinical data with a minimum of additional resources

CKD, chronic kidney disease; CKDu, chronic kidney disease of unknown etiology; ISN i3C, International Society of Nephrology International Consortium of Collaborators on Chronic Kidney Disease of Unknown Etiology.

in 18 low- and middle-income countries across 6 regions.[4] In comparison to a meta-analysis drawing the majority of its data from high-income countries, the biopsy complication rates were similar (Table 1).[5] Complication rates were lower with real-time ultrasound-guided biopsies, as compared to pre-marked and blind procedures (12.4% vs. 14.9% and 24.5%, respectively).

The ISN i3C Working Group discussants noted that typical patients with suspected CKDu are young, normotensive, and have normal or low body mass index: thus, they do not have the well documented risk factors for bleeding complications post-biopsy.[6] Furthermore, they also are less likely to be on antiplatelet or anticoagulant therapy or to have severe acute kidney injury needing hospitalization. Thus, the ISN i3C Working Group concluded that a kidney biopsy is likely to be as safe, if not safer, as it is for the traditional indications of kidney biopsy, as long as a trained nephrologist or a radiologist is performing the procedure with ultrasound guidance and using an automated biopsy gun.

Standardizing data collection during kidney biopsy

For cases in which the patient and treating nephrologist mutually agree to proceed with a kidney biopsy, the group discussed approaches to maximizing both the clinical and research benefit of a biopsy. Through consensus, we developed a case report form (Supplementary Appendix S1) to collect relevant clinical information before and after the procedure. We prioritized this form not only to be concise and practical for clinicians practicing in regions with a high prevalence of kidney disease, but also to enable research outputs when collated across multiple suspected CKDu hotspots.

Several benefits exist for such standardized data gathering, some of which will be directly and immediately relevant to patient care. For example, we could inform the pretest probability of kidney biopsy altering the diagnosis from primary tubulointerstitial kidney disease of unknown cause to a diagnosis attributable to specific cause or treatment. Also, the diagnostic certainty can conceivably affect prognosis; again, systematic clinical data matched to briefly collected outcome data could answer this question. Although available literature indicates that a higher degree of fibrosis will be associated with a worse prognosis, the precision with which we can make prognostic predictions will improve drastically with systematically available clinical data and standardized biopsy reporting. Finally, systematic approaches will elucidate the entire spectrum of pathology findings associated with the final clinical diagnosis of "CKDu," as both acute and severely chronic presentations with substantial secondary glomerulosclerosis have been described.

Standardizing biopsy reporting

The value of standardized biopsy reporting has been demonstrated in several disease entities: specifically, the Banff classification for reporting of kidney transplant biopsies and the MEST-C (for mesangial hypercellularity, endocapillary hypercellularity, segmental glomerulosclerosis, tubular atrophy/interstitial fibrosis, and the presence of crescents) score for IgA nephropathy scores are examples of standardized biopsy reporting that facilitated comparisons across sites and/or regions and have led to improved understanding of disease processes. Biopsy diagnosis and prognostication in presumed tubulointerstitial disease currently faces high interobserver and pathologist variability. Having a preconsensus overview with training sessions, and using standardized descriptors to document the pathologic findings in the kidney biopsy, has proven to be the best approach to improve concordance.[7] Thus, building on the pathology discussions at the National Institutes of Health (NIH)-sponsored Third International Workshop on Chronic Kidney Disease of Uncertain Etiology in 2019, templates introduced by Wijkstrom and colleagues,[8] and input of pathologists in the ISN Renal Pathology Working Group, we present a reporting form that facilitates the systematic description of each compartment in the biopsy (Supplementary Appendix S2). Electron microscopy

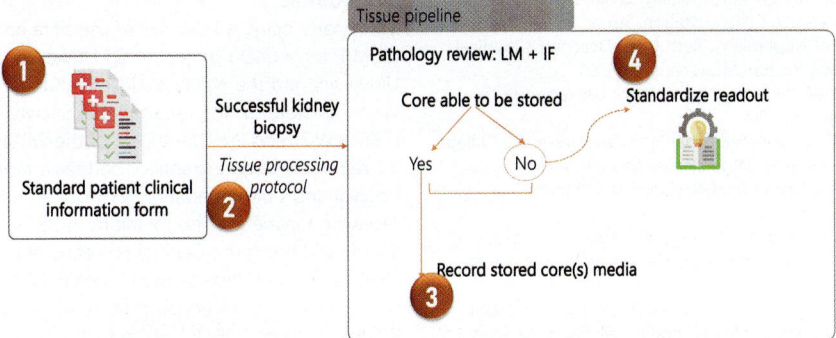

Figure 2 | Proposed work flow to maximize scientific output from kidney biopsies in chronic kidney disease of unknown etiology (CKDu) hotspots. We propose that the standard clinical data of patients undergoing kidney biopsies in CKDu-endemic regions be stored in a form amenable to aggregation across sites, and that the clinics note their standard biopsy-processing protocol, as well as cores obtained during the procedure. Pathologists working in these regions, or supporting these regions using telemedicine, should follow standard pathology reporting, again to enable rapid aggregation and discernment of patterns. IF, immunofluorescence; LM, light microscopy.

capability may not exist in a majority of settings, but technology enables later review of formalin-fixed paraffin-embedded (FFPE) tissue for electron microscopy, and increasingly, the application of additional molecular techniques. Careful record keeping of procedures and conditions of tissue storage would enable the creation of a core tissue bank with the potential to test multiple hypotheses.

Recommendations and the way forward

The clinical scenarios of persons with suspected CKDu represent outliers to conventional indications for kidney biopsy. No disease-specific treatment exists at the present time, and many believe that a reasonable probability exists of clinical and pathologic diagnostic concordance in CKDu hotspots. However, without systematic clinical data and pathology review of kidney biopsies, we cannot be certain of such an assumption. Until recently, biopsies in people with presumed diagnoses (such as diabetes and hypertension) had not been thought to be of clinical value. With the Kidney Precision Medicine Program, and the advent of increasingly sophisticated technologies for assessment of kidney tissue, nephrologists need to reexamine previous attitudes toward performing biopsies in CKD.

The ISN i3C Working Group thoroughly considered the various perspectives on the risks and benefits of performing kidney biopsy in people with suspected CKDu. The Working Group concluded that kidney biopsies for a clinical indication should be considered routinely in cases of suspected CKDu. Biopsies are justified given the need to both confirm a diagnosis and assess prognosis based on the acuity and severity of histologic features (Table 2). This justification was considered within the context of a low risk for complications in a "standard-of-care" setting of kidney biopsies performed by an ultrasound-guided nephrologist or a radiologist. The ISN i3C Working Group suggested that an informed patient-centered discussion be conducted so that patients are made aware of the current lack of disease-specific treatment, the potential patient-borne costs, and the individual risks for procedural complications.

Another major recommendation by the ISN i3C Working Group is for nephrology clinics in CKDu hotspots to standardize case report forms and pathology report forms. This standardization will enable collaborative approaches to advancing knowledge about the disease (Figure 2). At minimum, such an approach would facilitate large-scale intra- and cross-country comparisons on disease presentation, delineate a spectrum of pathology findings, and correlate specific findings in the tubulointerstitial compartment to outcomes.

Summary

CKDu remains an important problem in a number of regions around the world. This position statement prepared by the ISN i3C Working Group provides guidance to those working in endemic regions regarding clinical indications for kidney biopsies in individuals suspected of having CKDu.

APPENDIX
Members of the International Society of Nephrology's International Consortium of Collaborators on CKDu

Shuchi Anand, Division of Nephrology, Stanford University School of Medicine, Palo Alto, California, USA

Carmen Avila-Casado, Department of Laboratory Medicine & Pathology, University Health Network, University of Toronto, Toronto, Ontario, Canada

Sunita Bavanandan, Department of Nephrology, Hospital Kuala Lumpur, Kuala Lumpur, Malaysia

Divya Bajpai, Department of Nephrology, Seth G.S.M.C. and K.E.M. Hospital, Mumbai, India

Suman Behera, Division of Nephrology, McMaster University, Hamilton, Ontario, Canada; William Osler Health System, Brampton, Ontario, Canada

Jared M. Brown, Skaggs School of Pharmacy and Pharmaceutical Sciences, University of Colorado, Anschutz Medical Campus, Aurora, Colorado, USA

Ben Caplin, University College London Department of Renal Medicine, London, UK; Royal Free London NHS Foundation Trust, London, UK

Christoph Daniel, Department of Nephropathology, Friedrich-Alexander University Erlangen-Nürnberg (FAU), Erlangen, Germany

Marc de Broe, Department Physiopathology, University Antwerpen, Antwerpen, Belgium

Philipp Enghard, Department of Nephrology and Medical Intensive Care, Charité-Universitätsmedizin Berlin, Freie Universität Berlin and Humboldt-Universität Zu Berlin, Berlin, Germany; Deutsches Rheumaforschungszentrum, and Institute of the Leibniz Foundation, Berlin, Germany

Alejandro Ferreiro Fuentes, Centro de Nefrología, Universidad de la República, Montevideo, Uruguay

Andrew Z. Fire, Departments of Pathology and Genetics, Stanford University School of Medicine, Palo Alto, California, USA

Rebecca S.B. Fischer, Department of Epidemiology & Biostatistics, School of Public Health, Texas A&M University, College Station, Texas, USA

David Friedman, Division of Nephrology, Beth Israel Deaconess Medical Center, Harvard Medical School, Boston, Massachusetts, USA

Pablo Garcia, Department of Medicine (Nephrology), University of New Mexico, Albuquerque, New Mexico, USA

Marvin González-Quiroz, Department of Renal Medicine, University College London, London, UK; WUQU' KAWOQ, Maya Health Alliance, Tecpán, Guatemala; School of Medicine, Universidad Nacional de Chimborazo, Riobamba, Ecuador

Chula Herath, Sri Lanka Society of Nephrology, Colombo, Sri Lanka

Eva Honsova, Unilabs Pathology and Charles University, Prague, Czech Republic

Vivekanand Jha, George Institute for Global Health, UNSW, New Delhi, India; School of Public Health, Imperial College, London, UK; Prasanna School of Public Health, Manipal Academy of Medical Education, Manipal, India

Richard J. Johnson, University of Colorado, Anschutz Medical Campus, Aurora, Colorado, USA

Talerngsak Kanjanabuch, Division of Nephrology, Department of Medicine and Center of Excellence in Kidney Metabolic Disorders, Faculty of Medicine, Chulalongkorn University, Bangkok, Thailand; PD Excellent Center, King Chulalongkorn Memorial Hospital, Bangkok, Thailand

Neeraja Kambham, Department of Pathology, Stanford University School of Medicine, Palo Alto, California, USA

Varun Kumar Bandi, Dr. Pinnamaneni Siddharatha Institute of Medical Sciences & RF, Andhra Pradesh, India

Adeera Levin, Division of Nephrology, Department of Medicine, University of British Columbia, Vancouver, British Columbia, Canada

Magdalena Madero, Instituto Nacional de Cardiologia Ignacio Chávez, Mexico City, Mexico

Sreedhar Mandayam, Dialysis Services, University of Texas, MD Anderson Cancer Center, Houston, Texas, USA

Alexei Mikhailov, Atrium Wake Forest Baptist Medical Center, Medical Center Drive, Winston-Salem, North Carolina, USA

Nishantha Nanayakkara, National Hospital Kandy Sri Lanka, Kandy, Sri Lanka

Nadeesha Nishanthi, ESE Nephrology, TH Anuradahpura dialysis and transplant Center, North Central Province, Sri Lanka

Yannick M. Nlandu, Nephrology Unit, Kinshasa University Hospital, University of Kinshasa, Kinshasa, Democratic Republic of The Congo

Maria Pippias, Population Health Sciences, Bristol Medical School, University of Bristol, Bristol, UK; North Bristol NHS Trust, Renal Unit, Bristol, UK

Narayan Prasad, Sanjay Gandhi Postgraduate Institute of Medical Sciences, Lucknow, India

Muhammad Rafiqul Alam, Bangabandhu Sheikh Mujib Medical University, Dhaka, Bangladesh; ISN South Asia Regional Board, International Society of Nephrology, Brussels, Belgium; Bangladesh Renal Journal, Dhaka, Bangladesh

Vicente Sanchez Polo, Nephrology and Kidney Transplant Division, Social Security Guatemalan Institute, Concepción, Guatemala

Surya V. Seshan, Weill Cornell Medicine, New York, New York, USA

David Sheikh-Hamad, Selzman Institute for Kidney Health, Division of Nephrology, Department of Medicine, Baylor College of Medicine, Houston, Texas, USA

Geetika Singh, Renal Pathology and Electron Microscopy Laboratory, All India Institute of Medical Sciences, New Delhi, India

Anna Strasma, Division of Nephrology, Department of Medicine, Duke University School of Medicine, Durham, North Carolina, USA

Carmen Tzanno-Martins, Renalclass, São Paulo, Brazil

Ifeoma Ulasi, Renal Unit, Department of Medicine, College of Medicine, University of Nigeria, Nsukka , Enugu , Nigeria

Benjamin A. Vervaet, Institute of Pathology, RWTH Aachen University Hospital, Aachen, Germany; Laboratory of Pathophysiology, University Antwerp, Antwerp, Belgium

Sushrut S. Waikar, Section of Nephrology, Boston Medical Center and Boston University Chobanian & Avedisian School of Medicine, Boston, USA

Eranga Wijewickrama, Department of Clinical Medicine, Faculty of Medicine, University of Colombo, Colombo, Sri Lanka

Julia Wijkström, Division of Renal Medicine, Department of CLINTEC, Karolinska Institutet, Solna, Stockholm, Sweden

Chih-Wei Yang, Department of Nephrology, Chang Gung Memorial Hospital, Linkou, Taiwan; College of Medicine, Chang Gung University, Taoyuan, Taiwan

DISCLOSURE

EW reports being a member of the data and safety monitoring board (DSMB) for a CKDu project in Sri Lanka conducted by Stanford University and the National Hospital Kandy; Deputy Chair of the i3C Working Group of the International Society of Nephrology (ISN i3C [CKDu] WG), and President-Elect of the Sri Lanka Society of Nephrology. BC reports receiving grants or contracts from UK Medical Research Council and Colt Foundation (both paid to his institution). VSP reports receiving payment or honoraria from Bayer, AstraZeneca, Novartis, and Sanofi; and being the General Secretary of the Latin American Society of Nephrology and Hypertension (unpaid role). DF reports receiving grants or contracts from National Institute of Diabetes and Digestive and Kidney Diseases (NIDDK), National Institute on Minority Health and Health Disparities (NIMHD), the Department of Defense, royalties or licenses from Beth Israel Deaconess Medical Center, consulting fees from Vertex; payment or honoraria from Sanofi; having patents related to APOL1; and participating as a member for DSMB for the National Institutes of Health (NIH). MM reports receiving payment, grants, contracts, honoraria, and/or support for travelling and/or meetings from AztraZeneca and Boehringer; and having a leadership role at International Society of Peritoneal Dialysis (ISPD) Council, the Kidney Disease: Improving Global Outcomes (KDIGO) writing group for the CKD Guideline; being the KDIGO Chair Executive Committee and *Kidney International* editor. VJ reports receiving grants, contracts, payment and/or consulting fees from GlaxoSmith Klein, Baxter Healthcare, Biocon, Vera, Biocryst, GSK, Bayer, Astrazeneca, Boehringer, Ingelheim, NephroPlus, Zydus, and Cadilla (all paid directly to his institution); and participating as a member for DSMB for Zydus Cadilla. NK reports receiving all support for this article from 5R01DK12713803: NIH (Stanford University), grants or contracts from 5U01DK13006002: NIH (Stanford University), and payment from Elsevier for Amirsys series book on renal pathology. AL reports receiving support for attending meetings and/or travelling by International Society of Nephrology and NIH; participating as a member for DSMB for NIH Chronic kidney disease of UnceRtain Etiology in Agricultural Communities (CURE) Consortium; and having a leadership role on the ISN Research Committee and in the ISN Advocacy Working Group. SA reports that all support for this article comes from US NIH NIDDK R01DK127138, Doris Duke Charitable Fund, Stanford Center for Innovation in Global Health and King Center; serving as medical director for a Satellite Healthcare Dialysis unit; receiving consulting fees from Vera Therapeutics (Consultancy) and HealthPals; and participating as a member for a DSMB for NIA funded clinical trial on metabolic acidosis and CKD; serving as Chair of the ISN i3C Working Group and as a Board Member of the ISN US NIH NIAID U01, and as Executive Committee member for American Nephrologists of Indian Origin; and that Ascend Clinical and Abbott lab funds testing for US NIH NIAID funded U01. SB reports receiving payment or honoraria for educational purposes from Baxter, Astra Zeneca, and Boehringer Ingleheim; participating on the Astra Zeneca advisory board for hyperkalaemia management; being a Member of the Board of Directors (National Kidney Foundation of Malaysia), the Chair of ISN Oceania and South East Asia (OSEA) Regional Board, Executive Committee member of the Asian Pacific Society of Nephrology (APSN), and a KDIGO Executive Committee member. JB reports receiving grants or contracts from NIH (NIH R01 DK125351). PE reports receiving grants or contracts from the Federal Ministry of Education and Research (BMBF) and Deutsche Gesellschaft für Internationale Zusammenarbeit (GIZ). AFF reports being President (2019–2021) of the Latin American Society of Nephrology and Hypertension, with no payments made, and being Deputy Chair (2023–2025) of the ISN Latin America Regional Board. AZF reports receiving grants or contracts (R01DK127138 [to SA]), and participating on the Advisory group for NIH Program Project U01DK130060. RSBF reports receiving all support for the present article from the Texas A&M University School of Public Health, and receiving grants or contracts from NIH Fogarty International Center. RJJ reports receiving grants or contracts from NIH (NIH R01 DK125351), payment or honoraria from Horizon Pharma and Dinora LLC (paid to him), stocks from XORTX Therapeutics (to him); and having financial or nonfinancial interests in Colorado Research Partners (Equity). All the other authors declared no competing interests.

ACKNOWLEDGMENTS
This work was supported by in-kind administrative support from the International Society of Nephrology.

SUPPLEMENTARY MATERIAL
Supplementary File (Word)
Supplementary Appendix S1. Case report form.
Supplementary Appendix S2. Standardized biopsy report form.

REFERENCES
1. John O, Gummudi B, Jha A, et al. Chronic kidney disease of unknown etiology in India: What do we know and where we need to go. *Kidney Int Rep*. 2021;6:2743–2751.
2. Gifford FJ, Gifford RM, Eddleston M, Dhaun N. Endemic nephropathy around the world. *Kidney Int Rep*. 2017;2:282–292.
3. Johnson RJ, Wesseling C, Newman LS. Chronic kidney disease of unknown cause in agricultural communities. *N Engl J Med*. 2019;380:1843–1852.
4. Kajawo S, Ekrikpo U, Moloi MW, et al. A systematic review of complications associated with percutaneous native kidney biopsies in adults in low- and middle-income countries. *Kidney Int Rep*. 2021;6:78–90.
5. Poggio ED, McClelland RL, Blank KN, et al. Systematic review and meta-analysis of native kidney biopsy complications. *Clin J Am Soc Nephrol*. 2020;15:1595–1602.
6. Hogan JJ, Mocanu M, Berns JS. The native kidney biopsy: update and evidence for best practice. *Clin J Am Soc Nephrol*. 2016;11:354–362.
7. Barisoni L, Troost JP, Nast C, et al. Reproducibility of the NEPTUNE descriptor-based scoring system on whole-slide images and histologic and ultrastructural digital images. *Modern Pathol*. 2016;29:671–684.
8. Wijkstrom J, Annadata KC, Elinder CG, et al. Clinical findings and kidney morphology in chronic kidney disease of unknown cause in India. *J Intern Med*. 2023;294:492–505.

mini review

www.kidney-international.org

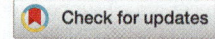

Pretransplant screening for coronary artery disease: data are required before practice change

John S. Gill[1] and Steven J. Chadban[2,3]

[1]Division of Nephrology, University of British Columbia, Vancouver, British Columbia, Canada; [2]Department of Renal Medicine, Royal Prince Alfred Hospital, Sydney, New South Wales, Australia; and [3]Kidney Node, Charles Perkins Centre, University of Sydney, New South Wales, Australia

Declining rates of peritransplant cardiovascular death, an increasing burden of pretransplant tests, and concerns about the effectiveness of screening candidates for coronary artery disease have led many transplant programs to de-escalate screening protocols. Recent Kidney Disease: Improving Global Outcomes and American Heart Association scientific statements and guidelines neatly summarize current evidence, but also identify areas of need. Here, we argue that key questions should be addressed by adequately powered clinical trials before our long-held screening paradigms are completely rewritten.

Kidney International (2024) **105,** 470–472; https://doi.org/10.1016/j.kint.2023.09.026

KEYWORDS: coronary artery disease; guidelines; kidney transplantation; screening; transplant candidate

Copyright © 2023, International Society of Nephrology. Published by Elsevier Inc. All rights reserved.

Correspondence: *Steven J. Chadban, Department of Renal Medicine, Royal Prince Alfred Hospital, Missenden Road, Camperdown, Sydney, New South Wales 2050, Australia.* E-mail: Steve.chadban@health.nsw.gov.au

Received 17 July 2023; revised 7 September 2023; accepted 25 September 2023; published online 31 October 2023

A deceased donor kidney transplant is uniquely an elective surgical procedure performed under emergent conditions. Surgery is further differentiated by the fact that a significant proportion of transplant candidates will have known or clinically occult coronary artery disease (CAD).[1] Accordingly, there are unique perioperative safety considerations that include the well-being of transplant recipients as well as the short- and long-term viability of scarcely available donated kidneys. Kidney transplant recipients experience a high rate of perioperative myocardial infarction, and cardiovascular disease is the leading cause of death within the first 3 months of kidney transplantation.[1] Therefore, identification of patients at risk for peritransplant CAD events remains an important clinical consideration in transplant medicine. Beyond seeking to minimize peritransplant CAD events, the rationale for screening wait-list candidates also includes maintaining the medical suitability of increasingly older candidates facing longer waiting times on dialysis.

For over a quarter century, transplant programs have implemented a strategy of screening candidates for clinically occult CAD before and during wait-listing followed by coronary angiography in patients with positive screening tests and either preemptive revascularization or exclusion from transplantation for those with critical disease. The balance between revascularization and exclusion has varied by program and over time and is influenced by external factors including risk appetite and funding implications. Challenges with this strategy include the limited sensitivity and specificity of noninvasive screening tests[2] and that perioperative myocardial infarctions may occur in a vessel territory with angiographically nonocclusive disease due to plaque instability and rupture rather than in a vessel territory detected by screening. The strategy of screening is also challenged by randomized trials in the general population that have consistently shown a lack of effectiveness of screening asymptomatic patients for CAD before noncardiac surgery. The recent ISCHEMIA-CKD (International Study of Comparative Health Effectiveness with Medical and Invasive Approaches–Chronic Kidney Disease) trial, which showed no benefit to coronary artery revascularization in patients with chronic kidney disease with a positive stress test and clinically stable CAD, did not specifically examine the role of screening before transplantation.[3] However, the absence of a benefit to revascularization in the trial indirectly challenges the rationale of the current transplant screening paradigm. Recent observations in transplant recipients showing no association between the use of pretransplant screening tests and death and myocardial infarction within 30 days of transplantation suggest that screening may be unnecessary, but do not consider the possibility that screening tests may have excluded high-risk patients from transplantation.[4] The lack of controlled data on the efficacy of screening transplant candidates, coupled with the challenges and costs associated with regular screening, have led to increased clinical practice variation.[5] Some centers have embraced clinical algorithms to facilitate a reduction in the use of screening tests before and during candidate wait-listing. Others simply withhold full candidate workup and wait-listing until the predicted waiting time for an individual is ∼12 months. Although these approaches may minimize the work and cost of wait-list management, their impact on health maintenance of candidates facing longer wait times for transplantation is uncertain.

Although well-intentioned, the transplant screening paradigm may cause harm. Tests are inconvenient, intrusive, and potentially expensive for patients and health care institutions. A positive screening test may lead to delays in wait-listing, temporary deactivation of already wait-listed candidates, or even exclusion of asymptomatic patients from transplantation. Coronary revascularization procedures and the use of anticoagulants including dual antiplatelet therapy that are required after revascularization are associated with an increased risk of adverse events, particularly in dialysis-treated patients, and many transplant programs will delay transplantation until these medications are withdrawn. Loss of residual kidney function with exposure to radiocontrast agents and during revascularization procedures is a further consideration.

The relative paucity of controlled evidence to inform the efficacy and safety of pretransplant screening identifies this as an area of unmet need in contemporary transplantation. Accumulating indirect evidence challenging the screening paradigm further highlights our need for robust data. Such clinical uncertainty is reflected in recent authoritative international guidelines.

The 2020 Kidney Disease: Improving Global Clinical Practice Guideline on the Evaluation and Management of Candidates for Kidney Transplantation softened recommendations made in previous guidelines regarding protocolized screening.[6] Clinical assessment by history, examination, and electrocardiography was advocated for all candidates, reserving noninvasive screening for asymptomatic patients who are either deemed to be at high risk for CAD (including those with diabetes, those with known vascular disease, smokers, "older candidates," and those with prolonged dialysis exposure) or who have poor exercise tolerance. This was a suggestion only (grade 2C), given the lack of evidence that coronary revascularization subsequent to a positive screening test reduces perioperative events in asymptomatic patients submitted to major surgery (grade 1B). The guidelines also suggest that candidates with a positive screening test and subsequent coronary angiography that demonstrates advanced triple vessel disease be excluded from transplantation unless they have an estimated post-transplant survival that is acceptable by national standards. Inclusion of a cardiologist experienced in transplant candidate management is recommended for evaluations and decisions. In the absence of evidence, no recommendations were made regarding periodic screening of wait-listed candidates.

In 2022, the American Heart Association updated their scientific statement and guidelines for screening kidney and liver transplant candidates.[7] The statement noted a wide variation in wait-list CAD screening practices in the United States[4] as well as the failure to demonstrate a reduction in the incidence of myocardial infarction or death for people with advanced chronic kidney disease and a positive cardiac stress, as compared to guideline-directed medical therapy in the ISCHEMIA-CKD trial.[3] As noted, the ISCHEMIA-CKD trial was not primarily designed to assess whether prophylactic revascularization reduces peritransplant cardiac events: a subgroup of ISCHEMIA-CKD participants who were wait-listed for transplantation (194 of 777) were studied *post hoc* including 51 patients who underwent transplantation.[8] This analysis found no difference between invasive and noninvasive strategies in the primary or secondary outcomes, consistent with the full study. However, the crossover rate from noninvasive to invasive of 33% was 7-fold greater than for the overall study, generating further uncertainty.

A similar approach to Kidney Disease: Improving Global Outcomes was advocated by the American Heart Association for candidates without known CAD, consisting of a clinical assessment to identify symptomatic patients, with asymptomatic patients subsequently referred for electrocardiography and transthoracic echocardiography and then noninvasive screening, preferably by stress echocardiography, only if there is echocardiographic (left ventricular ejection fraction <40%, regional wall motion abnormalities) or electrocardiographic (previous infarct) evidence of CAD or if deemed to be at high risk on clinical grounds. The American Heart Association differed from Kidney Disease: Improving Global Outcomes in recommending invasive coronary angiography for those with known CAD but no angiography for over 2 years and for those deemed to be at high risk with or without prior noninvasive screening. Justification for angiography included potentially increased utility to provide definitive anatomic and functional assessment in order to guide prognosis, to stratify access to transplantation or not, and to expedite access to revascularization for those who "may" benefit. Some aspects of utility here are questionable. Because angiography is typically preceded by echocardiography to avoid left ventriculography and contrast load, additional functional information may not be provided. Moreover, expedited access to revascularization may not be of benefit given the findings of the ISCHEMIA-CKD trial. Also noted were the increased risks of periprocedural events and the usual requirement for dual-antiplatelet therapy post-revascularization with consequent delays in transplantation. The issue of regular screening of wait-listed patients was discussed, and given existing uncertainties, no recommendation was made.

Overall, Kidney Disease: Improving Global Outcomes and American Heart Association guidelines synthesize the current evidence and, subject to adaptation to local context, outline rational pathways for pretransplant screening for CAD. Both highlight the importance of guideline-directed medical therapy for all patients. Both also highlight key areas of uncertainty that require assessment by well-designed, adequately powered clinical trials.

The guidelines focus attention on the main research questions related to the use of noninvasive CAD screening tests in transplant candidates: (i) Before wait-listing and (ii) after wait-listing, is periodic screening for CAD safe and effective? and (iii) Does revascularization of candidates with screen-detected CAD improve outcomes during wait-listing, peritransplant, and in the longer term. Question (i) has never been directly addressed. Question (ii) has been subjected to a cost-utility modeling study that found regular surveillance to be more expensive and detrimental to overall patient survival.[9] Seeking to definitively answer this question, the Canadian Australasian Randomized Trial of Screening Kidney Transplant Candidates for Coronary Artery Disease (ClinicalTrials.gov identifier NCT03674307) has randomized 2050 of the target 3300 participants to determine costs, benefits, and harms of regular screening versus no screening for wait-listed candidates using a noninferiority design. The results of the Canadian Australasian Randomized Trial of Screening Kidney Transplant Candidates for Coronary Artery Disease have been called for in both guidelines. Should no screening be found noninferior, this would likely lead to de-escalation of wait-list screening but would also bring greater focus on the utility of pretransplant screening. Question (iii) has in part been addressed by the ISCHEMIA-CKD trial; however, questions remain, including whether outcomes of revascularization for transplant candidates may differ from others with advanced chronic kidney disease and whether revascularization outcomes differ according to severity and specific anatomical location of CAD, particularly the patient with triple vessel disease and poor left ventricular function.

We have highlighted key uncertainties and evidence gaps in considering the role of pretransplant screening for CAD. In doing so, it is important to reflect on gains made despite our knowledge gaps. Cardiovascular death remains the most common cause of death within 3 months of kidney transplantation, and when this occurs, it costs the candidate their life, the community a donated kidney, and family, carer, and transplant team grief and stress. Temporal changes over the past 50 years of transplantation have seen substantial reductions in the incidence of early post-transplant cardiovascular death: declining from a rate of over 7 deaths per 100 patient-years in 1980 to 1.18 per 100 patient-years between 2015 and 2018 in Australia and New Zealand.[1] The reasons for such improvement, despite progressive increases in recipient age and cardiovascular risk factor burden, are not known. That screening programs have contributed to such improvement is plausible. It would therefore seem wise to provide evidence before we de-escalate current practice.

DISCLOSURE
JSG (Canadian Institute for Health Research [CIHR]) and SJC (National Health and Medical Research Council of Australia [NHMRC]) are recipients of research grant funding as chief investigators of the Canadian Australasian Randomized Trial of Screening Kidney Transplant Candidates for Coronary Artery Disease from the Canadian and Australian Commonwealth governments, respectively.

REFERENCES
1. Ying T, Shi B, Kelly PJ, et al. Death after kidney transplantation: an analysis by era and time post-transplant. *J Am Soc Nephrol*. 2020;31:2887–2899.
2. Wang LW, Masson P, Turner RM, et al. Prognostic value of cardiac tests in potential kidney transplant recipients: a systematic review. *Transplantation*. 2015;99:731–745.
3. Bangalore S, Maron DJ, O'Brien SM, et al., ISCHEMIA-CKD Research Group. Management of coronary disease in patients with advanced kidney disease. *N Engl J Med*. 2020;382:1608–1618.
4. Cheng XS, Liu S, Han J, et al. Association of pretransplant coronary heart disease testing with early kidney transplant outcomes. *JAMA Intern Med*. 2023;183:134–141.
5. Cheng XS, Mathew RO, Parasuraman R, et al. Coronary artery disease screening of asymptomatic kidney transplant candidates: a web-based survey of practice patterns in the United States. *Kidney Med*. 2020;2:505–507.
6. Chadban SJ, Ahn C, Axelrod DA, et al. KDIGO Clinical Practice Guideline on the evaluation and management of candidates for kidney transplantation. *Transplantation*. 2020;104(suppl 1):S11–S103.
7. Cheng XS, VanWagner LB, Costa SP, et al. Emerging evidence on coronary heart disease screening in kidney and liver transplantation candidates: a scientific statement from the American Heart Association. *Circulation*. 2022;146:e299–e324.
8. Herzog CA, Simgen MA, Xu Y, et al. Kidney transplant list status and outcomes in the ISCHEMIA-CKD trial. *J Am Col Cardiol*. 2021;78:348–361.
9. Ying T, Tran A, Webster AC, et al. Screening for asymptomatic coronary artery disease in waitlisted kidney transplant candidates: a cost-utility analysis. *Am J Kidney Dis*. 2020;75:693–704.

review

Complement activation and effector pathways in membranous nephropathy

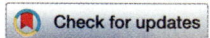

Andreas D. Kistler[1,2] and David J. Salant[3]

[1]Department of Medicine, Cantonal Hospital Frauenfeld, Spital Thurgau AG, Frauenfeld, Switzerland; [2]Faculty of Medicine, University of Zurich, Zurich, Switzerland; and [3]Section of Nephrology, Department of Medicine, Boston Medical Center and Boston University Chobanian and Avedisian School of Medicine, Boston, Massachusetts, USA

Complement activation has long been recognized as a central feature of membranous nephropathy (MN). Evidence for its role has been derived from the detection of complement products in biopsy tissue and urine from patients with MN and from mechanistic studies primarily based on the passive Heymann nephritis model. Only recently, more detailed insights into the exact mechanisms of complement activation and effector pathways have been gained from patient data, animal models, and *in vitro* models based on specific target antigens relevant to the human disease. These data are of clinical relevance, as they parallel the recent development of numerous specific complement therapeutics for clinical use. Despite efficient B-cell depletion, many patients with MN achieve only partial remission of proteinuria, which may be explained by the persistence of subepithelial immune complexes and ongoing complement-mediated podocyte injury. Targeting complement, therefore, represents an attractive adjunct treatment for MN, but it will need to be tailored to the specific complement pathways relevant to MN. This review summarizes the different lines of evidence for a central role of complement in MN and for the relevance of distinct complement activation and effector pathways, with a focus on recent developments.

Kidney International (2024) **105**, 473–483; https://doi.org/10.1016/j.kint.2023.10.035

KEYWORDS: complement; glomerulonephritis; glomerulus; membranous nephropathy; proteinuria

Copyright © 2023, International Society of Nephrology. Published by Elsevier Inc. All rights reserved.

Correspondence: *Andreas D. Kistler, Department of Medicine, Cantonal Hospital Frauenfeld, Pfaffenholzstrasse 4, 8501 Frauenfeld, Switzerland. E-mail: andreas.kistler@stgag.ch*

Received 1 August 2023; revised 25 September 2023; accepted 5 October 2023; published online 21 December 2023

Membranous nephropathy (MN), one of the most common causes of nephrotic syndrome in adults, is characterized by extensive alterations in podocyte structure and function, glomerular basement membrane (GBM) expansion, and the presence of subepithelial (subpodocyte) immune deposits. Traditionally subclassified into primary and secondary causes based on the association with systemic immunological and infectious diseases in the latter, recent advances in human MN and the identification of several target autoantigens have blurred this distinction. A common finding in almost all forms of MN is the presence of complement C3 in the immune deposits. Although studies in experimental animal models have clearly established that complement plays an important role in inducing the characteristic alterations in podocyte morphology and GBM expansion that characterize MN and underlie the development of proteinuria, the mechanisms of complement activation by human MN autoantibodies and the downstream mediators of podocyte injury have only recently begun to come to light from clinical and experimental observations. Given the proliferation of complement therapeutics that have been developed in recent years, identifying such mechanisms and mediators is much more than an academic exercise. Here, we will review evidence implicating a pathogenic role for complement in MN and the critical points at which intervention may be beneficial.

Brief primer on the complement system

The complement cascade can be activated via 3 distinct pathways, the classical, lectin, and alternative pathways, each converging on the same effector pathways[1] (Figure 1). The classical pathway is activated upon binding of C1q to the Fc region of IgG or IgM or to 1 of several surface-bound molecules, such as C-reactive protein or pentraxins. Multiple IgG molecules are required for efficient binding and activation of C1, such that the density and distribution of the epitope and IgG density in immune complexes are crucial determinants of complement activation.[2] Importantly, complement binding capacity depends on IgG subclass. Specifically, IgG4 has been shown not to activate complement via the classical pathway and may even act as competitive inhibitor of C1q binding to IgG1.[3] Similar to the classical pathway, the lectin pathway is activated by binding of a pattern-recognition molecule (mannose-binding lectin [MBL], collectin, or ficolin) to carbohydrate moieties. Upon binding of a pattern-recognition

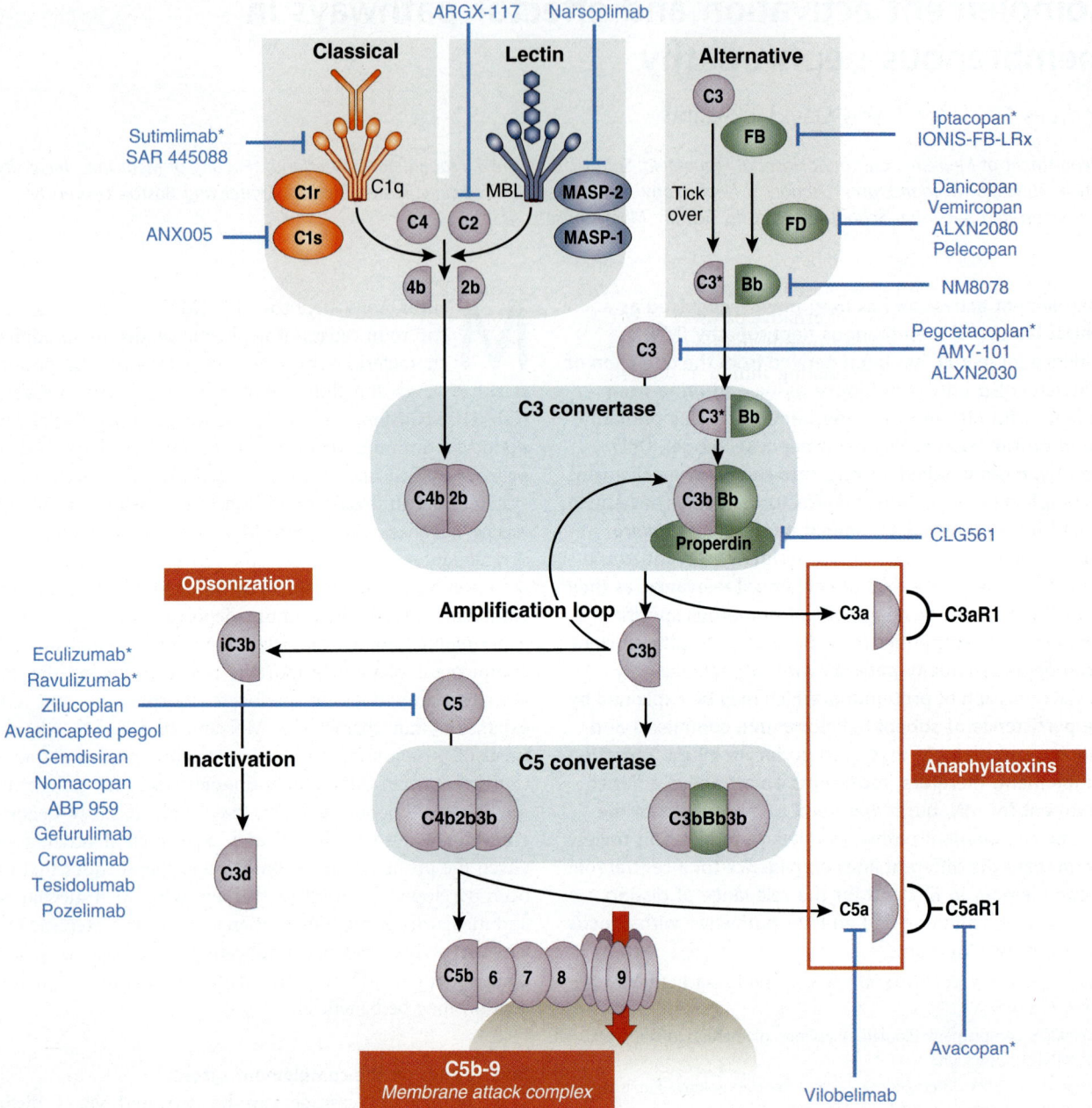

Figure 1 | Schematic drawing of the complement cascade and complement inhibitors currently in development or approved for clinical use with their sites of action. Factors specific to the classical pathway are depicted in orange, those specific to the lectin pathway are depicted in blue, and those specific to the alternative pathway are depicted in green. Factors common to multiple activation pathways are shown in purple. Complement effector mechanisms are highlighted in red. Specific complement inhibitors currently in clinical trials or approved (the latter marked by an asterisk) for indications other than membranous nephropathy are shown in cyan. FB, factor B; FD, factor D; MASP, mannose-binding lectin–associated serine protease; MBL, mannose-binding lectin.

molecule to its respective binding partner, serine proteases (C1r and C1s in the classical pathway and the MBL-associated serine proteases [MASPs] 1 and 2 in the lectin pathway) attached to the pattern-recognition molecule in a calcium-dependent manner become activated and cleave C2 and C4. This results in the formation of the multimeric protein complex C4b2b, the C3 convertase of the classical and lectin pathway. The alternative pathway, in contrast, does not involve pattern-recognition molecules and is constantly active at low levels through spontaneous hydrolysis of a thioester bond within C3, a process known as "tick over." After hydrolysis, $C3(H_2O)$ undergoes a conformational change and binds factor B (FB), which is then cleaved by factor D (FD), resulting in a C3-FB complex with enzymatic activity to cleave native C3 into C3a and C3b. The resulting C3b again associates with cleaved FB to form C3bBb, the alternative pathway complement convertase, leading to a positive feedback mechanism. Thus, the alternative pathway results in the generation of a protein complex with the same enzymatic activity (C3 convertase) but of a different molecular composition and structure than that of the classical and lectin pathways. Under physiological conditions, small amounts of C3b are constantly generated. Autohydrolysis of C3 and assembly of C3bBb can be enhanced by certain proteins, lipids, and carbohydrate surfaces present on pathogens and damaged host cells. On the other hand, alternative pathway activation is tightly controlled by protective membrane-bound factors on normal host cells and by circulating inhibitory factors. The alternative pathway serves not only as a third, independent pathway for complement activation, but also as an amplification loop to enhance complement activation initially triggered by the classical and lectin pathways.[4,5]

Once C3 convertase has assembled and C3 cleavage proceeds, all 3 pathways converge on a common downstream cascade with 3 distinct effector mechanisms: (i) opsonization of pathogens by complement fragments (primarily iC3b, a fragment of C3b); (ii) anaphylatoxin signaling via binding of C3a and C5a to their respective G-protein–coupled cell surface receptors C3aR1 and C5aR1; and (iii) assembly of the pore-forming terminal complement complex C5b-9, also termed membrane attack complex (MAC).

Evidence for a central role of complement in MN

Human MN biopsy samples. Numerous studies have shown the presence of C3 and C5b-9 in glomeruli of patients with MN by immune fluorescence (IF),[6–9] immune histochemistry,[9–13] and, more recently, mass spectrometry of laser-captured microdissected glomeruli.[12,14,15] This feature is shared by nearly all forms of human MN, irrespective of the target autoantigen, with the notable exception of protocadherin 7–associated MN.[16] Upon activation, C3 and C4 bind covalently to biological surfaces[17] and are immobilized at the site of activation, which facilitates detection by IF or immune histochemistry. C3d, a degradation product of C3b, may persist even longer in tissue[10,18] and is recognized by specific antibodies. Likewise, C5b-9 remains mostly at the site of its assembly, because it builds a pore within the cell membrane,[19] and detection by IF or immune histochemistry relies on neoepitopes formed during MAC assembly. Therefore, detection of C3 and C5b-9 in tissue mirrors local complement activation. Some studies have found the intensity of glomerular C3 staining to correlate with proteinuria and hypoalbuminemia,[8,10] and some have found glomerular C5b-9 staining to predict remission probability and renal survival in MN.[13]

Complement products in human urine and blood. Complement activation products are also detectable in urine of patients with MN.[12,20–31] In some studies, high urinary C3 and C5b-9 levels at baseline[22] or their persistence over time[23,27–29] predicted negative outcomes. However, although this was specific to MN in 1 study,[20] urinary excretion of complement products was found in other glomerular and tubulointerstitial diseases in other studies[21,24,28,30–32] and may reflect tubular complement activation.[26,32]

Serum levels of C3 and C4, which are routinely measured in clinical practice, are typically not reduced in MN, probably because of the chronic, slowly progressive nature of the disease and the local as opposed to systemic complement activation. Nevertheless, recent studies have detected C3a[30,33] and C5a[30,34] in the blood of patients with MN, and serum C3 levels in the lower range have been linked to worse outcomes in patients with MN.[35,36]

Together, these data from human samples provide compelling evidence that complement is activated in the glomeruli in virtually all forms of MN and that its degree of activation reflects disease activity. However, they do not formally prove that complement activation is causative of GBM alterations, podocyte damage, and proteinuria and, if so, whether it represents the sole mechanism of antibody-induced glomerular damage in MN.

Animal models of MN. Evidence that complement is responsible for the structural and functional changes that characterize MN is derived primarily from the Heymann nephritis model in rats.[37,38] Proteinuria in this model is the result of complement activation by the aggregated complement-fixing antibodies that bind to the target antigen, megalin, on the soles of the podocyte foot processes. Depletion of complement at the level of C3 with cobra venom factor completely prevents the development of proteinuria during the heterologous phase of passive Heymann nephritis (PHN) induced with sheep (or other) antisera containing anti-megalin antibodies.[39] In active Heymann nephritis, additional neutralizing antibodies are produced during immunization that are able to neutralize local complement regulatory factors and expose the podocytes to the full effects of uncontrolled complement activation.[40]

Animal studies on the role of complement in MN have been limited by the fact that M-type phospholipase A2 receptor (PLA2R1) is not expressed by rodent podocytes, and megalin, the target antigen in PHN, is not expressed on human podocytes. To overcome these limitations, studies have been done in minipigs that do express PLA2R1 on podocytes, and in mice that endogenously express thrombospondin type-1 domain-containing 7A (THSD7A) on podocytes, which are reactive with human MN-derived anti-PLA2R1 and anti-THSD7A, respectively.[41,42] These studies have convincingly shown that the transferred antisera form subepithelial immune deposits with the target antigens and cause podocyte injury and proteinuria, but both models have significant limitations with regard to the potential role of complement. Although mass spectrometry analysis of glomeruli obtained from 1 of the minipigs injected with human anti-PLA2R1 revealed classical, alternative, and terminal complement components, this might have been the result of the host (autologous) response to the injected human IgG.[41] In addition, the large size of the minipigs makes it difficult to

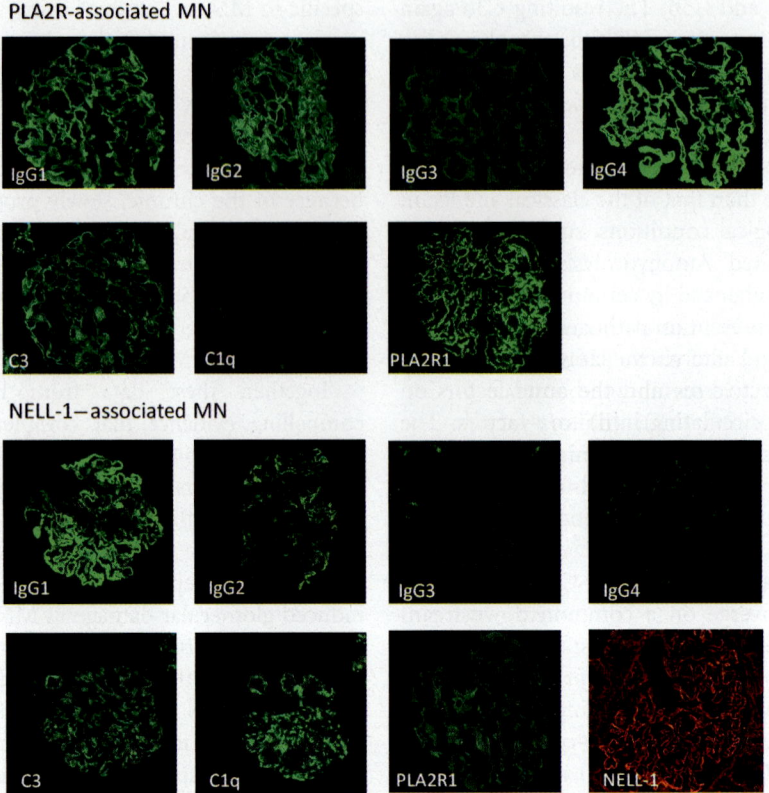

Figure 2 | Representative examples of an IgG4-predominant M-type phospholipase A2 receptor (PLA2R1)–positive membranous nephropathy (MN) (top 7 panels) and an IgG1-predominant neural epidermal growth factor-like 1 protein (NELL-1)–positive MN (bottom 8 panels). The PLA2R1-positive case was not associated with a systemic disease, whereas the NELL-1–positive case was associated with small-cell lung cancer. Note the positivity for C3 in both cases, but absent C1q staining in the PLA2R1-associated, IgG4-predominant case, whereas C1q stained strongly in the PLA2R1-negative, NELL-positive, IgG1-predominant case.

deliver adequate amounts of patient-derived serum to perform studies to establish if complement is necessary for injury. Likewise, the deposition of complement in the mice injected with human anti-THSD7A was found well after the onset of the autologous response.[42] The advent of transgenic mice that express human PLA2R1 on podocytes holds promise to test if murine antibodies to human PLA2R1 cause podocyte injury by activating complement.[43,44] A podocyte-specific human PLA2R1 transgenic mouse model was reported recently in which the mice spontaneously develop murine anti-human PLA2R1 antibodies, MN, and proteinuria at the age of 4 to 6 weeks, progressing to severe nephrotic syndrome, together with deposition of C1q, C4d, C3, factors B and H, and C5b-9.[44] Wild-type mice actively immunized with mouse THSD7A fragments developed a similar disease, and proteinuria was reduced, but not absent, in $C3^{-/-}$ mice.[45] Interestingly, in both models, the dominant murine antibody isoform was mIgG1, which is equivalent to human IgG4 and does not activate the classical complement pathway. However, there was also substantial mIgG2a and mIgG2b, which do activate the classical pathway and probably explain the presence of C1q in the glomerular deposits. Human PLA2R1-expressing recombination activating gene 2 $(Rag2)^{-/-}$ mice, used as negative controls because they are unable to produce antibodies, may prove useful for transfer experiments of human anti–PLA2R1-positive sera without interference from an autologous phase. Although some limitations of these rodent models remain, they do offer the potential to explore the role of complement through cross-breeding with factor-deficient mice and therapeutic studies with complement inhibitors.

Complement activation pathways in MN

Notwithstanding the strong evidence for complement activation in almost all forms of MN, the activation pathway(s) involved are less clear and may vary between different forms of MN. Distinct histologic patterns of MN were recognized decades ago. Isolated or dominant IgG4 positivity by IF and deposits confined to the subepithelial space by electron microscopy have been considered characteristic of primary MN. In contrast, IgG1- and/or IgG3-dominant IF (Figure 2) and electron-dense deposits in the mesangium and subendothelial space have been thought to be indicative of secondary MN. However, the lines distinguishing MN into primary and secondary forms have become blurred by the identification of several novel target antigens in MN that may or may not be associated with a systemic disease. Thus, MN might be better classified by both the target antigen (if identified) and the associated systemic disease (if present/identified).[46] IF and electron microscopy patterns may associate with the target antigen rather than with the "primary" or "secondary" nature of the disease. The IgG4-restricted or IgG4-dominant pattern is characteristic of autoantibodies against PLA2R1,[47] THSD7A,[48] high-temperature requirement A serine peptidase 1 (HTRA1),[49] and contactin-1.[50] Because IgG4 is considered not to bind C1q,[3] this raises the question how complement is activated in these forms of MN. The following explanations have been proposed: (i) although IgG4 is the predominant isoform, it is not the mechanistically relevant one (i.e., complement is activated via the classical pathway by autoantibodies of other subclasses and the absence of C1q staining is a methodological quirk); (ii) contrary to the common belief, IgG4 is able to activate complement via the classical pathway in MN; (iii) IgG4 is able to activate complement via the lectin and/or the alternative pathway. Although we find no evidence of the second explanation, the other 2 possibilities are discussed below.

IgG subclasses of autoantibodies in the circulation and tissue. The first hypothesis (i) would require that relevant amounts of non-IgG4 autoantibodies are present. In the original reports of both, anti–PLA2R1-associated and anti–THSD7A-associated MN, only faint bands were visible on Western blots of the target antigen probed with patient serum and secondary antibodies against IgG1-3, whereas secondary antibody against IgG4 showed strong reactivity.[47,48] Subsequent studies tested serum from large MN cohorts using Western blotting,[51] subclass-specific enzyme-linked immunosorbent assay,[52–55] and indirect IF[53,56] and confirmed a clear predominance of the IgG4 subclass among anti-PLA2R1 and anti-THSD7A antibodies, although other subclasses were also detectable at lower levels in a significant proportion of patients. Interestingly, in 1 study, anti-PLA2R1 IgG4 levels correlated better with baseline proteinuria than anti-PLA2R1 total IgG.[53] In addition, anti-PLA2R1 IgG4, but not IgG1 and IgG3 levels, correlated with outcomes.[53] This latter observation would argue for a direct pathogenic role of IgG4 and against explanation (i) above. The amount of IgG subclasses deposited in the subepithelial space may be influenced by factors other than their plasma concentration (namely, by their avidity to the target antigen and accessibility of the antigen). Several studies have analyzed the IgG isoform distribution of deposited antibodies in biopsy samples. By IF, a predominance of IgG4 or even isolated IgG4 staining was recognized as a characteristic of primary MN decades ago[10,57–60] and recently reproduced for PLA2R1-MN and THSD7A-MN.[6,7,61] The same has been shown by immune histochemistry[45] and mass spectrometry,[14] where IgG4 was also the predominant isoform in glomeruli of PLA2R1-associated MN, although these latter studies also detected considerable amounts of IgG1 and IgG3.

Complement products in glomeruli of patients with MN. Given that the classical, lectin, and alternative pathways include different proteins, detection of their respective cleavage products can point to the pathway(s) involved in complement activation. Detection of C1q, C1r, and C1s in tissue strongly indicates activation of the classical pathway; detection of C2 and C4 or their cleavage products indicates activation of either the classical or the lectin pathway; detection of MBL, other lectins, and MASP-1/2 reflects activation of the lectin pathway; and detection of FB and FD indicates activation of the alternative pathway. Several studies have reported staining for complement proteins in MN kidney biopsies. A typical finding in IgG4-dominant "primary" MN was little or absent C1q staining, arguing against activation of the classical pathway, whereas C4d was strongly positive, a constellation that would be consistent with lectin pathway activation (hypothesis [iii] above).[7,12,13,62–64] Supporting this explanation, several studies identified components of the lectin pathway (MBLs, ficolins, and MASPs) in MN patient biopsies,[7,12,35] and their abundance correlated with disease severity and outcomes in 2 studies.[7,35] In some contrast to these results, a recent study detected C1q in 5 of 5 and MBL in only 2 of 5 patients with PLA2R1-positive MN.[45] C1q was detected by these authors in paraffin-embedded tissue sections after antigen retrieval but not in frozen biopsy sections. This suggests that C1q may be masked and accessible to detection only after specific tissue treatment. However, other studies that also used paraffin-embedded tissue and antigen retrieval detected C1q in only a minority of patients at low levels.[12,13] Furthermore, the above-cited studies that failed to detect C1q in frozen tissue from patients with "primary" MN readily detected it in "secondary" forms using the same technique.[62,63]

By mass spectrometry, which should not experience "antigen masking," high spectral counts were found for C3 and C4.[14] However, the same study detected neither C1q, C1r, or C1s nor proteins of the lectin pathway in relevant amounts, and spectral counts of FB and FD were low, meaning that, paradoxically, abundant amounts of central complement pathway products pointed to strong complement activation but none of the activation pathways could be identified.

The previously cited study[45] further used proximity ligation assays to detect complement components in proximity to each other. They found signals for C3b close to FBb (indicative of the alternative pathway convertase) in 26 of 39 patients (67%) with PLA2R1- or THSD7A-positive MN; C4b close to C2b (indicative of the classical or lectin pathway C3 convertase) in all patients; signals of IgG close to C1q (indicative of classical pathway activation) in 87% of patients; and IgG close to MBL (indicative of lectin pathway activation, but note that other lectins than MBL were not assayed) in 60% of patients. Notably, in several studies, detection of IgG1 (and IgG3) correlated with C1q staining and detection of IgG4 with staining for lectin pathway components.[7,35,45,59] This is in line with preferential activation of the classical pathway by IgG1 (and IgG3) and activation of the lectin pathway by IgG4.

In vitro models to decipher complement pathways in MN. Whereas detection of complement products in human tissue experiences some technical limitations and represents only a snapshot in time, *in vitro* models allow for the modulation of specific complement components to study their roles. Recently, models using human anti–PLA2R1-positive MN sera and either HEK cells[54] or cultured human podocytes[65] expressing PLA2R1 have been developed. In an *in vitro* model based on cultured human podocytes expressing PLA2R1, addition of anti–PLA2R1-positive patient sera together with cryopreserved normal human serum as a source of complement led to complement fixation on cells and degradation of the essential podocyte structural proteins synaptopodin and Neph1.[65] This effect was lost after specific depletion of IgG4 from patient serum, whereas purified patient IgG4 was sufficient for complement fixation and to induce cleavage of synaptopodin and Neph1, strongly arguing for a pathogenic role of IgG4 antibodies (and against hypothesis [i] above). Synaptopodin and Neph1 degradation was prevented by adding ethylenediamine tetraacetic acid to the assay, which inhibits the classical and lectin pathways, and by specific MASP-1 and MASP-2 inhibitors that block the lectin pathway, pointing to a central role of the lectin pathway. Another group found a stronger cytotoxic effect of sera from patients with IgG1, IgG3, and IgG4 antibodies compared with patient sera with only IgG4 against PLA2R1.[54] However, these latter experiments were performed in HEK cells, not in podocytes, and specific IgG4 depletion of sera was not performed.

Additional evidence of lectin- and alternative-pathway activation by MN patient sera was obtained in a cell-free enzyme-linked immunosorbent assay in which immobilized THSD7A was exposed to anti–THSD7A-positive MN patient sera and normal human serum as a source of complement.[55] High-titer anti-THSD7A sera bound C3b/iC3b, C4, FB, and properdin but not C1q, which argues in favor of lectin and alternative, but not classical, pathway activation. The alternative pathway was essential for C3b/iC3b deposition as its deposition was almost completely abolished in FB-deficient serum, partially reduced in C4-deficient serum, and largely unaffected in C1q-deficient serum. These *in vitro* results suggest that MN autoantibodies activate complement through the lectin pathway but require amplification by the alternative pathway for full expression.[55]

Recently, a 3-dimensional co-culture system for human podocytes and glomerular endothelial cells ("glomerulus on a chip") has been reported.[66] Exposure of these cells to PLA2R1 antibody-positive MN sera led to albumin leakage through the artificial glomerular filtration barrier and C3d deposition. This model provides an opportunity to decipher the mechanisms of complement activation and podocyte injury in more detail.

Altered glycosylation of IgG4 in patients with MN and lectin pathway activation. MBL has been shown to directly bind affinity-purified anti–PLA2R1-IgG4 *in vitro*, and this binding was reduced after deglycosylation of IgG4, suggesting activation of the lectin pathway via glycosyl side chains of IgG4.[65] Human IgG is mainly glycosylated by N-linked glycans attached to asparagine 297 in the second domain of the constant region of each heavy chain (CH2 domain) close to the hinge region.[67] The glycans attached to Asn 297 consist of a default core structure to which additional sugar residues can be attached, resulting in a variety of glycan side chains. Glycosylation modulates IgG effector functions, and altered IgG glycosylation patterns have been associated with both normal aging and several autoimmune diseases.[67] Two independent studies have found reduced IgG4 galactosylation in MN.[65,68] Although a recent study reported no lectin pathway activation by glycoengineered recombinant IgG4 in an enzyme-linked immunosorbent assay, irrespective of the degree of galactosylation,[69] the hypothesis that alterations of IgG4 glycosylation affect complement activation could explain 2 observations. First, IgG galactosylation decreases with age in the normal population, and this mechanism might explain why primary MN is most prevalent after the age of 40 years. Second, both anti-PLA2R1 and anti-THSD7A antibodies have been found in asymptomatic subjects years before MN manifested clinically.[70,71] Thus, factors other than the presence and titer of antibodies in the circulation must contribute to disease manifestations (Figure 3), and antibody glycosylation patterns could be 1 of them. Notably, altered glycosylation patterns have been shown to modulate IgG function and to precede the clinical manifestation of various autoimmune diseases.[72]

Insights from exceptional patient cases. An index case and 4 additional patients with primary MN were found to be genetically MBL deficient.[73] The immunofluorescence pattern in these patients differed from 73 patients with primary MN without MBL deficiency: they exhibited less C4d staining, still only minimal C1q staining, but intense staining for the alternative pathway components FB and properdin. This indicates that MBL plays an important role in PLA2R1-positive MN but is dispensable for complement activation in some cases, where augmentation through the alternative pathway gains importance, whereas initiation of complement activation may occur through non-MBL lectins or through the classical pathway.

Another interesting observation has been made in alloimmune MN, where mothers genetically deficient of neutral endopeptidase (NEP) become immunized during pregnancy, and antibodies cross the placenta, bind to NEP expressed in fetal podocytes, and cause alloimmune neonatal nephrotic syndrome with a histologic pattern of MN.[74,75] Because of the short-lived nature of maternal IgG, the disease resolves spontaneously. Of interest, both IgG1- and IgG4-predominant alloimmunization has been observed in mothers, and the former caused much more severe disease in their children.[76] Strong complement activation via the classical pathway (with C1q deposition) occurred in the IgG1-predominant case, whereas anti–NEP-IgG4 may have been incapable to activate complement (although the IgG4-predominant case was not biopsied). This represents another hint that only altered IgG4 can activate complement, whereas normally glycosylated IgG4 may even act as a competitive inhibitor of complement-activating IgG1.

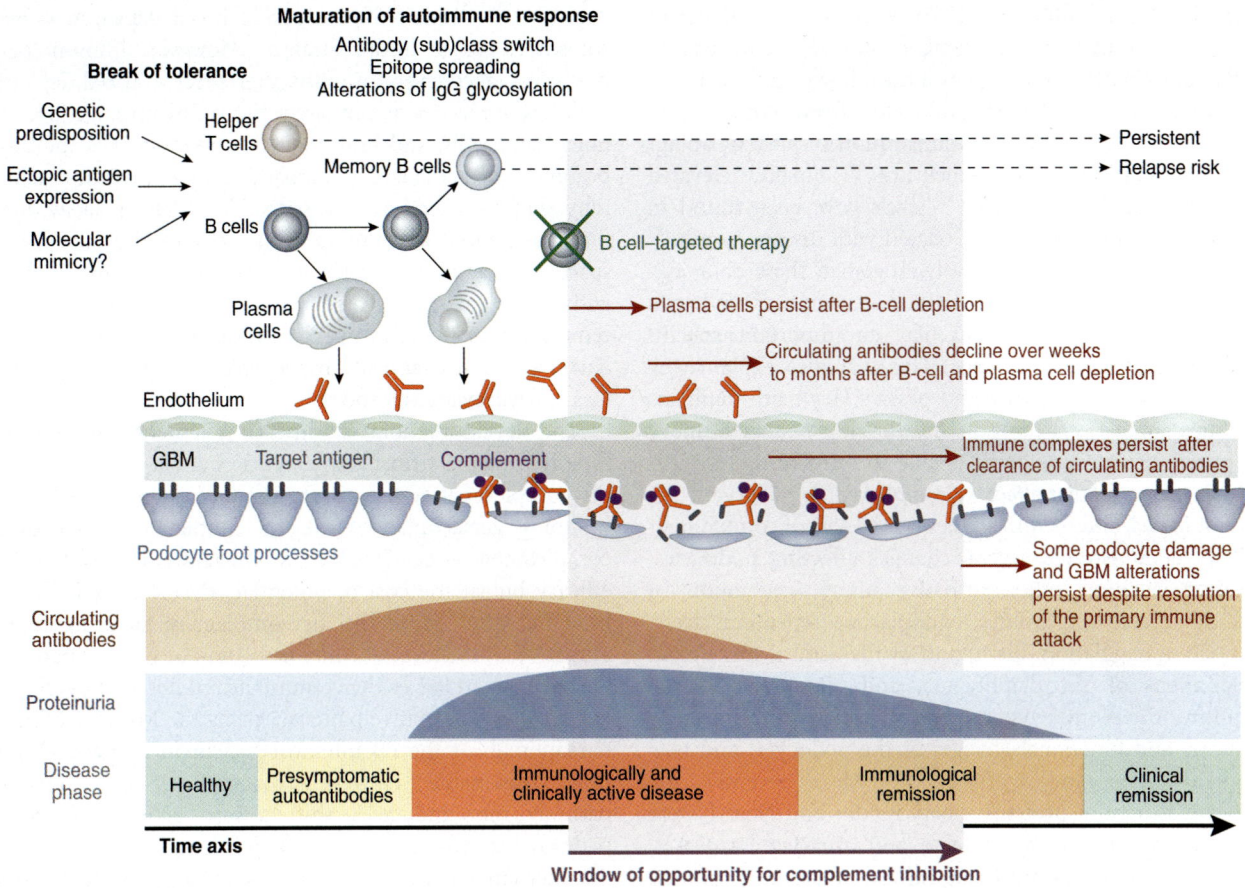

Figure 3 | Schematic drawing of the pathophysiology and temporal evolution of membranous nephropathy. GBM, glomerular basement membrane.

However, apart from complement activation, inhibition of NEP enzymatic activity may play a role in alloimmune anti-NEP MN, and only IgG1 but not IgG4 antibodies were found to inhibit NEP enzymatic activity, providing an alternative explanation for this observation.[77]

To summarize, IgG4 is clearly the predominant isoform of circulating autoantibodies against PLA2R1 and certain other MN antigens (including THSD7A) as well as in the corresponding glomerular immune complexes, but other isoforms are also present at lower levels in most, if not all, patients. Anti-PLA2R1 IgG1 and IgG3, if present, likely activate complement through the classical pathway. In contrast, IgG4 appears to activate the lectin pathway, which may depend on an altered glycosylation pattern. The alternative pathway probably serves as an amplification process. Thus, there is some evidence for both explanations (i) and (iii) mentioned above, and the relative contribution of each pathway likely differs between patients. Finally, one pathway may become more active if another one is defective or inhibited.

Complement effector pathways in MN

Once efficient C3 cleavage ensues through convergence of the 3 complement activation pathways, effector pathways involving anaphylatoxins (C3a and C5a) and the MAC (C5b-9) become operative (Figure 1). Although the specific activation pathway varies with the target antigen, predominant IgG subclass, and patient factors, complement effector pathways may be more uniform across various forms of MN.

MAC assembly and sublytic podocyte damage. Cell membrane insertion of the pore-forming terminal complement complex C5b-9 induces rapid osmotic lysis of bacteria[78] and erythrocytes.[79] In contrast, nucleated, metabolically active cells are more resistant to complement-mediated lysis.[79,80] In these cells, MAC insertion can trigger diverse events apart from cell lysis (called sublytic complement-induced damage).[80] Studies in the PHN model of MN[81,82] and in rabbits with cationized bovine serum albumin–induced MN,[83] as well as *in vitro* cytotoxicity experiments,[84] clearly documented MAC-induced podocyte injury using depletion techniques or factor-deficient animals and correspond to the presence of C5b-9 in the glomerular deposits and urine of patients with MN.[11,13,14,20–27] However, these studies were not designed to determine if activated C3 or C5 might also have a role through their cognate receptors, C3aR1 and/or C5aR1, on podocytes.

Anaphylatoxin-induced effects of complement in MN. Podocytes express both, C3aR1[33,65,85,86] and C5aR1,[65,85,86] and their expression levels were increased in MN.[33,65] In the human podocyte-based *in vitro* model of MN mentioned earlier,[65] not only inhibition of C5b-9 (by using C6-deficient serum as a source of complement) but also blockade of C3aR1 and C5aR1 signaling (by knockdown or pharmacologic inhibition) protected podocytes from complement injury. In the PHN model, administration of a C3aR antagonist markedly reduced proteinuria.[33] Finally, elevated circulating C3a[30,33] and C5a[30,34] levels have been found in patients with MN, and they correlated with disease severity[33] and remission rate,[34] respectively. Together, these data suggest that apart from MAC insertion, activation of podocyte C3a and C5a receptors might play an important role in mediating complement damage. This may also explain why C6-deficient rats with active and passive Heymann nephritis have substantial C3 deposition and develop podocyte injury and proteinuria despite being unable to form MAC.[87,88]

Downstream cellular effects of complement in podocytes. A series of *in vivo* and *in vitro* studies on the role of complement in PHN demonstrated several changes affecting podocytes, including calcium influx, oxidative injury, generation of arachidonic acid metabolites, endoplasmic reticulum stress, cell cycle dysregulation, disruption of the actin cytoskeleton, displacement of slit diaphragms, and alterations in the ubiquitin-proteasome system, all of which contribute to structural and functional changes in the podocytes and new basement membrane synthesis.[89–92] More recently, the podocyte structural proteins synaptopodin and Neph1 were shown to be cleaved by cysteine and aspartate proteases, respectively, upon complement injury in cultured human podocytes exposed to PLA2R1-positive patient sera, and their levels were reduced in glomeruli of biopsy specimens of patients with MN.[65] Together, these mostly preclinical studies provide insight into the mechanisms underlying the alterations in podocyte foot process and slit diaphragm morphology and GBM expansion that are characteristic of human MN.

Therapeutic targeting of complement in MN: future directions

The pathophysiology and clinical course of MN are complex (Figure 3). Mechanisms leading to a break of tolerance likely involve a genetic predisposition in some cases[93,94] and an immunizing stimulus, such as ectopic expression of the target antigen in tumor tissue,[95] molecular mimicry by a pathogen,[96] toxin exposure,[97] or other, as yet unidentified factors. Upon autoimmunization, maturation of the immune response results in antibody subclass switch,[59] epitope spreading,[98] and alterations of Ig glycosylation,[65,68] which may help explain the latency between autoimmunization and clinical manifestations of nephrotic syndrome.[70,71] Once clinically apparent and diagnosed, the disease may spontaneously remit or persist and progress. The discovery of target antigens and routine availability of quantitative testing for anti-PLA2R1 antibodies have revolutionized monitoring and treatment of MN.[99,100] Whereas "classical" treatment approaches for severe cases included broadly acting immunosuppressive drugs, like chlorambucil,[101] cyclophosphamide,[102] and calcineurin inhibitors,[103] current approaches put more emphasis on specific B-cell depletion,[99,104] and antigen-specific B-cell depletion is being considered as a future strategy. However, immunological remission takes several months after effective B-cell depletion, as these approaches do not target circulating immune globulins nor plasma cells, and immunologic remission (i.e., the disappearance of circulating autoantibodies) precedes clinical remission by several more months.[105–107] This is likely due to the persistence of immune complexes in the subepithelial space. As a result, podocytes are exposed to ongoing antibody- and complement-mediated injury, leading to substantial remodeling of the GBM, persistent distortion of podocyte architecture, and eventually irreversible damage (i.e., podocyte loss and glomerulosclerosis).

The development of specific complement inhibitors is a rapidly evolving field.[108] Intervention at the central point of the complement system, using the recently approved C3 inhibitor pegcetacoplan, results in complete blockade of the complement system (Figure 1), which should result in high efficacy but at the cost of potential adverse events.[109,110] To limit the latter, more specific complement targeting appears attractive, at the level of either activation or effector pathways. On the basis of the evidence summarized herein, targeting the lectin or the alternative pathway (using the MASP-2 inhibitor narsoplimab or the FB inhibitor iptacopan, respectively) appears reasonable. However, blockade of one activation pathway may induce a shift toward activity of another pathway (as seen in genetic MBL deficiency).[73] Also, although the alternative pathway is an important amplification system, it may be redundant if sufficient antibody-dependent activation of complement via the classical or lectin pathway takes place.[111] Eculizumab efficiently inhibits both MAC assembly as well as C5a signaling, but an early trial was halted for lack of efficacy. However, inadequate dosing of the monoclonal antibody and loss in the nephrotic urine may have been the cause. On the basis of recent data on C3a and C5a signaling in MN, specific blockade of their respective receptors might offer another option. The C5aR1 blocker avacopan has been approved for anti-neutrophil cytoplasmic autoantibody–associated vasculitis,[112] whereas we are not aware of a C3aR1 inhibitor under development for clinical use. On the basis of *in vitro* data, concurrent C3aR1 and C5aR1 blockade may be required but could be sufficient without simultaneous inhibition of MAC formation,[65] but this requires clinical confirmation.

Given all these open questions and uncertainties, how should specific complement inhibition be tested in MN? Because of the complexity of complement activation and the differences regarding IgG subclasses and complement regulatory proteins between rodents and humans, animal models will likely not be able to provide definitive answers. When considering clinical trials, their design will be crucial. Patients may need to be selected on the basis of their individual complement pattern identified on kidney biopsy (e.g., relative intensity of staining for C1q, C3, C4d, FB, FD, and MBL). In the future, measurement of complement cleavage products in blood and urine or an efficient *in vitro* cytotoxicity assay that relies on antigen-expressing podocytes and patient sera may enable selection of the most effective complement inhibitor for each patient. Furthermore, choosing the right time point for complement blockade (i.e., before irreversible GBM and podocyte remodeling have ensued) will be important (Figure 3), and a careful selection of surrogate end points, including measures of complement activation, such as blood and urinary levels of complement or staining for complement products in repeated biopsies, may be important in proof-of-concept studies.

Conclusions

Robust evidence supports a central role of complement as the mediator of antibody-dependent podocyte injury in MN. Although definitive treatment of MN ultimately depends on elimination of the offending antibodies, the time to immunologic remission and clearance of immune deposits from tissue provides a window of opportunity to protect podocytes from ongoing complement-mediated injury. Which one of an array of inhibitors acting at specific points in the complement cascade will ultimately prove to be most effective may be patient-dependent and will likely be guided in the near future from ongoing basic studies with newly developed cell-based and animal models, analysis of patient specimens using advanced technologies, and, finally, clinical trials.

DISCLOSURE

ADK declares receiving travel support and advisory board fees from Alexion Pharmaceutics and CSL Vifor; and grant support from Alexion Pharmaceutics and Novartis. All the other authors declared no competing interests.

ACKNOWLEDGMENTS

Images of IgG and complement for the 2 cases shown in Figure 2 are courtesy of Dr. Joel Henderson, Pathology Department, Boston Medical Center. Neural epidermal growth factor-like 1 protein (NELL-1) staining on the second case was done by A. Bernard Collins, Pathology Department, Massachusetts General Hospital.

REFERENCES

1. Merle NS, Church SE, Fremeaux-Bacchi V, et al. Complement system part I - molecular mechanisms of activation and regulation. *Front Immunol*. 2015;6:262.
2. Diebolder CA, Beurskens FJ, de Jong RN, et al. Complement is activated by IgG hexamers assembled at the cell surface. *Science*. 2014;343:1260–1263.
3. van der Zee JS, van Swieten P, Aalberse RC. Inhibition of complement activation by IgG4 antibodies. *Clin Exp Immunol*. 1986;64:415–422.
4. Harboe M, Mollnes TE. The alternative complement pathway revisited. *J Cell Mol Med*. 2008;12:1074–1084.
5. Lachmann PJ. The amplification loop of the complement pathways. *Adv Immunol*. 2009;104:115–149.
6. Song YS, Min KW, Kim JH, et al. Differential diagnosis of lupus and primary membranous nephropathies by IgG subclass analysis. *Clin J Am Soc Nephrol*. 2012;7:1947–1955.
7. Hayashi N, Okada K, Matsui Y, et al. Glomerular mannose-binding lectin deposition in intrinsic antigen-related membranous nephropathy. *Nephrol Dial Transplant*. 2018;33:832–840.
8. Zhang XD, Cui Z, Zhang MF, et al. Clinical implications of pathological features of primary membranous nephropathy. *BMC Nephrol*. 2018;19:215.
9. Stangou MJ, Marinaki S, Papachristou E, et al. Histological grading in primary membranous nephropathy is essential for clinical management and predicts outcome of patients. *Histopathology*. 2019;75:660–671.
10. Doi T, Kanatsu K, Nagai H, et al. Demonstration of C3d deposits in membranous nephropathy. *Nephron*. 1984;37:232–235.
11. Papagianni AA, Alexopoulos E, Leontsini M, et al. C5b-9 and adhesion molecules in human idiopathic membranous nephropathy. *Nephrol Dial Transplant*. 2002;17:57–63.
12. Ayoub I, Shapiro JP, Song H, et al. Establishing a case for anti-complement therapy in membranous nephropathy. *Kidney Int Rep*. 2021;6:484–492.
13. Teisseyre M, Beyze A, Perrochia H, et al. C5b-9 glomerular deposits are associated with poor renal survival in membranous nephropathy. *Kidney Int Rep*. 2023;8:103–114.
14. Ravindran A, Madden B, Charlesworth MC, et al. Proteomic analysis of complement proteins in membranous nephropathy. *Kidney Int Rep*. 2020;5:618–626.
15. Kawata N, Kang D, Aiuchi T, et al. Proteomics of human glomerulonephritis by laser microdissection and liquid chromatography-tandem mass spectrometry. *Nephrology (Carlton)*. 2020;25:351–359.
16. Sethi S, Madden B, Debiec H, et al. Protocadherin 7-associated membranous nephropathy. *J Am Soc Nephrol*. 2021;32:1249–1261.
17. Law SK, Dodds AW. The internal thioester and the covalent binding properties of the complement proteins C3 and C4. *Protein Sci*. 1997;6:263–274.
18. Zhang R, Zheng ZY, Lin JS, et al. The continual presence of C3d but not IgG glomerular capillary deposition in stage I idiopathic membranous nephropathy in patients receiving corticosteroid treatment. *Diagn Pathol*. 2012;7:109.
19. Bubeck D. The making of a macromolecular machine: assembly of the membrane attack complex. *Biochemistry*. 2014;53:1908–1915.
20. Schulze M, Donadio JV Jr, Pruchno CJ, et al. Elevated urinary excretion of the C5b-9 complex in membranous nephropathy. *Kidney Int*. 1991;40:533–538.
21. Kusunoki Y, Akutsu Y, Itami N, et al. Urinary excretion of terminal complement complexes in glomerular disease. *Nephron*. 1991;59:27–32.
22. Brenchley PE, Coupes B, Short CD, et al. Urinary C3dg and C5b-9 indicate active immune disease in human membranous nephropathy. *Kidney Int*. 1992;41:933–937.
23. Coupes BM, Kon SP, Brenchley PE, et al. The temporal relationship between urinary C5b-9 and C3dg and clinical parameters in human membranous nephropathy. *Nephrol Dial Transplant*. 1993;8:397–401.
24. Honkanen E, Teppo AM, Meri S, et al. Urinary excretion of cytokines and complement SC5b-9 in idiopathic membranous glomerulonephritis. *Nephrol Dial Transplant*. 1994;9:1553–1559.
25. Praga M, Paz Artal E, Hernández E, et al. Antiproteinuric effect of angiotensin-converting enzyme inhibition and C5b-9 urinary excretion in membranous glomerulonephritis. *Nephrol Dial Transplant*. 1997;12:2576–2579.
26. Montinaro V, Lopez A, Monno R, et al. Renal C3 synthesis in idiopathic membranous nephropathy: correlation to urinary C5b-9 excretion. *Kidney Int*. 2000;57:137–146.
27. Cattran DC, Wald R, Brenchley PE, et al. Clinical correlates of serial urinary membrane attack complex estimates in patients with idiopathic membranous nephropathy. *Clin Nephrol*. 2003;60:7–12.
28. Branten AJ, Kock-Jansen M, Klasen IS, et al. Urinary excretion of complement C3d in patients with renal diseases. *Eur J Clin Invest*. 2003;33:449–456.
29. Kon SP, Coupes B, Short CD, et al. Urinary C5b-9 excretion and clinical course in idiopathic human membranous nephropathy. *Kidney Int*. 1995;48:1953–1958.
30. Zhang MF, Huang J, Zhang YM, et al. Complement activation products in the circulation and urine of primary membranous nephropathy. *BMC Nephrol*. 2019;20:313.
31. Cumming AD, Thomson D, Davidson AM, et al. Significance of urinary C3 excretion in glomerulonephritis. *J Clin Pathol*. 1976;29:601–607.
32. Morita Y, Ikeguchi H, Nakamura J, et al. Complement activation products in the urine from proteinuric patients. *J Am Soc Nephrol*. 2000;11:700–707.
33. Gao S, Cui Z, Zhao MH. Complement C3a and C3a receptor activation mediates podocyte injuries in the mechanism of primary membranous nephropathy. *J Am Soc Nephrol*. 2022;33:1742–1756.

34. Chi JN, Lai TS, Wu CF, et al. The relationship of anti-phospholipase A2 receptor antibody and C5a complement with disease activity and short-term outcome in idiopathic membranous nephropathy. *J Formos Med Assoc.* 2019;118:898–906.
35. Li J, Zhang J, Wang X, et al. Lectin complement pathway activation is associated with massive proteinuria in PLA2R-positive membranous nephropathy: a retrospective study. *Int J Gen Med.* 2023;16:1879–1889.
36. Tsai SF, Wu MJ, Chen CH. Low serum C3 level, high neutrophil-lymphocyte-ratio, and high platelet-lymphocyte-ratio all predicted poor long-term renal survivals in biopsy-confirmed idiopathic membranous nephropathy. *Sci Rep.* 2019;9:6209.
37. Cybulsky AV, Quigg RJ, Salant DJ. Experimental membranous nephropathy redux. *Am J Physiol Renal Physiol.* 2005;289:F660–F671.
38. Beck LH Jr, Salant DJ. Membranous nephropathy: from models to man. *J Clin Invest.* 2014;124:2307–2314.
39. Salant DJ, Belok S, Madaio MP, et al. A new role for complement in experimental membranous nephropathy in rats. *J Clin Invest.* 1980;66:1339–1350.
40. Schiller B, He C, Salant DJ, et al. Inhibition of complement regulation is key to the pathogenesis of active Heymann nephritis. *J Exp Med.* 1998;188:1353–1358.
41. Reinhard L, Wiech T, Reitmeier A, et al. Pathogenicity of human anti-PLA 2 R1 antibodies in minipigs: a pilot study. *J Am Soc Nephrol.* 2023;34:369–373.
42. Tomas NM, Hoxha E, Reinicke AT, et al. Autoantibodies against thrombospondin type 1 domain-containing 7A induce membranous nephropathy. *J Clin Invest.* 2016;126:2519–2532.
43. Jaber S, Goehrig D, Bertolino P, et al. Generation of a conditional transgenic mouse model expressing human phospholipase A2 receptor 1. *Sci Rep.* 2020;10:8190.
44. Tomas NM, Dehde S, Meyer-Schwesinger C, et al. Podocyte expression of human phospholipase A2 receptor 1 causes immune-mediated membranous nephropathy in mice. *Kidney Int.* 2023;103:297–303.
45. Seifert L, Zahner G, Meyer-Schwesinger C, et al. The classical pathway triggers pathogenic complement activation in membranous nephropathy. *Nat Commun.* 2023;14:473.
46. Bobart SA, Tehranian S, Sethi S, et al. A target antigen-based approach to the classification of membranous nephropathy. *Mayo Clin Proc.* 2021;96:577–591.
47. Beck LH Jr, Bonegio RG, Lambeau G, et al. M-type phospholipase A2 receptor as target antigen in idiopathic membranous nephropathy. *N Engl J Med.* 2009;361:11–21.
48. Tomas NM, Beck LH Jr, Meyer-Schwesinger C, et al. Thrombospondin type-1 domain-containing 7A in idiopathic membranous nephropathy. *N Engl J Med.* 2014;371:2277–2287.
49. Al-Rabadi LF, Caza T, Trivin-Avillach C, et al. Serine protease HTRA1 as a novel target antigen in primary membranous nephropathy. *J Am Soc Nephrol.* 2021;32:1666–1681.
50. Fehmi J, Davies AJ, Antonelou M, et al. Contactin-1 links autoimmune neuropathy and membranous glomerulonephritis. *PLoS One.* 2023;18: e0281156.
51. von Haxthausen F, Reinhard L, Pinnschmidt HO, et al. Antigen-specific IgG subclasses in primary and malignancy-associated membranous nephropathy. *Front Immunol.* 2018;9:3035.
52. Kanigicherla D, Gummadova J, McKenzie EA, et al. Anti-PLA2R antibodies measured by ELISA predict long-term outcome in a prevalent population of patients with idiopathic membranous nephropathy. *Kidney Int.* 2013;83:940–948.
53. Hofstra JM, Debiec H, Short CD, et al. Antiphospholipase A2 receptor antibody titer and subclass in idiopathic membranous nephropathy. *J Am Soc Nephrol.* 2012;23:1735–1743.
54. Lateb M, Ouahmi H, Payré C, et al. Anti-PLA2R1 antibodies containing sera induce in vitro cytotoxicity mediated by complement activation. *J Immunol Res.* 2019;2019:1324804.
55. Manral P, Caza TN, Storey AJ, et al. The alternative pathway is necessary and sufficient for complement activation by anti-THSD7A autoantibodies, which are predominantly IgG4 in membranous nephropathy. *Front Immunol.* 2022;13:952235.
56. Hoxha E, Kneißler U, Stege G, et al. Enhanced expression of the M-type phospholipase A2 receptor in glomeruli correlates with serum receptor antibodies in primary membranous nephropathy. *Kidney Int.* 2012;82:797–804.
57. Kuroki A, Shibata T, Honda H, et al. Glomerular and serum IgG subclasses in diffuse proliferative lupus nephritis, membranous lupus nephritis, and idiopathic membranous nephropathy. *Intern Med.* 2002;41:936–942.
58. Segawa Y, Hisano S, Matsushita M, et al. IgG subclasses and complement pathway in segmental and global membranous nephropathy. *Pediatr Nephrol.* 2010;25:1091–1099.
59. Huang CC, Lehman A, Albawardi A, et al. IgG subclass staining in renal biopsies with membranous glomerulonephritis indicates subclass switch during disease progression. *Mod Pathol.* 2013;26:799–805.
60. Imai H, Hamai K, Komatsuda A, et al. IgG subclasses in patients with membranoproliferative glomerulonephritis, membranous nephropathy, and lupus nephritis. *Kidney Int.* 1997;51:270–276.
61. Dong HR, Wang YY, Cheng XH, et al. Retrospective study of phospholipase A2 receptor and IgG subclasses in glomerular deposits in Chinese patients with membranous nephropathy. *PLoS One.* 2016;11: e0156263.
62. Jennette JC, Hipp CG. Immunohistopathologic evaluation of C1q in 800 renal biopsy specimens. *Am J Clin Pathol.* 1985;83:415–420.
63. Custódio FB, Silva CAD, Helmo FR, et al. Complement system and C4d expression in cases of membranous nephropathy. *J Bras Nefrol.* 2017;39:370–375.
64. Zhang MF, Cui Z, Zhang YM, et al. Clinical and prognostic significance of glomerular C1q deposits in primary MN. *Clin Chim Acta.* 2018;485:152–157.
65. Haddad G, Lorenzen JM, Ma H, et al. Altered glycosylation of IgG4 promotes lectin complement pathway activation in anti-PLA2R1-associated membranous nephropathy. *J Clin Invest.* 2021;131:e140453.
66. Petrosyan A, Cravedi P, Villani V, et al. A glomerulus-on-a-chip to recapitulate the human glomerular filtration barrier. *Nat Commun.* 2019;10:3656.
67. Gudelj I, Lauc G, Pezer M. Immunoglobulin G glycosylation in aging and diseases. *Cell Immunol.* 2018;333:65–79.
68. Chinello C, de Haan N, Capitoli G, et al. Definition of IgG subclass-specific glycopatterns in idiopathic membranous nephropathy: aberrant IgG glycoforms in blood. *Int J Mol Sci.* 2022;23:4664.
69. Oskam N, Damelang T, Streutker M, et al. Factors affecting IgG4-mediated complement activation. *Front Immunol.* 2023;14:1087532.
70. Burbelo PD, Joshi M, Chaturvedi A, et al. Detection of PLA2R autoantibodies before the diagnosis of membranous nephropathy. *J Am Soc Nephrol.* 2020;31:208–217.
71. Burbelo PD, Olson SW, Keller JM, et al. Prediagnostic appearance of thrombospondin type-1 domain 7A autoantibodies in membranous nephropathy. *Kidney360.* 2023;4:217–225.
72. Seeling M, Brückner C, Nimmerjahn F. Differential antibody glycosylation in autoimmunity: sweet biomarker or modulator of disease activity? *Nat Rev Rheumatol.* 2017;13:621–630.
73. Bally S, Debiec H, Ponard D, et al. Phospholipase A2 receptor-related membranous nephropathy and mannan-binding lectin deficiency. *J Am Soc Nephrol.* 2016;27:3539–3544.
74. Debiec H, Guigonis V, Mougenot B, et al. Antenatal membranous glomerulonephritis due to anti-neutral endopeptidase antibodies. *N Engl J Med.* 2002;346:2053–2060.
75. Debiec H, Nauta J, Coulet F, et al. Role of truncating mutations in MME gene in fetomaternal alloimmunisation and antenatal glomerulopathies. *Lancet.* 2004;364:1252–1259.
76. Vivarelli M, Emma F, Pellé T, et al. Genetic homogeneity but IgG subclass-dependent clinical variability of alloimmune membranous nephropathy with anti-neutral endopeptidase antibodies. *Kidney Int.* 2015;87:602–609.
77. Beck LH. Lessons from a rare disease: IgG subclass and disease severity in alloimmune antenatal membranous nephropathy. *Kidney Int.* 2015;87:494–497.
78. Bhakdi S, Kuller G, Muhly M, et al. Formation of transmural complement pores in serum-sensitive *Escherichia coli*. *Infect Immun.* 1987;55:206–210.
79. Koski CL, Ramm LE, Hammer CH, et al. Cytolysis of nucleated cells by complement: cell death displays multi-hit characteristics. *Proc Natl Acad Sci U S A.* 1983;80:3816–3820.
80. Cole DS, Morgan BP. Beyond lysis: how complement influences cell fate. *Clin Sci (Lond).* 2003;104:455–466.

81. Cybulsky AV, Rennke HG, Feintzeig ID, et al. Complement-induced glomerular epithelial cell injury: role of the membrane attack complex in rat membranous nephropathy. *J Clin Invest*. 1986;77:1096–1107.
82. Baker PJ, Ochi RF, Schulze M, et al. Depletion of C6 prevents development of proteinuria in experimental membranous nephropathy in rats. *Am J Pathol*. 1989;135:185–194.
83. Groggel GC, Adler S, Rennke HG, et al. Role of the terminal complement pathway in experimental membranous nephropathy in the rabbit. *J Clin Invest*. 1983;72:1948–1957.
84. Cybulsky AV, Quigg RJ, Salant DJ. The membrane attack complex in complement-mediated glomerular epithelial cell injury: formation and stability of C5b-9 and C5b-7 in rat membranous nephropathy. *J Immunol*. 1986;137:1511–1516.
85. Braun MC, Reins RY, Li TB, et al. Renal expression of the C3a receptor and functional responses of primary human proximal tubular epithelial cells. *J Immunol*. 2004;173:4190–4196.
86. Liu L, Zhang Y, Duan X, et al. C3a, C5a renal expression and their receptors are correlated to severity of IgA nephropathy. *J Clin Immunol*. 2014;34:224–232.
87. Leenaerts PL, Hall BM, Van Damme BJ, et al. Active Heymann nephritis in complement component C6 deficient rats. *Kidney Int*. 1995;47:1604–1614.
88. Spicer ST, Tran GT, Killingsworth MC, et al. Induction of passive Heymann nephritis in complement component 6-deficient PVG rats. *J Immunol*. 2007;179:172–178.
89. Takano T, Elimam H, Cybulsky AV. Complement-mediated cellular injury. *Semin Nephrol*. 2013;33:586–601.
90. Saran AM, Yuan H, Takeuchi E, et al. Complement mediates nephrin redistribution and actin dissociation in experimental membranous nephropathy. *Kidney Int*. 2003;64:2072–2078.
91. Minto AW, Kalluri R, Togawa M, et al. Augmented expression of glomerular basement membrane specific type IV collagen isoforms (alpha3-alpha5) in experimental membranous nephropathy. *Proc Assoc Am Physicians*. 1998;110:207–217.
92. Nangaku M, Shankland SJ, Couser WG. Cellular response to injury in membranous nephropathy. *J Am Soc Nephrol*. 2005;16:1195–1204.
93. Stanescu HC, Arcos-Burgos M, Medlar A, et al. Risk HLA-DQA1 and PLA(2)R1 alleles in idiopathic membranous nephropathy. *N Engl J Med*. 2011;364:616–626.
94. Xie J, Liu L, Mladkova N, et al. The genetic architecture of membranous nephropathy and its potential to improve non-invasive diagnosis. *Nat Commun*. 2020;11:1600.
95. Hoxha E, Wiech T, Stahl PR, et al. A mechanism for cancer-associated membranous nephropathy. *N Engl J Med*. 2016;374:1995–1996.
96. Wiech T, Reinhard L, Wulf S, et al. Bacterial infection possibly causing autoimmunity: *Tropheryma whipplei* and membranous nephropathy. *Lancet*. 2022;400:1882–1883.
97. Cremoni M, Agbekodo S, Teisseyre M, et al. Toxic occupational exposures and membranous nephropathy. *Clin J Am Soc Nephrol*. 2022;17:1609–1619.
98. Seitz-Polski B, Dolla G, Payré C, et al. Epitope spreading of autoantibody response to PLA2R associates with poor prognosis in membranous nephropathy. *J Am Soc Nephrol*. 2016;27:1517–1533.
99. Kidney Disease: Improving Global Outcomes (KDIGO) Glomerular Diseases Work Group. KDIGO 2021 clinical practice guideline for the management of glomerular diseases. *Kidney Int*. 2021;100(4S):S1–S276.
100. Bomback AS. Management of membranous nephropathy in the PLA(2)R era. *Clin J Am Soc Nephrol*. 2018;13:784–786.
101. Ponticelli C, Zucchelli P, Imbasciati E, et al. Controlled trial of methylprednisolone and chlorambucil in idiopathic membranous nephropathy. *N Engl J Med*. 1984;310:946–950.
102. Ponticelli C, Altieri P, Scolari F, et al. A randomized study comparing methylprednisolone plus chlorambucil versus methylprednisolone plus cyclophosphamide in idiopathic membranous nephropathy. *J Am Soc Nephrol*. 1998;9:444–450.
103. Cattran DC, Greenwood C, Ritchie S, et al. Canadian Glomerulonephritis Study Group. A controlled trial of cyclosporine in patients with progressive membranous nephropathy. *Kidney Int*. 1995;47:1130–1135.
104. Fervenza FC, Appel GB, Barbour SJ, et al. Rituximab or cyclosporine in the treatment of membranous nephropathy. *N Engl J Med*. 2019;381:36–46.
105. Beck LH Jr, Fervenza FC, Beck DM, et al. Rituximab-induced depletion of anti-PLA2R autoantibodies predicts response in membranous nephropathy. *J Am Soc Nephrol*. 2011;22:1543–1550.
106. Hoxha E, Thiele I, Zahner G, et al. Phospholipase A2 receptor autoantibodies and clinical outcome in patients with primary membranous nephropathy. *J Am Soc Nephrol*. 2014;25:1357–1366.
107. Ruggenenti P, Debiec H, Ruggiero B, et al. Anti-phospholipase A2 receptor antibody titer predicts post-rituximab outcome of membranous nephropathy. *J Am Soc Nephrol*. 2015;26:2545–2558.
108. Lamers C, Ricklin D, Lambris JD. Complement-targeted therapeutics: an emerging field enabled by academic drug discovery. *Am J Hematol*. 2023;98(suppl 4):S82–S89.
109. Hillmen P, Szer J, Weitz I, et al. Pegcetacoplan versus eculizumab in paroxysmal nocturnal hemoglobinuria. *N Engl J Med*. 2021;384:1028–1037.
110. Gerber GF, Brodsky RA. Pegcetacoplan for paroxysmal nocturnal hemoglobinuria. *Blood*. 2022;139:3361–3365.
111. de Boer EC, Thielen AJ, Langereis JD, et al. The contribution of the alternative pathway in complement activation on cell surfaces depends on the strength of classical pathway initiation. *Clin Transl Immunol*. 2023;12:e1436.
112. Jayne DRW, Merkel PA, Schall TJ, et al. Avacopan for the treatment of ANCA-associated vasculitis. *N Engl J Med*. 2021;384:599–609.

basic research

www.kidney-international.org

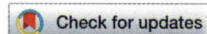

A proteomic atlas of kidney amyloidosis provides insights into disease pathogenesis

see commentary on page 427

Charalampos Charalampous[1], Surendra Dasari[2], Ellen McPhail[3], Jason D. Theis[3], Julie A. Vrana[3], Angela Dispenzieri[1], Nelson Leung[1], Eli Muchtar[1], Morie Gertz[1], Marina Ramirez-Alvarado[4] and Taxiarchis Kourelis[1]

[1]Division of Hematology, Mayo Clinic, Rochester, Minnesota, USA; [2]Department of Quantitative Health Sciences, Mayo Clinic, Rochester, Minnesota, USA; [3]Department of Laboratory Medicine and Pathology, Mayo Clinic, Rochester, Minnesota, USA; and [4]Department of Biochemistry and Molecular Biology, Mayo Clinic, Rochester, Minnesota, USA

The mechanisms of tissue damage in kidney amyloidosis are not well described. To investigate this further, we used laser microdissection-mass spectrometry to identify proteins deposited in amyloid plaques (expanded proteome) and proteins overexpressed in plaques compared to controls (plaque-specific proteome). This study encompassed 2650 cases of amyloidosis due to light chain (AL), heavy chain (AH), leukocyte chemotactic factor-2-type (ALECT2), secondary (AA), fibrinogen (AFib), apo AIV (AApoAIV), apo CII (AApoCII) and 14 normal/disease controls. We found that AFib, AA, and AApoCII have the most distinct proteomes predominantly driven by increased complement pathway proteins. Clustering of cases based on the expanded proteome identified two ALECT2 and seven AL subtypes. The main differences within the AL and ALECT2 subtypes were driven by complement proteins and, for AL only, 14-3-3 family proteins (a *family* of structurally similar phospho-binding proteins that regulate major cellular functions) widely implicated in kidney tissue dysfunction. The kidney AL plaque-specific proteome consisted of 24 proteins, including those implicated in kidney damage (α1 antitrypsin and heat shock protein β1). Hierarchical clustering of AL cases based on their plaque-specific proteome identified four clusters, of which one was associated with improved kidney survival and was characterized by higher overall proteomic content and 14-3-3 proteins but lower levels of light chains and most signature proteins. Thus, our results suggest that there is significant heterogeneity across and within amyloid types, driven predominantly by complement proteins, and that the plaque protein burden does not correlate with amyloid toxicity.

Kidney International (2024) 105, 484–495; https://doi.org/10.1016/j.kint.2023.11.023

KEYWORDS: amyloidosis; protein aggregation; proteomics

Copyright © 2023, International Society of Nephrology. Published by Elsevier Inc. All rights reserved.

Translational Statement

We present the amyloid proteome of 2650 kidney amyloid cases from 8 different types of kidney amyloidosis. We find that complement pathway proteins are deposited across all amyloid types. We identify that secondary amyloidosis (AA), fibrinogen amyloidosis (Afib), and apolipoprotein C-II amyloidosis (AApoCII) are the most distinct proteomically, compared to other types, and that light chain (AL) and leukocyte chemotactic factor-2-type (ALECT2) have significant proteomic heterogeneity. A subset of AL patients with high amyloid plaque proteomic content but low amounts of light chains and proteins involved in kidney fibrosis were found to have improved kidney survival. Our results suggest that the deposition dynamics of the amyloidogenic protein are decoupled to that of other proteins and that the kidney toxicity in this disease may not be explained by merely amyloid abundance. Exploring the role of key proteins identified herein in the role of disease pathogenesis may serve as a starting point for the development of novel therapies.

Kidney amyloidosis is a heterogeneous disease caused by the deposition of several different types of amyloidogenic proteins.[1] Ig light chain (AL) is the most common type of kidney amyloidosis, and the goal of therapy is to control the underlying plasma cell clone. For other amyloid types, such as secondary amyloidosis (AA), in which the precursor protein is serum amyloid A (SAA), treatment focuses on controlling the inflammatory disease driving amyloid deposition. Despite such treatment, kidney function deterioration can continue even after achieving optimal control of the underlying cause. Finally, for other types, such as ALECT2 (leukocyte chemotactic factor-2-type), no disease-specific therapies exist. To develop novel therapies, we need to better understand the mechanisms of tissue damage in this disease.

The kidney amyloid plaque proteome is an untapped source of information that can provide insights into the

Correspondence: Kourelis Taxiarchis, Division of Hematology, Mayo Clinic, 200 First Street SW, Rochester, Minnesota 55906, USA. E-mail: Kourelis.taxiarchis@mayo.edu

Received 28 March 2023; revised 4 October 2023; accepted 5 November 2023; published online 12 December 2023

mechanisms of tissue damage. Our center has extensive expertise in amyloid typing using laser microdissection (LMD) and mass spectrometry (MS),[2–6] during which amyloid plaques are microdissected and analyzed by MS. In addition to the amyloidogenic protein, several other proteins are identified that could inform disease physiology. For instance, the amyloid signature proteins (clusterin, vitronectin, apolipoprotein (Apo)E, ApoA4, and serum amyloid P-component [SAP]) are seen with every amyloid type and across all tissues. Some (e.g., clusterin) can act as amyloid chaperones,[7] inhibiting amyloidogenicity, whereas others (e.g., SAP) can promote amyloidogenicity. In addition, several proteins of the involved tissue are represented within the plaque proteome. Although amyloid plaques do not consist of live cells, their proteome can provide information about amyloid burden, mechanisms of cellular toxicity, or physiologic tissue responses to amyloid deposition. This study aimed to comprehensively characterize the kidney amyloid proteome and its correlation with patient characteristics and outcomes.

METHODS

This study was approved by Mayo Clinic's institutional review board (07-000988). Given that most cases included were from outside institutions, the research could not have been completed otherwise, and the nature of the project posed minimal risk to the patients, so a waiver of consent was granted. All newly diagnosed internal and external cases of the most common types submitted to Mayo Clinic for typing between 2008 and 2020 were included. A case had to be Congo red–positive to be analyzed. We also included 9 disease controls (membranous nephropathy) with diagnostic biopsies, and 5 normal controls (day-zero kidney transplant biopsy) from between 2008 and 2013. Our methodology has abided by the Declaration of Helsinki and the Declaration of Istanbul guidelines. Peptide identification was performed using LMD/MS[3] of Congo red–positive amyloid deposits in amyloidosis cases, and glomeruli in control cases. All cases were analyzed by MS within approximately 1 week of receiving the biopsy sample. The amyloid typing assay is a College of American Pathologists/Clinical Laboratory Improvement Amendments (CAP/CLIA)–validated assay. Stringent, periodic quality control occurs to ensure consistent proteomic outputs from the instrument. A single change in MS instrumentation occurred during the study period. This change was meticulously validated by comparing the old and new proteomes of hundreds of samples and proving that the new method/change did not alter the proteomic output (a requirement for the above validation). Therefore, batch effects were not a concern, despite the retrospective nature of the study. Protein spectral counts, normalized to the total number of spectral counts per LMD, were used as a semiquantitative measure of abundance. The existing kidney staging system[8] was used to risk-stratify patients with AL amyloidosis.

Statistical and bioinformatic analyses

Statistical analyses were performed using JMP (SAS Institute Inc.) and the omiq.ai online platform. All identified proteins were considered part of the expanded amyloid proteome, and comparisons across groups considered a false detection rate–corrected P value of < 0.05, except for protein comparisons and clinical parameters when considering the plaque-specific proteome, for which a P value of < 0.05 was considered significant, given the limited number of comparisons. Proteins were considered part of the plaque-specific proteome if their abundance in the amyloid plaque was increased by 50% compared to pooled normal and disease controls, using an false detection rate–corrected P value < 0.05 for consistency with prior work.[9] For dimensionality reduction and visualization, we used uniform manifold approximation and projection (UMAP),[10] and to cluster the UMAP dataset, we used phenograph[11] with the expanded proteome as input features for both methods, and the default parameters within omiq.ai. To cluster AL patients using their plaque-specific proteome, we used hierarchical clustering in JMP using 'Ward's minimum variance method to calculate distances between clusters. Overrepresentation analyses were performed in WebGestalt[12] and using the Reactome database and a false detection rate–corrected $P < 0.05$ when identifying significantly overrepresented pathways. Patient overall and kidney survival (OS and RS, respectively) were calculated from the time of diagnosis to the time of death or initiation of dialysis, respectively, using the Kaplan–Meier method. For kidney survival, the composite endpoint of transition to hemodialysis or patient death was considered. A Cox proportional hazards model was used to determine outcome differences. The Fisher exact test was used to compare categorical variables, and the Wilcoxon rank-sum test was used for continuous variables.

RESULTS

We included a total of 2650 kidney amyloidosis cases. The distribution of the cases is shown in Table 1. Given that most cases were referred to our institution for amyloid typing, no other clinical information was available in our database, except that for a subset of AL patients.

The total protein content varies across amyloidosis types

We identified 498 distinct proteins across all types. The most overrepresented pathway was the complement cascade (Supplementary Figure S1). AL and AApoAIV (apolipoprotein A-IV amyloidosis) had the lowest proteomic burden (defined as the total abundance of all identified proteins in normalized spectral counts), whereas AFib (fibrinogen

Table 1 | Amyloid cases included in the study

Disease type	N = 2650	%	Female sex, n (%)[a]	Age, yr, median (range)[a]
Ig	618	35.52	640 (40)	66 (25–93)
Lambda	1075	25.68	417 (39)	66 (25–90)
Kappa	412	9.84	165 (40)	66 (32–93)
IGH	73	1.74	36 (49)	65 (34–92)
AH	58	1.39	22 (44)	70 (41–88)
ALECT2	474	11.32	220 (46)	67 (18–92)
AA	418	9.99	186 (44)	60 (20–94)
AFib	80	1.91	26 (33)	63 (34–81)
AApoAIV	38	0.91	9 (24)	69 (47–86)
AApoCII	22	0.53	14 (64)	70 (53–98)
Controls	N = 14			
Normal controls	5	36	2 (40)	52 (51–67)
Membranous nephropathy controls	9	64	2 (22)	55 (48–86)

AA, secondary amyloidosis; AApoAIV, apo A-IV amyloidosis; AApoCII, Apo C-II amyloidosis; Afib, fibrinogen amyloidosis; AH, heavy chain amyloidosis; ALECT2, LECT2 amyloidosis; IGH, mix of heavy and light chain amyloid.
[a]Fifty-seven patients (2%) did not have available gender and/or age information.

amyloidosis) and AApoCII (apolipoprotein C-II amyloidosis) had the highest burden (Supplementary Figure S1). Compared to the previously published cardiac proteome,[9] the kidney proteome appeared to be more diverse (498 vs. 161 distinct proteins). Pathway analyses of proteins unique to the heart and/or kidney or common across organs are shown in Supplementary Figure S2. Protein pathways that were increased in both organs reflected processing of lipoproteins (e.g., uptake of ligands by scavenger receptors),[13] fibrosis pathways (e.g., "extracellular matrix proteoglycans," and "degradation of the extracellular matrix"), and keratinization pathways, which reflect patterns of organ damage shared across the 2 organs.[14,15] Pathways unique to heart tissue were muscle contractility and keratinization pathways. Pathways unique to the kidneys included the complement cascade and pathways driven by high tubulin superfamily protein expression (e.g., all 4 top pathways for kidney-specific proteins; Supplementary Figure S2), which reflect distinct physiological responses to kidney damage.[16,17] Of note, complement proteins C3, C4B, and C9, as well as the complement regulatory proteins CFH and CFHR1 were present in both organs, suggesting that the complement pathway was activated from early to late components in amyloid plaques of hearts and kidneys across various amyloid types. The top 3% of the most abundant proteins in the kidney proteome (excluding the amyloidogenic protein) across all types included amyloid signature proteins,[18,19] serum, and structural proteins (Supplementary Figure S3). Signature proteins accounted for 19% of the proteomic abundance of kidney plaques (interquartile range 12.6%–25%). APOAIV had the largest relative expression of signature proteins despite the lowest overall proteomic count, whereas AH/ALH had the lowest (Supplementary Figure S4). The abundance trends for each signature protein were similar across proteomic subtypes, with 2 exceptions. Kappa-restricted AL had the highest clusterin abundance, and APOAIV was nearly absent in ALECT2 (Supplementary Figure S4). Similar relative signature protein abundance (median 17%, interquartile range 2%–55%) was seen in cardiac amyloid plaques.[9] These data suggest that the protein deposition dynamics for signature proteins are decoupled to that of other proteins in amyloid plaques but are preserved across tissues, and that AL-K has high levels of protective chaperone clusterin. To understand the major drivers of variability across the entire dataset, we performed principal component (PC) analysis (PCA). PCs 1 through 5 explained 20.5% of the variability in the data (not shown). The top 5% of proteins (25) with the highest absolute loading values for each of the first 5 PCs were involved in pathways relating to apoptotic cleavage of cell adhesion proteins (e.g., DSG1 and PKP1) and laminin family proteins, likely reflecting the differential breakdown of structural integrity caused by the various amyloid types.

AFib, AA, and AApoCII have distinct proteomes
To appreciate how the different amyloid types relate to one another based on their expanded proteomes, we used UMAP to visualize this dataset. This analysis positioned AFib, AA, and AApoCII separately, whereas the other types seemed to congregate in the center of the map (Figure 1). These data suggest that AFib, AA, and AApoCII have very distinct proteomes.

Phenograph identifies 2 ALECT2 and 7 AL proteomic subtypes
We used phenograph to identify proteomic subtypes (Figure 1). As expected, AFib, AA, and AApoCII formed distinct clusters in the periphery of the map, as did AApoAIV in the center. However, AL was characterized by significant heterogeneity, forming 7 distinct clusters. The expected distribution of lambda and kappa cases in AL is approximately 70:30 for lambda:kappa. In 4 of the 7 identified AL clusters, this distribution was largely maintained. However, 2 clusters showed lambda predominance (lambda-like 1,2 with 95% and 89% lambda cases, respectively), and 1 cluster showed kappa predominance (kappa-like, with 99.5% kappa cases). AH, and in some cases ALECT2 and AA, cases were included in some of the AL-rich clusters (Supplementary Figure S5), which suggests that some ALECT2 and AL/AH cases are characterized by some proteomic overlap.

Complement and collagens are the main proteins differentially expressed across various types
We evaluated what drives the AA, AFib, and AApoCII proteomes to be so distinct (Supplementary Spreadsheet; Supplementary Figures S6–S8). Several complement proteins were increased across all 3 types, and for AA, fibrinogen proteins were also increased, consistent with a more inflammatory phenotype. Among the most differentially expressed proteins, some structural proteins, such as fibulin (*FBLN1*), were increased in AA, which could reflect the different amyloid deposition pattern (interstitial/vascular vs. glomerular). Others, such as midkine (*MDK*) in AA, could reflect its more inflammatory phenotype. Collagen proteins were decreased compared to the central clusters. Proteins relating to proteostasis (ubiquitins) were increased in AApoCII only.

We then compared ALECT2 to AL/AH and identified that complement proteins were increased, along with various collagen proteins (Supplementary Figure S9; Supplementary Spreadsheet), whereas various structural proteins, fibrinogen, and 14-3-3 family proteins (gene names *YWHA*) were decreased. However, the differences in structural/collagen proteins seen here and in the case of AA, AFib, and AApoCII could be explained by the different deposition pattern in ALECT2 (predominantly interstitial). Finally, we compared AApoAIV to AL/AH and identified several apolipoproteins that were increased in the former, whereas fibrinogen and several collagen proteins were increased in the latter (Supplementary Figure S10; Supplementary Spreadsheet).

In AL/AH amyloidosis, AL had decreased complement pathway proteins and increased collagen proteins (Supplementary Figure S11; Supplementary Spreadsheet). Comparison of kappa to lambda cases showed that

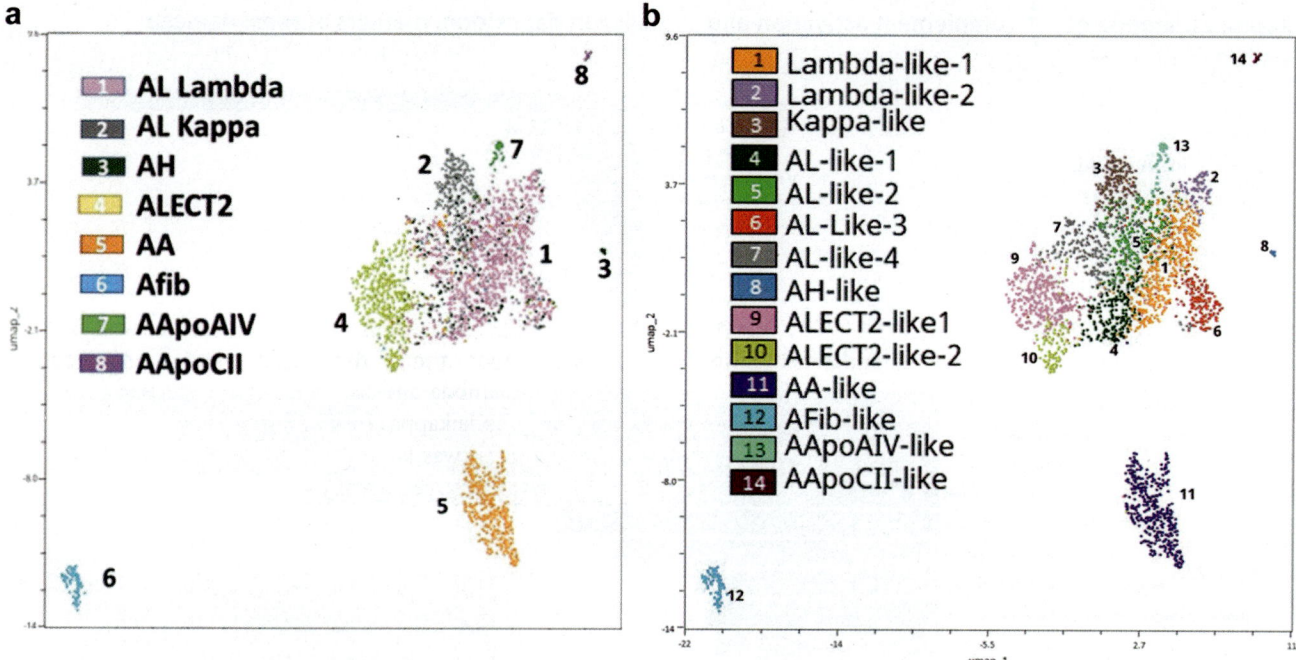

Figure 1 | Uniform manifold approximation and projection (UMAP)–based dimensionality reduction and clustering of most common amyloid types. (**a**) Each dot represents a unique amyloid case. Cases are organized based on proteomic similarity so that cases with more similar proteomes appear closer on the map. This suggests that fibrinogen amyloidosis (AFib), secondary amyloidosis (AA) and Apo C-II amyloidosis (AApoCII) have more distinct proteomes than all other types. (**b**) Phenograph clustering (projected onto the UMAP map) identifies 2 subtypes of LECT2 amyloidosis (ALECT2) and 7 subtypes of light chain amyloidosis (AL). AApoAIV, apo A-IV amyloidosis; AH, heavy chain amyloidosis.

complement pathway proteins were increased, and 14-3-3 family proteins, well-described markers of kidney damage,[20] were decreased (Figures 2 and 3). Of note, the top increased protein in kappa cases was DnaJ heat shock protein (Hsp40) family member B9 (*DNAJB9*), which has been implicated in the development of fibrillary glomerulonephritis,[21–23] suggesting that this protein may be implicated in other diseases in which Ig-based fibrils are present. After lambda Ig genes, plasminogen (*PLG*) was the most increased protein in lambda cases and has been implicated in kidney fibrosis by promoting the epithelial-to-mesenchymal transition.[24]

We then focused on the difference between the 2 ALECT2 subtypes (cluster #9 vs. #10 in Figure 1). Pathways overrepresented within the increased proteins were related to the complement pathway and collagen formation and/or degradation (Supplementary Figure S12; Supplementary Spreadsheet). Pathways overrepresented within the decreased proteins included common serum proteins such as albumin, hemoglobin, haptoglobin, transferrin, serum amyloid A-4 protein (*SAA4*), protein S100-A8, which may reflect a loss of these proteins in the kidney interstitium in cluster 9 or an acute phase reaction *in situ* in cluster 10. Of note, alpha-1-acid glycoprotein 1 (*ORM1*) was the second most increased protein in cluster 10 after *SAA4*; it has been associated with protection from kidney inflammation and fibrosis[25,26] and could represent a compensatory mechanism. *DNAJB9* was again noted to be one of the most increased in cluster 9.

Having described major differences between kappa and lambda AL cases, we evaluated potential differences between the mixed AL-like subclusters. We considered the mixed AL-like clusters 4,5,7 together, because they congregated closer in the UMAP (Figure 1), and compared them with the more distal, mixed AL-like cluster 6. Complement, collagen, and keratin proteins, well-characterized markers of kidney epithelial damage, were overrepresented in clusters 4,5,7.[15] Laminin family and cytoskeletal proteins, heat shock proteins (HSPs), which are thought to have a protective role in various forms of kidney injury,[27] and tubulin family proteins (Supplementary Figure S13; Supplementary Spreadsheet) were decreased. Of note, clusters 4, 5, and 7 were twice as likely to have kidney stage 3 compared to cluster 6 (34% vs. 15%, respectively; $P = 0.03$), which suggests that *HSP* activation may have protective effects in a subset of AL cases.

Finally, to evaluate the impact of deposition patterns (glomerular vs. interstitial vs. perivascular), we evaluated AL cases that had pathology information available and identified 108 cases with glomerular but no interstitial involvement, as well as 32 cases with glomerular but no perivascular involvement, and 11 cases with perivascular but no glomerular involvement, and compared their proteomes. Only 12 proteins were significantly increased in cases with interstitial involvement (Supplementary Spreadsheet). Reassuringly, only collagen alpha-1,2(I) overlapped with some of the proteins seen differentially expressed in the comparisons above. No significant differences were identified between glomerular and

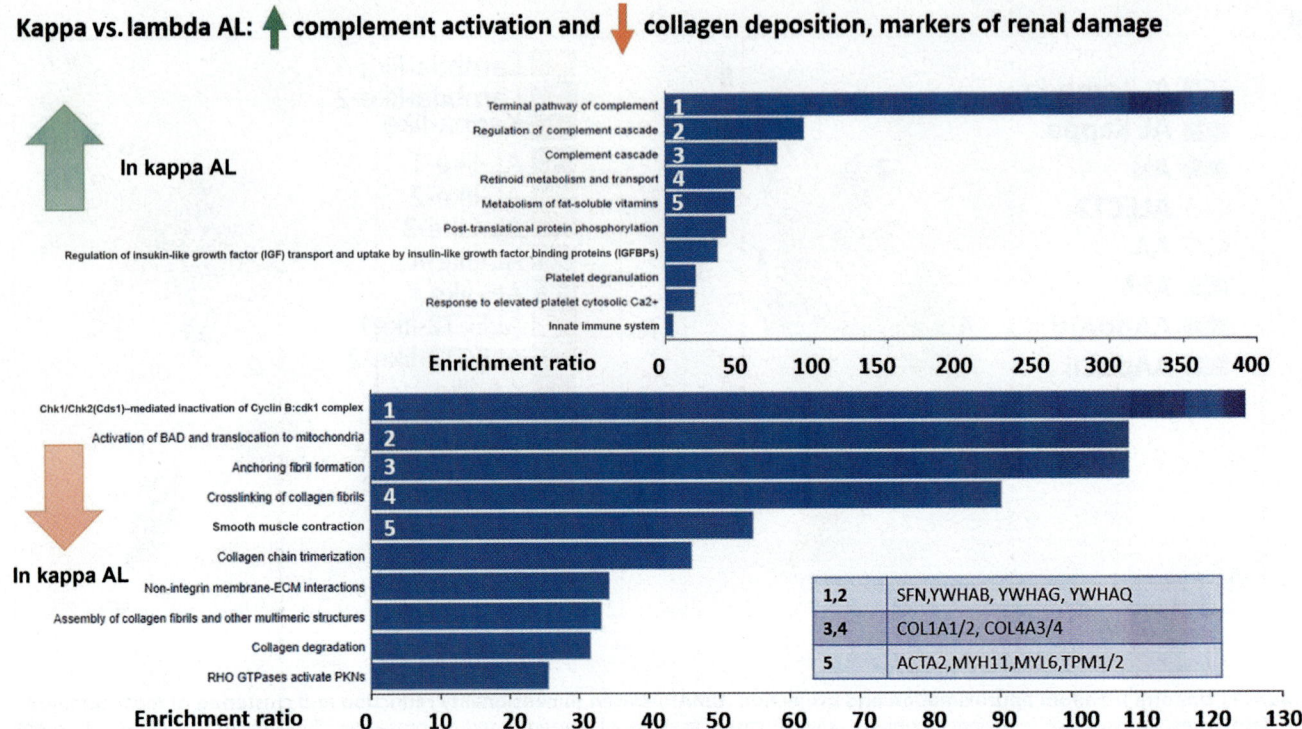

Figure 2 | Pathway analyses (reactome) of proteins that are differentially expressed between kappa and lambda amyloidosis. For kappa, we found increased complement activation and decreased collagen deposition, as well as markers of renal damage. AL, light chain amyloidosis; BAD, BCL2 associated agonist of cell death; Cds1, CDP-diacylglycerol synthase 1; Cdk1, cyclin dependent kinase 1; Chk, choline kinase; ECM, extracellular matrix; GTPase, guanosine triphosphate; PKN, protein kinase N.

perivascular cases, possibly due to the limited number of samples.

The plaque-specific proteomes of kidney AL and AH are highly restricted

Given that many of the proteins identified in amyloid plaques could be part of normal tissue background or nonspecific nephrotic syndrome markers, we compared the expanded proteomes of AL, AH, AApoCII, and AFib to pooled cases from normal controls and from patients with membranous nephropathy. We limited ourselves to these subtypes because of their predominantly glomerular distribution, and LMD samples were taken from controls. The plaque-specific proteome of AL consisted of 24 proteins (Table 2[20,28–37]). The AH plaque proteome was identical to that of AL except for *AHNAK*, Ig heavy constant mu (*IGHM*), and secreted phosphoprotein 2 (*SPP2*), which were unique to AH, and the absence of apolipoprotein A-I (*APOA1*), myosin heavy chain 11 (*MYH11*), H1.0 linker histone (*H1-0*), Ig lambda constant 3 (*IGLC3*), and metallopeptidase inhibitor 3 (*TIMP3*), which were unique to AL (Supplementary Table S1). AFib and AApoCII had a less-restricted plaque proteome with a total of 51 and 43 identified proteins, respectively (Supplementary Spreadsheet), with a predominance of complement pathway proteins (Supplementary Figures S14 and S15). When considering proteins decreased in AL or AH compared to controls (Supplementary Figure S16), ubiquitin-related proteins were among the most decreased in AL compared to controls, suggesting impaired protein processing in AL (Supplementary Spreadsheet). For AFib and AApoCII, heat shock and collagen proteins were decreased (Supplementary Spreadsheet; Supplementary Figures S14 and S15).

The plaque-specific proteome of kappa AL is different from that of lambda AL

Kappa cases had a higher proteomic content than lambda cases (Supplementary Figure S17), including higher ($P < 0.001$ for all) amyloidogenic, complement C6, and signature proteins, except for serum amyloid P-component and *ApoA4*. Plaque-specific proteins significantly lower ($P < 0.001$ for all) in kappa included the following: Tyrosine 3-Monooxygenase/Tryptophan 5-Monooxygenase Activation Protein Beta (*YWHAB*), Alpha-1 antitrypsin, Laccase-3, *IGLC3*, *MYH11*, transgelin, and all the collagen proteins except for *COL6A1* (not shown).

The plaque-specific and expanded proteomes of AL differ according to kidney stage and gender

Of 2650 cases, only 353 were evaluated at our institution and had some clinical information available. Of these, we analyzed the 228 kidney AL patients who had complete clinical follow-up and adequate demographic and clinical data available (Supplementary Table S2). Regarding the plaque-specific proteome, and despite similar overall proteomic content, we found that *YWHAB*, *H1-0*, and moesin (*MSN*) were higher in patients with stage 1 or 2 versus stage

Protein (gene symbol)	Log2 fold change	Protein (gene symbol)	Log2 fold change	Protein (gene symbol)	Log2 fold change
DNAJB9	7.766106	ALB	0.42499	COL4A3	−0.51984
IGKC	4.801048	H2BC1	0.412236	YWHAQ	−0.50284
APOB	3.837124	HSPG2	0.326402	PRDX1	−0.50087
C7	2.186334	APOE	0.297083	FLNA	−0.48534
C8A	2.141322	VTN	0.296005	SERPINA1	−0.4827
C5	1.999357	C3	0.251701	TPM2	−0.45821
C8B	1.596573	IGLC7	−7.45081	APCS	−0.45001
SPP2	1.23396	IGLC1	−4.83142	YWHAB	−0.44653
IGHG4	1.230476	IGLC3	−4.29387	COL3A1	−0.39656
CXCL14	1.189888	IGLC3	−3.94362	EEF1A1	−0.39427
C6	1.161839	IGLC2	−3.8245	HSPB1	−0.38764
APOA2	1.158891	PLG	−1.58155	COL1A2	−0.34061
TTR	1.110925	ATP5F1A	−1.17429	EEF1A1P5	−0.32894
AMBP	1.107204	GATM	−1.12204	COL1A1	−0.32412
CLU	1.027796	MLRN	−1.03058	MYL6	−0.28277
FN1	0.863618	LAC3	−1.02334	APOA4	−0.26459
IGHG1	0.842007	ATP5F1B	−0.99087	LMNA	−0.2545
CFHR5	0.817226	SFN	−0.74861	H3-4	−0.23036
NPNT	0.785676	TPM1	−0.66684	H4C1	−0.22728
TF	0.757747	MYH11	−0.65196	H1-4	−0.21333
MFGE8	0.749248	TAGLN	−0.64567	H3C13	−0.21215
C9	0.669253	ACTA2	−0.57452	H3C1	−0.2106
MDK	0.65542	YWHAG	−0.57195	H2BC13	−0.16476
FGA	0.623313	COL4A4	−0.52514	VIM	−0.10963

Figure 3 | List of proteins differentially expressed between kappa versus lambda light chain AL amyloidosis. Proteins in green are increased and in red decreased in kappa compared to lambda cases. A false detection rate–corrected P value of < 0.05 was considered significant for all proteins.

3 disease; these proteins are associated with amyloid fibrils in other types of amyloid[38,39] (false detection rate $P < 0.05$ for all, not shown). Clusterin was higher in patients with stage 3. In the expanded proteome, patients with kidney stage 3 had higher levels of fibrinogen and alpha-2-microglobulin (Figure 4; Supplementary Spreadsheet), all markers of progressive kidney dysfunction,[40–42] and higher levels of complement pathway proteins. Despite a similar protein burden, several proteins were increased in female versus male patients, including several histone proteins, complement C8b, and clusterin (Supplementary Spreadsheet). Except for complement, no other pathways were significantly over or underrepresented (not shown). Whether these are amyloid-specific differences or generally observed differences between male and female patients is unclear, although complement proteins are generally higher in male patients.[43]

A plaque-specific proteomic signature is associated with improved kidney survival

To identify patterns of plaque-specific deposition, we used hierarchical clustering to group AL cases with available clinical data based on their plaque-specific proteome. We identified 4 major clusters (Figure 5). The distribution of the expanded proteome clusters (Figure 1) within the amyloid-specific proteome clusters (Figure 5) is shown in Supplementary Figure S18. AL-like-3 cluster (expanded proteome) and Lambda-like-2 cluster (expanded proteome) were overrepresented in cluster 1 (33.1% vs. 16.6%, $P < 0.001$, and 44.8% vs. 8%, $P < 0.001$, respectively). The major differences in (amyloid-specific) protein abundance are shown in Supplementary Figure S19A–C. Clusters 1 and 4 had the highest protein abundance but the lowest light chain deposition, suggesting that the dynamics of the light chain deposition differ from those of the total proteome, similar to what we have shown in the heart.[9] We explored whether any of these groups correlated with different kidney outcomes and found that cluster 1 was associated with improved kidney survival compared to the rest (Figure 6). In a multivariable analysis (not shown) that includes cluster 1 status and kidney stage, this effect was not independent ($P > 0.05$) of kidney stage, and indeed, cluster 1 was more likely to have a lower kidney stage (97% kidney stage 1 or 2 vs. 72%, $P = 0.001$). Cluster 1 had the highest levels of YWHAB, H1-0, MSN, S100A6, Thymosin beta-4 (TMSB4X), and Usherin (USH2A), and the lowest levels of TIMP3 and vitronectin. Collagen proteins and TIMP3 clustered predominantly in clusters 3 and 4 and transgelin (TAGLN) in cluster 4, whereas complement 6 was deposited at very low levels in cluster 4 (Figure 5; Supplementary Figure S19B and

Table 2 | The plaque-specific proteome of AL amyloidosis (proteins increased in AL vs. normal or disease controls)

Protein	Function in kidneys	Log2 fold change	FDR corrected P value
COL1A2 Collagen alpha-2(I) chain	Collagen protein.	22.74	<0.0001
COL1A1 Collagen alpha-1(I) chain	Collagen protein.	22.43	<0.0001
APOA4 Apolipoprotein A-IV	Signature protein.	22.35	<0.0001
TAGLN Transgelin	Implicated in several types of kidney disease.[28]	21.92	0.009
COL3A1 Collagen alpha-1(III) chain	Collagen protein.	21.82	<0.0001
TIMP3 Metallopeptidase Inhibitor 3	Implicated in several types of kidney disease.[29,30]	21.59	0.008
H1-0 Histone H1.0	Unclear.	21.52	0.02
C6 Complement component 6	Complement activation.	21.5	0.03
MYH11 Myosin heavy chain 11	Structural.	21.45	0.02
HSPB1 Heat shock protein beta-1	Increased in response to kidney insults. Chaperone activity. Protects from complement-mediated kidney epithelial injury.[31,32]	21.23	0.005
USH2A Usherin	Unclear.	20.94	0.0007
TMSB4X Thymosin beta 4	Implicated in several types of kidney disease.[33]	20.6	0.01
MSN Moesin	Implicated in several types of kidney disease.[34,35]	20.4	0.02
IGLC3 Ig lambda constant 3	Amyloidogenic protein.	5.45	0.0003
SERPINA1 Alpha-1 antitrypsin	Marker of kidney damage in other nephrotic syndromes.[36]	5.24	0.02
COL6A1 Collagen alpha-1(VI) chain	Collagen protein.	4.64	0.04
LAC3 Laccase-3	Unclear.	4.61	0.007
APCS Serum amyloid P-component	Signature protein.	4.54	<0.0001
APOE Apolipoprotein E	Signature protein.	4.39	<0.0001
VTN Vitronectin	Signature protein.	4.06	<0.0001
APOA1 Apolipoprotein A-I	Unclear.	3.79	0.02
CLU Clusterin	Signature protein.	3.56	<0.0001
S100A6 Protein S100-A6	Kidney damage marker.[37]	3.22	<0.0001
YWHAB Tyrosine 3-Monooxygenase/tryptophan 5-monooxygenase activation protein beta	Regulates large spectrum of signaling pathways, including several implicated in kidney disease.[20]	2.9	0.04

AL, light chain; FDR, false detection rate.

C). When considering the expanded proteome of cluster 1 compared to the other clusters, 14-3-3 family proteins (*YWHA*) were increased, whereas collagen proteins were decreased (Supplementary Figure S20; Supplementary Spreadsheet). *TMSB4X* was the most increased protein in cluster 1, and its loss has been implicated in accelerated kidney fibrosis.[44] Galectin-1 (*LGALS1*) was among the highest expressed proteins and has anti-ischemic and anti-inflammatory effects in the kidney.[45,46] These data suggest that proteins relating to matrix remodeling (collagens, TIMP3) deposit in different patterns and that lower levels of matrix fibrosis may be responsible for the improved kidney survival seen in cluster 1.

DISCUSSION

This study is the first to comprehensively examine the proteomic content of the amyloidosis plaque in the kidney. Key findings include that the more indolent (non-AL) amyloid types have a higher proteomic content than AL. The complement cascade was the most overrepresented pathway across all types, and was responsible for most of the differences across various disease types. We show that AA, AFib,

basic research

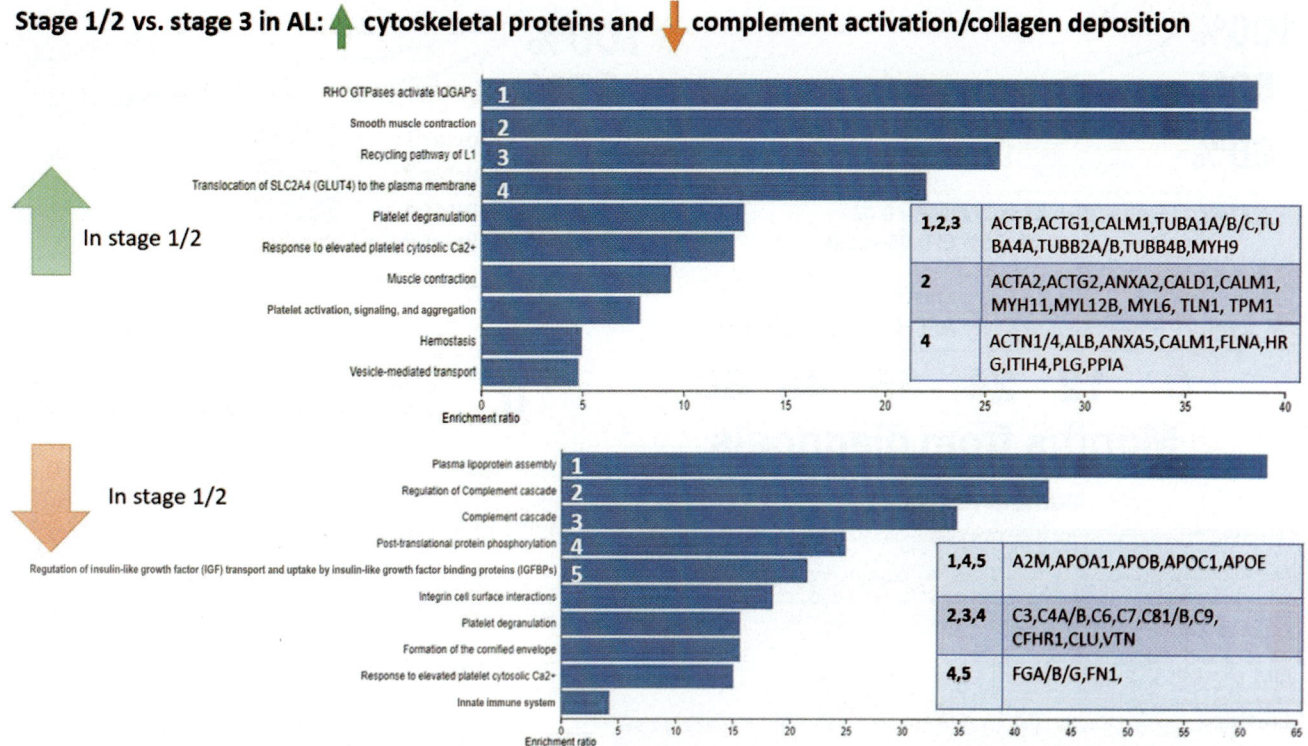

Figure 4 | Pathway analyses (reactome) of differentially expressed proteins between light chain amyloidosis (AL) kidney stage 1/2 compared to kidney stage 3. For kidney stage 1/2, we found increased cytoskeletal proteins and decreased collagen activation, as well as markers of kidney damage. GTPase, guanosine triphosphate; IQGAPs, IQ motif containing GTPase activating protein.

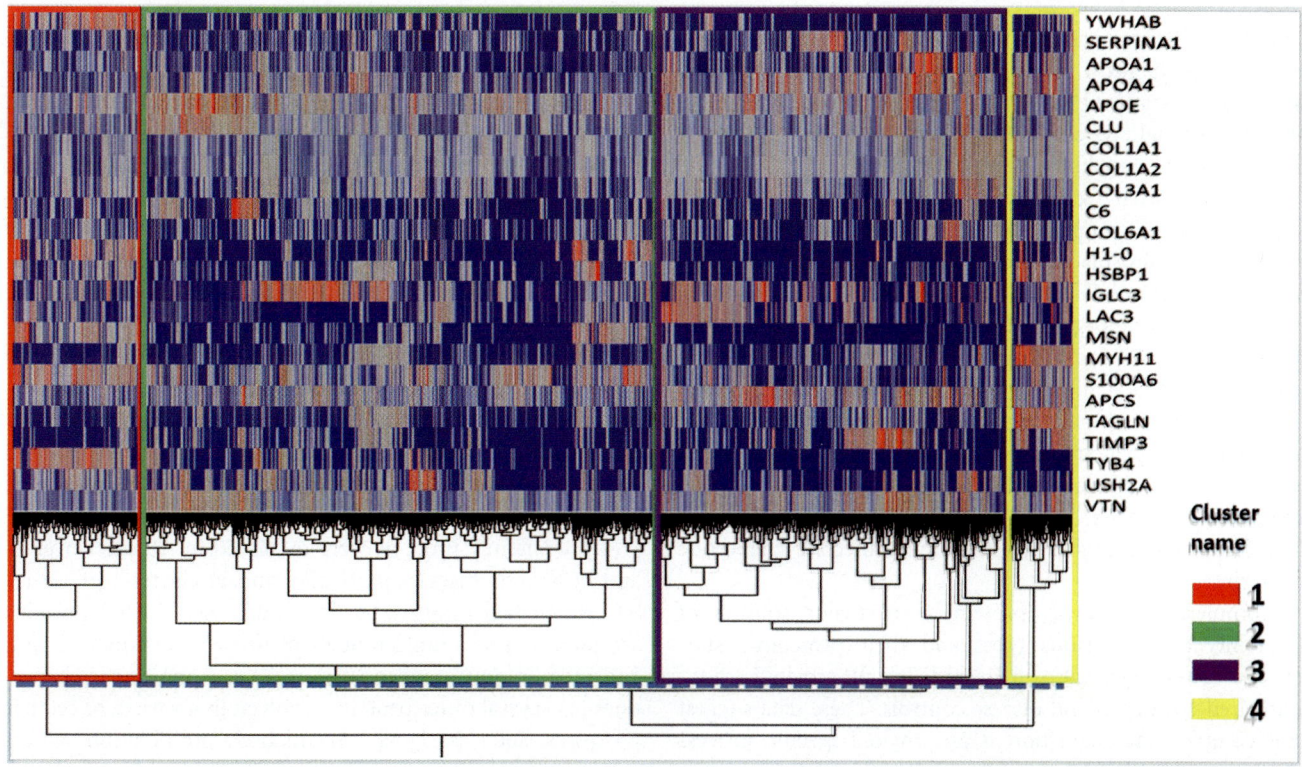

Figure 5 | Hierarchical clustering of light chain amyloidosis (AL) cases with available clinical data, based on their plaque-specific proteome. We identified 4 major clusters. Cluster 1 had increased proteomic burden and increased levels of 14-3-3 family proteins.

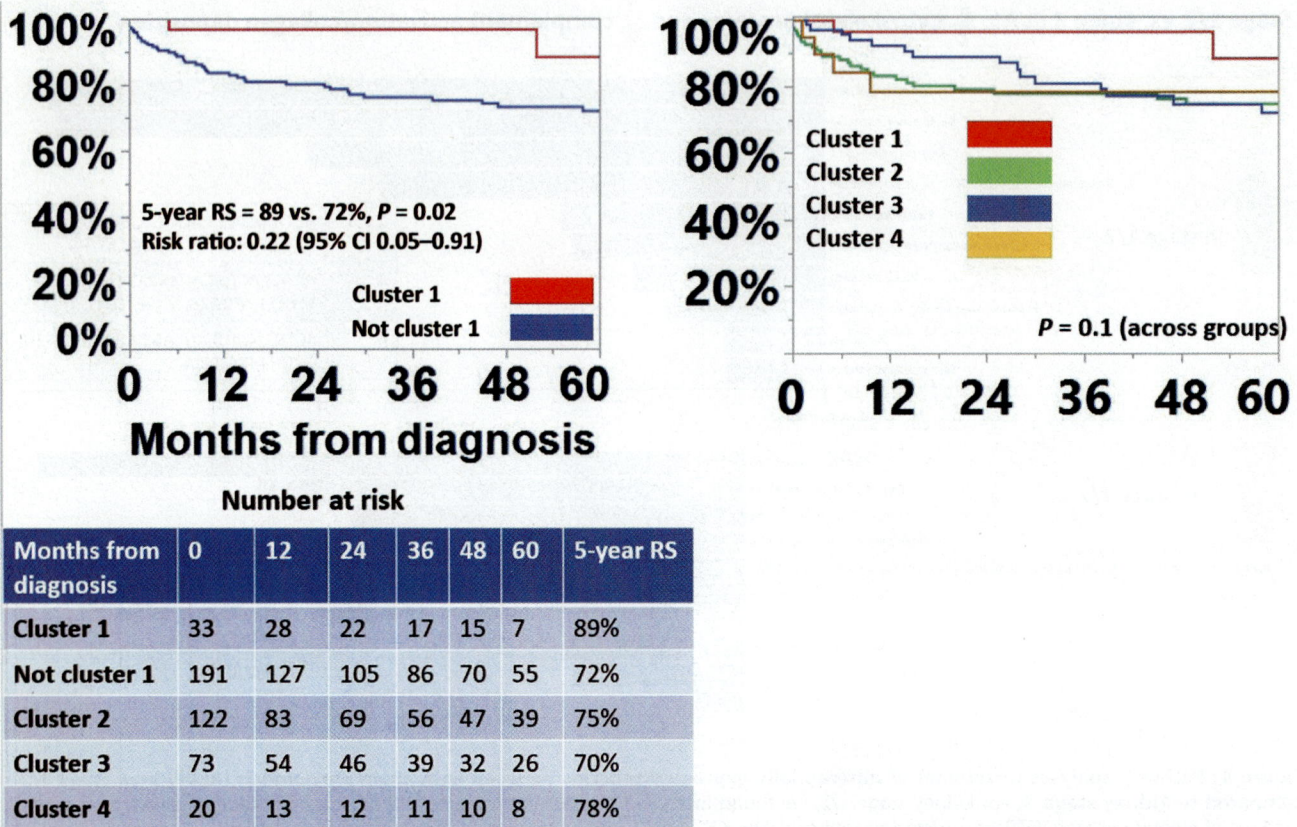

Figure 6 | Kaplan-Meier curve comparing kidney survival (time to dialysis or patient death) between patients in cluster 1 and all other clusters. Cluster 1 had improved kidney survival, compared to other proteomic clusters. CI, confidence interval; RS, renal survival.

and AApoCII are distinct proteomically and that AL and ALECT2 are the most heterogeneous. Finally, we show that a subset of AL patients with high proteomic content but low amounts of light chains and proteins involved in kidney fibrosis has the best kidney survival.

Similar to what we have shown for cardiac transthyretin amyloid (ATTR) compared to AL, the more rapidly evolving AL had the lowest plaque proteomic content, which suggests that the proteomic "density" of amyloid plaques may be a surrogate of more indolent disease progression.[9] In addition, patients with AL and worse kidney outcomes had higher levels of amyloidogenic light chains but lower overall proteomic content, suggesting that the deposition dynamics of amyloidogenic proteins are decoupled from that of other proteins. Kappa AL cases, associated with improved survival compared to lambda,[47] also had a higher proteomic burden than lambda and higher levels of the protective chaperone clusterin.

Complement pathway proteins were major sources of variability across various types and their proteomic subgroups. They were also increased in all amyloid cases, compared to normal and disease controls. These data suggest that complement deposition is an amyloid-specific process seen in most amyloid types. In addition to systemic deposition, our group previously has shown upregulation of complement genes after exposure to AL fibrils in cultured cardiomyocytes in vitro.[48] This finding suggests that complement may be produced in situ and may represent a form of an atypical response to pathogen. To what extent complement activation is responsible for kidney tissue damage is unclear.

We noted a relative decrease of ubiquitins and heat shock proteins in AL, AH, AApoCII, and AFib patients, compared to controls. Indeed, amyloid proteins cause a reduction of free ubiquitin levels in in vitro models of Alzheimer's disease.[49] This reduction may reflect the overutilization of these proteins by the ubiquitin–proteasome system. The same may be true for heat shock proteins, a well-described group of "anti-amyloid" chaperones that could be amenable to pharmacologic interventions.[50] Ubiquitins and heat shock proteins can be directly sequestered within misfolded protein aggregates, further contributing to the cell's proteostatic collapse.[51-53]

14-3-3 family proteins were increased in AL cases overall, and in lambda cases in particular, and in cluster 1 of kidney AL, which had improved kidney outcomes. 14-3-3 proteins are increased in animal models of ureteric obstruction, IgA, and membranous nephropathy and act as molecular chaperones for several other proteins involved in a variety of cellular processes, such as signal transduction, proliferation, differentiation, apoptosis, and autophagy.[54] They have been shown to interact directly with other amyloid types where they promote amyloid clearance.[55,56]

The AL-specific proteome was enriched in some proteins of interest to kidney pathologies, such as HSPB1, S100A6, TAGLN, and TIMP3. HSPB1 increases and induces autophagy in acute kidney injury,[31] which also is induced in response to misfolded proteins. S100A6, a calcium-binding protein, is increased in acute kidney injury and may decrease beta-amyloid deposition in animal models of Alzheimer's disease.[37,57] TAGLN interacts with cytoskeletal proteins and is induced by amyloid precursor protein in Alzheimer's disease.[58] Finally, TIMP3, also a component of the cardiac amyloid proteome, could be related to matrix remodeling and fibrosis in AL.[9]

We found that proteins associated with the protection from oxidative stress were increased in the early stages. Glutathione-S transferase (GST) and phosphatidylethanolamine-binding protein 1 (PEB1) were the most upregulated proteins in the proteome of early-stage amyloidosis. Both proteins act as antioxidants, with PEB1 being a major regulator of the ferroptosis pathway.[59,60] Studies from cardiomyocytes demonstrate that AL fibrils induce cell death through oxidative stress,[61,62] which suggests an organ-wide mechanism of cellular toxicity. On the other hand, we did not note proteins associated with autophagy, unlike what we have noted in the heart[9] and in *in vitro* models,[63] suggesting that this is a cardiac-specific mechanism of tissue damage.

Our study had limitations. Our definition of amyloid-specific proteome was conservative. In addition, although LMD/MS has high accuracy and has been extensively validated, the risk of contamination by normal tissue or serum proteins was possible, though unlikely. We generally expect kidney tissue to have several thousands of proteins identified,[64,65] and not the less than 500 proteins identified here. Therefore, if any samples were significantly contaminated by adjacent normal tissue, this would have been reflected in the identified proteomic diversity. Similarly, the lack of proteomic information from adjacent kidney tissue containing live cellular material is another limitation. Indeed, the kidney proteome presents us with only remnant proteins of dying kidney cells that adhere to amyloid plaques. Therefore, they are not fully representative of the complex physiological responses occurring in the tissue. Many of the identified differences in structural proteins could be attributed to differences in amyloid deposition patterns across the various types (e.g., interstitial, perivascular, glomerular). However, only a limited number of AL cases had complete pathology information and pure glomerular/interstitial/perivascular involvement to be used to compare these compartments proteomically. Finally, we did not have enough clinical data for comparisons for all the amyloid types, and thus, clinical correlations were restricted to AL. Even within this subtype, only a small number of patients had enough clinical information to perform additional analyses based on proteomic subtypes, which limited the statistical power of this study. Our analyses in relationship to some of these outcomes should, therefore, be considered exploratory and in need of additional validation.

DISCLOSURE
All the authors declared no competing interests.

DATA STATEMENT
All raw and proccessed, anonymized proteomic data used for this article have been deposited to zenodo in 9 separate batches, available at https://zenodo.org/record/8347058, https://zenodo.org/record/8350517, https://zenodo.org/record/8350765, https://zenodo.org/record/8351623, https://zenodo.org/record/8352367, https://zenodo.org/record/8352939, https://zenodo.org/record/8353759, https://zenodo.org/record/8355053, and https://zenodo.org/record/8357105.

ACKNOWLEDGMENTS
The authors acknowledge the patients for allowing use of their biopsy data for research purposes.

FUNDING
This work was supported by the Paul Calabresi K12 Career Development Award (CA90628-21), the Mayo Clinic Myeloma SPORE, and an Amyloidosis Research Foundation research grant.

SUPPLEMENTARY MATERIAL
Supplementary File (PowerPoint)
Supplementary Figure S1. Total proteomic burden across types and pathways associated with identified proteins.
Supplementary Figure S2. Overlap of kidney and cardiac amyloid proteomes.
Supplementary Figure S3. Top 3% (N = 15) most abundant proteins (excluding amyloidogenic protein).
Supplementary Figure S4. Relative abundance of signature proteins compared to total proteomic count by amyloid type.
Supplementary Figure S5. Relative proportions of various amyloid types identified within phenograph clusters.
Supplementary Figure S6. Pathway analyses (reactome) of differentially expressed proteins between the secondary amyloidosis (AA) cluster and all the central clusters (non-fibrinogen amyloidosis [AFib]/Apo C-II amyloidosis [AApoCII]).
Supplementary Figure S7. Pathway analyses (reactome) of differentially expressed proteins between the fibrinogen amyloidosis (AFib) cluster and all the central clusters (non-secondary amyloidosis [AA]/Apo C-II amyloidosis [AApoCII]).
Supplementary Figure S8. Pathway analyses (reactome) of differentially expressed proteins between the Apo C-II amyloidosis (AApoCII) cluster and all the central clusters (non-secondary amyloidosis [AA]/fibrinogen amyloidosis [AFib]).
Supplementary Figure S9. Pathway analyses (reactome) of differentially expressed proteins between the leukocyte chemotactic factor-2-type (ALECT2) cluster and light chain/heavy chain amyloidosis (AL/AH).
Supplementary Figure S10. Pathway analyses (reactome) of differentially expressed proteins between apo AIV (AApoAIV) cluster and light chain/heavy chain amyloidosis (AL/AH).
Supplementary Figure S11. Pathway analyses (reactome) of differentially expressed proteins between the light chain (AL) and heavy chain (AH) amyloidosis.

Supplementary Figure S12. Pathway analyses (reactome) of differentially expressed proteins between the leukocyte chemotactic factor-2-type (ALECT2) clusters.
Supplementary Figure S13. Pathway analyses (reactome) of differentially expressed proteins between the clusters 4,5,7 and cluster 6 in light chain amyloidosis (AL).
Supplementary Figure S14. Pathway analyses (reactome) of differentially expressed proteins between the fibrinogen amyloidosis (AFib) versus normal and disease controls.
Supplementary Figure S15. Pathway analyses (reactome) of differentially expressed proteins between the Apo C-II amyloidosis (AApoCII) versus normal and disease controls.
Supplementary Figure S16. Pathway analyses (reactome) of differentially decreased proteins between the light chain/heavy chain amyloidosis (AL/AH) versus normal and disease controls.
Supplementary Figure S17. Total protein abundance, amyloidogenic, and signature protein abundance of kappa versus lambda light chain amyloidosis (AL).
Supplementary Figure S18. Relative proportions of expanded amyloid proteome clusters identified within amyloid-specific clusters.
Supplementary Ffigure S19 (**A**) Major differences in protein abundance among the 4 clusters. (**B**) Major differences in protein abundance between the four clusters. (**C**) Major differences in protein abundance among the 4 clusters.
Supplementary Figure S20. Pathway analyses (reactome) of differentially expressed proteins between cluster 1 and the remaining light chain amyloidosis (AL) clusters.
Supplementary Table S1. The plaque-specific proteome of heavy chain amyloidosis (AH; proteins increased in AH compared to normal/disease controls).
Supplementary Table S2. Baseline demographic and clinical data of 228 kidney light chain amyloidosis (AL) patients with clinical information.
Supplementary File (Excel)
Supplementary Spreadsheet. This spreadsheet contains all the proccessed, anonymized proteomic data and clinicolaboratory information required to recreate the study. The unique ID column is a unique identifier linked to the raw proteomic data that have been deposited to zenodo.

REFERENCES

1. Benson MD, Buxbaum JN, Eisenberg DS, et al. Amyloid nomenclature 2020: update and recommendations by the International Society of Amyloidosis (ISA) Nomenclature Committee. *Amyloid*. 2020;27:217–222.
2. Dasari S, Theis JD, Vrana JA, et al. Amyloid typing by mass spectrometry in clinical practice: a comprehensive review of 16,175 samples. *Mayo Clin Proc*. 2020;95:1852–1864.
3. Vrana JA, Gamez JD, Madden BJ, et al. Classification of amyloidosis by laser microdissection and mass spectrometry-based proteomic analysis in clinical biopsy specimens. *Blood*. 2009;114:4957–4959.
4. Sethi S, Theis JD, Leung N, et al. Mass spectrometry-based proteomic diagnosis of renal immunoglobulin heavy chain amyloidosis. *Clin J Am Soc Nephrol*. 2010;5:2180–2187.
5. Vrana JA, Theis JD, Dasari S, et al. Clinical diagnosis and typing of systemic amyloidosis in subcutaneous fat aspirates by mass spectrometry-based proteomics. *Haematologica*. 2014;99:1239–1247.
6. Sethi S, Vrana JA, Theis JD, et al. Laser microdissection and mass spectrometry-based proteomics aids the diagnosis and typing of renal amyloidosis. *Kidney Int*. 2012;82:226–234.
7. Poon S, Easterbrook-Smith SB, Rybchyn MS, et al. Clusterin is an ATP-independent chaperone with very broad substrate specificity that stabilizes stressed proteins in a folding-competent state. *Biochemistry*. 2000;39:15953–15960.
8. Palladini G, Hegenbart U, Milani P, et al. A staging system for renal outcome and early markers of renal response to chemotherapy in AL amyloidosis. *Blood*. 2014;124:2325–2332.
9. Kourelis TV, Dasari SS, Dispenzieri A, et al. A proteomic atlas of cardiac amyloid plaques. *JACC CardioOncol*. 2020;2:632–643.
10. Becht E, McInnes L, Healy J, et al. Dimensionality reduction for visualizing single-cell data using UMAP. *Nat Biotechnol*. 2019;37:38–44.
11. Levine JH, Simonds EF, Bendall SC, et al. Data-driven phenotypic dissection of AML reveals progenitor-like cells that correlate with prognosis. *Cell*. 2015;162:184–197.
12. Liao Y, Wang J, Jaehnig EJ, et al. WebGestalt 2019: gene set analysis toolkit with revamped UIs and APIs. *Nucleic Acids Res*. 2019;47:W199–w205.
13. Canton J, Neculai D, Grinstein S. Scavenger receptors in homeostasis and immunity. *Nat Rev Immunol*. 2013;13:621–634.
14. Papathanasiou S, Rickelt S, Soriano ME, et al. Tumor necrosis factor-alpha confers cardioprotection through ectopic expression of keratins K8 and K18. *Nat Med*. 2015;21:1076–1084.
15. Djudjaj S, Papasotiriou M, Bülow RD, et al. Keratins are novel markers of renal epithelial cell injury. *Kidney Int*. 2016;89:792–808.
16. Manissorn J, Khamchun S, Vinaiphat A, Thongboonkerd V. Alpha-tubulin enhanced renal tubular cell proliferation and tissue repair but reduced cell death and cell-crystal adhesion. *Sci Rep*. 2016;6:28808.
17. Han SJ, Kim JH, Kim JI, Park KM. Inhibition of microtubule dynamics impedes repair of kidney ischemia/reperfusion injury and increases fibrosis. *Sci Rep*. 2016;6:27775.
18. Rognoni P, Mazzini G, Caminito S, et al. Dissecting the molecular features of systemic light chain (AL) amyloidosis: contributions from proteomics. *Medicina (Kaunas)*. 2021;57:916.
19. Mollee P, Boros S, Loo D, et al. Implementation and evaluation of amyloidosis subtyping by laser-capture microdissection and tandem mass spectrometry. *Clin Proteomics*. 2016;13:30.
20. Rizou M, Frangou EA, Marineli F, et al. The family of 14-3-3 proteins and specifically 14-3-3σ are up-regulated during the development of renal pathologies. *J Cell Mol Med*. 2018;22:4139–4149.
21. Dasari S, Alexander MP, Vrana JA, et al. DnaJ heat shock protein family b member 9 is a novel biomarker for fibrillary GN. *J Am Soc Nephrol*. 2018;29:51–56.
22. Nasr SH, Vrana JA, Dasari S, et al. DNAJB9 is a specific immunohistochemical marker for fibrillary glomerulonephritis. *Kidney Int Rep*. 2017;3:56–64.
23. Andeen NK, Yang HY, Dai DF, et al. DnaJ homolog subfamily B member 9 is a putative autoantigen in fibrillary GN. *J Am Soc Nephrol*. 2018;29:231–239.
24. Zhang G, Kernan KA, Collins SJ, et al. Plasmin(ogen) promotes renal interstitial fibrosis by promoting epithelial-to-mesenchymal transition: role of plasmin-activated signals. *J Am Soc Nephrol*. 2007;18:846–859.
25. Bi J, Watanabe H, Fujimura R, et al. A downstream molecule of 1,25-dihydroxyvitamin D3, alpha-1-acid glycoprotein, protects against mouse model of renal fibrosis. *Sci Rep*. 2018;8:17329.
26. Watanabe H, Fujimura R, Hiramoto Y, et al. An acute phase protein α(1)-acid glycoprotein mitigates AKI and its progression to CKD through its anti-inflammatory action. *Sci Rep*. 2021;11:7953.
27. Nayak Rao S. The role of heat shock proteins in kidney disease. *J Transl Int Med*. 2016;4:114–117.
28. Marshall CB, Krofft RD, Blonski MJ, et al. Role of smooth muscle protein SM22alpha in glomerular epithelial cell injury. *Am J Physiol Renal Physiol*. 2011;300:F1026–F1042.
29. Fiorentino L, Cavalera M, Menini S, et al. Loss of TIMP3 underlies diabetic nephropathy via FoxO1/STAT1 interplay. *EMBO Mol Med*. 2013;5:441–455.
30. Wang Z, Famulski K, Lee J, et al. TIMP2 and TIMP3 have divergent roles in early renal tubulointerstitial injury. *Kidney Int*. 2014;85:82–93.
31. Matsumoto T, Urushido M, Ide H, et al. Small heat shock protein beta-1 (HSPB1) is upregulated and regulates autophagy and apoptosis of renal tubular cells in acute kidney injury. *PLoS One*. 2015;10:e0126229.
32. Sanchez-Nino MD, Sanz AB, Sanchez-Lopez E, et al. HSP27/HSPB1 as an adaptive podocyte antiapoptotic protein activated by high glucose and angiotensin II. *Lab Invest*. 2012;92:32–45.
33. Mason WJ, Vasilopoulou E. The pathophysiological role of thymosin beta4 in the kidney glomerulus. *Int J Mol Sci*. 2023;24:7684.
34. Caster DJ, Korte EA, Merchant ML, et al. Patients with proliferative lupus nephritis have autoantibodies that react to moesin and demonstrate increased glomerular moesin expression. *J Clin Med*. 2021;10:793.
35. Chen YX, Zhang W, Wang WM, et al. Role of moesin in renal fibrosis. *PLoS One*. 2014;9:e112936.

36. Candiano G, Musante L, Bruschi M, et al. Repetitive fragmentation products of albumin and alpha1-antitrypsin in glomerular diseases associated with nephrotic syndrome. *J Am Soc Nephrol*. 2006;17:3139–3148.
37. Cheng CW, Rifai A, Ka SM, et al. Calcium-binding proteins annexin A2 and S100A6 are sensors of tubular injury and recovery in acute renal failure. *Kidney Int*. 2005;68:2694–2703.
38. Duce JA, Smith DP, Blake RE, et al. Linker histone H1 binds to disease associated amyloid-like fibrils. *J Mol Biol*. 2006;361:493–505.
39. Darmellah A, Rayah A, Auger R, et al. Ezrin/radixin/moesin are required for the purinergic P2X7 receptor (P2X7R)-dependent processing of the amyloid precursor protein. *J Biol Chem*. 2012;287:34583–34595.
40. Randles M, Lausecker F, Kong Q, et al. Identification of an altered matrix signature in kidney aging and disease. *J Am Soc Nephrol*. 2021;32:1713–1732.
41. Yang AH, Chen JY. Glomerular deposition of alpha 2-macroglobulin in glomerular diseases. *Nephrol Dial Transplant*. 1997;12:465–469.
42. Motojima M, Matsusaka T, Kon V, Ichikawa I. Fibrinogen that appears in Bowman's space of proteinuric kidneys in vivo activates podocyte Toll-like receptors 2 and 4 in vitro. *Nephron Exp Nephrol*. 2010;114:e39–e47.
43. Gaya da Costa M, Poppelaars F, van Kooten C, et al. Age and sex-associated changes of complement activity and complement levels in a healthy Caucasian population. *Front Immunol*. 2018;9:2664.
44. Vasilopoulou E, Kolatsi-Joannou M, Lindenmeyer MT, et al. Loss of endogenous thymosin β(4) accelerates glomerular disease. *Kidney Int*. 2016;90:1056–1070.
45. Gu M, Mei X, Zhao Y. Galectins as potential pharmacological targets in renal injuries of diverse etiology. *Eur J Pharmacol*. 2020;881:173213.
46. Carlos CP, Silva AA, Gil CD, Oliani SM. Pharmacological treatment with galectin-1 protects against renal ischaemia-reperfusion injury. *Sci Rep*. 2018;8:9568.
47. Sidiqi MH, Aljama MA, Muchtar E, et al. Light chain type predicts organ involvement and survival in AL amyloidosis patients receiving stem cell transplantation. *Blood Adv*. 2018;2:769–776.
48. Jordan TL, Maar K, Redhage KR, et al. Light chain amyloidosis induced inflammatory changes in cardiomyocytes and adipose-derived mesenchymal stromal cells. *Leukemia*. 2020;34:1383–1393.
49. Park CW, Jung BK, Ryu KY. Reduced free ubiquitin levels and proteasome activity in cultured neurons and brain tissues treated with amyloid beta aggregates. *Mol Brain*. 2020;13:89.
50. Balana AT, Levine PM, Craven TW, et al. O-GlcNAc modification of small heat shock proteins enhances their anti-amyloid chaperone activity. *Nat Chem*. 2021;13:441–450.
51. Park SH, Kukushkin Y, Gupta R, et al. PolyQ proteins interfere with nuclear degradation of cytosolic proteins by sequestering the Sis1p chaperone. *Cell*. 2013;154:134–145.
52. Boronat S, Cabrera M, Hidalgo E. Spatial sequestration of misfolded proteins as an active chaperone-mediated process during heat stress. *Curr Genet*. 2021;67:237–243.
53. Eisele F, Eisele-Burger AM, Hao X, et al. An Hsp90 co-chaperone links protein folding and degradation and is part of a conserved protein quality control. *Cell Rep*. 2021;35:109328.
54. Aghazadeh Y, Papadopoulos V. The role of the 14-3-3 protein family in health, disease, and drug development. *Drug Discov Today*. 2016;21:278–287.
55. Williams DM, Thorn DC, Dobson CM, et al. The amyloid fibril-forming β-sheet regions of amyloid β and α-synuclein preferentially interact with the molecular chaperone 14-3-3ζ. *Molecules*. 2021;26:6120.
56. Herod SG, Dyatel A, Hodapp S, et al. Clearance of an amyloid-like translational repressor is governed by 14-3-3 proteins. *Cell Rep*. 2022;39:110753.
57. Tian ZY, Wang CY, Wang T, et al. Glial S100A6 degrades β-amyloid aggregation through targeting competition with zinc ions. *Aging Dis*. 2019;10:756–769.
58. Müller T, Concannon CG, Ward MW, et al. Modulation of gene expression and cytoskeletal dynamics by the amyloid precursor protein intracellular domain (AICD). *Mol Biol Cell*. 2007;18:201–210.
59. Wenzel SE, Tyurina YY, Zhao J, et al. PEBP1 wardens ferroptosis by enabling lipoxygenase generation of lipid death signals. *Cell*. 2017;171:628–641.e26.
60. Pasten C, Herrera-Luna Y, Lozano M, et al. Glutathione S-transferase and clusterin, new players in the ischemic preconditioning renal protection in a murine model of ischemia and reperfusion. *Cell Physiol Biochem*. 2021;55:635–650.
61. Imperlini E, Gnecchi M, Rognoni P, et al. Proteotoxicity in cardiac amyloidosis: amyloidogenic light chains affect the levels of intracellular proteins in human heart cells. *Sci Rep*. 2017;7:15661.
62. Shi J, Guan J, Jiang B, et al. Amyloidogenic light chains induce cardiomyocyte contractile dysfunction and apoptosis via a non-canonical p38alpha MAPK pathway. *Proc Natl Acad Sci U S A*. 2010;107:4188–4193.
63. Zhang Y, Yu W, Chang W, et al. Light chain amyloidosis-induced autophagy is mediated by the Foxo3a/Beclin-1 pathway in cardiomyocytes. *Lab Invest*. 2023;103:100001.
64. Kim MS, Pinto SM, Getnet D, et al. A draft map of the human proteome. *Nature*. 2014;509:575–581.
65. Wilhelm M, Schlegl J, Hahne H, et al. Mass-spectrometry-based draft of the human proteome. *Nature*. 2014;509:582–587.

basic research

In vivo base editing rescues primary hyperoxaluria type 1 in rats

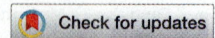

see commentary on page 430

Zhoutong Chen[1,5], Dexin Zhang[2,5], Rui Zheng[3,5], Lei Yang[4], Yanan Huo[4], Dan Zhang[4], Xiaoliang Fang[1], Yueyan Li[3], Guofeng Xu[3], Dali Li[4] and Hongquan Geng[1]

[1]Department of Urology, Children's Hospital of Fudan University, Shanghai, China; [2]Department of Urology, Xinhua Hospital Affiliated to Shanghai Jiao Tong University School of Medicine, Shanghai, China; [3]Department of Pediatric Urology, Xinhua Hospital Affiliated to Shanghai Jiao Tong University School of Medicine, Shanghai, China; and [4]Shanghai Key Laboratory of Regulatory Biology, Institute of Biomedical Sciences and School of Life Sciences, East China Normal University, Shanghai, China

Primary hyperoxaluria type 1 (PH1) is a childhood-onset autosomal recessive disease, characterized by nephrocalcinosis, multiple recurrent urinary calcium oxalate stones, and a high risk of progressive kidney damage. PH1 is caused by inherent genetic defects of the alanine glyoxylate aminotransferase (AGXT) gene. The in vivo repair of disease-causing genes was exceedingly inefficient before the invention of base editors which can efficiently introduce precisely targeted base alterations without double-strand DNA breaks. Adenine base editor (ABE) can precisely convert A·T to G·C with the assistance of specific guide RNA. Here, we demonstrated that systemic delivery of dual adeno-associated virus encoding a split-ABE8e could artificially repair 13% of the pathogenic allele in $Agxt^{Q84X}$ rats, a model of PH1, alleviating the disease phenotype. Specifically, ABE treatment partially restored the expression of alanine-glyoxylate-aminotransferase (AGT), reduced endogenous oxalate synthesis and alleviated calcium oxalate crystal deposition. Western blot and immunohistochemistry confirmed that ABE8e treatment restored AGT protein expression in hepatocytes. Moreover, the precise editing efficiency in the liver remained stable six months after treatment. Thus, our findings provided a prospect of in vivo base editing as a personalized and precise medicine for PH1 by directly correcting the mutant Agxt gene.

Kidney International (2024) 105, 496–507; https://doi.org/10.1016/j.kint.2023.11.029

KEYWORDS: adeno-associated virus; base editing; gene repair; primary hyperoxaluria

Copyright © 2023, International Society of Nephrology. Published by Elsevier Inc. All rights reserved.

Correspondence: Hongquan Geng, Department of Urology, Children's Hospital of Fudan University, No. 399, Wanyuan Road, Shanghai, China. E-mail: genghongquan@fudan.edu.cn; or Dali Li, Shanghai Key Laboratory of Regulatory Biology, Institute of Biomedical Sciences and School of Life Sciences, East China Normal University, No. 500, Dongchuan Road, Shanghai, China. E-mail: dlli@bio.ecnu.edu.cn; or Guofeng Xu, Department of Pediatric Urology, Department of Urology, Xinhua Hospital Affiliated to Shanghai Jiao Tong University School of Medicine, No. 1665, Kongjiang Road, Shanghai, China. E-mail: xuguofeng@xinhuamed.com.cn

[5]ZC, DeZ, and RZ are joint first authors.

Received 7 February 2023; revised 1 November 2023; accepted 16 November 2023; published online 21 December 2023

Translational Statement

Primary hyperoxaluria type 1 (PH1) is a genetic disorder caused by alanine glyoxylate aminotransferase (AGXT) gene mutations, leading to glyoxylate metabolism dysfunction and increased urinary oxalate. Patients can develop nephrocalcinosis and recurrent, multiple urinary stones as well as a high risk of progressive kidney failure and systemic oxalosis. Here, we used adeno-associated viruses to deliver a split adenine base editor 8e and single-guide RNA to target the mutant Agxt gene in PH1 rats. This therapy achieved an average of 13% precise correction and effectively reduced urinary oxalate levels and kidney crystal deposition. Our findings suggest that the adeno-associated virus base editor strategy shows promise as an efficient treatment option for PH1.

Primary hyperoxaluria type 1 (PH1) is a childhood-onset autosomal recessive disease caused by an inherent genetic defect of the alanine glyoxylate aminotransferase (AGXT) gene. Patients fail to encode the liver peroxisomal alanine glyoxylate aminotransferase (AGT) to convert glyoxylate to glycine.[1,2] In this instance, the overproduced glyoxylate is converted to oxalate by lactate dehydrogenase. Because kidneys function as the primary site for oxalate, hyperoxaluria results in calcium oxalate (CaOx) crystal formation and deposition in the kidney parenchyma, a condition known as nephrocalcinosis, and recurrent and multiple calcium oxalate calculi in the urinary tract. Without effective treatment, patients with PH1 would ultimately succumb to kidney failure[3] and/or complications of systemic oxalosis.[4,5]

Reducing hepatic oxalate overproduction is a primary treatment strategy for PH1. Pyridoxine, an essential cofactor of AGT, proves effectiveness for specific AGXT mutation types in patients with PH1 by facilitating the peroxisomal import of mislocated AGT.[6,7] A breakthrough in the treatment of PH1 is RNA interference (RNAi) therapeutics.[8,9] Two different RNAi therapy agents, lumasiran and nedosiran, effectively reduce hepatic oxalate overproduction by targeting the liver-specific glycolate oxidase enzyme and lactate dehydrogenase, respectively, thereby repairing PH1 phenotypes. ERKNet and OxalEurope guidelines state that patients who progress to the stage of kidney failure are eligible for kidney transplantation only if they have responsiveness to vitamin B6 and/or lumasiran.[10,11] However, pyridoxine treatment is only effective for a subset of patients with PH1,[12] and the life-long administration of RNAi places a heavy financial burden on some patients. Hence, restoration of endogenous AGT expression through a single permanent treatment may surmount the limitations of current PH1 therapies.

Base editors have emerged as a breakthrough for precise and efficient point mutation correction in recent years. By combining a cytidine or adenosine deaminase to Cas9 nickase, base editors can efficiently introduce precise targeted C·G to T·A (cytosine base editor [CBE])[13] or A·T to G·C (adenine base editor [ABE])[14] base alterations without double-strand DNA breaks. Base editors can theoretically correct >30% of human pathogenic single-nucleotide polymorphisms by targeting the 4 transition mutations.[15] Base editors have shown effectiveness in treating various genetic diseases in the past few years.[16–18] However, the efficacy of base editors in PH1 has not been investigated. Point mutations account for 84.5% of pathogenic *AGXT* mutations in patients with PH1. ABE and CBE have shown potential for repairing 39.4% and 14.2% (https://www.ncbi.nlm.nih.gov/clinvar) of these mutations, respectively. This highlights the significant promise of base editors, especially ABE, in the treatment of PH1. By adenosine deaminase engineering, a novel evolved version of ABE known as ABE8e has demonstrated exceptional deamination kinetics.[19] Consequently, we hypothesized that the ABE8e would permanently and preciously correct the mutations associated with PH1.

Herein, we demonstrated an efficient ABE-mediated repair of clinically reported *AGXT* mutants *in vitro*. Furthermore, we reported the effective *in vivo* delivery of a split-inter ABE8e using adeno-associated virus (AAV) in a PH1 rat model[20] with a nonsense mutation in *Agxt* (c.250C>T, p.Q84X). The treatment led to a precise correction of 13% *Agxt*^{Q84X}, resulting in the restoration of AGT expression and a substantial reduction in oxalate production and kidney CaOx deposition in PH1 rats. These findings provided a feasible therapeutic approach for PH1 that directly corrected the causative mutation *in vivo* and held potential for achieving the goals of precision medicine.

METHODS
Animal experiments
All experiments in live animals were approved by the Institutional Animal Care and Use Committee of the Ethics Committee of Xinhua Hospital Affiliated to Shanghai Jiao Tong University School of Medicine, the Shanghai Laboratory Animal Commission, and the East China Normal University Public Platform for innovation (011). The male *Agxt*^{Q84X} rats were obtained as previously described,[20] with age-matched male commercial Sprague-Dawley rats used as wild-type (WT) controls. Rats were housed in the East China Normal University vivarium and maintained on a normal chow diet and a 12-hour/12-hour light/dark cycle. For systematic recombinant adeno-associated virus (rAAV) delivery, 7-day-old rats were injected with 5×10^{11} viral vector genomes (for each of the 2 rAAVs packaging ABE8e-N and ABE8e-C) per rat via the tail vein; a safe dosage and time course have been used in earlier studies.[21,22] Three weeks after treatment, a liver biopsy was performed to detect AGT expression and deep sequencing. Six months after the treatment, all 3 groups of rats were given water containing 1% (vol/vol) ethylene glycol (EG). After 2 weeks of EG challenge, rats were humanely killed, and organs (liver, kidney, skeletal muscle, heart, spleen, testicle, and lung) were collected for analyses. Urine was collected regularly.

Plasmid construction
The plasmids encoding ABEmax, ABE8e, ABEmax-N, and ABEmax-C were purchased from Addgene (plasmid numbers 102919, 112095, 138489, 137173, and 137174). The VQR-spCas9 (D1135V/R1335Q/T1337R), spG-spCas9, and spRY-spCas9 variants were installed via overlap extension polymerase chain reaction (PCR), as previously described.[23,24] Fragments TadA-8e (template: ABE8e) were amplified and assembled into the ABEmax-N (digested with Nhe1 and BglII) using ClonExpress MultiS One Step Cloning Kit (Vazyme) to generate plasmid ABE8e-N. The C-terminal ABEs required the installation of VQR mutations (D1135V, R1335Q, and T1337R) and the single-guide RNA (sgRNA) sequence targeting *Agxt*^{Q84X}. Analogous to C-terminal ABEs, ABE8e-VQR-C were generated. The sgRNA targeting *Agxt*^{Q84X} was cloned into C-terminal ABEs using the BbsI restriction site. The plasmids targeting the *Agxt*^{Q84X} allele in the reporter HEK293T cell line contain the sgRNA driven by the U6 promoter and enhanced green fluorescent protein driven by the elongation factor 1 alpha (EF1-a) promoter. The N- and C-terminal AAV expression vectors were constructed by Gibson cloning of PCR-amplified inserts into restriction enzyme–digested backbones. For constructing a lentiviral vector plasmid to generate the reporter HEK293T cell line, we used the lentiCRISPRv2 (Addgene 52961) plasmid as the backbone vector. Exons 1 and 2 of the *Agxt* Q84X allele and DsRed cassette were inserted into the lentiCRISPRv2 vector via restriction cloning.

AAV production
The AAV production procedure was described in our previous study.[22] Briefly, HEK293T cells were transfected with AAV8 capsid plasmid, AAV helper plasmid, and AAV expression vector. Three days after transfection, cells were resuspended in lysis buffer (150 mM NaCl and 20 mM Tris [pH 8.0]) and lysed by 3 freeze-thaw cycles between liquid nitrogen and a 37 °C water bath, followed by incubation with $MgCl_2$ (1 mM) and benzonase (25 U/mL; Merck). Then, cell lysates were centrifuged at 5500 rpm, 4 °C, for 20 minutes to harvest the supernatant. Viruses were isolated by iodixanol gradient ultracentrifugation (60,000 rpm for 90 minutes at 16 °C) and concentrated. The virus genomic titer was determined by quantitative real-time PCR using SYBR Green (Sigma-Aldrich).

Serum and urine analysis
Rats' blood was minimally collected via retro-orbital bleeding, and serum was prepared by centrifugation after blood clotting. Creatinine, blood urea nitrogen, aspartate aminotransferase, alanine aminotransferase, and total bilirubin levels were measured in serum samples using a commercial colorimetric assay (Servicebio). For urine collection, animals were acclimated in metabolic cages for 24 hours. Urine samples were acidified, and oxalate concentrations were measured by ion-exchange chromatography using a Dionex ICS-5000 (Thermo Scientific).

Histologic evaluation and tubular injury assessment
Rats were humanely killed after EG challenge. The kidneys and livers were fixed and embedded as described above. Hematoxylin/eosin

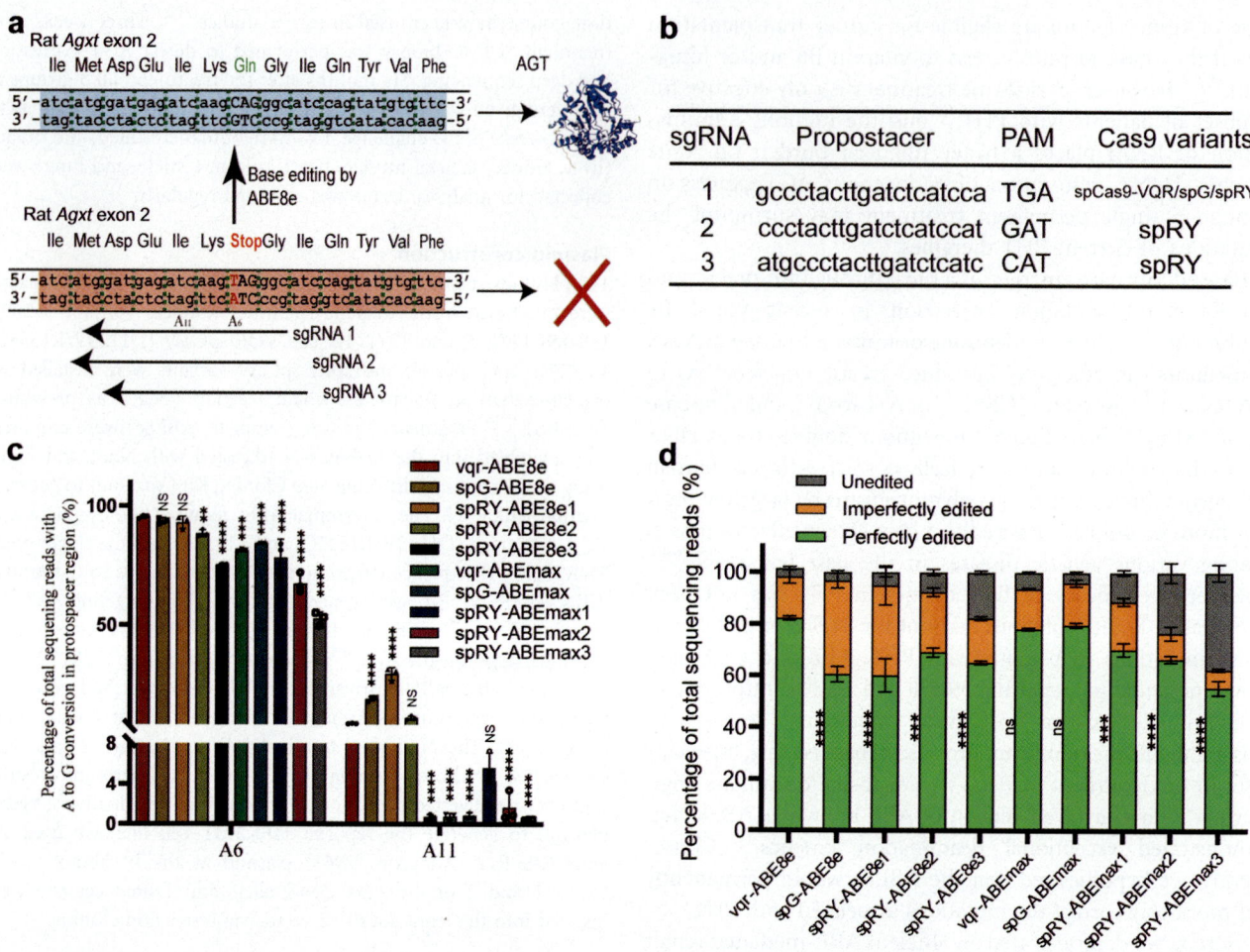

Figure 1 | Adenine base editor (ABE)–mediated correction of the alanine glyoxylate aminotransferase (*Agxt*) mutation in the *Agxt*-Q84X cell line. (**a**) The *Agxt* c.250 C>T mutation introduced a stop codon in the exon 2 of the *Agxt* gene, resulting in alanine-glyoxylate-aminotransferase (AGT) expression loss. (**b**) Three single-guide RNAs (sgRNAs) were identified to position the pathogenic *Agxt* mutation within the ABE activity window. (**c**) Editing efficiencies of target adenine (A6) and a bystander adenine (A11) in the *Agxt* gene in the *Agxt*-Q84X cell line by high-throughput sequencing. spRY-ABE8e/ABEmax1/2/3 represents different sgRNAs and spRYABE8e/ABEmax combinations. Each base editor was compared with vqr-ABE8e. (**d**) The percentage of unedited, imperfectly edited, and perfectly edited targeted adenine (A6) indicated that the vqr-ABE8 mediated the highest correction efficiency. For perfectly edited reads, each base editor was compared with vqr-ABE8e. Imperfectly edited reads meant any other base conversions (expect perfect A6>G) and insertions/deletions in target windows. Data are presented as means ± SD (n = 3). *$P < 0.05$, **$P < 0.01$, ***$P < 0.001$, ****$P < 0.0001$. NS, nonsignificant; PAM, protospacer-adjacent motif.

staining was performed in liver and kidney for structural analysis. Pizzolato staining was used to visualize CaOx crystals and crystal deposit formation in the kidney. Renal cell death was assessed through terminal deoxynucleotidyl transferase–mediated dUTP nick-end labeling staining using a commercial kit (Promega). Positive cells in terminal deoxynucleotidyl transferase–mediated dUTP nick-end labeling assays were counted in 9 randomly chosen magnification fields (×200) for each group.

Lentiviral production, lentiviral transduction, cell culture, Western blot, immunohistochemistry, quantitative real-time PCR, deep sequencing and off-target analysis, whole-genome sequencing, and data analysis and statistical analysis are detailed in the Supplementary Methods.

RESULTS
Screening of *Agxt* base editing *in vitro*

Around the c.250T>C mutation in *Agxt*, we identified 3 sgRNAs with different protospacer and protospacer-adjacent motif (PAM) sequences (Figure 1a). To target these PAMs, we first developed ABE8e/ABEmax-spNG, ABE8e/ABEmax-VQR, and ABE8e/ABEmax-SpRY systems by combining ABE8e/ABEmax and the corresponding Cas variants: SpCas9-VQR variant (NGA),[25] SpG variant (NGN),[23] and SpRY variant (NRN, NYN).[23] Specifically, ABE8e/ABEmax-spRY can recognize all 3 PAMs: ABE8e/ABEmax-spRY1, ABE8e/ABEmax-spRY2, and ABE8e/ABEmax-spRY3 (Figure 1b).

To test the base-editing efficacy *in vitro*, we generated a reporter HEK293T cell line by stably integrating the *Agxt*-Q84X mutant gene, referred to as the *Agxt*-Q84X cell line. We transfected *Agxt*-Q84X cells with ABE8e-VQR, ABE8e-spNG, ABE8e-SpRY1,2,3 and ABEmax-VQR, ABEmax-spNG, ABEmax-SpRY1,2,3, along with the corresponding sgRNA expression plasmids targeting the *Agxt*-Q84X mutation and observed an average of 95.3%, 93.7%, 92.9%, 88.4%, 75.2%, 81.3%, 84.4%, 82.3%, 67.3%, and 52.7% correction of the

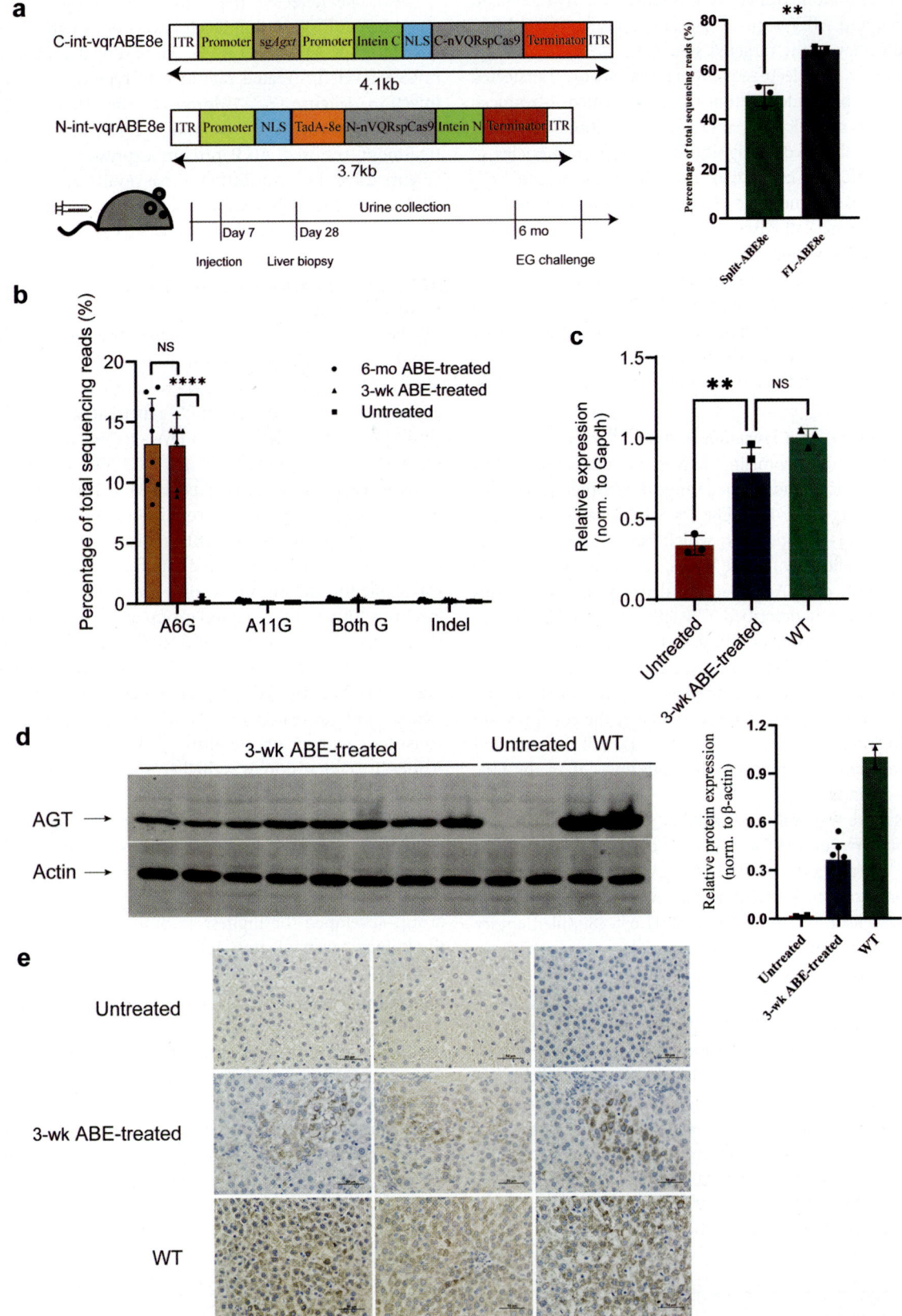

Figure 2 | The *in vivo* base editing corrected the disease-causing alanine glyoxylate aminotransferase (*Agxt*) mutation and restored AGT expression in *Agxt*[Q84X] rats. (a) Schematic of 2 vector genomes for adeno-associated virus (AAV) 8 delivery (adenine base editor [ABE] 8e–AAV8) and an overview of animal experiments. (b) DNA-editing efficiencies for correcting *Agxt* c.250 from A (pathogenic) to G (wild type [WT]) 3 weeks and 6 months after tail vein injection with ABE8e-expressing AAV8. (c) Real-time polymerase chain reaction (continued)

pathogenic mutation, respectively (Figure 1c). ABE8e-VQR, ABE8e-spG, and ABE8e-spRY1 presented similar A>G base-editing efficiency at the targeted site.

Nevertheless, the deep-sequencing analysis on transfected cells showed a bystander editing (A_{11}>G), which introduced an Ile to Thr mutation at amino acid position 82. These variants were observed at significantly lower frequencies in ABEmax-transfected cells than in ABE8e-transfected cells (Figure 1d). We defined the perfect correction as the proportion of sequences of correct conversion without unwanted bystander editing within the editing windows. The ABE8e-VQR–mediated perfect correction had an efficiency of ≈82.2%, which was higher than VQR-ABEmax (78.2%) and spG-ABEmax (79.7%). These results demonstrated that ABE8e-VQR could efficiently and specifically correct the Agxt-Q84X mutation; thus, it was selected for further studies.

ABE corrected the Agxt mutation in Agxt^{Q84X} rats

AAV is 1 of the most promising delivery vectors because of its low immunogenicity and a broad range of serotype specificity. However, the large size of ABE8e (≈5.4 kilobases) precludes the packaging in 1 single AAV, which has a limited carrying capacity (<4.7 kilobases).[26] We leveraged a split-intein ABE8e compatible with dual AAV particle delivery to surpass this barrier, as previously described.[27] Briefly, we split ABE8e into 2 halves with the corresponding split-intein moiety, called ABE8e-N and ABE8e-C (Figure 2a), and, on coexpression, the full ABE8e was reconstituted, mediated by the intein trans-splicing. According to the deep sequencing, the coexpression of the split-intein ABE8e in the Agxt-Q84X cell line resulted in significant editing efficiency, although lower than the full-length base editor (Figure 2a).

Furthermore, we evaluated whether the split-intein ABE8e system could rescue AGT and harbor disease progression in the Agxt^{Q84X} rat model of PH1. First, viral transduction efficiency was examined, revealing that AAV8 efficiently transduced liver cells at an average rate of 41.6% (Supplementary Figure S1). To quantify Agxt gene correction rates in vivo, we performed a liver biopsy and high-throughput sequencing in the liver genome 3 weeks after treatment. The A_6 to G correction rate was 13.3% (range, 9.1%–15.9%; n = 8; Figure 2b). Considering position A_{11} to G conversion generated by ABE8e in vitro, we also detected the editing efficiency at this position. The high-throughput sequencing showed that the simultaneous conversion of A_6 to G and A_{11} to G was rare (≈0.3%), with precise A_6 to G correction (13.0%±2.5%) in vivo (Supplementary Figure S2). Moreover, the precise editing efficiency in the liver remained stable 6 months after treatment (Figure 2b).

Next, we detected the expression of Agxt at the transcription and translation levels. Consistent with the genomic correction of Agxt c.250 A>G, we observed similar liver Agxt mRNA levels in treated rats to wild-type ones 3 weeks after injection (Figure 2c). Moreover, the Western blot and immunohistochemistry staining confirmed that ABE8e treatment restored AGT protein expression in hepatocytes (Figure 2d and e). Altogether, these results demonstrated that ABE could precisely correct the Agxt c.250 A>G mutation in vivo and rescue the absent AGT expression.

AGT partial restoration led to a decrease in oxalate excretion in Agxt^{Q84X} rats

Furthermore, we evaluated whether the split-intein ABE8e could slow disease progression in Agxt^{Q84X} rats. One-month-old Agxt^{Q84X} rats presented hyperoxaluric compared with WT expression. Meanwhile, Agxt^{Q84X} rats treated with ABE8e had similar urinary oxalate (UOx) levels to WT rats (7.70 ± 2.08 vs. 5.54 ± 1.05 μmol/24 h; $P = 0.1260$) and significantly lower levels than untreated rats (10.84 ± 1.92 μmol/24 h; $P = 0.0214$), suggesting near normalization of UOx in the first month. The UOx in the ABE8e-treated group was significantly lower than in untreated rats from 1 month. The effect was stable throughout the whole experiment because the UOx level was lower in the treated group at every checkpoint until 6 months (47.3%, 40.9%, and 48.5% lower in the second, fourth, and sixth months of the experiment, respectively; Figure 3a). We observed an overall increasing trend in UOx in treated and untreated rats from 1 month old (Figure 3b), consistent with prior literature.[20] However, the UOx in the ABE8e-treated group was higher than in WT rats from 2 months (Figure 3a and b). Overall, base editing effectively reduced the oxalate excretion in the treated group during 6 months of follow-up (Supplementary Table S1). Pizzolato staining of the kidney after 2 weeks of 1% EG challenge revealed CaOx deposition in all 3 groups. The untreated group developed the highest amount of CaOx deposition in the kidney cortex (Figure 3c).

AGT partial restoration alleviated kidney phenotype in Agxt^{Q84X} rats

Progressive decline of kidney function is a typical characteristic of PH1. By measuring blood urea nitrogen and serum creatinine after 2 weeks of EG challenge, the treated group showed a serum creatinine level comparable to that of the WT group, whereas the untreated group exhibited a significantly elevated creatinine level (Figure 4a). Hematoxylin/eosin staining revealed tubular CaOx deposition in all 3 groups, with no other kidney lesion in WT group. Tubular CaOx

---

Figure 2 | (continued) showed the relative Agxt mRNA expression in the liver tissue 3 weeks after injection. (**d**) Western blot of AGT expression in the liver of Agxt^{Q84X} rats 3 weeks after injection via tail vein with ABE8e-AAV8. (**e**) Representative immunohistochemistry images of AGT. Bars = 100 μm. *$P < 0.05$, **$P < 0.01$, ***$P < 0.001$, ****$P < 0.0001$ by 1-way analysis of variance. Gapdh, glyceraldehyde-3-phosphate dehydrogenase; ITR, internal terminal repeat; NLS, nuclear localization signal; NS, nonsignificant. To optimize viewing of this image, please see the online version of this article at www.kidney-international.org.

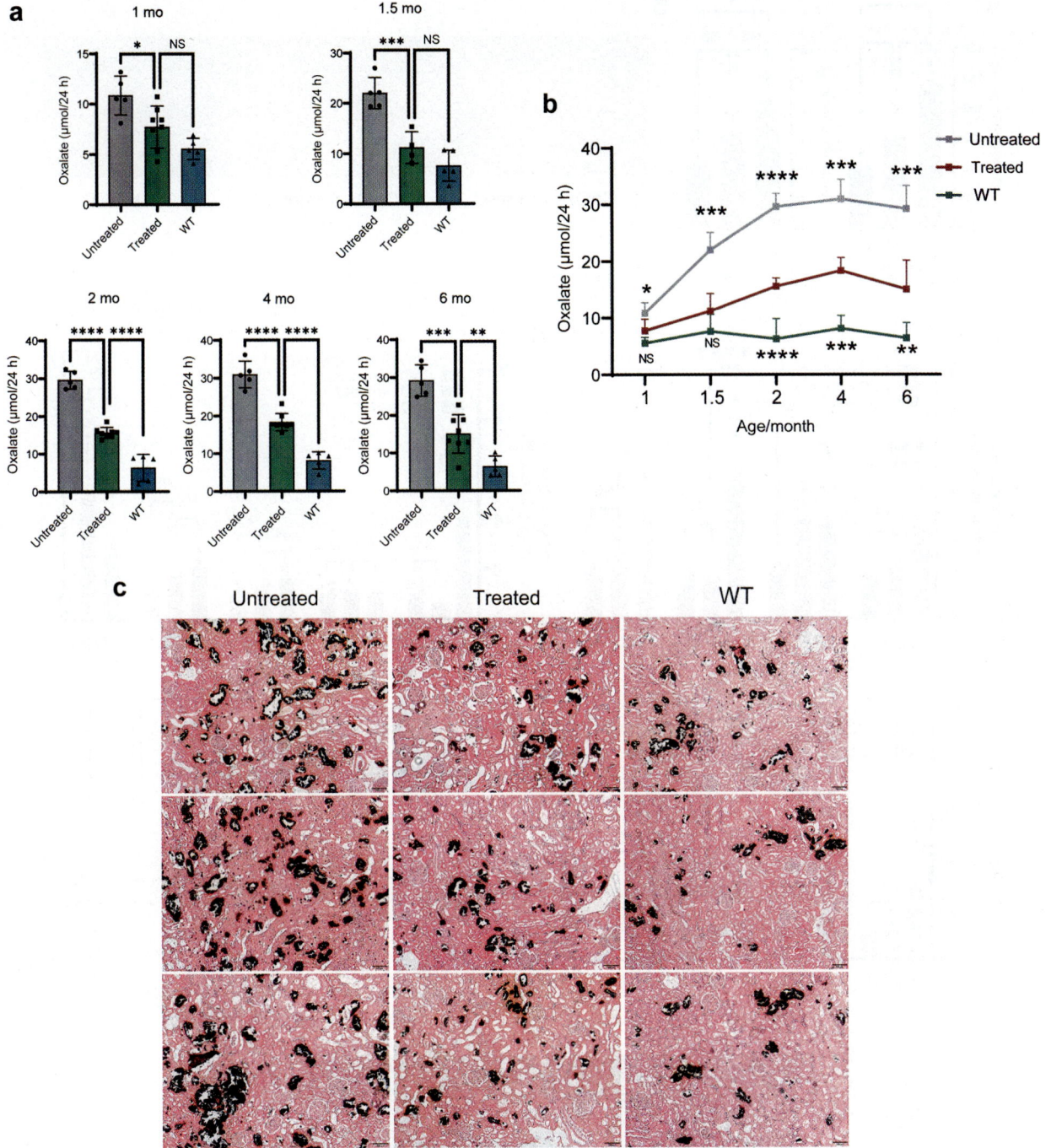

Figure 3 | Therapeutic efficacy of adenine base editor 8e–mediated alanine glyoxylate aminotransferase correction in primary hyperoxaluria type 1 rats. (a) Quantification of 24-hour urinary oxalate levels at different times throughout the experiment (n = 5 in the untreated group, n = 8 in the treated group, and n = 5 in the wild-type [WT] group). (b) Trends in urinary oxalic acid at different times. (c) Representative Pizzolato staining of kidney cortex from untreated, treated, and WT rats after 2 weeks of 1% ethylene glycol challenge. Bar = 200 μm. $*P < 0.05$, $**P < 0.01$, $***P < 0.001$, $****P < 0.0001$. To optimize viewing of this image, please see the online version of this article at www.kidney-international.org.

deposition, tubular casts, intratubular erythrocyte casts, tubular dilation, and tubular epithelial cell abscission were observed in both the treated and the untreated groups, with a more severe degree of CaOx deposition and tubular dilation in the untreated group. Kidney interstitial edema and inflammation, as well as tubular atrophy, were also observed in the untreated group (Figure 4b). Quantitative real-time PCR analysis revealed that after 2 weeks of 1% EG challenge, the relative expression levels of kidney genes, such as inflammation-related CD68 and interleukin-1β (Figure 4c), necroptosis-related caspase-1 (Figure 4d), and fibrosis-related transforming growth factor-β and α-smooth muscle actin

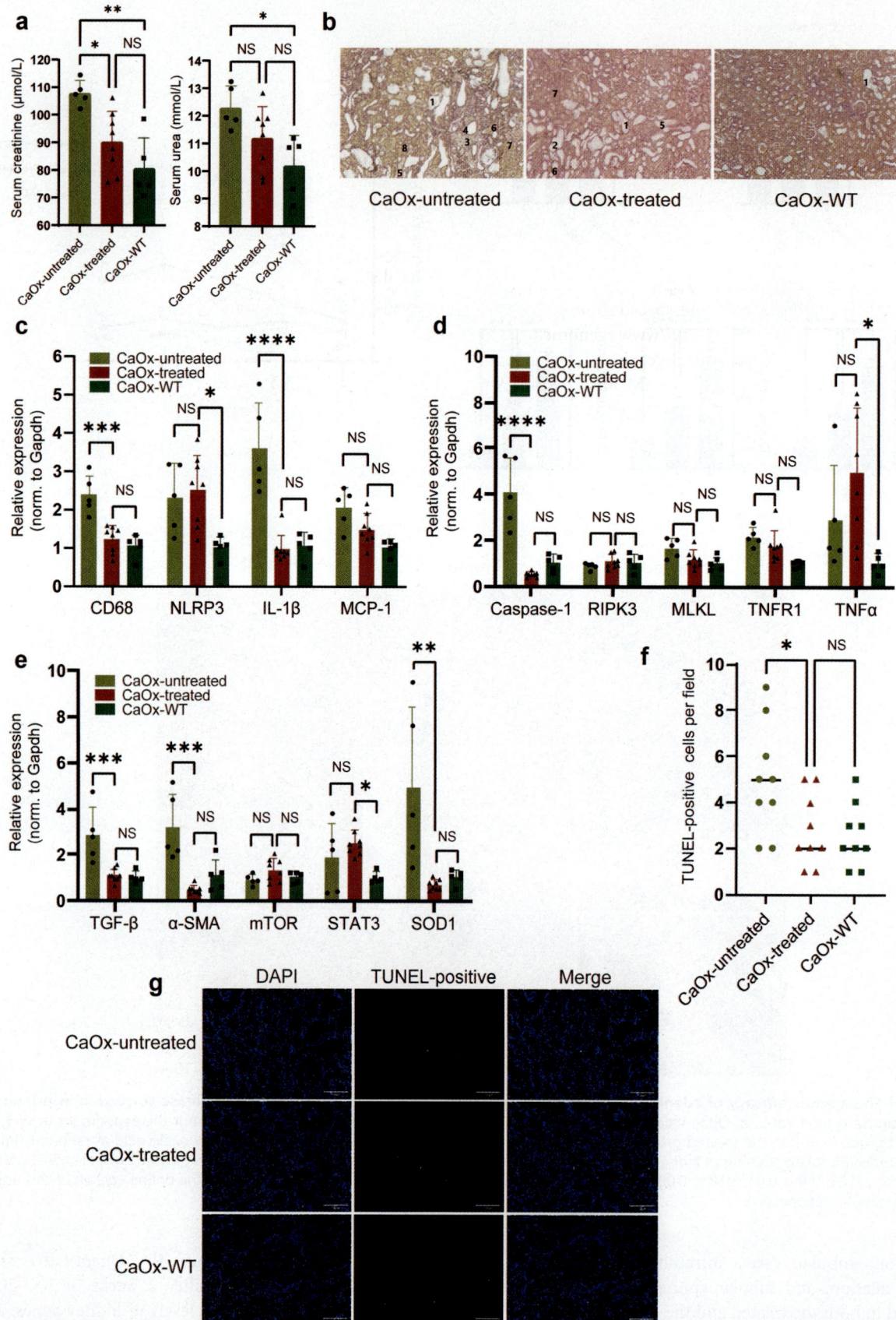

Figure 4 | *In vivo* adeno-associated virus–adenine base editor 8e treatment alleviated kidney injury in primary hyperoxaluria type 1 rats. (**a**) Comparison of serum urea and serum creatinine levels between untreated (n = 5), treated (n = 8), and wild-type (WT; n = 5) rats after 2 weeks of 1% ethylene glycol challenge. (**b**) Hematoxylin/eosin staining of kidney cortex of WT, treated, and untreated rats. (**c–e**) Relative expression of (**c**) inflammation-related genes, (**d**) necroptosis-related genes, and (**e**) fibrosis- and other calcium oxalate (CaOx) (continued)

(Figure 4e), were closer to the normal WT level in the treated group compared with the untreated group. Quantification of terminal deoxynucleotidyl transferase–mediated dUTP nick-end labeling fluorescence indicated more apoptotic cells in untreated rats than in treated ones (Figure 4f and g). The above results indicate that ABE treatment can partially alleviate kidney injury.

Safety assessment of the ABE8e-mediated genome editing therapy *in vivo*

To identify the off-target effects of split-intein ABE8e *in vivo*, we used the clustered regularly interspaced short palindromic repeats (CRISPR) software (http://www.rgenome.net/) to screen out the top 20 potential off-target sites (Supplementary Table S2), with a functional NGA PAM and up to 4 base mismatches compared with the on-target site. The deep sequencing of the rat liver genome revealed no increased A·T to G·C conversions or insertion/deletion formation in predicted off-target sites in treated versus control groups (Figure 5a), indicating that the *Agxt*-targeting sgRNA and split-intein ABE8e did not induce significant off-target effects *in vivo*. To further unbiasedly explore potential off-target effects, we performed whole-genome sequencing at an average depth of 50× with liver tissues from the treated and untreated rats. Treated and untreated rats exhibited a similar distribution of mutation types, and no off-target mutation was observed in the treated rat after deep analysis (Figure 5b).

Besides the safety concerns associated with the underlying off-target risk, vector-dependent hepatotoxicity is another potential safety hazard.[28] Therefore, we evaluated potential hepatotoxicity by histologic examination, serum biochemistry, and inflammatory marker detection. The hematoxylin/eosin staining of liver sections from treated rats showed similar histologic morphology to controls (Figure 5c). Consistently, alanine aminotransferase, aspartate aminotransferase, and total bilirubin levels in treated rats did not increase 3 weeks after treatment (Figure 5d), indicating that AAV injection had a negligible impact on liver function at this dose. Furthermore, cytokine mediators of inflammation, including interleukin 6, interferon-β1, and interleukin 10, did not differ between treated and untreated groups (Figure 5e).

Genome editing in other organs might pose unexpected risks for gene therapy. Thus, we collected samples from various organs (testes, spleen, lung, heart, kidney, and skeletal muscle) and evaluated the hepatotropism of the applied delivery vector. We found that the editing rates in these organs remained <1%, indicating great tissue specificity of the AAV8 capsid (Figure 5f). In summary, these results demonstrated that AAV-ABE8e–mediated genome editing therapy would not cause significant off-target activity, liver damage, or extrahepatic organ tropism.

Evaluation of the translational application of ABE-mediated gene therapy in patients with PH1

To expand the scope and explore the application in PH1 clinical scenes, we investigated whether our findings could be generalized to pathogenic *AGXT* point mutations in patients. Over 200 different mutations in the *AGXT* gene have been reported in patients with PH1[29] (https://www.ncbi.nlm.nih.gov/clinvar; Figure 6a), and 84.5% are point mutations. Theoretically, by targeting the 4 transition mutations, 53.7% of associated point mutations can be corrected by base editing. Limited by the requirement of suitable PAMs, we selected 39 transition mutations and constructed them into HEK293T cell lines for base editing efficiency examination (Supplementary Table S3).

The high-throughput sequencing results showed that the average editing efficiency for these point mutations corrected by ABE and CBE was 64.1% and 48.4%, respectively (Figure 6b). Although some unwanted bystander editing was observed, base editing–mediated perfect correction achieved a mean editing rate of 32.4%. Notably, some common *AGXT* mutations, including c.508G>A (Gly170Arg) and c.32C>T (Pro11Leu),[30] can be precisely corrected by ABE at an efficiency of 55.5% and 31.9%, respectively (Figure 6c). Our results demonstrated the feasibility of base editing, especially ABE, in pathogenic *AGXT* mutation correction and raised the prospect of personalized and precision medicine for patients with PH1.

DISCUSSION

In this study, we demonstrated that systemic delivery of dual AAV vector particles encoding a split-ABE8e could directly correct 13% pathogenic allele in the $Agxt^{Q84X}$ rat model. The partial rectification of the *Agxt* mutation via base editing restated the AGT expression, reduced the endogenous oxalate synthesis, alleviated kidney injury, and diminished CaOx deposition within kidney tubules. To enhance the applicability of this therapeutic strategy, we investigated 39 pathogenic *AGXT* single-nucleotide variations and found most of them

---

Figure 4 | (continued) precipitation-related genes in WT (n = 5), treated (n = 8), and untreated (n = 5) rats after 2 weeks of 1% ethylene glycol challenge. (**f**) Tubular epithelial cell death was quantified by counting terminal deoxynucleotidyl transferase–mediated dUTP nick-end labeling (TUNEL)–positive cells. In each group, 3 animals were selected; for each animal, 3 random sections were analyzed. (**g**) Representative pictures of TUNEL staining in kidney tissues. Results are means ± SD. Significance was determined with (**a,c–e**) 1-way analysis of variance and (**f**) an unpaired Mann-Whitney test. *P < 0.05, **P < 0.01, ***P < 0.001. Bar = 100 μm. 1 = CaOx; 2 = kidney tubular dilation; 3 = kidney interstitial edema; 4 = kidney interstitial inflammation; 5 = tubular casts; 6 = tubular epithelial cell abscission; 7 = intratubular erythrocyte casts; and 8 = kidney tubular atrophy. Gapdh, glyceraldehyde-3-phosphate dehydrogenase; IL, interleukin; MCP-1, monocyte chemoattractant protein-1; MLKL, mixed lineage kinase domain-like protein; mTOR, mammalian target of rapamycin; NLRP3, NOD-like receptor thermal protein domain associated protein 3; NS, nonsignificant; RIPK3, receptor-interacting protein kinase 3; α-SMA, α-smooth muscle actin; SOD1, superoxide dismutase 1; STAT3, signal transducer and activator of transcription 3; TGF-β, transforming growth factor-β; TNF-α, tumor necrosis factor-α; TNFR1, tumor necrosis factor receptor 1. To optimize viewing of this image, please see the online version of this article at www.kidney-international.org.

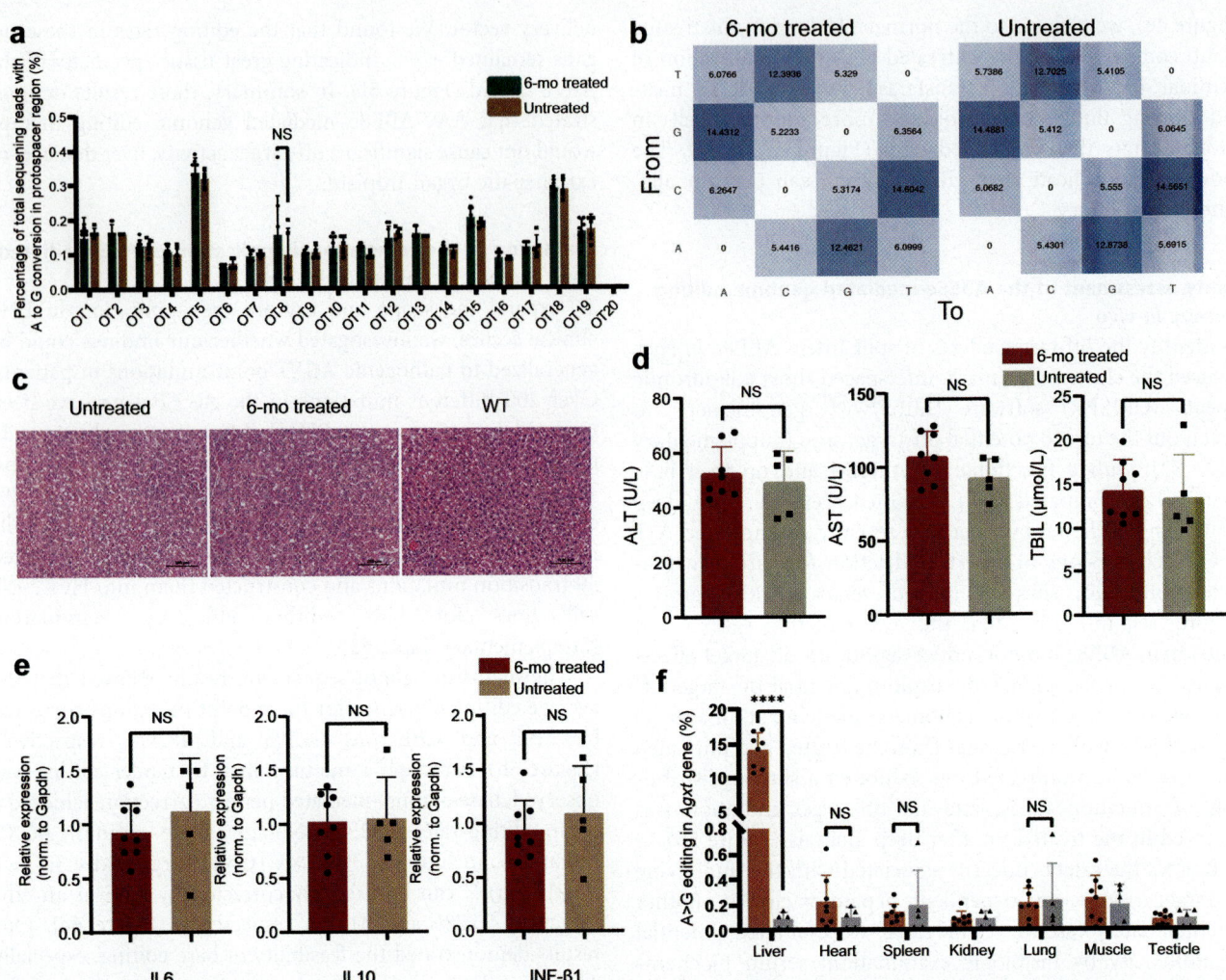

Figure 5 | Adeno-associated virus–mediated adenine base editor 8e delivery did not induce substantial off-target (OT) editing, liver toxicity, and extrahepatic organ tropism. (a) DNA sequencing for the top 20 computationally predicted off-target loci from treated and untreated rat livers 6 months after injection. (b) Mutation types of treated and untreated rat livers 6 months after injection by whole-genome sequencing. (c) Hematoxylin/eosin staining of liver tissue sections from treated and untreated rats. n = 8 in the treated group, and n = 5 in the untreated group and wild-type group. (d) Levels of serum transaminases (aspartate aminotransferase [AST], alanine aminotransferase [ALT], and total bilirubin [TBIL]) in peripheral blood from treated and untreated rat livers 6 months after injection. (e) Relative interleukin (IL)-6, IL-10, and interferon (INF)-β mRNA levels in the liver tissue 6 months after injection. (f) A>G editing efficiency of the *Agxt* gene in DNA isolated from other tissues than the liver. Bar =100 μm. *$P < 0.05$, **$P < 0.01$, ***$P < 0.001$, ****$P < 0.0001$ by 1-way analysis of variance. Gapdh, glyceraldehyde-3-phosphate dehydrogenase; NS, nonsignificant. To optimize viewing of this image, please see the online version of this article at www.kidney-international.org.

could be efficiently corrected. Consequently, our outcomes suggested that CRISPR base editors might be a promising and efficient therapeutic approach for PH1.

The primary goal of PH1 treatment is to reduce endogenous oxalate production. The latest European Association of Urology (EAU) guidance especially recommended pyridoxine and lumasiran because of their effectiveness in reducing UOx.[31] Pyridoxine can restore AGT mistargeting from the mitochondrion to the peroxisome, although responsiveness is mutation dependent.[12] RNAi therapeutics, like lumasiran (targeting glycolate oxidase) and nedosiran (targeting hepatic lactate dehydrogenase A), are promising treatments for PH1. Early clinical trials demonstrated normal or near-normal UOx levels in most patients 6 months after lumasiran or nedosiran treatment.[8,32] RNAi therapy was unquestionably a breakthrough in PH1 treatment. But at the same time, RNAi therapy implies lifelong treatment and high financial burden.[33]

The CRISPR/Cas9-mediated *Hao1* or *Ldha* gene knockout is a tactic to cure PH1 by disrupting key enzymes in oxalate metabolism.[21,22,34,35] However, knockout of upstream genes, like *Hao1* and *Ldha*, requires a high insertion/deletion rate (at least 20%–40%), and double-stranded DNA breaks caused by CRISPR/Cas9 pose safety concerns, such as chromosomal rearrangements and tumorigenic risk.[36] In contrast, the restoration of AGT expression through *in vivo* gene editing appears to be an ideal strategy for PH1, as it can reestablish normal glyoxylate metabolism and is more

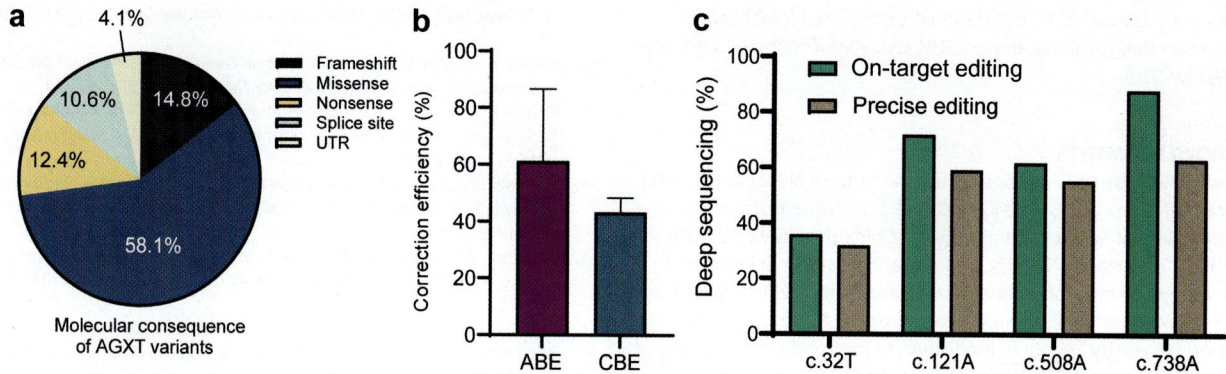

Figure 6 | Pathogenic human alanine glyoxylate aminotransferase (*AGXT*) variants might be efficiently corrected by base editing. (a) The 291 known pathogenic human *AGXT* variants in ClinVar (https://www.ncbi.nlm.nih.gov/clinvar/), classified by molecular consequence. Most of them are point mutations. (b) Correction efficiency of *AGXT* variants using adenine base editor (ABE) and cytosine base editor (CBE). (c) Correction efficiency of some common pathogenic variants. UTR, untranslated region.

ethically viable for patients with PH1. CRISPR base editors, with their potential to correct deleterious point mutations without double-stranded DNA breaks, open up new possibilities for genetic disorder treatment.[37] Previous studies have shown promising *in vivo* therapeutic effects of base editing in accurately modifying disease-related genes for genetic disorders.[16,17,38] However, there has been limited experimental evidence supporting the effects of functional *Agxt* correction. We found a significant reduction in UOx levels, despite the genome-editing efficiency of the mutant *Agxt* gene being only 13%. This discrepancy could be attributed to several factors. One explanation is that the actual repair rate might be underestimated by genomic DNA sequencing from whole liver extracts, as nonparenchymal cells account for 30% to 40% of total liver cells,[39] which could not be transfected. Furthermore, our study showed that a low repair rate could lead to relatively higher mRNA and protein restoration, consistent with findings from several studies on gene repair for metabolic liver diseases.[17,40,41] This may relate to the high catalytic activity of the AGT enzyme with low Michaelis constant (Km) for glyoxylate, which means even a relatively low level of protein can efficiently catalyze the conversion from glyoxylate to glycine.[42] UOx excretion was considered an independent risk factor for the decline in kidney function,[43] consistent with our previous findings in the PH1 rat model.[20] This study suggests that the severity of kidney function impairment is positively associated with the extent of calcium oxalate deposition in the kidneys. Furthermore, this reinforces the evidence that inflammation, fibrosis, and necroptosis-related pathways play a primary role in kidney injury associated with kidney calcium oxalate crystal formation.

Careful evaluation of the safety of AAVs and CRISPR-associated base editors is essential to ensure the translational applicability of this platform. First, we observed no off-target editing through high-throughput sequencing analysis of the top 20 predicted sites and through whole-genome sequencing analysis. Second, we did not observe any signs of potential hepatotoxicity by monitoring AAV-induced liver injury and inflammation. However, because of the current lack of a protocol for detecting single hepatocytes *in vitro*, the possibility of off-target effects, potential carcinogenesis,[44] and immunogenicity,[45] induced by AAVs, cannot be completely ruled out.

Efficient *in vivo* base editing is crucial for successful treatments of genetic disorders. Although we achieved a therapeutic effect for PH1, a higher and more precise level of correction is necessary to fully rectify the PH1 phenotype. A growing number of engineered base editor variants[46–50] have been developed, which can recognize more PAM sites and accurately edit the specific position within the protospacer sequence. These novel base editor variants may enhance the clinical utility of base-editing treatment for PH1. On the other hand, because of humoral responses,[51] redosing of AAV vector is challenging, whereas nonviral vectors, such as lipid nanoparticles, have lower immunogenicity and a larger packaging capacity. Several studies have recently proven the *in vivo* therapeutic potential of lipid nanoparticle–based delivery of mRNA encoding an ABE and a single-guide RNA.[52,53] A second lipid nanoparticle dose may also aid in improving editing efficiency.[52] In summary, the novel base editor variants, as well as the mRNA–lipid nanoparticle platform, hold promise in facilitating the accelerated application of gene therapy.

In conclusion, our study demonstrated the efficient and precise correction of single-nucleotide *Agxt* loss-of-function mutations using AAV-mediated *in vivo* delivery of split-inter base editing agents. Our findings revealed that partial correction of the mutant *Agxt* gene could lead to a significant reduction in UOx and alleviate CaOx deposition, thereby establishing the potential for personalized medicine in PH1.

DISCLOSURE
All the authors declared no competing interests.

DATA STATEMENT
The data that support the findings of this study are available from the corresponding author on reasonable request. The sequencing data of

all rats were uploaded to the National Center for Biotechnology Information BioProject database (PRJNA1019886, PRJNA1025298, and PRJNA1025830).

ACKNOWLEDGMENTS
This work was partially supported by grants from National Key R&D Program of China (2023YFC3403400 and 2023YFE0209200 to DL), the National Natural Science Foundation of China (No. 32025023, No. 32230064, and No. 81770702), and a grant from the Science and Technology Commission of Shanghai Municipality (22YF1426900). We thank Jia Wang and Kailun Xu (Xinhua Hospital Affiliated to Shanghai Jiaotong University School of Medicine) for interpreting the lesions of hematoxylin/eosin staining of kidney sections.

SUPPLEMENTARY MATERIAL
Supplementary File (Word)
Supplementary Methods.
Supplementary File (PDF)
Supplementary Figure S1. Frozen sections of livers from rats injected with adeno-associated virus (AAV) green fluorescent protein (GFP) or phosphate-buffered saline (PBS).
Supplementary Figure S2. Specific alleles with base substitution in each vqrABEe-treated rat after recombinant adeno-associated virus (rAAV) injection. Top 10 alleles are listed.
Supplementary File (Word)
Supplementary Table S1. The 24-hour urinary oxalate at different times after treatment.
Supplementary Table S2. Potential off-target sites and A-to-G editing frequency.
Supplementary Table S3. A total of 39 pathogenic transition mutations of patients' alanine glyoxylate aminotransferase (*AGXT*) and corresponding editing efficiency.
Supplementary Table S4. Primers used in this study.

REFERENCES
1. Purdue PE, Lumb MJ, Fox M, et al. Characterization and chromosomal mapping of a genomic clone encoding human alanine:glyoxylate aminotransferase. *Genomics*. 1991;10:34–42.
2. Hopp K, Cogal AG, Bergstralh EJ, et al. Phenotype-genotype correlations and estimated carrier frequencies of primary hyperoxaluria. *J Am Soc Nephrol*. 2015;26:2559–2570.
3. Cochat P, Rumsby G. Primary hyperoxaluria. *N Engl J Med*. 2013;369:649–658.
4. Demoulin N, Aydin S, Gillion V, et al. Pathophysiology and management of hyperoxaluria and oxalate nephropathy: a review. *Am J Kidney Dis*. 2022;79:717–727.
5. Harambat J, van Stralen KJ, Espinosa L, et al. Characteristics and outcomes of children with primary oxalosis requiring renal replacement therapy. *Clin J Am Soc Nephrol*. 2012;7:458–465.
6. Miyata N, Steffen J, Johnson ME, et al. Pharmacologic rescue of an enzyme-trafficking defect in primary hyperoxaluria 1. *Proc Natl Acad Sci U S A*. 2014;111:14406–14411.
7. Cellini B, Montioli R, Oppici E, et al. The chaperone role of the pyridoxal 5′-phosphate and its implications for rare diseases involving B6-dependent enzymes. *Clin Biochem*. 2014;47:158–165.
8. Garrelfs SF, Frishberg Y, Hulton SA, et al. Lumasiran, an RNAi therapeutic for primary hyperoxaluria type 1. *N Engl J Med*. 2021;384:1216–1226.
9. Hoppe B, Koch A, Cochat P, et al. Safety, pharmacodynamics, and exposure-response modeling results from a first-in-human phase 1 study of nedosiran (PHYOX1) in primary hyperoxaluria. *Kidney Int*. 2022;101:626–634.
10. Sellier-Leclerc A-L, Metry E, Clave S, et al. Isolated kidney transplantation under lumasiran therapy in primary hyperoxaluria type 1: a report of five cases. *Nephrol Dial Transplant*. 2023;38:517–521.
11. Groothoff JW, Metry E, Deesker L, et al. Clinical practice recommendations for primary hyperoxaluria: an expert consensus statement from ERKNet and OxalEurope. *Nat Rev Nephrol*. 2023;19:194–211.
12. Mandrile G, Beck B, Acquaviva C, et al. Genetic assessment in primary hyperoxaluria: why it matters. *Pediatr Nephrol*. 2023;38:625–634.
13. Komor AC, Kim YB, Packer MS, et al. Programmable editing of a target base in genomic DNA without double-stranded DNA cleavage. *Nature*. 2016;533:420–424.
14. Gaudelli NM, Komor AC, Rees HA, et al. Programmable base editing of A*T to G*C in genomic DNA without DNA cleavage. *Nature*. 2017;551:464–471.
15. Anzalone AV, Randolph PB, Davis JR, et al. Search-and-replace genome editing without double-strand breaks or donor DNA. *Nature*. 2019;576:149–157.
16. Suh S, Choi EH, Leinonen H, et al. Restoration of visual function in adult mice with an inherited retinal disease via adenine base editing. *Nat Biomed Eng*. 2021;5:169–178.
17. Villiger L, Grisch-Chan HM, Lindsay H, et al. Treatment of a metabolic liver disease by *in vivo* genome base editing in adult mice. *Nat Med*. 2018;24:1519–1525.
18. Koblan LW, Erdos MR, Wilson C, et al. *In vivo* base editing rescues Hutchinson-Gilford progeria syndrome in mice. *Nature*. 2021;589:608–614.
19. Richter MF, Zhao KT, Eton E, et al. Phage-assisted evolution of an adenine base editor with improved Cas domain compatibility and activity. *Nat Biotechnol*. 2020;38:883–891.
20. Li Y, Zheng R, Xu G, et al. Generation and characterization of a novel rat model of primary hyperoxaluria type 1 with a nonsense mutation in alanine-glyoxylate aminotransferase gene. *Am J Physiol Renal Physiol*. 2021;320:F475–F484.
21. Zheng R, Fang X, Chen X, et al. Knockdown of lactate dehydrogenase by adeno-associated virus-delivered CRISPR/Cas9 system alleviates primary hyperoxaluria type 1. *Clin Transl Med*. 2020;10:e261.
22. Zheng R, Li Y, Wang L, et al. CRISPR/Cas9-mediated metabolic pathway reprogramming in a novel humanized rat model ameliorates primary hyperoxaluria type 1. *Kidney Int*. 2020;98:947–957.
23. Walton RT, Christie KA, Whittaker MN, et al. Unconstrained genome targeting with near-PAMless engineered CRISPR-Cas9 variants. *Science*. 2020;368:290–296.
24. Xin GW, Hu XX, Wang KJ, et al. [Cas9 protein variant VQR recognizes NGAC protospacer adjacent motif in rice]. *Yi Chuan*. 2018;40:1112–1119 [in Chinese].
25. Kleinstiver BP, Prew MS, Tsai SQ, et al. Engineered CRISPR-Cas9 nucleases with altered PAM specificities. *Nature*. 2015;523:481–485.
26. van Haasteren J, Li J, Scheideler OJ, et al. The delivery challenge: fulfilling the promise of therapeutic genome editing. *Nat Biotechnol*. 2020;38:845–855.
27. Chew WL, Tabebordbar M, Cheng JK, et al. A multifunctional AAV-CRISPR-Cas9 and its host response. *Nat Methods*. 2016;13:868–874.
28. Nidetz NF, McGee MC, Tse LV, et al. Adeno-associated viral vector-mediated immune responses: understanding barriers to gene delivery. *Pharmacol Ther*. 2020;207:107453.
29. Williams EL, Acquaviva C, Amoroso A, et al. Primary hyperoxaluria type 1: update and additional mutation analysis of the AGXT gene. *Hum Mutat*. 2009;30:910–917.
30. Milliner DS, Harris PC, Sas DJ, et al. Primary hyperoxaluria type 1. Last revised February 10, 2022. Accessed January 17, 2024. https://www.ncbi.nlm.nih.gov/books/NBK1283/
31. EAU Guidelines Office. EAU Guidelines. Edn. presented at the EAU Annual Congress Milan. 2023. ISBN 978-94-92671-19-6.
32. Baum MA, Langman C, Cochat P, et al. PHYOX2: a pivotal randomized study of nedosiran in primary hyperoxaluria type 1 or 2. *Kidney Int*. 2023;103:207–217.
33. Drugs.com. Accessed January 22, 2024. https://www.drugs.com/
34. Martin-Higueras C, Luis-Lima S, Salido E. Glycolate oxidase is a safe and efficient target for substrate reduction therapy in a mouse model of primary hyperoxaluria type I. *Mol Ther*. 2016;24:719–725.
35. Zheng R, Zhang D-X, Shao Y-J, et al. Multiplex gene editing reduces oxalate production in primary hyperoxaluria type 1. *Zool Res*. 2023;44:993–1002.
36. Choi PS, Meyerson M. Targeted genomic rearrangements using CRISPR/Cas technology. *Nat Commun*. 2014;5:3728.
37. Porto EM, Komor AC, Slaymaker IM, et al. Base editing: advances and therapeutic opportunities. *Nat Rev Drug Discov*. 2020;19:839–859.

38. Song CQ, Jiang T, Richter M, et al. Adenine base editing in an adult mouse model of tyrosinaemia. *Nat Biomed Eng*. 2020;4:125–130.
39. Friedman SL. Hepatic stellate cells: protean, multifunctional, and enigmatic cells of the liver. *Physiol Rev*. 2008;88:125–172.
40. Zhao H, Li Y, He L, et al. *In vivo* AAV-CRISPR/Cas9-mediated gene editing ameliorates atherosclerosis in familial hypercholesterolemia. *Circulation*. 2020;141:67–79.
41. Yin H, Song C-Q, Dorkin JR, et al. Therapeutic genome editing by combined viral and non-viral delivery of CRISPR system components *in vivo*. *Nat Biotechnol*. 2016;34:328–333.
42. Ichiyama A. Studies on a unique organelle localization of a liver enzyme, serine:pyruvate (or alanine:glyoxylate) aminotransferase. *Proc Jpn Acad Ser B Phys Biol Sci*. 2011;87:274–286.
43. Ermer T, Nazzal L, Tio MC, et al. Oxalate homeostasis. *Nat Rev Nephrol*. 2023;19:123–138.
44. Baum C, Kustikova O, Modlich U, et al. Mutagenesis and oncogenesis by chromosomal insertion of gene transfer vectors. *Hum Gene Ther*. 2006;17:253–263.
45. Bessis N, GarciaCozar FJ, Boissier MC. Immune responses to gene therapy vectors: influence on vector function and effector mechanisms. *Gene Ther*. 2004;11(suppl 1):S10–S17.
46. Miller SM, Wang T, Randolph PB, et al. Continuous evolution of SpCas9 variants compatible with non-G PAMs. *Nat Biotechnol*. 2020;38:471–481.
47. Collias D, Beisel CL. CRISPR technologies and the search for the PAM-free nuclease. *Nat Commun*. 2021;12:555.
48. Wang J, Teng Y, Zhang R, et al. Engineering a PAM-flexible SpdCas9 variant as a universal gene repressor. *Nat Commun*. 2021;12:6916.
49. Goldberg GW, Spencer JM, Giganti DO, et al. Engineered dual selection for directed evolution of SpCas9 PAM specificity. *Nat Commun*. 2021;12:349.
50. Chen L, Zhang S, Xue N, et al. Engineering a precise adenine base editor with minimal bystander editing. *Nat Chem Biol*. 2023;19:101–110.
51. Kuranda K, Jean-Alphonse P, Leborgne C, et al. Exposure to wild-type AAV drives distinct capsid immunity profiles in humans. *J Clin Invest*. 2018;128:5267–5279.
52. Rothgangl T, Dennis MK, Lin PJC, et al. *In vivo* adenine base editing of PCSK9 in macaques reduces LDL cholesterol levels. *Nat Biotechnol*. 2021;39:949–957.
53. Musunuru K, Chadwick AC, Mizoguchi T, et al. *In vivo* CRISPR base editing of PCSK9 durably lowers cholesterol in primates. *Nature*. 2021;593:429–434.

basic research

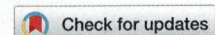

OPEN

Fibroblastic reticular cell-derived exosomes are a promising therapeutic approach for septic acute kidney injury

Yiming Li[1,2,9], Chang Hu[1,2,9], Pan Zhai[3,9], Jing Zhang[1,2], Jun Jiang[1,2], Jinmeng Suo[1], Bo Hu[1,2], Jing Wang[1,2], Xiaocheng Weng[4], Xiang Zhou[4], Timothy R. Billiar[5], John A. Kellum[6], Meihong Deng[7] and Zhiyong Peng[1,2,6,8]

[1]Department of Critical Care Medicine, Zhongnan Hospital of Wuhan University, Wuhan, China; [2]Clinical Research Center of Hubei Critical Care Medicine, Wuhan, China; [3]Department of Integrated Traditional Chinese and Western Medicine, Union Hospital, Tongji Medical College, Huazhong University of Science and Technology, Wuhan, China; [4]College of Chemistry and Molecular Sciences, Wuhan University, Wuhan, China; [5]Department of Surgery, University of Pittsburgh, Pittsburgh, Pennsylvania, USA; [6]Department of Critical Care Medicine, University of Pittsburgh, Pittsburgh, Pennsylvania, USA; [7]Center for Immunology and Inflammation, Feinstein Institutes for Medical Research, Manhasset, New York, USA; and [8]Intensive Care Unit of the second affiliated Hospital of Hainan Medical College, Haikou, Hainan, China

Sepsis-induced acute kidney injury (S-AKI) is highly lethal, and effective drugs for treatment are scarce. Previously, we reported the robust therapeutic efficacy of fibroblastic reticular cells (FRCs) in sepsis. Here, we demonstrate the ability of FRC-derived exosomes (FRC-Exos) to improve C57BL/6 mouse kidney function following cecal ligation and puncture-induced sepsis. *In vivo* imaging confirmed that FRC-Exos homed to injured kidneys. RNA-Seq analysis of FRC-Exo-treated primary kidney tubular cells (PKTCs) revealed that FRC-Exos influenced PKTC fate in the presence of lipopolysaccharide (LPS). FRC-Exos promoted kinase PINK1-dependent mitophagy and inhibited NLRP3 inflammasome activation in LPS-stimulated PKTCs. To dissect the mechanism underlying the protective role of Exos in S-AKI, we examined the proteins within Exos by mass spectrometry and found that CD5L was the most upregulated protein in FRC-Exos compared to macrophage-derived Exos. Recombinant CD5L treatment *in vitro* attenuated kidney cell swelling and surface bubble formation after LPS stimulation. FRCs were infected with a CD5L lentivirus to increase CD5L levels in FRC-Exos, which were then modified *in vitro* with the kidney tubular cell targeting peptide LTH, a peptide that binds to the biomarker protein kidney injury molecule-1 expressed on injured tubule cells, to enhance binding specificity. Compared with an equivalent dose of recombinant CD5L, the modified CD5L-enriched FRC-Exos selectively bound PKTCs, promoted kinase PINK-ubiquitin ligase Parkin-mediated mitophagy, inhibiting pyroptosis and improved kidney function by hindering NLRP3 inflammasome activation, thereby improving the sepsis survival rate. Thus, strategies to modify FRC-Exos could be a new avenue in developing therapeutics against kidney injury.

Kidney International (2024) **105**, 508–523; https://doi.org/10.1016/j.kint.2023.12.007

KEYWORDS: CD5L; exosome; mitophagy; NLRP3 inflammasome; sepsis-induced acute kidney injury

Copyright © 2023, International Society of Nephrology. Published by Elsevier Inc. This is an open access article under the CC BY-NC-ND license (http://creativecommons.org/licenses/by-nc-nd/4.0/).

Translational Statement

Although much has been learned about the mechanisms underlying sepsis-induced acute kidney injury, successful translation of this knowledge to clinical application is very limited. This study highlights that the fibroblastic reticular cell derived exosomes (FRC-Exos) homed in injured kidneys and influenced the fate of primary kidney tubular cells. Further examination of FRC-Exos identified CD5L as the critical protein that improved kidney function by promoting mitophagy and inhibiting NOD-like receptor protein 3 (NLRP3) inflammasome activation. These findings provide a solid foundation for developing innovative strategies to use modified FRC-Exos as a potential therapeutic approach for kidney injury and offer a promising avenue for improving outcomes in septic patients.

Correspondence: ZhiYong Peng, Department of Critical Care Medicine, Zhongnan Hospital of Wuhan University, Wuhan, Hubei, China. E-mail: pengzy5@hotmail.com and pengzy5@whu.edu.cn

[9]YL, CH, and PZ are co–first authors.

Received 4 August 2023; revised 4 November 2023; accepted 1 December 2023; published online 30 December 2023

Acute kidney injury (AKI) is a common condition linked to various etiologies that has unacceptable rates of morbidity and mortality.[1,2] Notably, up to 60% of patients with sepsis develop AKI. Nevertheless, the pathophysiology of sepsis-induced AKI (S-AKI) remains incompletely understood.[3] Therefore, current treatments are reactive and nonspecific, and preventive therapies for S-AKI are not yet available.

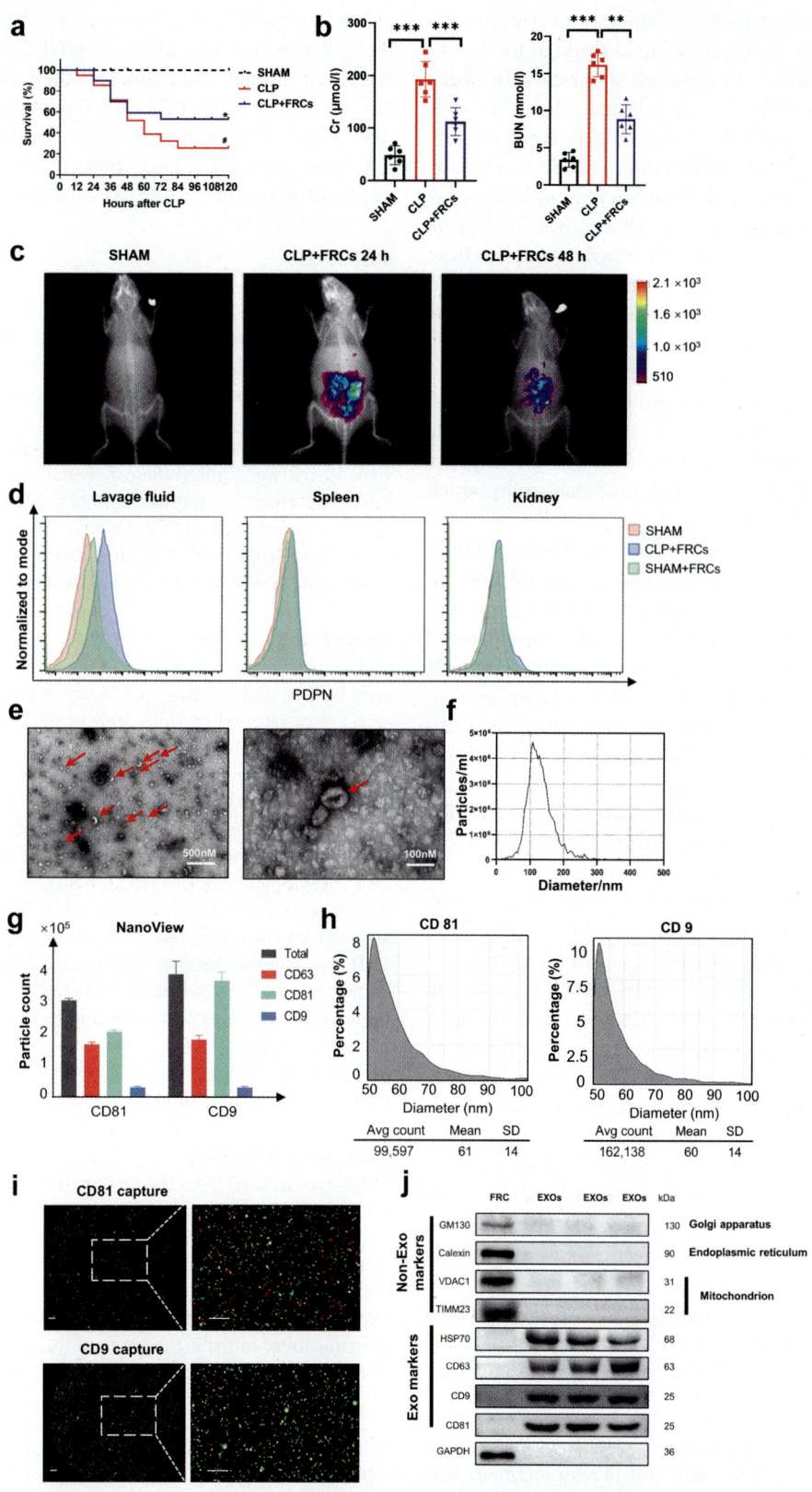

Figure 1 | Fibroblastic reticular cells (FRCs) improve kidney function and secrete extracellular vesicles (EVs), which have characteristics that are consistent with those of exosomes (Exos). (**a**) The 120-hour survival rate was determined after i.p. FRC injection into mice 1 hour after cecal ligation and puncture (CLP). (**b**) Serum creatinine (Scr) and blood urea nitrogen (BUN) levels were measured 24 hours after CLP; $n = 6$ per group. (**c**) Fluorescence-labeled FRCs were injected i.p. Optical *in vivo* imaging was performed at 24 hours and 48 hours after CLP. (**d**) FRCs were injected i.p. 1 hour after CLP. Flow cytometric analysis of FRC accumulation in peritoneal lavage fluid, spleen, (continued)

The conduit network, which is a hallmark of lymph node (LN) microanatomy, is widely distributed through the LN T-cell zones and B follicles. The network is enriched in fibroblastic reticular cells (FRCs) and follicular dendritic cells (FDCs).[4] FRCs are specialized stromal cells in lymphoid organs and actively interact with immune cells.[5] The interactions between FRCs and lymphocytes promote LN lymphangiogenesis[6] and improve T-cell survival in murine LNs.[7] In recent years, stromal cell–based therapies have gained substantial clinical attention due to their ability to reduce inflammation and promote tissue healing. LN FRC transplantation showed robust therapeutic efficacy in a high-mortality murine sepsis model.[8] We previously demonstrated that FRCs regulate peritoneal immunity through toll-like receptor 9 (TLR9) signaling in sepsis.[9] Furthermore, a single injection of ex vivo–expanded allogeneic FRCs could improve survival after S-AKI. However, the exact mechanism by which FRCs attenuate S-AKI remains unknown.

Exosomes (Exos), which are a heterogeneous group of double membrane-bound vesicles, play a crucial role in mediating intercellular communication by shuttling molecular cargo from donor cells to recipient cells. Exos released from different cells exert distinct effects and can be selectively taken up by neighboring or distant cells, thereby reprogramming the recipient cells based on their bioactive compounds.[10] Motivated by these findings, we examined the function of FRC-derived Exos (FRC-Exos) in S-AKI to determine whether FRC-Exos exert therapeutic effects similar to those of FRCs in a sepsis model, and we found that FRC-Exos protect the kidneys from sepsis-induced injury.

CD5L is an immunoregulatory protein secreted mainly by macrophages. CD5L exhibits a broad pathogen recognition spectrum and is involved in the early response to microbes.[11] In an ischemia-induced mouse model of AKI, CD5L in cellular debris was found to bind to kidney injury molecule-1 (KIM-1) and enhance the phagocytic removal of debris by epithelial cells, thus promoting the repair of kidney tissue.[12] In serum, CD5L binds to the IgM pentamer of the crystallizable fragment (Fc) region, preventing its renal excretion. However, only IgM-free CD5L promotes disease repair.[13] Efficient delivery of CD5L to primary kidney tubular cells (PKTCs) may contribute to the treatment of AKI and avoid adverse reactions induced by high concentrations of CD5L in the circulation.

In this study, we demonstrated that FRC-Exos improved kidney function in S-AKI. FRC-Exos, which are rich in CD5L, promoted PINK-Parkin–mediated mitophagy in primary kidney epithelial cells, resulting in the degradation of the NOD-like receptor protein 3 (NLRP3) inflammasome and improved kidney function. Furthermore, modification of FRC-Exos with LTH (LTHVVWL peptide), a targeting peptide that targets KIM-1, can enhance the therapeutic efficacy of Exo-based therapies. This study reveals the therapeutic potential of managing S-AKI via modified FRC-Exos.

METHODS

Study protocol approval

The animal experiments were conducted at Zhongnan Hospital of Wuhan University (Wuhan, China). All experiments were performed in accordance with the protocol approved by the Animal Care and Use Committee of Wuhan University (approval number: WP2020-08022).

The clinical cohort study was approved by the Institutional Review Board for Clinical Research and the Ethics Committee of Zhongnan Hospital (approval number: 2020045-1K). All septic patients were enrolled at the Critical Care Medicine Department, Zhongnan Hospital of Wuhan University. All patients provided written informed consent to participate before inclusion in the study.

Animal study design

To construct sepsis models, 25–30-gram C57/BL6 mice underwent cecal ligation and puncture (CLP) surgery. Following the procedure, septic mice received i.p. injections of FRCs (2×10^5 per mouse) 1 hour later. In addition, other septic mice were injected with FRC-Exos (300 ug per mouse), recombinant CD5L (rCD5L; 2 μg per mouse), CD5L-293T-Exos (300 ug per mouse), and CD5L-FRC-Exos (300 ug per mouse) via tail vein, respectively. Quantification of proteins in Exos was performed using the bicinchoninic acid assay kit (Thermo Scientific). After 24 hours, blood samples and kidney tissues were harvested from the mice. The blood samples were analyzed for creatinine, blood urea nitrogen (BUN, interleukin (IL)-1, IL-18, malondialdehyde and lactate dehydrogenase levels. The kidney tissues were subjected to hematoxylin and eosin staining, immunohistochemistry, immunofluorescence, TdT-mediated dUTP nick-end labeling (TUNEL) assay, transmission electron microscopy, and western blotting. The survival rate of the mice in various treatment groups was monitored closely for 5–7 days.

Isolation of FRC-Exos

FRCs were isolated from the mesenteric tissue of wild-type C57BL/6 mice (male, 8–12 weeks), cultured, and identified according to the protocol reported by our team.[9] Furthermore, FRCs were cultured in serum-free medium without Exos for 48 hours. After collection of the cell supernatant, filtration was performed using a 0.2-μM filter. Exosomes were isolated from the cell culture medium using ultracentrifugation. Initially, the medium was centrifuged at 300 g for 10 minutes at 4 °C to remove cells. The resulting supernatant was

Figure 1 | (continued) and kidney tissue was performed at 24 hours after CLP. (**e**) Observation of EV morphology by transmission electron microscopy (TEM); bar = 500 nm (left) and 100 nm (right). (**f**) Nanoparticle tracking analysis (NTA) of EV diameter. (**g–i**) An automatic EV fluorescent detection analysis system (Nanoview) was used to detect CD81 and CD9. The chips contained spots printed with anti-CD81 and anti-CD9, which captured Exos expressing homologous antibodies. The particle count, diameter, and fluorescence of EVs captured by the anti-CD81 and anti-CD9 chip are shown. Bar = 10 μm (left and right). (**j**) Western blot analysis of the expression of Exo markers (HSP70, CD63, CD9, and CD81) and non-Exo markers (GM130, calnexin, VDAC1, and TIM23) in FRCs and FRC-Exos. For (**a**) $n = 13$ in the SHAM group; $n = 19$ in the CLP group; $n = 21$ in the CLP + FRCs group; $*P < 0.05$, CLP + FRC vs. CLP; $^\#P < 0.01$, CLP + FRCs vs. SHAM, log-rank test. For (**b**) the data are shown as the mean ± SD. Symbols represent individual mice. $*P < 0.05$, $**P < 0.01$, $***P < 0.001$, unpaired, 2-tailed Student's t test. Avg, average; BUN, blood urea nitrogen; Cr, creatinine; PDPN, podoplanin.

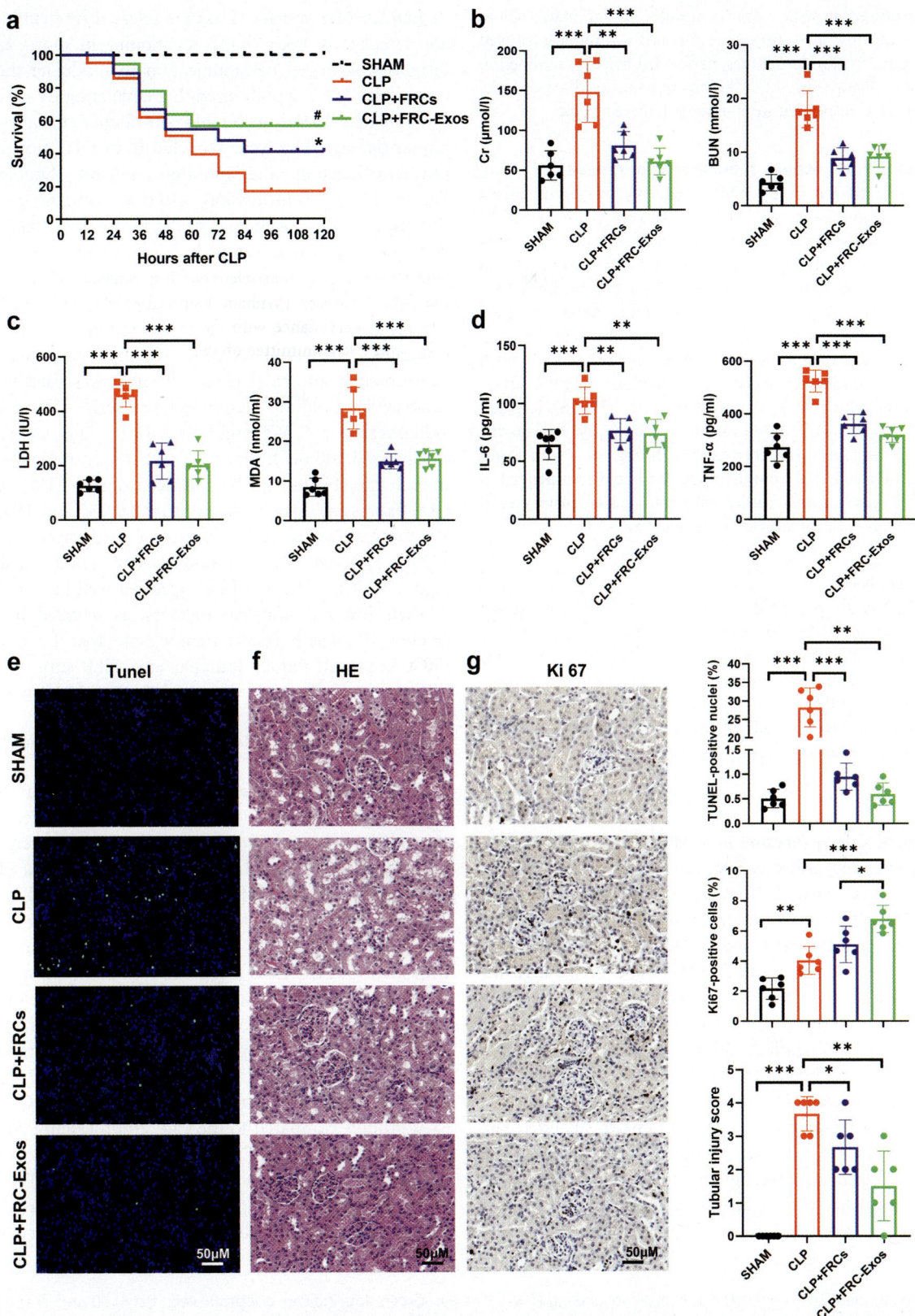

Figure 2 | Fibroblastic reticular cells (FRCs) protect the kidneys from sepsis-induced injury by secreting exosomes (Exos). (a–g) Mice were subjected to cecal ligation and puncture (CLP). FRCs (2×10^5 per mouse) were injected i.p., or an equivalent amount of FRC-released Exos (300 μg per mouse) were injected via the caudal vein 1 hour after CLP. (**a**) The 120-hour survival of each group was determined. (**b–d**) The serum concentrations of creatinine (Cr), blood urea nitrogen (BUN), lactate dehydrogenase (LDH), malondialdehyde (MDA), interleukin (IL)-6, and tumor necrosis factor (TNF)-α were measured 24 hours after CLP. (**e**) The apoptosis rate in the kidneys was analyzed by (continued)

further centrifuged at 3000 g for 10 minutes, to eliminate cellular debris. Subsequently, the supernatant obtained was ultracentrifuged at 100,000 g at 4 °C for 70 minutes, performed twice, as outlined in Supplementary Figure S1C. After the supernatant was discarded, the FRC-Exos were resuspended in phosphate buffered saline.

Isolation of primary kidney tubular cells of mouse
Kidneys were extracted from C57/BL6 mice that were euthanized using inhalation anesthesia of isoflurane. The kidneys were carefully decapsulated and bisected, removing the medulla. The remaining cortical tissue was finely diced using a scalpel and transferred into Dulbecco's modified Eagle's medium (DMEM)–F12 medium containing 1 mg/ml collagenase type II. The kidney tissue was then incubated with collagenase at 37 °C for 15 minutes. The resulting kidney digest was washed through the sieves using primary cell wash buffer (1 × Hanks balanced salt solution [HBSS], N-2-hydroxyethylpiperazine-N′-2-ethanesulfonic acid [HEPES], 0.45 μg/ml sodium bicarbonate, 50 ug/ml sodium hydroxide, 2% fetal bovine serum), and the filtrate was then passed through a 40-μm nylon mesh. Cells were collected from the nylon mesh and resuspended in medium. The cells were then seeded onto tissue culture plates coated with 1% gelatin and incubated at 37 °C with 5% CO_2.

Statistical analysis
All numeric data are presented as mean ± SD. Unpaired, 2-tailed Student's t tests were used for comparisons between 2 groups. Survival data were analyzed using the log-rank test. A P value <0.05 was considered significant. All tests were performed using Prism software (version 8.11, GraphPad).

Additional details for all methods are provided in the Supplementary Methods.

RESULTS
FRCs improve kidney function in sepsis and secrete Exos
We first confirmed previous findings that *ex vivo*–expanded allogeneic FRCs isolated from pooled mesenteric tissues reduced mortality in a CLP-induced murine model of sepsis (Supplementary Figure S1A and B; Figure 1a).[8] Remarkably, the elevations in serum creatinine (Scr) and blood urea nitrogen (BUN) levels after CLP surgery were significantly suppressed after a single i.p. injection of FRCs (Figure 1b). To investigate how FRCs affect kidney function, fluorescently labeled FRCs were injected into the peritoneal cavity, the animals were subjected to small animal imaging, and the major organs were subjected to flow cytometric analysis. The expression of the FRCs marker podoplanin (PDPN) indicated that FRCs accumulated mainly in the peritoneal cavity 24 hours and 48 hours after injection, whereas few FRCs accumulated in the spleen or kidneys (Figure 1c and d).

Extracellular vesicles (EVs) are released by many cell types and circulate in body fluids, functioning in short- and long-distance cell-to-cell communication to modulate the fate of target cells.[14] We hypothesized that circulating EVs released by FRCs mediate kidney repair and contribute to the alleviation of kidney damage. EVs were extracted from FRC medium by an ultracentrifugation and filtration method (Supplementary Figure S1C). Transmission electron microscopy images showed that the morphology of the FRC-derived nanoparticles was typical of Exos, as round, bulging structures were observed (Figure 1e). Nanoparticle tracking analysis (NTA) revealed that the cellular particles were approximately 110 nm in size (Figure 1f). EVs, such as Exos, are known to express tetraspanins, including CD81, CD63, and CD9. The Leprechaun platform (Unchained Labs) was used to capture extracellular immune images to characterize EVs at the individual vesicle level. We found that CD81, CD63, and CD9 were coexpressed, although they were not strictly evenly distributed in each Exo (Figure 1g). The diameter of anti-CD81- and anti-CD9-expressing Exos was approximately 55 nm (Figure 1h). We present representative images of Exos captured by anti-CD81 and anti-CD9 antibodies in FRCs medium in Figure 1i. The extracted EVs expressed well known Exo biomarkers but not non-Exo markers, as revealed by blotting (Figure 1j). These results demonstrate that treatment with FRCs improved kidney function after CLP surgery and that FRCs secreted EVs with characteristics consistent with Exos.

The renoprotective role of FRCs in S-AKI is mediated by FRC-derived Exos
Next, we investigated whether FRC-Exos, similar to FRCs, could improve the survival rates in septic mice. *Ex vivo*–expanded FRCs and Exos isolated from FRCs were injected caudally 1 hour after CLP. As shown in Figure 2a, FRC-Exos significantly increased the survival rate of septic mice. The kidney function of septic mice, reflected by Scr and BUN levels, was significantly improved 24 hours after treatment with FRCs or FRC-Exos (Figure 2b). In addition, we observed significantly decreased lactate dehydrogenase and malondialdehyde levels in the FRC and FRC-Exos groups, indicating lower levels of oxidative stress (Figure 2c). Moreover, production of the proinflammatory cytokines IL-6 and tumor necrosis factor α was significantly lower in the FRC and FRC-Exos groups, compared to the CLP group (Figure 2d). In line with this finding, FRC-Exos treatment was found to suppress cell death in the kidneys, as revealed by the TdT-mediated dUTP nick-end labeling (TUNEL) assay (Figure 2e), and effectively improved kidney histopathologic injury, reducing

Figure 2 | (continued) TdT-mediated dUTP nick-end labeling (TUNEL) assays. Green dots indicate apoptotic cells. Bar = 50 μm. (**f**) The collected kidneys from the 4 groups were stained with hematoxylin and eosin (H&E). Bar = 50 μm. (**g**) Photomicrograph of kidney tissue sections that were immunohistochemically stained for Ki67. Dense brown nuclear immunohistochemical staining indicates Ki67-positive status. Bar = 50 μm. For (**a**) $n = 16$ in the SHAM group; $n = 21$ in the CLP group; $n = 19$ in the CLP + FRCs group; $n = 19$ in the CLP + exosome-derived FRC (FRC-Exos) group; *$P < 0.05$, CLP + FRC-Exos vs. CLP; #$P < 0.05$, CLP + FRCs vs. CLP, log-rank test. The data are from 3 separate experiments. Significant differences were determined using the log-rank test. For (**b–d**), the data are shown as the mean ± SD. Symbols represent individual mice. *$P < 0.05$, **$P < 0.01$, ***$P < 0.001$, unpaired, 2-tailed Student's t test. To optimize viewing of this image, please see the online version of this article at www.kidney-international.org.

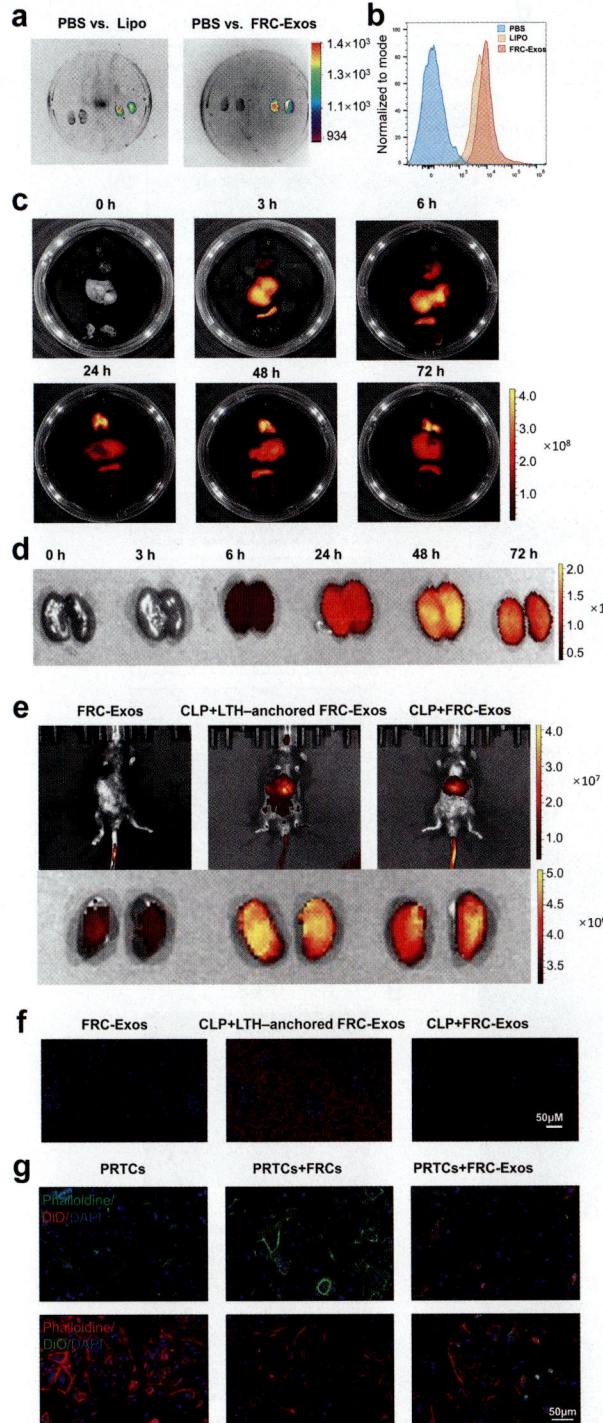

tubular cell swelling and vacuolization (Figure 2f). Furthermore, FRCs and FRC-Exos promoted kidney cell proliferation, as indicated by an increase in the number of Ki67-positive cells (Figure 2g), suggesting augmented injury repair. Together, these findings suggest that Exos derived from FRCs were able to alleviate kidney injury induced by sepsis.

Exos derived from FRCs aggregate to injured kidneys

To further investigate whether FRC-Exos could be taken up by kidney tubular cells, we labeled FRC-Exos with the fluorescent dye DiD (1,1′-dioctadecyl-3,3,3′,3′-tetramethylindodicarbocyanine,4-chlorobenzenesulfonate salt) and injected them into the tail veins of mice immediately after CLP surgery, with labeled liposomes as positive controls. Whole-kidney fluorescence was then observed by small animal imaging. We found fluorescence throughout the kidney tissue 24 hours after the injection of FRC-Exos (Figure 3a). The kidney tissue was then minced and digested with collagenase. Flow cytometric analysis of the kidney cell suspension showed significantly enhanced DiD fluorescence after FRC-Exos injection (Figure 3b). To detect the distribution of FRC-Exos, 1,1-dioctadecyl-3,3,3,3-tetramethylindotricarbocyaine iodide (DiR)–labeled FRC-Exos were injected from tail vein labeled in septic mice. FRC-Exos was distributed mainly in the liver and lung, with lower amounts in the kidneys (Figure 3c). The fluorescence intensity of FRC-Exos in the kidney is difficult to observe at high-intensity fluorescence in the liver and lung, and we observed the fluorescence in the kidney, individually. The fluorescence of FRC-Exos in the kidney was found to be strongest at 48 hours (Figure 3d). An interesting point to note is that, compared with healthy mice after FRC-Exos injection, kidney DiR fluorescence was significantly higher in the kidneys from septic mice (Figure 3e).

We then utilized LTH, a targeting peptide obtained through bacteriophage screening that targets KIM-1, to enhance the targeting specificity of the FRCs-Exos. We intravenously injected LTH-anchored and DiR-labeled FRC-Exos into mice and observed a higher intensity of red fluorescence in the kidney tissues after injection for 24 hours, compared to that in the group treated with FRC-Exos without LTH anchoring (Figure 3e). DiD fluorescence was higher after LTH-anchored FRC-Exos injection, indicating that LTH significantly enhanced the kidney-targeting capability (Figure 3f).

Furthermore, we isolated PKTCs from the mouse kidneys and added DiD- or 3,3′-dioctadecyloxacarbocyanine

Figure 3 | Exosomes (Exos) derived from fibroblastic reticular cells (FRCs) aggregate to injured kidneys. (a) DiD-labeled liposome (Lipo) and FRC-derived exosomes (FRC-Exos) were injected via the tail vein. Optical *in vivo* imaging of the kidneys was performed 24 hours after cecal ligation and puncture (CLP). (b) DiD fluorescence in kidney tissue was measured by flow cytometry. (c) For *in vivo* distribution, septic mice were injected intravenously with DiR-labeled FRC-Exos. Imaging of fluorescence intensity of indicated organs at 0, 3, 6, 24, 48, and 72 hours after injection. (d) Imaging of fluorescence intensity at indicated time in kidneys. (e) Healthy and septic mice were injected intravenously with DiR-labeled FRC-Exos or LTH-anchored FRC-Exos. (f) Observation of kidney tissue sections under a fluorescence microscope for DiD

Figure 3 | (continued) fluorescence. (g) In the (continued)FRC group, DiD/DiO-labeled FRCs were cocultured with kidney tubular cells in Transwell chambers for 24 hours. In the FRC-Exos group, DiD/DiO-labeled FRC-Exos were added to PKTC culture medium, and the cells were incubated for 24 hours. The kidney tubular cell cytoskeleton was stained with phalloidin, and 4′,6-diamidino-2-phenylindole (DAPI) was used to stain the nuclei. Red: DiD; green: DiO. The fluorescence of kidney tubular cells was observed under a confocal microscope. Bar = 50 μm. The experiments were performed 3 times. LTH, LTHVVWL peptide; PBS, phosphate buffered saline. To optimize viewing of this image, please see the online version of this article at www.kidney-international.org.

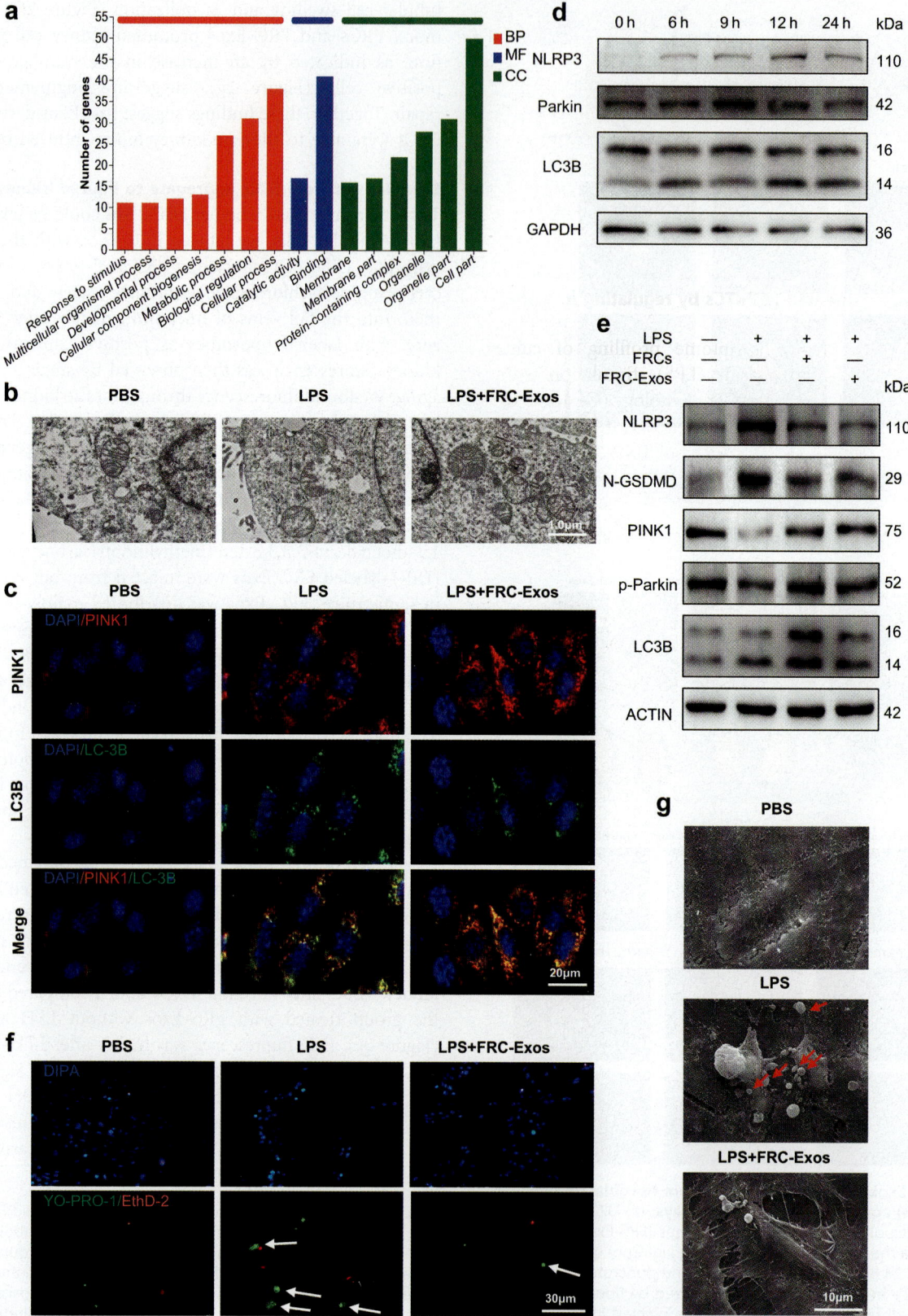

Figure 4 | Role of fibroblastic reticular cells derived exosomes (FRC-Exos) in the fate of kidney tubular epithelial cells. (a–g) PKTCs were treated with lipopolysaccharide (LPS; 10 μg/ml) or LPS and FRC-Exos for 24 hours. (a) Gene ontology (GO) annotation analysis of differentially expressed genes in primary kidney cells in the LPS and LPS FRC-Exos groups. BP, biological process; MF, molecular function; CC, cell component. (b) Observations of mitochondrial ultrastructure changes in PKTCs by transmission electron microscopy (TEM). Bar = 1.0 μm. (c) Immunofluorescence staining of PINK1 (red), LC3 (green), and nuclei (blue) in PKTCs. Bar = 10 μm. (d) Representative western (continued)

perchlorate (DiO)–labeled FRC-Exos to the media of these cells; fluorescently labeled FRCs also were cocultured with PKTCs as controls (Figure 3g). Only a few PKTCs exhibited fluorescence after coculture with FRCs for 24 hours, whereas significantly more PKTCs showed fluorescence in the FRC-Exos group. These results suggest that FRC-Exos derived from FRCs could aggregate to injured kidneys. Thus, in vivo and in vitro experiments confirmed that FRC-derived Exos homed to injured kidneys and were taken up by kidney tubular cells.

FRC-Exos affect the fate of PKTCs by regulating mitophagy and pyroptosis in S-AKI

We then performed transcriptome profiling of cultured PKTCs after lipopolysaccharide (LPS) stimulation with or without FRC-Exos treatment. Gene ontology (GO) analysis of differentially expressed genes revealed that the immune system, signal transduction, and metabolism were the top 3 pathways affected by LPS treatment (Supplementary Figure S2). Furthermore, we added FRC-Exos to the medium of PKTCs stimulated with LPS, and performed GO analysis to determine the biological functions of FRC-Exos in the kidneys (Figure 4a). Mitochondria are central to cellular energy metabolism and are closely related to multiple cell-death pathways, including mitophagy, pyroptosis, and apoptosis. We found that mitochondria were intact in the absence of stimulation, but they were fragmented and exhibited disappearance of cristae after LPS stimulation. This effect was largely reversed by FRC-Exos treatment (Figure 4b). We also found that intracellular LC3B-positive puncta colocalized with PINK1 in PKTCs, which was markedly enhanced after FRC-Exos treatment, suggesting the upregulation of mitophagy (Figure 4c). Western blot analysis demonstrated that the expression of NLRP3, Parkin, and LC3B increased in a time-dependent manner after LPS stimulation (Figure 4d). Furthermore, the expression of NLRP3 and the pyroptosis executor N-terminal gasdermin D (N-GSDMD) was suppressed in the FRC and FRC-Exos groups compared to the LPS alone, and the expression levels of PINK1, Parkin, and p-Parkin were preserved after coculture with FRCs or FRC-Exos (Figure 4e). YO-PRO-1 (a pyroptotic pore-permeable dye) and EthD-2 staining were used to examine PKTC pyroptosis, and we observed less pyroptosis in the presence of FRC-Exos after LPS stimulation (Figure 4f). After LPS treatment for 24 hours, numerous pores of varying sizes were distributed over the entire cell surface, and typical characteristics of pyroptosis, including cell swelling and large bubbles on the cell membrane surface, were observed using scanning electron microscopy (SEM). FRC-Exos significantly reduced PKTC pyroptosis (Figure 4g). Together, these results demonstrate that FRC-Exos affected the fate of PKTCs by regulating mitophagy and pyroptosis in S-AKI.

FRC-Exos restrict NLRP3 inflammasome activation by promoting PINK1-dependent mitophagy in S-AKI

To investigate the effects of FRC-Exos on septic mice, FRC-Exos were injected via the tail vein immediately after CLP surgery. The ultrastructure of the kidneys was observed by transmission electron microscopy. We found that the numbers of autophagosomes in the kidney tubular cells were significantly increased after FRC-Exos injection (Figure 5a). In the sham group, kidney tissue exhibited low levels of LC3b, whereas FRC-Exos injection in the CLP group increased LC3-II levels. Moreover, the expression of the mitophagy-related proteins PINK1, Parkin, and p-Parkin in kidney tissue was also increased after FRC-Exos treatment, compared to that in the CLP group. In line with the ex vivo results regarding PKTCs stimulated with LPS, FRC-Exos downregulated the expression of NLRP3, GSDMD, N-GSDMD, CASPASE-1, and CASPASE-1/P20 (Figure 5b). Additionally, serum levels of the cytokines IL-1 and IL-18 were decreased in the FRC-Exos group (Figure 5c). Reactive oxygen species (ROS) generation was significantly increased in the kidney tissue after CLP, as indicated by an increase in dihydroethidium (DHE) intensity, and it was decreased by FRC-Exos injection (Figure 5d). ML385, a specific nuclear factor erythroid 2-related factor 2 (NRF2) inhibitor, was used to inhibit the production of ROS. Notably, we found that FRC-Exos had a powerful antioxidant effect. NLRP3 and N-GSDMD levels were similar between the FRC-Exos and FRC-Exos+ML385 groups (Figure 5e). We used the oxidative phosphorylation (OXPHOS) uncoupling agent FCCP, which is known to induce mitophagy, and the mitochondrial fission antagonist Mdivi-1, which is known to inhibit autophagy. FCCP induced PINK1 activation and promoted Parkin phosphorylation. Normally, PINK1 is constitutively imported into the inner membrane via the TIMM-TOMM complex. FCCP reduces the expression of TOMM20 and TIMM23. Parkin mediates the ubiquitination of mitochondrial substrates, whereas PINK1- and Parkin-dependent mitophagy activation downregulates receptor-mediated mitophagy-related proteins, including BNIP3/BNIP3L and FUNDC1, indicating that receptor-mediated mitophagy and PINK1-mediated mitophagy compete to some extent. Mdivi-1 was used to inhibit mitochondrial fission and suppress mitophagy. LPS stimulation significantly reduced the accumulation of TOMM20 and TIMM23, which was abolished by FRC-Exos treatment. We

Figure 4 | (continued) blots showing NLRP3, Parkin, and LC3 expression in PKTCs at different times after LPS (10 μg/ml) treatment. (**e**) The levels of NLRP3, N-terminal gasdermin D (N-GSDMD), PINK1, p-Parkin, and LC3 in PKTCs were analyzed by western blotting. (**f**) Fluorescence staining of YO-PRO-1, Eth-D2, and 4′,6-diamidino-2-phenylindole (DAPI). YO-PRO-1: pyroptotic cells, Eth-D2: dead cells, DAPI: nuclei. Arrow: pyroptotic cells. Bar = 1.0 μm. (**g**) Scanning electron microscopy was used to observe the membrane morphology of PKTCs. Bar = 50 μm. The data are from 3 separate experiments. GAPDH, glyceraldehyde-3-phosphate dehydrogenase; PBS, phosphate buffered saline. To optimize viewing of this image, please see the online version of this article at www.kidney-international.org.

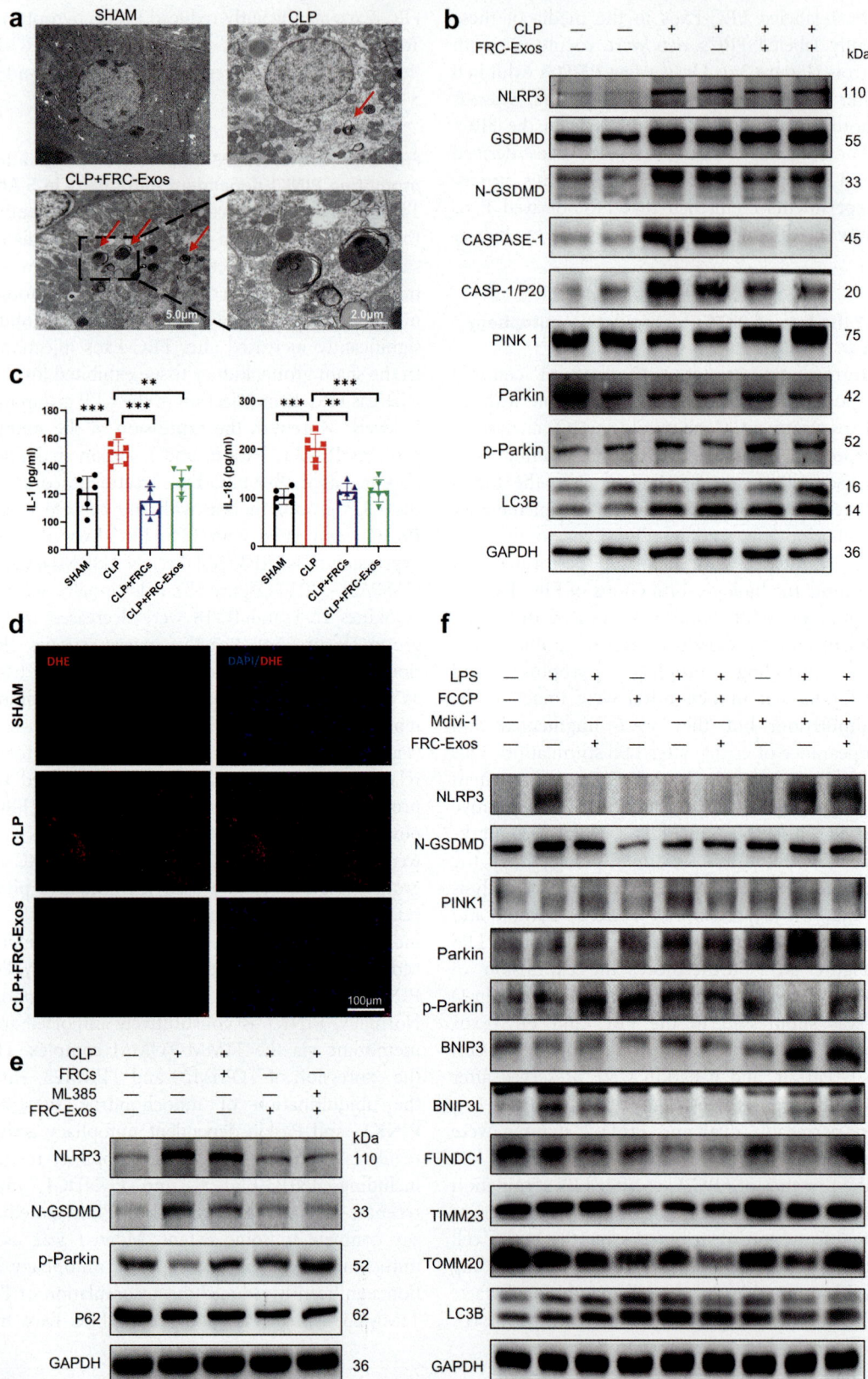

Figure 5 | Fibroblastic reticular cells derived exosomes (FRC-Exos) restrict NLRP3 inflammasome activation by promoting PINK1-dependent mitophagy in Sepsis-induced acute kidney injury (S-AKI). (a–d) FRC-Exos were injected into C57BL/6 mice via the tail vein 1 hour after cecal ligation and puncture (CLP). Kidney tissue and serum were harvested 24 hours after CLP. (a) Transmission electron microscopy (TEM) was used to observe the ultrastructure of mitochondrial autophagy in the kidneys of the SHAM, CLP, and CLP + FRC-Exos groups. (b) Representative western blots showing NLRP3, GSDMD, N-GSDMD, CASPASE-1, CASP-1/P20, PINK1, p-Parkin, and LC3 (continued)

found that the levels of LC3-II were increased in PKTCs after FCCP treatment but decreased in response to Mdivi-1 treatment. Furthermore, mitophagy blockade by Mdivi led to the formation of the NLRP3 inflammasome (Figure 5f). Collectively, these data indicate that FRC-Exos prevented NLRP3 inflammasome activation by promoting mitophagy in S-AKI.

FRC-Exos ameliorate septic kidney injury by promoting mitophagy and inhibiting pyroptosis through CD5L

Our data indicate a protective effect of FRC-Exos against S-AKI. A previous study reported that macrophage-derived Exos impaired tubular epithelial cells in AKI mice.[15] To further clarify the mechanism responsible for the protective role of FRC-Exos, we used classically activated macrophage-derived Exos (M1-Exos) as controls. Flow cytometry and western blotting confirmed that the RAW264.7 cells treated by interferon (IFN)-γ and LPS expressed the M1 markers iNOS and CD80 (Supplementary Figure S3A and B). LPS-stimulated PKTCs were then treated with M1-Exos or FRC-Exos for 24 hours. We found that FRC-Exos, as opposed to M1-Exos, activated the PINK-Parkin pathway and reduced the formation of the NLRP3 inflammasome (Figure 6a). Mass spectrometry was used to identify the proteins in M1-Exos and FRC-Exos, and we found a series of proteins that were highly enriched in FRC-Exos (Figure 6b; Supplementary Figure S3C). KEGG (Kyoto Encyclopedia of Genes and Genomes) analysis showed that these differentially expressed proteins were involved in infection, carbon metabolism, lipid atherosclerosis, and autophagy (Supplementary Figure S3D). Among the proteins that were significantly enriched in FRC-Exos, CD5L exhibited the most expression difference. We further measured the levels of CD5L in the serum and urine of healthy individuals and septic patients and found that CD5L expression was significantly increased in septic patients (Figure 6c). Additional clinical characteristics of the patients are presented in Supplementary Table S1. CD5L levels in patient serum at 6 hours after sepsis diagnosis were positively correlated with creatinine levels measured at the same time (Figure 6d). Furthermore, we found that CD5L was elevated in septic AKI patients who showed improvement in their kidney function, whereas CD5L levels were decreased in septic AKI patients who experienced worsening kidney function (Figure 6e). Immunofluorescence (IF) confirmed that CD5L was widely distributed in the cytoplasm of FRCs (Figure 6f). An interesting finding is that when we treated LPS-stimulated PKTCs with FRC-Exos and an equimolar amount of recombinant mouse rCD5L, we found that rCD5L also effectively reduced the levels of NLRP3 and N-GSDMD (Figure 6g). Pyroptosis of PKTCs, as observed by SEM, was also apparently alleviated after FRC-Exos and rCD5L treatment, and this elevation was accompanied by decreased ROS levels (Figure 6h; Supplementary Figure S3E). Furthermore, we measured the mitochondrial membrane potential ($\Delta\psi$m) using tetramethylrhodamine ethyl ester (TMRE), a $\Delta\psi$m-dependent dye. Healthy mitochondria in the PKTCs accumulated TMRE, exhibiting high TMRE-derived fluorescence, whereas LPS-treated mitochondria with a depolarized mitochondrial membrane showed reduced TMRE fluorescence. FRC-Exos and rCD5L reversed the LPS-induced decline in $\Delta\psi$m (Figure 6i). After LPS stimulation, GSDMD colocalized with mitochondria in the PKTCs, an effect that was significantly reduced after FRC-Exos or rCD5L treatment (Figure 6j). Taken together, these results suggest that FRC-Exos alleviate septic kidney injury by promoting mitophagy and inhibiting pyroptosis through CD5L.

Modified FRC-Exos can effectively attenuate S-AKI

To enhance the expression of CD5L, FRCs and 293T were infected with a lentivirus expressing CD5L. The expression of CD5L in FRCs and 293T cells was significantly increased after lentivirus infection (Supplementary Figure S4A and B). We infected FRCs and 293T cells with a lentivirus expressing CD5L and incubated the extracted Exos with the peptide LTH; the resulting Exos are hereafter referred to as CD5L-FRC-Exos and CD5L-293T-Exos, respectively. We then intravenously administered rCD5L, CD5L-FRC-Exos, and CD5L-293T-Exos via the tail vein to septic mice. Notably, compared to both rCD5L and CD5L-293T-Exos treatment, FRC-CD5L-Exos treatment significantly reduced mortality in septic mice (Figure 7a). Important to note is that CD5L-FRC-Exos injection alleviated structural alterations in kidney tubular epithelial cells, including vacuolization, dilation, and loss of the brush border (Figure 7b). The CD5L-FRC-Exos group showed the highest levels of CD5L and PINK1 proteins in the kidney tissues and the lowest level of N-GSDMD protein (Figure 7c). Furthermore, Scr and BUN levels were dramatically lower after CD5L-FRC-Exos injection than they were in the CLP group (Figure 7d). Additionally, levels of MDA and lactate dehydrogenase also were significantly reduced in the CD5L-FRC-Exos group (Figure 7e). The IF results showed an increase in the content of PINK1 in kidney tissue after CD5L-FRC-Exo injection (Figure 7f). Furthermore, the CD5L-FRC-Exos group exhibited the lowest levels of IL-1 and IL-18 (Figure 7g). Together, these results support the idea that modified FRC-Exos can specifically target the

---

Figure 5 | (continued) in kidney tissues from the indicated mice. (**c**) Serum levels of interleukin (IL)-1 and IL-18 were measured by enzyme-linked immunosorbent assay (ELISA). All the statistical tests used in (**c**) were 2-sided, and a 2-sided $P < 0.05$ was considered to indicate statistical significance. **$P < 0.01$. ***$P < 0.001$. (**d**) Dihydroethidium (DHE) staining was used to label superoxide dismutase ($O2^-$). DHE staining of kidney tissue is shown. (**e**) ML385 was injected 1 hour before the CLP procedure. Western blot analysis of NLRP3, N-GSDMD, p-Parkin, and P62 in kidney tissues. (**f**) Mdivi-1 or FCCP was used to treat PKTCs for 24 hours. Western blot analysis of NLRP3, N-GSDMD, PINK1, Parkin, p-Parkin, BNIP3, BNIP3L, FUNDC1, TIMM23, TOMM20, and LC-3B in PKTCs was performed. FCCP, 10 μM, Mdivi, 10 μM. The data are from three separate experiments. To optimize viewing of this image, please see the online version of this article at www.kidney-international.org.

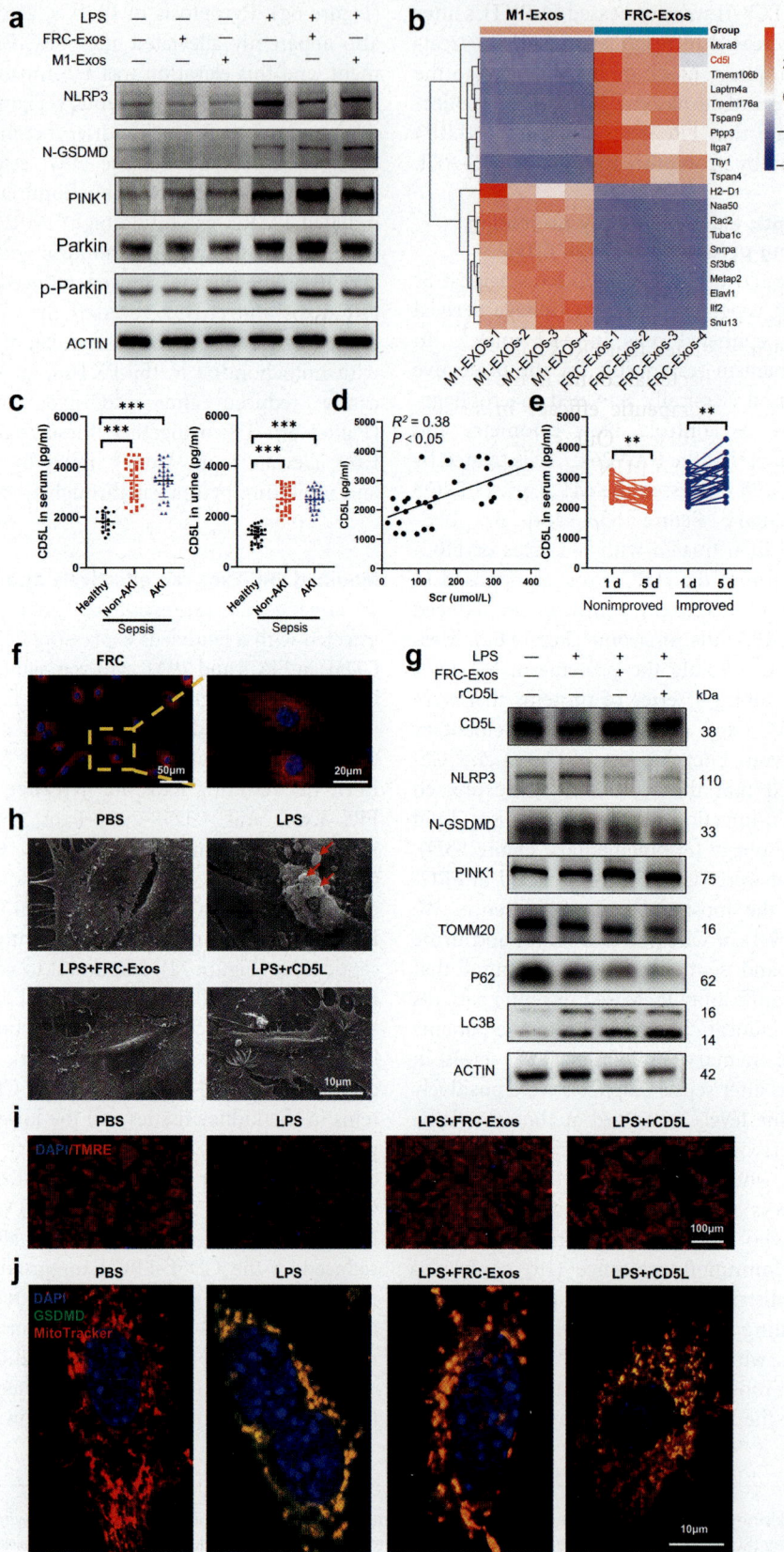

Figure 6 | Fibroblastic reticular cells derived exosomes (FRC-Exos) improve septic kidney injury through CD5L. (**a**) Representative western blots showing NLRP3, N-GSDMD, PINK1, Parkin, and p-Parkin in primary kidney tubular cells (PKTCs) after the indicated treatments. (**b**) Heatmap of differentially expressed proteins in FRC-Exos and M1-Exos. The top 20 proteins are shown. For the convenience of statistical analysis and visualization, extremely low protein content was assigned the minimum value. (**c**) The concentration of CD5L in the (*continued*)

kidneys in sepsis, transport CD5L content to injured kidney tubular cells, and promote mitophagy, ultimately leading to improved kidney function and reduced mortality.

DISCUSSION

S-AKI is common in critically ill patients and is strongly associated with adverse outcomes.[16] However, currently, no therapeutic drugs are available to treat it. Herein, we found that the modification of FRC-Exos with CD5L and the anchor of LTH resulted in a notable improvement of both kidney function and survival rate.

Our team previously demonstrated that FRCs could reduce mortality after septic insult and bacterial counts in the blood.[9] Whether FRCs show similar therapeutic efficacy in sepsis-induced organ failure remains unclear. Our study revealed that FRCs effectively reduced Scr and BUN levels after sepsis. As FRCs cannot be filtered by the glomerulus because of their size, how FRCs mediate their protective role in the kidneys remains a mystery. Given that EVs can alter the tissue micromilieu by transferring components to remote organs,[17,18] the hypothesis that FRCs play a protective role in S-AKI by secreting EVs was reasonable. Indeed, after administration of FRC-Exos to septic mice, Scr and BUN levels decreased, and the survival rate significantly improved.

Mitochondria are central to energy metabolism during S-AKI.[19] FRC-Exos treatment improved mitochondrial integrity. Mitophagy, which is rapidly induced in the early stage of injury, can remove damaged mitochondria, minimize cell injury, and accelerate the recovery of tubular epithelial cells in various models of AKI.[20–22] PINK1-Parkin– and BNIP3 (BCL2/adenovirus E1B interacting protein 3)-mediated mitophagy protects kidney tubular cells from damage by increasing ROS and subsequently NLRP3 inflammasome formation.[23,24] We provide in vitro and in vivo evidence that FRC-Exos promote PINK1-PARK2-mediated mitophagy in PKTCs. Here, we showed that mitophagy blockade by Mdivi-1 led to the accumulation of damaged, ROS-generating mitochondria, which in turn activated the NLRP3 inflammasome. In contrast, FRC-Exos treatment decreased the NLRP3 level in LPS-stimulated PKTCs, indicating that FRC-Exos disrupted NLRP3 inflammasome formation. Furthermore, the mitophagy agonist FCCP contributed to damaged mitochondrial clearance and reduced NLRP3 inflammasome formation. Mitophagy during sepsis also degrades CASPASE-1 and inflammatory cytokine through the clearance of damaged mitochondria.[25] Collectively, these findings suggest that FRC-Exos restrict NLRP3 inflammasome activation by promoting PINK1-dependent mitophagy in S-AKI.

The compositions of Exos from different cells are uniquely disparate and complex.[26] Proteomic analysis of Exos produced by FRCs and M1 cells identified CD5L as one of the most abundant proteins in FRC-Exos. FRCs naturally secreted CD5L-rich Exos and exhibited high CD5L specificity. CD5L is an important regulator of inflammatory responses that was initially named for its antiapoptotic role.[27] CD5L also has been shown to be involved in a variety of diseases, including infection, fatty liver disease atherosclerosis, and cancer.[28–30] In mice, CD5L enhances intraluminal debris clearance and ameliorates ischemia reperfusion–induced AKI.[12] CD5L levels in humans and mice are approximately 5 μg/ml in serum,[31–33] and the total amount of CD5L is approximately 7.5 μg per mouse, taking blood volume into consideration. In a study by Arai and colleagues, 1 mg of recombinant CD5L protein, which is 133 times the total amount in the whole mouse body, was injected into individual mice.[12] Although the authors reported that a high dose of CD5L did not induce a proinflammatory response,[12] CD5L has been found to contribute to plaque growth in cholesterol-rich diet-induced aortic atherosclerosis.[34] Moreover, the majority of circulating CD5L is associated with the IgM pentamer in the presence of the joining chain, which prevents kidney excretion of CD5L.[33] This high binding affinity with IgM-Fc pentamers contributes to less CD5L being released from IgM, which may increase susceptibility to kidney failure.[31] Therefore, whether a high dose of CD5L does not harm the body is unclear. In our study, rather than injecting exogenous recombinant CD5L, we delivered CD5L through FRC-Exos, effectively avoiding the binding of CD5L and IgM and the unpredictable adverse events caused by high doses of CD5L, to achieve a therapeutic effect.

Attempts to modify Exos to increase their targeting efficiency to specific tissue types are the current focus in the field of EVs. Exosomal transport is a novel pathway for intercellular communication during sepsis.[35] FRC-Exos specifically targeted damaged kidneys, as fluorescence was observed in PKTCs after coculture with FRC-Exos. Furthermore, the anchor of an LTH-targeting peptide segment, which specifically targets KIM-1

Figure 6 | (continued) serum or urine of patients or healthy controls was measured with an enzyme-linked immunosorbent assay (ELISA) kit. (**d**) The correlation between the CD5L level in serum and creatinine was analyzed by linear regression. (**e**) On day 1 and day 5, blood samples were obtained from patients diagnosed with sepsis-induced acute kidney injury (S-AKI). Kidney function improvement was defined as serum creatinine levels below 0.5 times the value of day 1 on day 5, whereas renal function nonimprovement was defined as levels above 1.5 times the value of the first day. ELISA was used to measure serum CD5L levels. (**f**) Immunofluorescence images of FRCs stained with CD5L antibodies (red). Left, bar = 50 μm. Right, bar = 20 μm. (**g**) Representative western blots showing CD5L, NLRP3, N-GSDMD, PINK1, TOMM20, P62, and LC3B in PKTCs. (**h**) After LPS treatment for 24 h, SEM was used to observe the membrane morphology of PKTCs. Bar = 10 μm. (**i**) Tetramethylrhodamine ethyl ester (TMRE) was used to measure the $\Delta\psi$m. TMRE: red; 4′,6-diamidino-2-phenylindole (DAPI): blue. Bar = 100 μm. (**j**) MitoTracker Red CMXRos was used to label mitochondria. Staining with xx (GSDMD) antibodies (green) was performed. Images were obtained using confocal microscopy. Bar = 10 μm. For (**c,d**), the graphs show the mean ± SD. Circles, squares, and triangles represent individual patients. $P < 0.05$ was considered to indicate statistical significance. $**P < 0.01$. $***P < 0.001$. The statistical tests used in (**c**) and (**d**) were 2-sided. The data are from 3 separate experiments. LPS, lipopolysaccharide; PBS, phosphate buffered saline; Scr, serum creatinine. To optimize viewing of this image, please see the online version of this article at www.kidney-international.org.

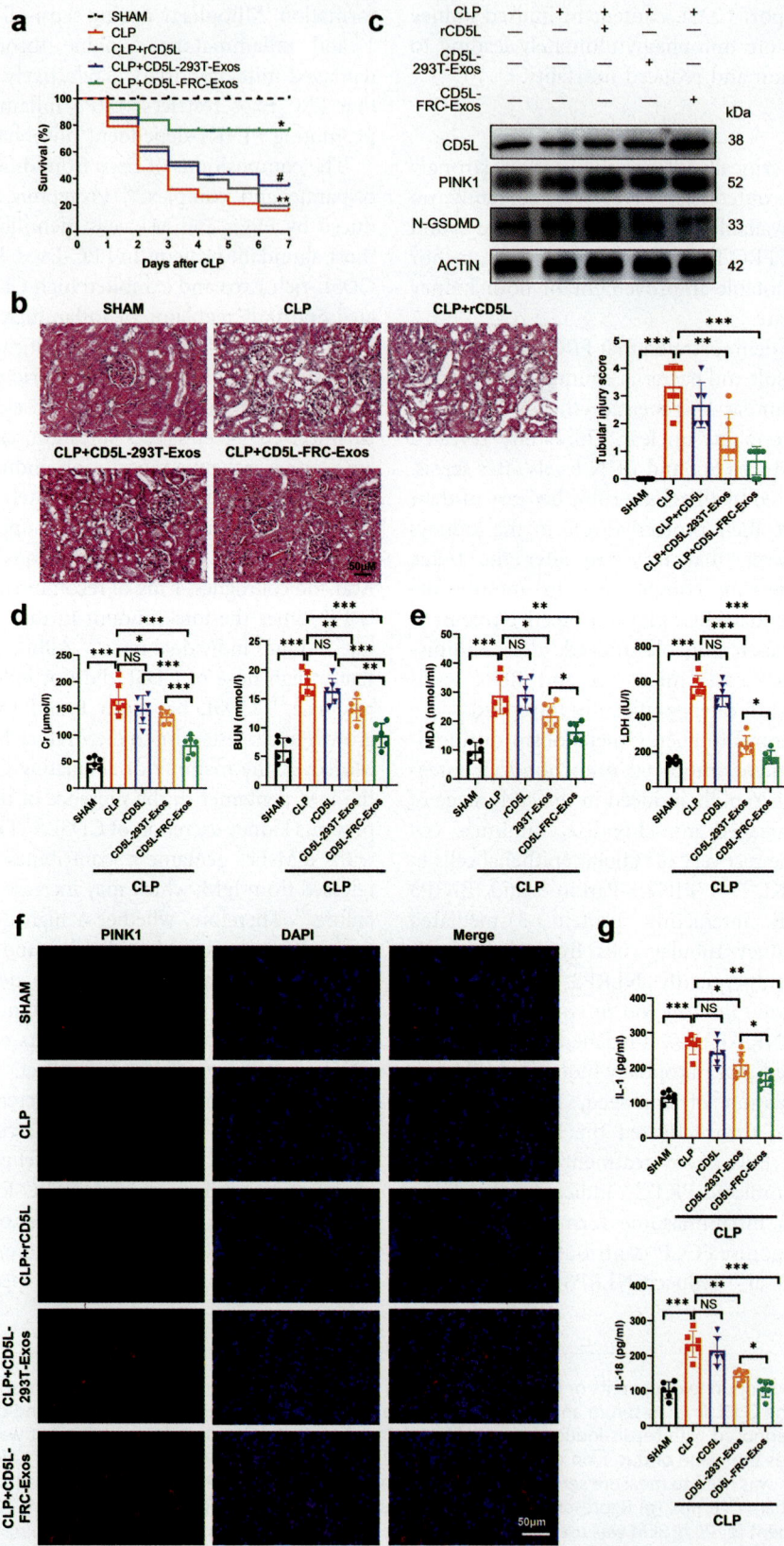

Figure 7 | Modified fibroblastic reticular cell–derived exosomes (FRC-Exos) can effectively attenuate sepsis-induced kidney injury. Wild-type (WT) mice were subjected to cecal ligation and puncture (CLP). Recombinant CD5L (rCD5L), CD5L-293T-Exos, and CD5L-FRC-Exos were all administered via tail vein injection to septic mice. Kidney tissue and serum were collected at 24 hours after CLP. (a) Seven-day survival after CLP. $*P <0.05$, CLP + CD5L-FRC-Exos vs. CLP + rCD5L; $**P <0.01$, CLP + CD5L-FRC-Exos vs. CLP; $^{\#}P <0.05$, CLP + CD5L-FRC-Exos vs. CLP + CD5L-293T-Exos; SHAM, $n = 12$, CLP, $n = 19$; CLP + rCD5L, $n = 20$; CLP + CD5L-293T-Exos, $n = 21$; CLP + CD5L-FRC-Exos, $n = 20$. (b) Hematoxylin (continued)

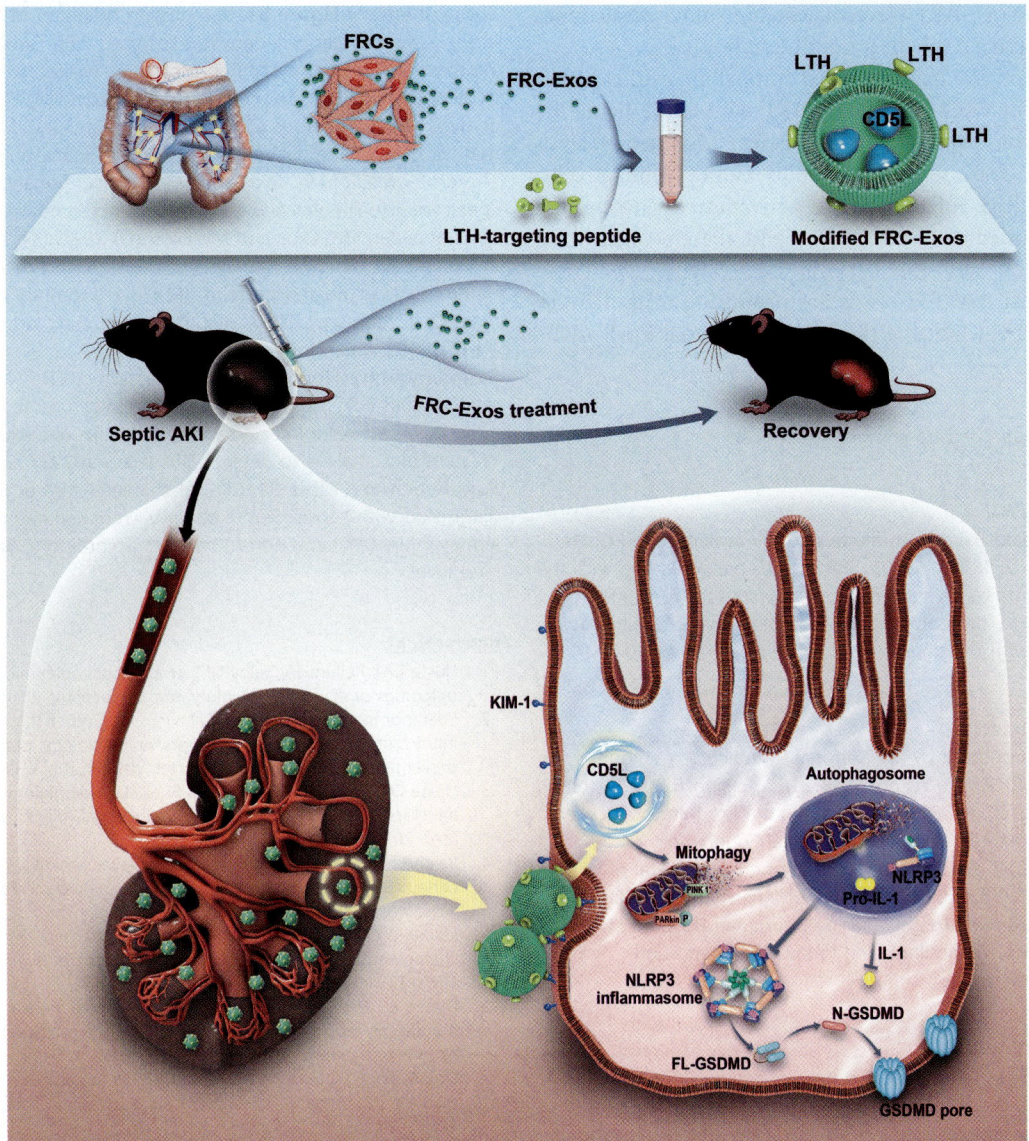

Figure 8 | Schematic diagram showing the potential mechanism by which modified fibroblastic reticular cell–derived exosomes (FRC-Exos) attenuate sepsis-induced acute kidney injury (S-AKI). Modifying the targeting peptide segment enhances the specificity of FRC-Exos binding to injured kidney tubular cells. CD5L degrades the NLRP3 inflammasome by promoting PINK1-Parkin–mediated mitophagy and improving kidney function, subsequently attenuating AKI pathogenesis. FL-GSDMD, full-length gasdermin D; GSDMD, gasdermin D; N-GSDMD, N-terminal gasdermin D; IL, interleukin; KIM-1, kidney injury molecule 1; LTH, LTHVVWL peptide.

expressed on injured kidney cells, significantly enhanced the targeting capabilities of the Exos towards kidney tubular cells. In the present study, FRC-Exos rich in CD5L were engulfed by PKTCs, which then promoted PINK-mediated mitophagy to minimize the damage. Exos have advantages over synthetic carriers such as liposomes or capsules because they contain active mediators of motility and homing.[36]

In our S-AKI model, we observed a statistically significant improvement in kidney function, but the function was not fully restored. This lack of function restoration could have been due to several factors, including the severity of sepsis, and the dose, timing, and frequency of FRC-Exos administration. Although CD5L was identified via mass spectrometry, other components, such as microRNAs and long, noncodingRNAs, may also play

Figure 7 | (continued) and eosin (H&E) staining of kidney tissue. (**c**) Western blot detection of CD5L, PINK1, and N-GSDMD levels in various groups of mouse kidney tissues. (**d,e**) Measurement of serum creatinine (Scr), blood urea nitrogen (BUN), malondialdehyde (MDA), and lactate dehydrogenase (LDH) levels. (**f**) Immunofluorescence observation of PINK1 content in kidney tissue. (**g**) Interleukin (IL)-1 and IL-18 levels in kidney tissue were detected with an enzyme-linked immunosorbent assay (ELISA) kit. The data are shown as the mean ± SD from 2 separate experiments. Symbols represent individual mice. *$P < 0.05$; **$P < 0.01$; ***$P < 0.001$, unpaired, 2-tailed Student's *t* tests. To optimize viewing of this image, please see the online version of this article at www.kidney-international.org.

protective roles in S-AKI. Nevertheless, our study revealed that CD5L plays a crucial role in promoting mitophagy.

In conclusion, we have provided compelling evidence that Exos secreted by FRCs attenuate S-AKI, with CD5L being the most abundant protein in FRC-Exos. Modified CD5L-enriched FRC-Exos selectively bound kidney tubular cells, inhibiting NLRP3 inflammasome activation by promoting PINK-Parkin–mediated mitophagy, and thereby improving kidney function and the survival rate (Figure 8). These findings suggest that FRC-Exos are promising drug-delivery vehicles with great targeted therapeutic potential for S-AKI.

DISCLOSURE
All the authors declared no competing interests.

DATA STATEMENT
All mRNA-Seq data have been made publicly available via PubMed with BioProject ID: PRJNA993005. SRA records are accessible with the following link: https://www.ncbi.nlm.nih.gov/sra/PRJNA993005. All mass spectrometry proteomics data have been made publicly available via PRIDE with the dataset identifier (Project ID) PXD041501.

ACKNOWLEDGMENTS
This work was supported by the National Natural Science Foundation of China (no. 82102273 to YL, no. 81971816 to ZP; no. 82272208 to ZP; no. 82241039 to ZP, no. 82202388 to JW); the Program of Excellent Doctoral (Postdoctoral); Wu Jieping Medical Foundation (no. 320.6750.2023-02-4 to YL); Research of Zhongnan Hospital of Wuhan University (no. ZNYB2020008 to YL); the Hainan Province Clinical Medical Center (project to ZP), and the Zhongnan Hospital of Wuhan University Science, Technology and Innovation Seed Fund (CXPY2020012 to YL).

AUTHOR CONTRIBUTIONS
YL conceived the project, designed the project, and approved the final manuscript. CH, PZ, JZ, and JS performed the experiments. ZJ provided clinical samples. BH and JW extracted and analyzed the data. XW, XZ, TB, JK, and MD revised the manuscript. YL, CH, and PZ contributed equally to this study. YL initiated this study and therefore is in the first position in the author list. ZP initiated and led this study, edited the manuscript, and approved the final version.

SUPPLEMENTARY MATERIAL
Supplementary File (Word)
Supplementary Methods: Detailed experimental materials and methods.
Supplementary Figure S1. The identification of fibroblastic reticular cells (FRCs) and extraction methods for derived exosomes (FRC-Exos). (A) FRCs were isolated from mesenteric tissues and expanded ex vivo. Observation of the morphology of FRCs under an optical microscope. FRCs had a spindle-like morphology with the formation of dendritic protrusions and veil-like extensions. (B) The purity of FRCs (CD45-CD31-PDPN+) was assessed using flow cytometry. (C) Illustration of the Exos extraction process by ultracentrifugation.
Supplementary Figure S2. Reactome annotation analysis of differentially expressed genes (DEGs) in lipopolysaccharide (LPS)-treated and untreated primary kidney tubular cells (PKTCs). Transcriptomic RNA-seq analysis of LPS-treated and untreated PKTCs. Reactome annotation analysis of the DEGs was performed.
Supplementary Figure S3. The protein profile of M1-Exos and fibroblastic reticular cell–derived exosomes (FRC-Exos) was identified via mass spectrometry. (A) Representative western blots showing iNOS and MINCLE in the treated macrophages. (B) Flow cytometric analysis of macrophages. CD80: classically activated (M1) macrophage marker; CD206: alternatively activated (M2) macrophage marker. (C) The proteomes of FRC-Exos and M1-Exos were analyzed by mass spectrometry. The volcano plot displays differentially expressed proteins between FRC-Exos and M1-Exos. (D) KEGG (Kyoto Encyclopedia of Genes and Genomes) analysis of the signaling pathways of the differentially expressed proteins. (E) Flow cytometry analysis of reactive oxygen species (ROS) content in primary kidney tubular cells (PKTCs). MFI, mean fluorescence intensity.
Supplementary Figure S4. The expression of CD5L in fibroblastic reticular cells (FRCs) and 293T cells after lentivirus infection. (A,B) 293T and FRCs. Cells were infected with a lentivirus overexpressing CD5L. Western blot analysis to detect CD5L levels in 293T cells and FRCs.
Supplementary Table S1. Clinical characteristics of patients diagnosed with sepsis. Septic patients were separated into acute kidney injury (AKI) and non-AKI groups according to serum creatinine (Scr) level.

REFERENCES
1. Hoste EAJ, Kellum JA, Selby NM, et al. Global epidemiology and outcomes of acute kidney injury. *Nat Rev Nephrol*. 2018;14:607–625.
2. Peerapornratana S, Manrique-Caballero CL, Gómez H, et al. Acute kidney injury from sepsis: current concepts, epidemiology, pathophysiology, prevention and treatment. *Kidney Int*. 2019;96:1083–1099.
3. Hoste EAJ, Bagshaw SM, Bellomo R, et al. Epidemiology of acute kidney injury in critically ill patients: the multinational AKI-EPI study. *Intens Care Med*. 2015;41:1411–1423.
4. Bajénoff M, Germain RN. B-cell follicle development remodels the conduit system and allows soluble antigen delivery to follicular dendritic cells. *Blood*. 2009;114:4989–4997.
5. Onder L, Cheng H-W, Ludewig B. Visualization and functional characterization of lymphoid organ fibroblasts. *Immunol Rev*. 2022;306:108–122.
6. Dubey LK, Karempudi P, Luther SA, et al. Interactions between fibroblastic reticular cells and B cells promote mesenteric lymph node lymphangiogenesis. *Nat Commun*. 2017;8:367.
7. Link A, Vogt TK, Favre S, et al. Fibroblastic reticular cells in lymph nodes regulate the homeostasis of naive T cells. *Nat Immunol*. 2007;8:1255–1265.
8. Fletcher AL, Elman JS, Astarita J, et al. Lymph node fibroblastic reticular cell transplants show robust therapeutic efficacy in high-mortality murine sepsis. *Sci Trans Med*. 2014;6:249ra109.
9. Xu L, Li Y, Yang C, et al. TLR9 signaling in fibroblastic reticular cells regulates peritoneal immunity. *J Clin Invest*. 2019;129:3657–3669.
10. Zhang Y, Liu Y, Liu H, et al. Exosomes: biogenesis, biologic function and clinical potential. *Cell Biosci*. 2019;9:19.
11. Martinez VG, Escoda-Ferran C, Tadeu Simões I, et al. The macrophage soluble receptor AIM/Api6/CD5L displays a broad pathogen recognition spectrum and is involved in early response to microbial aggression. *Cell Mol Immunol*. 2014;11:343–354.
12. Arai S, Kitada K, Yamazaki T, et al. Apoptosis inhibitor of macrophage protein enhances intraluminal debris clearance and ameliorates acute kidney injury in mice. *Nat Med*. 2016;22:183–193.
13. Yang H, Luo Y, Lai X. The comprehensive role of apoptosis inhibitor of macrophage (AIM) in pathological conditions. *Clin Exp Immunol*. 2023;212:184–198.
14. Chen C, Zhang Z, Gu X, et al. Exosomes: new regulators of reproductive development. *Mater Today Bio*. 2023;19:100608.
15. Xiang H, Xu Z, Zhang C, et al. Macrophage-derived exosomes mediate glomerular endothelial cell dysfunction in sepsis-associated acute kidney injury. *Cell Biosci*. 2023;13:46.
16. Zarbock A, Nadim MK, Pickkers P, et al. Sepsis-associated acute kidney injury: consensus report of the 28th Acute Disease Quality Initiative workgroup. *Nat Rev Nephrol*. 2023;19:401–417.
17. Raeven P, Zipperle J, Drechsler S. Extracellular vesicles as markers and mediators in sepsis. *Theranostics*. 2018;8:3348–3365.

18. Kalluri R, LeBleu VS. The biology, function, and biomedical applications of exosomes. *Science*. 2020;367:eaau6977.
19. Gómez H, Kellum JA, Ronco C. Metabolic reprogramming and tolerance during sepsis-induced AKI. *Nat Rev Nephrol*. 2017;13:143–151.
20. Kramann R, Humphreys BD. Kidney pericytes: roles in regeneration and fibrosis. *Semin Nephrol*. 2014;34:374–383.
21. Parikh SM, Yang Y, He L, et al. Mitochondrial function and disturbances in the septic kidney. *Semin Nephrol*. 2015;35:108–119.
22. Sun J, Zhang J, Tian J, et al. Mitochondria in sepsis-induced AKI. *J Am Soc Nephrol*. 2019;30:1151–1161.
23. Lin Q, Li S, Jiang N, et al. Inhibiting NLRP3 inflammasome attenuates apoptosis in contrast-induced acute kidney injury through the upregulation of HIF1A and BNIP3-mediated mitophagy. *Autophagy*. 2021;17:2975–2990.
24. Lin Q, Li S, Jiang N, et al. PINK1-parkin pathway of mitophagy protects against contrast-induced acute kidney injury via decreasing mitochondrial ROS and NLRP3 inflammasome activation. *Redox Biol*. 2019;26:101254.
25. Zhong Z, Umemura A, Sanchez-Lopez E, et al. NF-κB restricts inflammasome activation via elimination of damaged mitochondria. *Cell*. 2016;164:896–910.
26. Mathivanan S, Fahner CJ, Reid GE, et al. ExoCarta 2012: database of exosomal proteins, RNA and lipids. *Nucl Acids Res*. 2012;40:D1241–D1244.
27. Miyazaki T, Hirokami Y, Matsuhashi N, et al. Increased susceptibility of thymocytes to apoptosis in mice lacking AIM, a novel murine macrophage-derived soluble factor belonging to the scavenger receptor cysteine-rich domain superfamily. *J ExperMed*. 1999;189:413–422.
28. Wang C, Yosef N, Gaublomme J, et al. CD5L/AIM regulates lipid biosynthesis and restrains Th17 cell pathogenicity. *Cell*. 2015;163:1413–1427.
29. Wu X, Li M, Chen T, et al. Apoptosis inhibitor of macrophage/CD5L is associated with disease activity in rheumatoid arthritis. *Clin Exp Rheumatol*. 2021;39:58–65.
30. LaFargue CJ, Amero P, Noh K, et al. Overcoming adaptive resistance to anti-VEGF therapy by targeting CD5L. *Nat Commun*. 2023;14:2407.
31. Miyazaki T, Yamazaki T, Sugisawa R, et al. AIM associated with the IgM pentamer: attackers on stand-by at aircraft carrier. *Cell Mol Immunol*. 2018;15:563–574.
32. Arai S, Maehara N, Iwamura Y, et al. Obesity-associated autoantibody production requires AIM to retain the immunoglobulin M immune complex on follicular dendritic cells. *Cell Rep*. 2013;3:1187–1198.
33. Hiramoto E, Tsutsumi A, Suzuki R, et al. The IgM pentamer is an asymmetric pentagon with an open groove that binds the AIM protein. *Sci Adv*. 2018;4:eaau1199.
34. Galle-Treger L, Moreau M, Ballaire R, et al. Targeted invalidation of SR-B1 in macrophages reduces macrophage apoptosis and accelerates atherosclerosis. *Cardiovasc Res*. 2020;116:554–565.
35. Hashemian SM, Pourhanifeh MH, Fadaei S, et al. Non-coding RNAs and exosomes: their role in the pathogenesis of sepsis. *Mol Ther Nucl Acids*. 2020;21:51–74.
36. Herrmann IK, Wood MJA, Fuhrmann G. Extracellular vesicles as a next-generation drug delivery platform. *Nat Nanotechnol*. 2021;16:748–759.

basic research

Collectin 11 has a pivotal role in host defense against kidney and bladder infection in mice

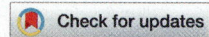

Kun-Yi Wu[1], Bo Cao[1], Wan-Bing Chen[1], Weiju Wu[2], Shujuan Zhao[1], Xiao-Yun Min[1], Jurong Yang[3], Jin Han[4], Xia Dong[5], Na Wang[1], Yi Wu[6], Peter Garred[7], Steven H. Sacks[2], Wuding Zhou[2,8] and Ke Li[1,8]

[1]Core Research Laboratory, Second Affiliated Hospital, Xi'an Jiaotong University, Xi'an, China; [2]Peter Gorer Department of Immunobiology, School of Immunology & Microbial Sciences, Faculty of Life Sciences & Medicine, King's College London, London, UK; [3]Department of Nephrology, The Third Affiliated Hospital of Chongqing Medical University, Chongqing, China; [4]Department of Nephrology, Second Affiliated Hospital, Xi'an Jiaotong University, Xi'an, China; [5]Department of Ophthalmology, The First Affiliated Hospital, Sun Yat-sen University, Guangdong, China; [6]MOE Key Laboratory of Environment and Genes Related to Diseases, School of Basic Medical Sciences, Xi'an Jiaotong University, Xi'an, China; and [7]Laboratory of Molecular Medicine, Department of Clinical Immunology, Rigshospitalet and University of Copenhagen, Copenhagen, Denmark

The urinary tract is constantly exposed to microorganisms. Host defense mechanisms in protection from microbial colonization and development of urinary tract infections require better understanding to control kidney infection. Here we report that the lectin collectin 11 (CL-11), particularly kidney produced, has a pivotal role in host defense against uropathogen infection. CL-11 was found in mouse urine under normal and pathological conditions. Mice with global gene ablation of *Colec11* had increased susceptibility to and severity of kidney and to an extent, bladder infection. Mice with kidney-specific *Colec11* ablation exhibited a similar disease phenotype to that observed in global *Colec11* deficient mice, indicating the importance of kidney produced CL-11 for protection against kidney and bladder infection. Conversely, intravesical or systemic administration of recombinant CL-11 reduced susceptibility to and severity of kidney and bladder infection. Mechanism analysis revealed that CL-11 can mediate several key innate defense mechanisms (agglutination, anti- adhesion, opsonophagocytosis), and limit local inflammatory responses to pathogens. Furthermore, CL-11-mediated innate defense mechanisms can act on clinically relevant microorganisms including multiple antibiotic resistant strains. CL-11 was detectable in eight of 24 urine samples from patients with urinary tract infections but not detectable in urine samples from ten healthy individuals. Thus, our findings demonstrate that CL-11 is a key factor of host defense mechanisms in kidney and bladder infection with therapeutic potential for human application.

Kidney International (2024) **105**, 524–539; https://doi.org/10.1016/j.kint.2023.11.031

KEYWORDS: collectin 11; cystitis; pyelonephritis; urinary tract infections; uropathogenic *E. coli*

Copyright © 2023, International Society of Nephrology. Published by Elsevier Inc. All rights reserved.

Translational Statement

In this study, by employing 2 collectin-11 (CL-11)– deficient mouse strains (global; kidney-specific) and pharmacologic treatment with recombinant CL-11 (rCL-11), we demonstrate that CL-11 has a pivotal role in host defense against uropathogenic *Escherichia coli* via reduction of susceptibility to and severity of the infection. We have validated the clinical relevance of these data with patient urine isolates. Taken together, our findings provide evidence for kidney-produced CL-11 as a key defense mechanism against urinary tract infection, with potential for therapeutic human application.

Correspondence: *Ke Li, Core Research Laboratory, The Second Affiliated Hospital, School of Medicine, Xi'an Jiaotong University, Xi'an, 710004 China. E-mail: ke.li@mail.xjtu.edu.cn; or Wuding Zhou, Peter Gorer Department of Immunobiology, School of Immunology & Microbial Sciences, King's College London, Guy's Hospital, London SE1 9RT, UK. E-mail: wuding.zhou@kcl.ac.uk*

[8]KL and WZ are senior/corresponding authors.

Received 24 February 2023; revised 11 November 2023; accepted 28 November 2023; published online 27 December 2023

Urinary tract infections (UTIs) are among the most common infectious diseases (150 million cases per year worldwide). They are especially frequent in women, children, and the elderly, and they are a particular problem for patients with diabetes and indwelling urinary catheters. Although antibiotics are available to treat UTI, a number of challenges remain, such as frequent recurrence, persistence of infection, and the increasing risk of resistance to antibiotics. An increasing prevalence of multidrug-resistant uropathogenic *Escherichia coli* (UPEC) strains has been reported globally, which has significant impact on overall antimicrobial resistance.[1,2] For these reasons, more research is needed, to improve our understanding of UTI pathogenesis and host defense, and to identify novel defense mechanisms and develop new treatment strategies that could be used to improve current treatment.

UTIs comprise a wide spectrum of diseases, including bladder infection (cystitis), kidney infection (pyelonephritis), and the kidney infection–caused sepsis and severe systemic infection that occurs with multi-organ failure.[3] UTIs usually start in the bladder and can spread to the kidney (called ascending UTI). The urinary tract is exposed constantly to microorganisms that inhabit the gastrointestinal tract. Therefore, effective natural and constitutive defense mechanisms are critical for providing protection from microbial colonization and preventing UTIs, such as epithelial surface barrier, antimicrobial peptides and proteins produced by urinary tract epithelial cells or immune cells.[4] If the infection is not controlled by those natural defense mechanisms, UPEC strains can persist within the urinary tract, which colonize and invade epithelium and worsen UTI. Upon contact with epithelial cells, UPEC liberate toxins that mediate direct injury of the cells, disrupting the mucosal barrier and opening access to the underlying tissue.[5] UPEC colonization and entry into the underlying tissue can initiate host immune responses, which are considered to be critical in fighting the infection. However, UPEC-mediated excessive inflammatory responses also can cause renal tissue inflammation and epithelial destruction, allowing bacteria to enter the underlying tissue.[3,6] Therefore, natural and constitutive defense mechanisms and fine-tuned induced immune responses are required for effective defense against UTI.

The collectins are a group of soluble C-type lectins; mannose-binding lectin (MBL) and lung surfactant proteins (SPs) are well known members of this group. They function as pattern-recognition receptors that bind to carbohydrate moieties on the surface of pathogens and host cells and accordingly have important roles in both host defense and the regulation of cellular responses.[7–9] Collectin-11 (CL-11; also known as CL-K1) is a recently described member of the collectin family and displays structural similarities with MBL, SP-A, and SP-D. CL-11 consists of a carbohydrate recognition domain, followed by a neck region. CD-11 is highly conserved among species; human and mice are 92% homologous at the amino-acid level.[10] Compared to other collectins, CL-11 has some unique characteristics, such as the following: (i) a wide tissue distribution with high-level expression was found in the kidney; (ii) relatively lower concentrations in the circulation ($\sim$300 ng/ml), often in complex with other serum proteins,[11] and thus potentially not sufficiently extravasated; and (iii) the ability to bind a wide range of biological molecules and microbes.[10,12–14] This set of characteristics has led to the suggestion that CL-11 is multifunctional molecule and that local production of CL-11 may play important roles in host defense at the sites of pathogen encounter. Given that the kidney is a major organ for synthesizing CL-11, that several well known collectins (e.g., MBL) may not be produced in the kidney, and that CL-11 has several biological functions related to host defense mechanisms (e.g., binding to microbes, acting as opsonin),[10,13,15] we hypothesized that CL-11, particularly kidney-produced CL-11, plays important roles in host defense against UTI.

To investigate the hypothesis, we employed a well-established murine model of ascending UTI,[16–18] which is induced by bladder inoculation with human UPEC strain CFT073 or J96.[16,19] The model, in combination with 2 CL-11-deficient mouse strains (global; kidney-specific), was used to determine the protective roles of CL-11 in kidney and bladder infection and evaluate the importance of renal production of CL-11 for defending against kidney and bladder infection. We also performed a series of *ex vivo* or *in vitro* analyses to address the mechanisms conferring the protection and validated its clinical relevance with patient urine isolates. The murine model in combination with intravesical or intraperitoneal administration of recombinant CL-11 (rCL-11) was used to further confirm the protective role of CL-11 in kidney and bladder infection.

METHODS

Mice

Global CL-11-deficient ($Colec11^{-/-}$) mice on a C57BL/6 (B6) background[20] were provided by Mutant Mouse Resource and Research Centers (UC Davis, Davis, CA) and have been back-crossed onto the B6 strain for least 8 generations. Wild-type (WT) littermates were used as controls for $Colec11^{-/-}$ (assigned to knockout [KO]) mice. Kidney CL-11-deficient mice (Six2-$Colec11^{-/-}$, assigned to K-KO) and a kidney CL-11-sufficient littermate (Six2-$Colec11^{+/+}$, assigned to K-WT littermate) were generated by crossbreeding Colec11$^{flox/flox}$ and Six2/cre mice; both strains are on a B6 background (see details in Supplementary Figure S1). Female mice (aged 8–10 weeks) were used in all experiments. All mice were maintained in specific pathogen-free conditions on a 12-hour reversed light–dark cycle. The Ethics Review Committee for Animal Experimentation at Xi'an Jiaotong University approved and oversaw all mouse experiments.

Bacterial strains

UPEC strains CFT073 (O6:H1:K2) and *E. coli* J96 (serotype O4; K6) were isolated from acute pyelonephritis patients; these are serum-resistant, hemolysin-secreting *E. coli* strains that express both type 1 and P fimbriae.[16,19] *E. coli* J96 was provided by Dr. R. Welch, University of Wisconsin, USA. CFT073 was provided by Professor S. Wigneshwera, Imperial College, UK. For clinical isolates, 6 clinical isolates were isolated from the urine of patients with UTIs and characterized in terms of their virulence and antibiotic resistance. Details are given in Supplementary Tables S1 and S2.

Induction of UTI

Murine UTI was induced in female mice by bladder inoculation with UPEC *per* urethra as previously described.[17,18] For assessing UTI infection rate, mice were inoculated with a low dose of UPEC (5 x 10^5 colony-forming units [cfu] in 50 μl phosphate-buffered saline [PBS]); for assessing severity of UTI, mice were inoculated with a high dose of UPEC (1 x 10^8 CFU in 50 μl PBS). Mice were killed at different time points up to 48 hours post-inoculation (hpi). Kidney and bladder tissues were collected and used for analyzing bacterial load, bacterial colonization, histopathology, immunohistochemical staining, and intrarenal gene expression. To avoid bias, we consistently use the left kidney to measure the bacterial load, and the right kidney is used for measuring other parameters. In some experiments, pharmacologic treatment with rCL-11 was employed. For local (intravesical) treatment, each mouse was inoculated with 50 μl of a mix of UPEC (2 x 10^9 CFU/ml) and rCL-11 or bovine serum albumin (BSA; 1200 ng/ml) in PBS. For systemic treatment, each mouse was given rCL-11 or BSA in saline (600 ng per mouse) by intraperitoneal (i.p.) injection at 2 hours before and 6 hours after inoculation. The dosages of rCL-11 used in pharmacological administration experiments were close to the range of serum concentrations of CL-11 in health and diseases (200–700 ng/ml).

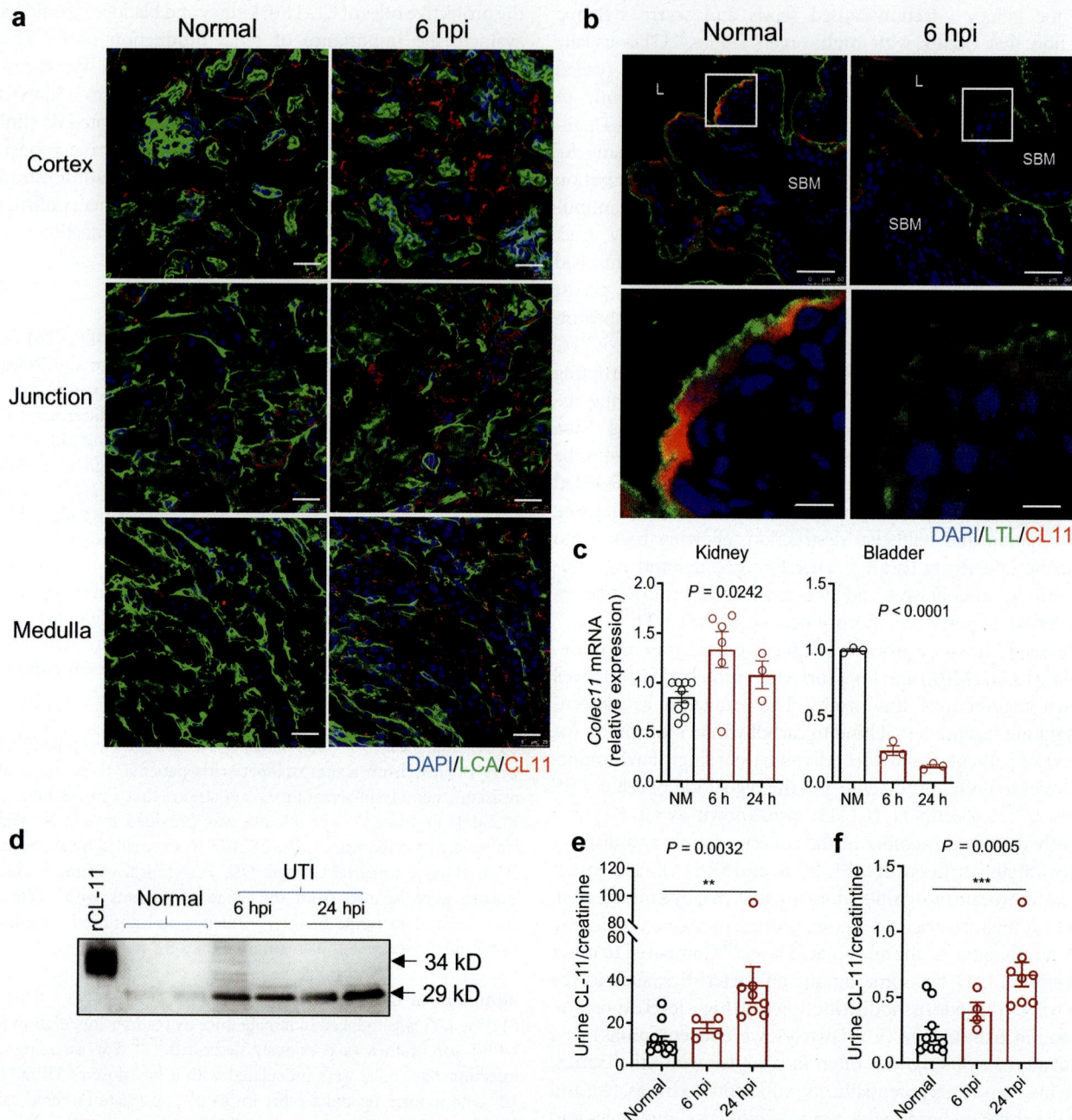

Figure 1 | Detection of collectin 11 (CL-11) in urinary tract and its relevance to urinary tract infection (UTI). (**a**) Representative images of immunofluorescence for CL-11 in the kidney of normal mice and mice at 6 hours post-infection (hpi). Images of cortex, corticomedullary junction, and medulla were taken from the kidney sections stained with anti-CL-11 (red), LCA (green; for illustrating tubules and glomeruli), and 4′,6-diamidino-2-phenylindole (DAPI; blue). Bars = 25 μm. (**b**) Representative images of immunofluorescence for CL-11 in the bladder of normal mice and mice at 6 hpi. Images were taken from the bladder sections stained with anti-CL-11 (red), LTL (green; for illustrating superficial uroepithelial cells), and DAPI (blue). Top panel: low-magnification images. Bars = 50 μm. Bottom panels: high-magnification images corresponding to the boxed regions in the top panel. Bars = 10 μm. (**a,b**) A representative of 3 experiments is shown. (**c**) Reverse transcription quantitative polymerase chain reaction for detecting *Colec*11 mRNA in kidney and bladder tissues of normal (NM) and infected mice. Data were analyzed by 1-way analysis of variance with multiple-comparison test (kidney: n = 9, 6, 3 mice per group for NM, 6 hpi and 24 hpi, respectively; bladder: n = 3 mice per group). (**d–f**) Western blot for detecting CL-11 in urine of NM (non-infected) and infected mice. (**d**) Representative immunoblots showing CL-11 protein (~29 kD) was detected in the urine. Each lane represents urine sample from an individual mouse. Recombinant CL-11 (rCL-11) used as positive control resulted in an ~34-kD band. (**e**) Estimated levels of CL-11 in urine samples using rCL-11 blot as a standard. (**f**) Normalized measurements of urine CL-11 (ng/ml) using urine creatinine levels (mg/ml). Data were analyzed by 1-way analysis of variance with multiple-comparison test (n = 11, 4, and 8 for NM, 6 hpi, and 24 hpi, respectively). **P < 0.005; ***P < 0.001. L, lumen; LCA, lens culinaris agglutinin; LTL, lotus tetragonolobus lectin; SBM, submucosa. To optimize viewing of this image, please see the online version of this article at www.kidney-international.org.

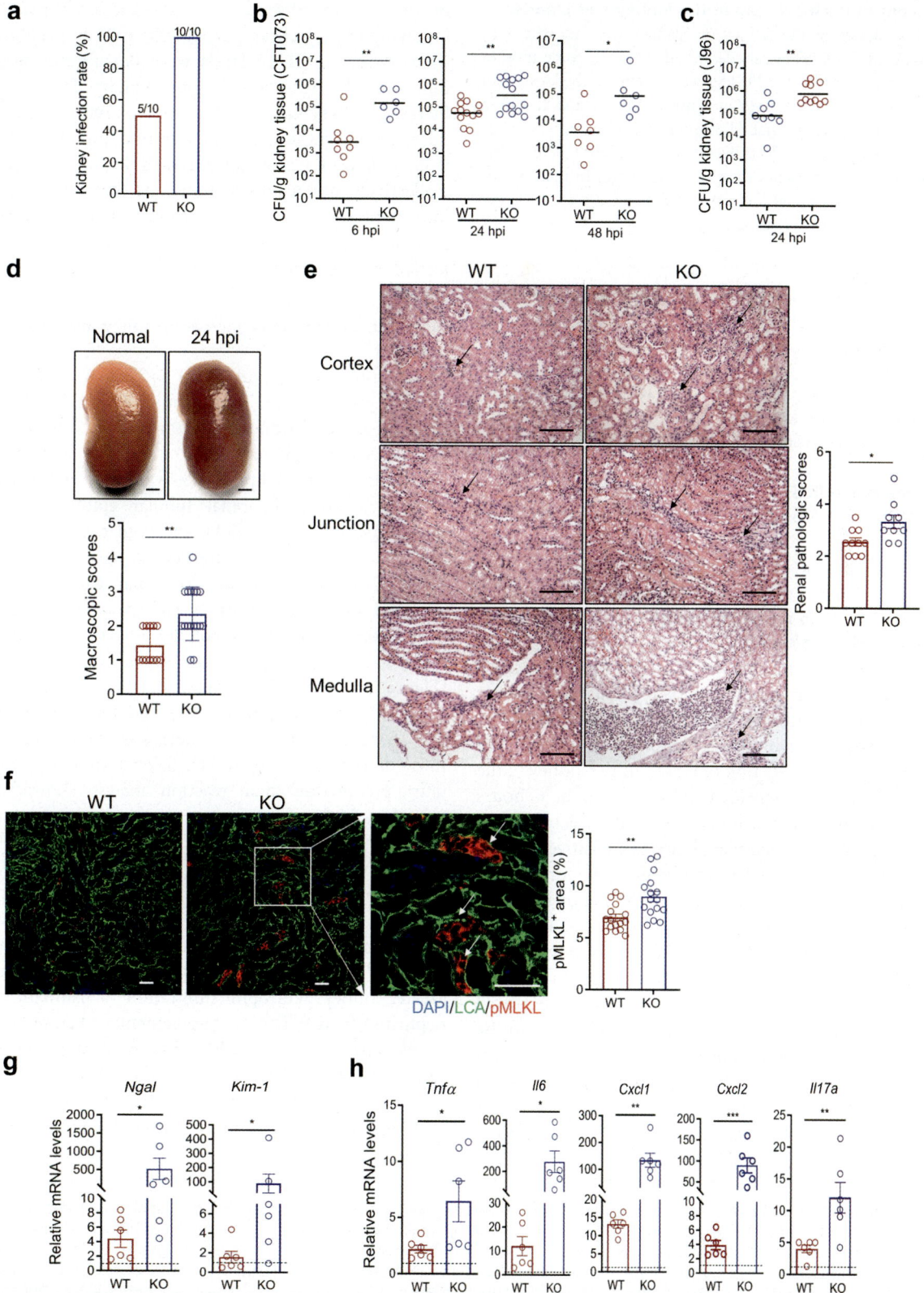

Figure 2 | Global collectin 11 (CL-11) deficiency increases kidney infection. (**a**) Kidney infection rate in wild-type (WT) and *Colec11−/−* knockout (KO) mice at 24 hours post-infection (hpi) with CFT073 (*n* = 10 mice per group). (**b**) Kidney bacterial load of WT and KO mice at 6, 24, and 48 hpi with CFT073. Data were analyzed by Mann-Whitney test (*n* = 6–8, 13–14, 6–7 mice per group for 6, 24, and 48 hpi, respectively). (**c**) Kidney bacterial loads of WT and KO mice at 24 hpi with J96. Data were analyzed by Mann-Whitney test (*n* = 8–10 mice per group). (**d**) Kidney macroscopic pathology analysis. Top panel: Representative macroscopic images of kidneys of normal and infected mice (with score: 2). Bars = 1 mm. Bottom panel: Macroscopic pathology scores at 24 hpi. Data were analyzed by unpaired *t* test (continued)

Measurement of bacterial load in the kidney and bladder

Bacterial load levels in the kidney or bladder were measured by bacterial CFU assay as previously described,[21,22] with some modifications. In brief, the kidney or bladder was weighted. The kidney (or bladder) tissue was homogenized in 1 ml of 0.1% Triton X-100 in sterile PBS, and 50 μl of a serial dilution of homogenates was plated on duplicate cystine lactose electrolyte deficient (CLED) plates. After incubation of plates for 24 hours at 37 °C, colonies formed on the plate were manually counted and expressed as an average CFU per gram of kidney (or bladder) tissue.

Statistical analysis

Data are shown as mean ± SEM. Unpaired t test or Mann-Whitney test was used to compare the means of two groups. A paired t-test was used to compare the means of matched-pairs. A 1-way or 2-way analysis of variance or a Kruskal-Wallis test with multiple comparison was used to compare the means of more than 2 independent groups. All the analyses were performed using GraphPad Prism 9 software. $P < 0.05$ was considered to be significant.

Supplementary methods

Reagents and extended methods are given in the Supplementary Methods.

RESULTS

Production of CL-11 in urinary tract and its relevance to kidney and bladder infection

We first examined the production of CL-11 in urinary tract and assessed whether its production is regulated in response to UPEC infection. Immunofluorescence (IF) for CL-11 showed that positive staining was observed in normal kidney, confirming the production of CL-11 in the kidney[12]; the positive staining was intensified in the kidney at 6 hours post-infection (hpi), with a broad distribution across 3 regions (cortex, junction, medulla; Figure 1a). Positive staining of CL-11 also was observed in the bladder of normal and infected mice, mainly in the urothelium; the staining appears more pronounced in normal mice than in infected mice at 6 hpi (Figure 1b). CL-11 mRNA was detected in normal kidney and bladder by reverse transcription polymerase chain reaction (RT-PCR); the levels in the kidney were increased after infection at 6 hpi and 24 hpi, whereas the levels in the bladder were decreased after infection (Figure 1c), consistent with the IF observations. The reduction of CL-11 expression in the bladder could be due to the shedding of uroepithelium. Western blot analysis showed that CL-11 was detected in normal and infected urine, and the levels were elevated following the infection, particularly at 24 hpi (Figure 1d–f), whereas serum CL-11 levels were not altered significantly following the infection (Supplementary Figure S2). The increased CL-11 in infected urine may reflect a net effect of upregulated synthesis and/or secretion and increased release from damaged tissues and/or cells within the renal tract. Collectively, our results demonstrate that urinary tract is an important source of CL-11 production under normal and pathologic conditions, which serves as an important protective mechanism against UTI.

Global CL-11 deficiency increases kidney and bladder infection

To determine the role of CL-11 in UTI, we induced UTI in WT and global $Colec11^{-/-}$ (KO) mice with UPEC (CFT073 or J96) and assessed kidney infection rate and infection severity. Compared with WT mice, KO mice had a higher kidney infection rate at 24 hpi (100% vs. 50%; Figure 2a), more bacterial colonies in renal tubular epithelium at 6 hpi (Supplementary Figure S3A), and higher renal bacterial load levels at all examined time points (6, 24, and 48 hpi; Figure 2b). Similar results of renal bacterial load were observed when the J96 strain was used (Figure 2c). Kidney macroscopic and histopathologic analysis showed that KO mice have higher pathology scores than do WT mice (Figure 2d and e). IF revealed that the kidney of KO mice exhibited more phosphorylated mixed lineage kinase domain-like (pMLKL, a marker of necrosis)–stained tubules than those of WT mice (Figure 2f). Reverse transcription quantitative polymerase chain reaction analysis showed that KO mice had higher intrarenal gene expression of renal injury markers (neutrophil gelatinase-associated lipocalin [NGAL], kidney injury molecule 1 [KIM-1]; Figure 2g), proinflammatory mediators (i.e., tumor necrosis factor alpha [TNFα], interleukin [IL]-6, CXCL1, CXCL2, IL-17A), but lower expression of IL-10, than WT mice (Figure 2h). Immunohistochemical staining showed that KO mice had greater kidney neutrophil infiltration (a hallmark of pyelonephritis) than WT mice (Supplementary Figure S4).

We also assessed bladder infection rate and infection severity in WT and KO mice. Compared with WT mice, KO mice displayed a higher bladder infection rate (83% vs. 60%) at 6 hpi (Figure 3a), more bacterial colonies in bladder

Figure 2 | (continued) ($n = 12$ [WT] or 17 [KO] mice per group). (**e**) Kidney histopathology analysis. Left panel: Representative images of hematoxylin and eosin–stained kidney sections at 24 hpi, taken at cortex, corticomedullary junction, and medulla. Arrows indicate renal lesions. Bar = 100 mm. Right panel: Histopathologic scores. Data were analyzed by unpaired t test ($n = 9$ mice per group). (**f**) Immunofluorescence staining for phosphorylated mixed lineage kinase domain-like (pMLKL) in kidney sections of WT and KO mice at 24 hpi. Left panel: Representative images taken at medulla. Arrows indicate pMLKL-positive tubules. Bars = 50 μm. Right panel: Quantification of pMLKL fluorescence intensity. Data were analyzed by unpaired Student t test ($n = 16$ images, at original magnification ×200, from 4 mice per group). (**g**) Reverse transcription quantitative polymerase chain reaction (RT-qPCR) for detecting *Ngal* and *Kim-1* in kidney tissues at 24 hpi. Data were analyzed by Mann-Whitney test ($n = 6$ mice per group). (**h**) RT-qPCR for detecting cytokine and/or chemokine expression in kidney tissues at 24 hpi. Data were analyzed by unpaired t test ($n = 6$ mice per group). The dotted line across each graph in (**g**) and (**h**) represents the gene expression level of normal kidney tissue, which is similar between WT and KO mice. *$P < 0.05$; **$P < 0.005$; ***$P < 0.001$. CFU, colony-forming unit; DAPI, 4′,6-diamidino-2-phenylindole; IL, interleukin; KIM-1, kidney injury molecule 1; LCA, lens culinaris agglutinin; NGAL, neutrophil gelatinase-associated lipocalin. To optimize viewing of this image, please see the online version of this article at www.kidney-international.org.

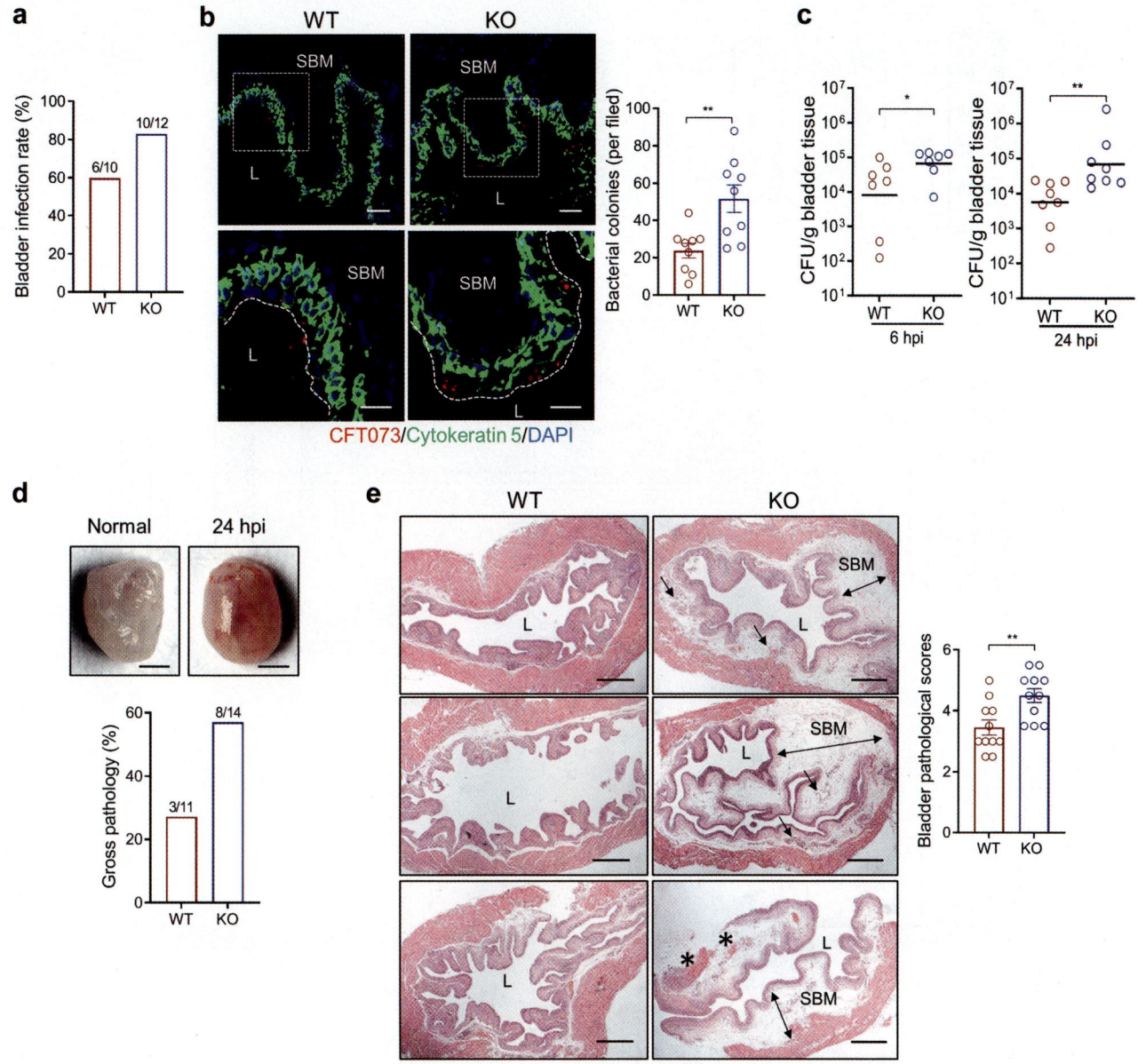

Figure 3 | Global collectin 11 (CL-11) deficiency increases bladder infection. (a) Bladder infection rate of wild-type (WT) and *Colec11−/−* knockout (KO) mice at 6 hours post-infection (hpi) with CFT073 (n = 10–12 mice per group). (b) Fluorescence microscope analysis of uropathogenic *Escherichia coli* (UPEC) colonization. Left panel: Representative microscope images of bladder sections of WT and KO mice at 3 hpi. Tetramethylrhodamine (TRITC)-labelled CFT073 (red) and cytokeratin 5 (green), 4′,6-diamidino-2-phenylindole (DAPI; blue) are shown. Top: low-magnification images. Bar = 50 μm. Bottom: high-magnification images corresponding to the boxed regions in the top images. Bar = 25 μm. Dotted lines indicate luminal surface of urothelium. Left panel: quantification of bacterial colonies in the bladders. Data were analyzed by unpaired t test (n = 9 fields [at original magnification ×200] from 3 mice per group). (c) Bacterial load in bladder tissues of WT and KO mice at 6 and 24 hpi with CFT073. Data were analyzed by Mann-Whitney test (n = 7–8 mice per group). (d) Bladder macroscopic pathology analysis. Top panel: Representative of macroscopic images of bladders of normal and infected mice with pathologic signs. Bottom panel: Frequencies of bladders exhibiting macroscopic signs of pathology in WT and KO mice at 24 hpi. Bars = 1 mm. (e) Bladder histopathology analysis. Left panel: Representative images of hematoxylin and eosin–stained bladder sections of WT and KO mice (n = 3 mice per group) at 24 hpi. Bars = 500 μm. Symbols: double arrows indicate edema in SBM; arrows indicate infiltrating cells; stars indicate hemorrhage. Left panel: Histologic scores. Data were analyzed by unpaired t test (n = 11 mice per group). CFU, colony-forming unit; L, lumen; SBM, submucosa. *$P < 0.05$; **$P < 0.005$. To optimize viewing of this image, please see the online version of this article at www.kidney-international.org.

epithelium at 3 hpi (Figure 3b), and higher bacterial load levels in the bladder at 24 and 48 hpi (Figure 3c). Macroscopic assessment showed that KO mice had higher frequencies of bladders that showed macroscopic signs of pathology than WT mice (Figure 3d). Histopathologic analysis showed that KO mice had more severe bladder injury with acute inflammatory lesions (i.e., edema, hemorrhage, and cellular infiltration) than WT mice at 24 hpi (Figure 3e). Collectively,

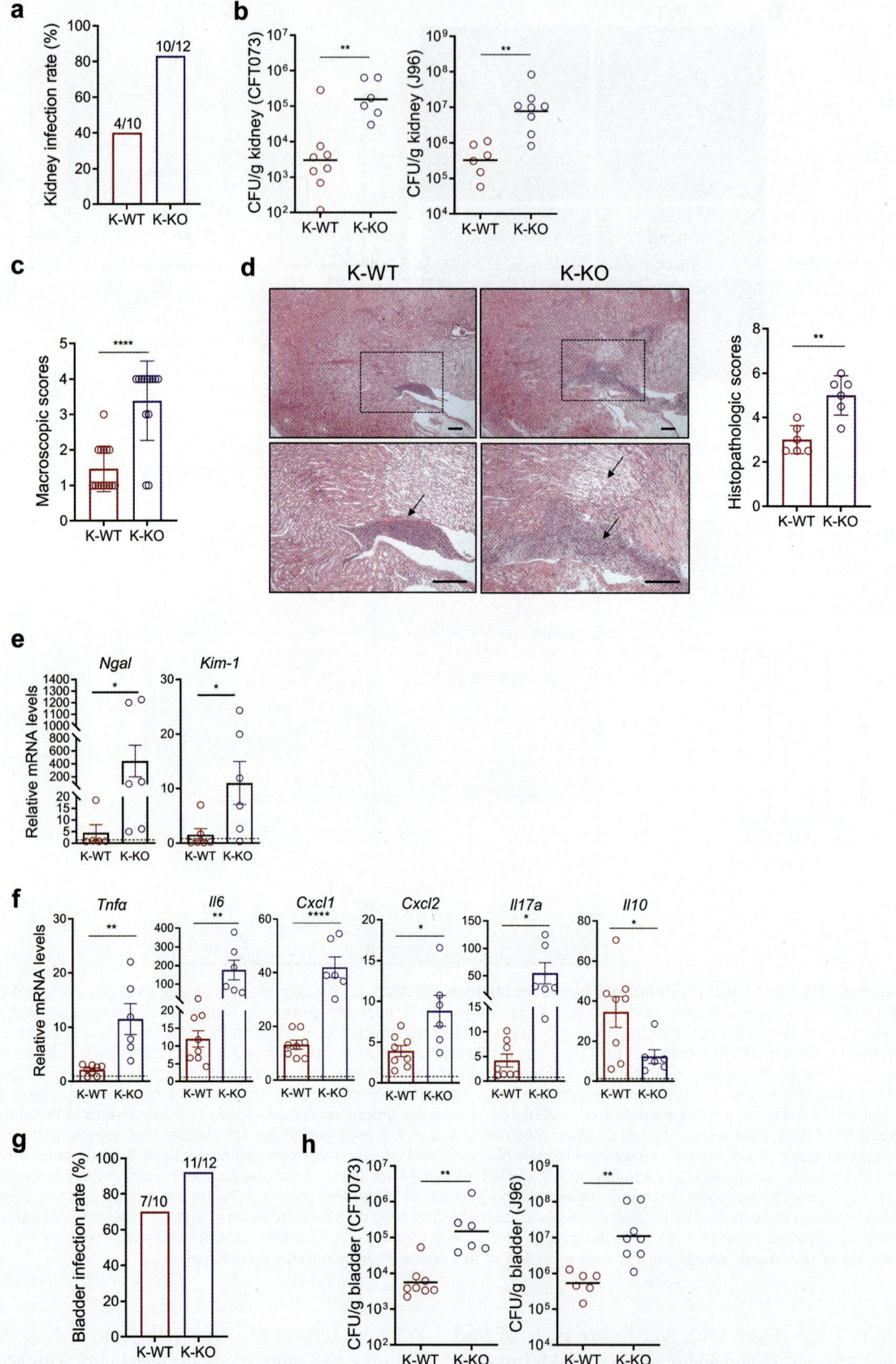

Figure 4 | Kidney-specific collectin-11 (CL-11) deficiency increases kidney and bladder infections. (a) Kidney infection rate in kidney CL-11-sufficient (K-WT) and kidney CL-11-deficient (K-KO) mice at 24 hours post-infection (hpi; $n = 10–12$ mice per group). (b–f) Kidney (continued)

these results demonstrate that CL-11 deficiency increases kidney and bladder infection rates and causes more severe kidney infection and tissue damage.

Kidney-specific CL-11 deficiency increases kidney and bladder infection

As kidney is an important source of CL-11 production, we hypothesized that local production of CL-11 in the kidney may play a dominant role in protection against UTI. To investigate this hypothesis, we induced UTI in kidney-specific CL-11-deficient mice (K-KO mice) and kidney CL-11-sufficient littermates (K-WT mice) using the same method as before. Compared with K-WT mice, K-KO mice displayed a higher kidney infection rate at 24 hpi (83% vs. 40%; Figure 4a), had higher kidney bacterial load levels at 24 hpi (Figure 4b), which was associated with pronounced kidney injury (evidenced by higher macroscopic and histopathologic scores and increased intrarenal gene expression of NGAL and KIM-1), and kidney inflammation (evidenced by increased intrarenal gene expression of proinflammatory mediators, i.e., TNFα, IL-6, CXCL1, CXCL2, and IL-17A, but decreased the expression of IL-10; [Figure 4c–f]). Besides kidney infection, we also assessed the impact of lack of kidney production of CL-11 on bladder infection. Interestingly, compared with K-WT mice, K-KO mice also displayed a higher bladder infection rate at 6 hpi (92% vs. 70%; Figure 4g), and higher bacterial load levels at 24 hpi (Figure 4h). Together, these results demonstrate that lack of CL-11 production in the kidney increases both kidney and bladder infection.

Pharmacologic administration of recombinant CL-11 reduces kidney and bladder infection

Our findings that CL-11 deficiency increases kidney and bladder infection suggest a protective role for CL-11 in this model. To further evaluate the protective role of CL-11, we employed pharmacologic treatment approaches in the murine model using murine rCL-11 (∼34 KD). Intravesical treatment is an appealing alternative to systemic treatment for urinary tract disorders.[23–26] We therefore first investigated whether intravesical administration was protective. WT mice were given a mix of UPEC and murine rCL-11 or a control agent (BSA) via the urethra. Mice receiving rCL-11 displayed a marked reduction in the infection rate, lower bacterial colonies in urinary tract epithelium, lower kidney and bladder bacterial load levels, and less kidney and bladder tissue injury, compared with the control group (Figure 5a; Supplementary Figure S3B). These results demonstrate that local (intravesical) administration of rCL-11 can provide good protection against kidney and infection in this model. We also investigated whether systemic administration was protective. Prior to performing the treatment experiments, we assessed the bioavailability of rCL-11 by examining the distribution of biotin-rCL-11 in the kidney and bladder, and found that the injected rCL-11 was present in kidney and bladder epithelium (Supplementary Figure S5). Next, we performed the systemic treatment experiments. WT mice were given rCL-11 or BSA by i.p. injection at 2 hours before and 6 hours after inoculation. Mice receiving rCL-11 displayed a significant reduction in kidney and bladder bacterial load levels and tissue injury, compared with the control group (Figure 5b). These results demonstrate that systemic administration of rCL-11 also can provide good protection in this model.

In addition to demonstrating that administration of rCL-11 is protective in WT mice, we performed rescue experiments by administrating rCL-11 in (global) CL-11 KO mice. Intravesical or systemic administration of rCL-11 in CL-11 KO mice provided good protection against kidney and bladder infections. The CL-11 KO mice receiving rCL-11 exhibited reduced kidney and bladder bacterial load, compared to that in the mice receiving the control agent (BSA). Important to note is that the level of protection achieved by administrating rCL-11 was close to that observed in WT mice (Figure 5c and d). These results demonstrate that rCL-11 administration can effectively rescue the phenotype of CL-11 KO mice.

CL-11 induces innate defense mechanisms against UPEC

To explore the underlying mechanisms by which CL-11 confers protection against UTI, we investigated the effects of CL-11 on several innate defense mechanisms (i.e., bacteria agglutination, prevention of bacterial adhesion to epithelium, phagocytosis). We first examined whether CL-11 binds to UPEC. Flow cytometry analysis showed that rCL-11 effectively bonds to UPEC (Figure 6a). Next, we examined whether CL-11 induces UPEC agglutination. Fluorescence microscopy showed that rCL-11 induced the agglutination in a dose-dependent (0–1200 ng/ml) and time-dependent (0–1.5 hours) manner (Figure 6b; Supplementary Figure S6).

Figure 4 | (continued) infection severity in K-WT and K-KO mice at 24 hpi with CFT073 or J96. (**b**) Bacterial load in kidney tissues. Data were analyzed by Mann-Whitney test ($n = 6–8$ mice per group). (**c**) Kidney macroscopic pathology analysis. Data were analyzed by unpaired t test ($n = 13–15$ mice per group). (**d**) Kidney histopathology analysis. Left panel: Representative images of hematoxylin and eosin–stained kidney sections; the high-magnification images (bottom) correspond to the boxed regions of low-magnification images (top). Bars = 500 μm. Arrows show renal lesions. Right panel: Histologic scores. Data were analyzed by unpaired t test ($n = 6$ mice per group). (**e**) Reverse transcription quantitative polymerase chain reaction (RT-qPCR) for detecting Ngal and Kim-1 in kidney tissues. Data were analyzed by Mann-Whitney test ($n = 6$ mice per group). (**f**) RT-qPCR for detecting cytokine and/or chemokine expression in kidney tissues. Data were analyzed by unpaired t test ($n = 6$ mice per group). (**g**) Bladder infection rate of K-WT and K-KO mice at 6 hpi ($n = 10–12$ mice per group). (**h**) Bacterial load in bladder tissues of K-WT and K-KO mice at 24 hpi with CFT073 or J96. Data were analyzed by unpaired t test ($n = 5–8$ mice per group). Each dot represents an individual mouse. The dotted line across each graph in (**e**) and (**f**) represents the gene expression level of normal kidney tissue, which is similar between K-WT and K-KO mice. *$P < 0.05$; **$P < 0.005$; ****$P < 0.0001$. CFU, colony-forming unit. To optimize viewing of this image, please see the online version of this article at www.kidney-international.org.

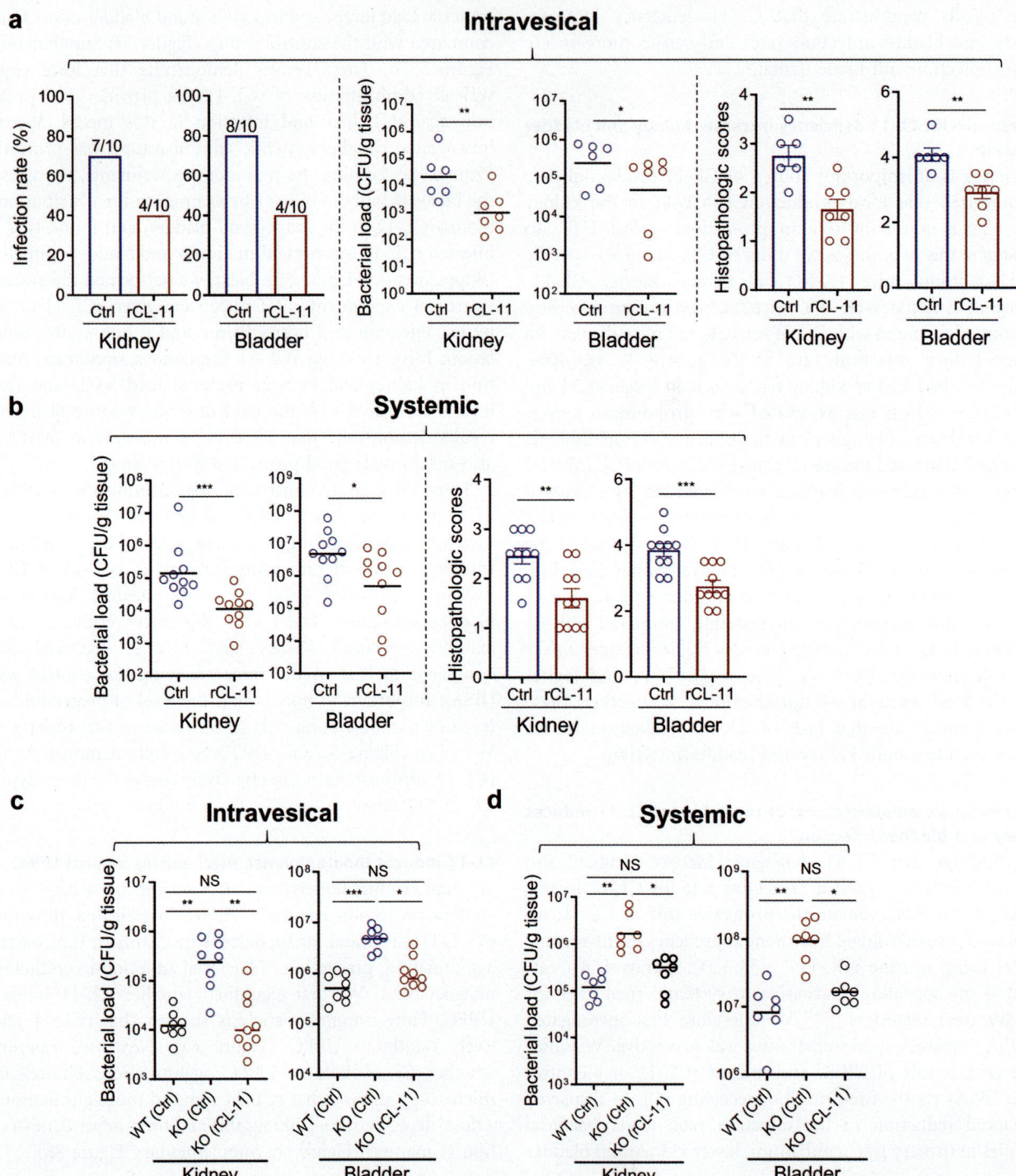

Figure 5 | Administration of recombinant collectin 11 (rCL-11) reduces infection rate and severity of urinary tract infection (UTI). (a) Effects of intravesical administration of rCL-11 on protecting kidney and bladder infections in wild-type (WT) mice. Left panel: Kidney and bladder infection rate in mice receiving rCL-11 or control (bovine serum albumin [BSA]) at 24 hours post-infection (hpi; $n = 10$ mice per group). Middle panel: Bacterial load in the kidney and bladder of mice receiving rCL-11 or control at 24 hpi. Data were analyzed by Mann-Whitney test ($n = 6$–7 mice per group). Right panel: Histologic scores in kidney and bladder corresponding to the 2 groups of mice. Data were analyzed by unpaired t test ($n = 6$–7 mice per group). (b) Effects of systemic administration of rCL-11 on protecting kidney and bladder infections in WT mice. Left panel: Bacterial load in kidney and bladder of mice receiving rCL-11 or control (Ctrl; by intraperitoneal injection) at 24 hpi. Data were analyzed by Mann-Whitney test ($n = 10$ mice per group). Right panel: Histologic scores in kidney and bladder corresponding to the 2 groups of mice. Data were analyzed by unpaired t test ($n = 10$ mice per group). (c,d) Rescue experiments were conducted in (global) CL-11 knockout (KO) and WT mice by (c) intravesical or (d) systemic administration of rCL-11 or control. Kidney and bacteria load were assessed at 24 hpi. Data were analyzed by Kruskal-Wallis test with multiple-comparison test ($n = 7$ mice per group). Each dot represents an individual mouse. *$P < 0.05$; **$P < 0.005$; ***$P < 0.001$; CFU, colony-forming unit; NS, not significant.

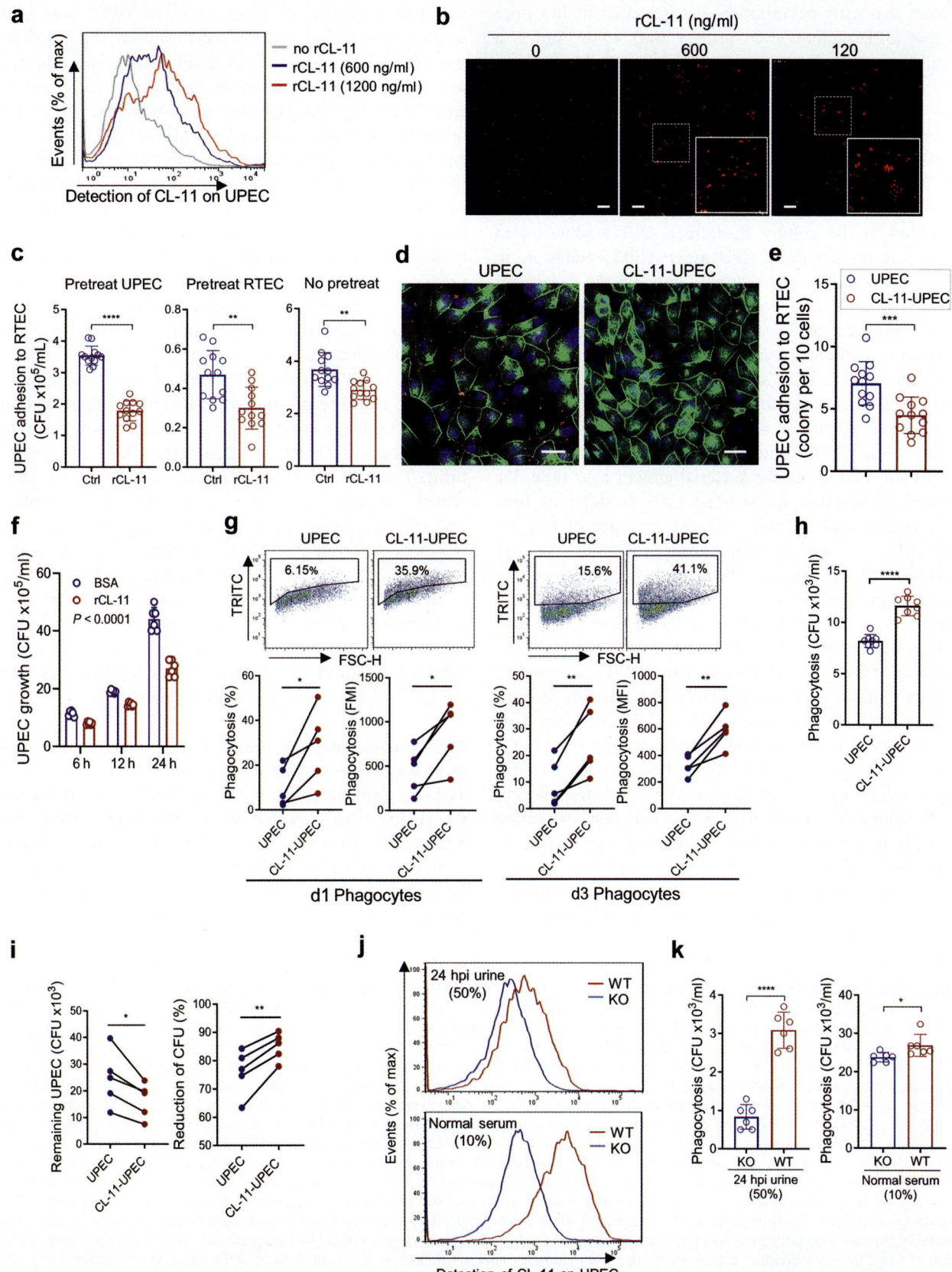

Figure 6 | Collectin-11 (CL-11) induces innate defense mechanisms against uropathogenic *Escherichia coli* (UPEC). (**a**) Flow cytometry analysis detecting CL-11 binding to UPEC following incubation of bacteria with recombinant CL-11 (rCL-11) or saline for 30 minutes at 37 °C. (**b**) Microscopy images of bacterial agglutination following incubation of tetramethylrhodamine (TRITC)-labelled UPEC with rCL- (continued)

Given that early colonization was increased in KO mice and that UPEC adhesion to urinary tract epithelium is a critical step in colonization, we reasoned that CL-11 may have a role in preventing UPEC adhesion to renal epithelium. To assess this possibility, we cultured murine primary renal tubular epithelial cells (RTECs) from WT mice and assessed the effects of CL-11 in preventing UPEC adhesion to RTECs using 3 different rCL-11 treatment protocols (i.e., pretreatment UPEC; pretreatment RTEC; no pretreatment [rCL-11 was added in the culture medium]). UPEC adhesion to RTECs was measured by CFU assay. UPEC adhesion to RTECs was significantly reduced with all the treatment protocols. Among those protocols, pretreatment UPEC with rCL-11 appeared to be more effective, causing a 50% reduction in UPEC adhesion (Figure 6c). The reduction of UPEC adhesion to RTECs by pretreatment of UPEC with rCL-11 was further demonstrated by fluorescence microscopy analysis (Figure 6d and e). We also assessed the effect of rCL-11 on UPEC growth by adding rCL-11 to UPEC cultures and monitored the bacterial growth over time. We observed a reduction in bacterial CFU at different time points (6, 12, and 24 hours) in the presence of rCL-11, compared to the control group without rCL-11 (Figure 6f). Taken together, these results demonstrate that CL-11 can prevent UPEC adhesion to renal epithelial cells, possibly through binding UPEC or RTEC, and CL-11 also has an inhibitory effect on UPEC growth.

Binding of CL-11 to UPEC suggests that CL-11 can function as an opsonin, enhancing phagocytosis. We therefore assessed the effect of CL-11 on phagocytosis of UPEC by using thioglycolate-elicited peritoneal cells or macrophages and CL-11-opsonized or non-opsonized UPEC. Flow cytometry–based phagocytosis assay was performed in d1 (neutrophil-rich) and d3 (monocyte and/or macrophage-rich cells) peritoneal cells with tetramethyl rhodamine isothiocyanate (TRITC)–labelled UPEC. Enhanced phagocytosis of UPEC was observed in the CL-11-opsonized group, in both gated neutrophils (d1) and macrophages (d3) (Figure 6g; Supplementary Figure S7). CL-11-enhancement of phagocytosis of UPEC was further confirmed by CFU-based phagocytosis assay using peritoneal macrophages (Figure 6h). In addition to phagocytosis, we assessed the biological relevance of CL-11 in pathogen clearance. Peritoneal macrophages were incubated with CL-11-opsonized or non-opsonized UPEC for 45 minutes; the amount of bacteria remaining in the supernatants was quantified by CFU assay. The amount of bacteria remaining was significantly lower in the CL-11-opsonized group than in the non-opsonized group, indicating that CL-11 mediates better bacterial clearance (Figure 6i). To assess whether natural CL-11 present in the serum or urine plays a crucial role in mediating opsonophagocytosis, we conducted additional sets of binding and phagocytosis assays using serum or urine from WT and CL-11 KO mice. CL-11 was detected on UPEC following incubation of UPEC with WT serum or urine, but not when using CL-11 KO serum and urine. Bacteria when preincubated with WT serum or urine were phagocytosed more efficiently by macrophages compared to when using CL-11 KO serum or urine. These results strongly indicate that natural CL-11 present in the serum or urine plays a crucial role in mediating opsonophagocytosis (Figure 6j and k). Taken together, these results demonstrate that CL-11 can enhance the phagocytosis of UPEC and contribute to the clearance of UPEC.

In addition to using the classical CFT073 UPEC strain, we performed a series of *in vitro* experiments (i.e., binding, agglutination, phagocytosis) using the J96 strain. The observations with the J96 strain were similar to those made using the CFT073 strain (Supplementary Figure S8).

CL-11 provides defense against kidney infection irrespective of its involvement in complement activation

The complement system is a major host defense mechanism; CL-11 has been reported to be able trigger complement activation.[27] However, most UPEC strains are resistant to complement-mediated killing.[28,29] Next, we assessed whether CL-11's defense against kidney infection requires complement activation in this UTI model. We first conducted additional

Figure 6 | (continued) 11 or bovine serum albumin (BSA) for 1 hour at 37 °C (original magnification ×200). Bar = 25 μm. (**c**) Colony-forming unit (CFU)–based assay detecting UPEC adhesion to primarily cultured murine renal tubular epithelial cells (RTECs) under 3 conditions of rCL-11 treatment, as follows: (i) pretreat UPEC; (ii) pretreat RTECs; (iii) no pretreatment. Data analyzed by unpaired *t* test (*n* = 12 wells per group, pooled from 3 independent experiments). (**d**) Representative microscopy images showing binding of tetramethyl rhodamine isothiocyanate (TRITC)–labelled UPEC (CL-11-opsonized or non-opsonized) to RTECs. Bar = 25 μm. (**e**) Quantification of UPEC binding to RTECs illustrated in (**d**). Data were analyzed by unpaired *t* test (*n* = 12 images per group, 3 images per well, 4 wells from 2 individual experiments). (**f**) CFU assay measuring bacterial growth following the incubation of bacteria (5 × 10^5 per ml) with rCL-11 or control agent (BSA, 600 ng/ml) for the indicated hours at 37 °C. Data were analyzed by 2-way analysis of variance (*n* = 6 wells, from 2 individual experiments). (**g**) Flow cytometry–based phagocytosis assay detecting phagocytosis of TRITC-labelled UPEC (CL-11 opsonized or non-opsonized), in thioglycolate-induced d1 and d3 peritoneal cells. Stepwise gating strategy used in flow cytometric analysis of bacterial phagocytosis is given in Supplementary Figure S7. Top panels: Representative flow cytometry scatter plots. Bottom panels: Quantification of rhodamine + phagocytes (number [%] and intensity [FMI]). Data were analyzed by paired *t* test (*n* = 5 individual experiments). (**h**) CFU-based phagocytosis assay detecting phagocytosis of UPEC (CL-11-opsonized or non-opsonized) in peritoneal macrophages. Data were analyzed by unpaired *t* test (*n* = 8 wells, from 2 individual experiments). (**i**) Bacterial clearance by peritoneal macrophages. Data were expressed as remaining *E. coli* (CFU) and reduction of CFU (%) and were analyzed by paired *t* test (*n* = 5 individual experiments). (**j**) Flow cytometry analysis detecting CL-11 binding to UPEC following incubation of bacteria with pooled 24 hours post-infection (hpi) urine or normal serum from 3 of wild-type (WT) or CL-11 knockout (KO) mice. (**k**) CFU-based phagocytosis assay detecting phagocytosis of UPEC (preincubated with the 24 hpi urine or normal serum mentioned in (**j**)) in peritoneal macrophages. Data were analyzed by unpaired *t* test (*n* = 6 wells per group). (**j,k**) Representative results of 3 independent experiments are shown. CL-11-UPEC, CL-11 opsonized UPEC. FSC-H, forward scatter height; UPEC, non-opsonised UPEC. *$P < 0.05$; **$P < 0.005$; ***$P < 0.001$; ****$P < 0.0001$. To optimize viewing of this image, please see the online version of this article at www.kidney-international.org.

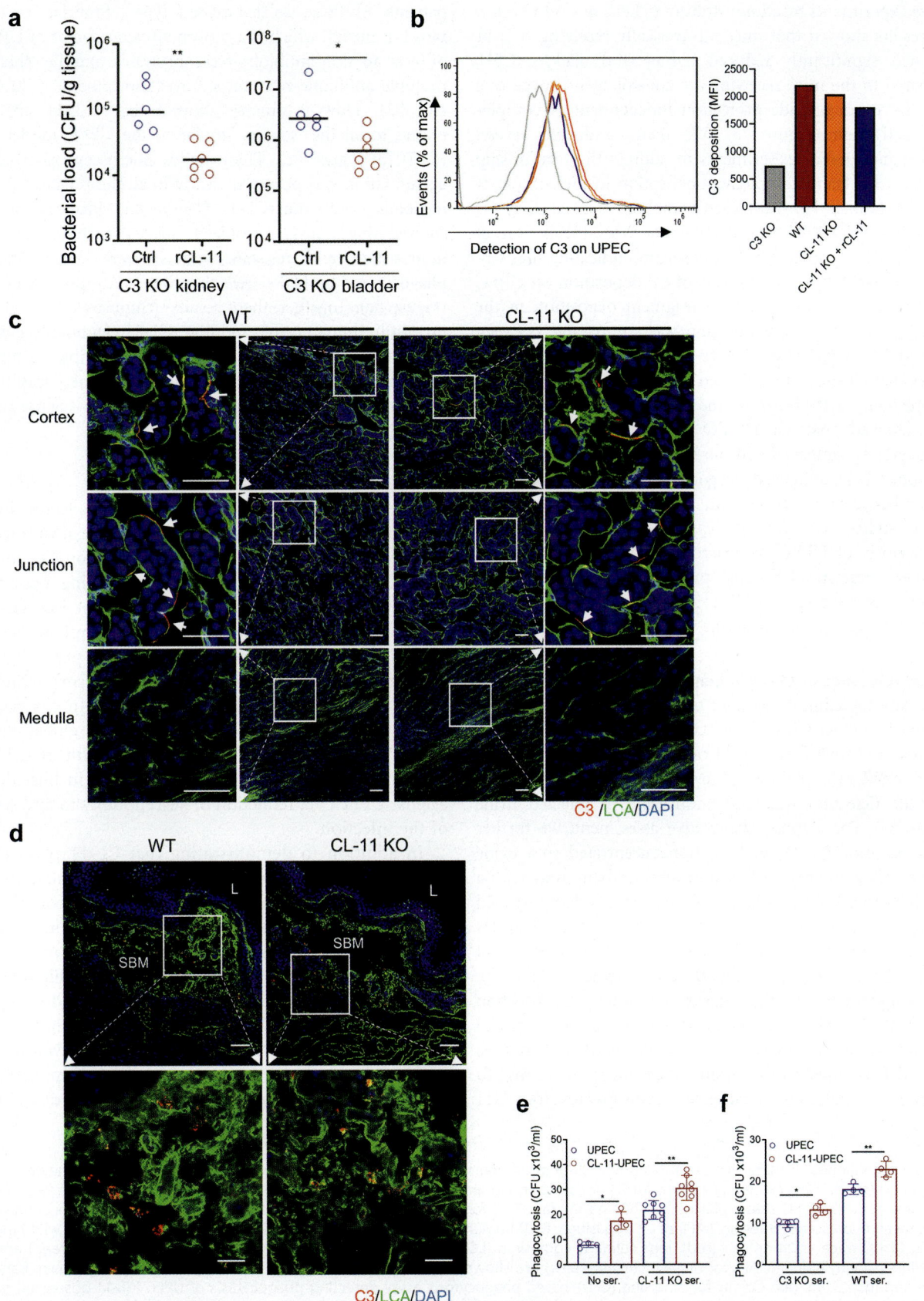

Figure 7 | Collectin-11 (CL-11) provides defense against kidney infection irrespective of its involvement in complement activation. (a) Kidney and bladder bacterial load in C3 knockout (KO) mice receiving recombinant CL-11 (rCL-11) or control (continued)

in vivo experiments by administrating rCL-11 in C3 KO mice. The results showed that mice intravesically receiving rCL-11 exhibited significantly reduced kidney and bladder CFU, compared to the mice receiving the control agent, suggesting that CL-11 can provide protection independent of complement activation (Figure 7a). We then conducted several *in vitro* and *ex vivo* experiments to address the relationship between CL-11 and complement activation in the context of the UTI model. Flow cytometry analysis showed that C3 deposition on UPEC was comparable with incubation of UPEC with WT versus CL-11 KO serum, indicating that CL-11 is not essential for the process of C3 deposition on UPEC (Figure 7b). IF showed that C3 fragment deposition in the kidney and bladder after infection was comparable between WT and CL-11 KO mice (Figure 7c and d). This finding indicates that CL-11 is not required for C3 fragment deposition (complement activation) in the UTI model. Phagocytosis assay showed that CL-11 KO or WT serum enhanced phagocytosis, compared with no serum or C3 KO serum. In addition, CL-11 enhanced phagocytosis of UPEC, regardless of whether serum was present, indicating that CL-11 and serum and/or complement can independently enhance phagocytosis of UPEC by macrophages (Figure 7e and f). Together, these novel findings provide compelling evidence for the protective role of CL-11, irrespective of its involvement in complement activation.

Clinical relevance of CL-11 in human UTI

To explore the clinical relevance of CL-11 in human UTI, we examined whether CL-11 is present in human urine. Western blot analysis showed that CL-11 can be detected in spot urine, concentrated x10, of both healthy subjects and patients with UTI; the detection was more noticeable in infected urine (Figure 8a). For a more quantitative assessment, we further evaluated urine CL-11 levels in nonconcentrated spot urine samples using an enzyme-linked immunosorbent assay with a sensitivity threshold of 29.6 pg/ml. The results demonstrated that CL-11 was detectable in 33% of urine samples (8 of 24) from UTI patients, with levels ranging from 30 to 2530 pg/ml (Figure 8b). Conversely, we found no detectable CL-11 in the urine samples from healthy subjects, indicating a 0% detection rate (0 of 10). Next, we examined whether CL-11 binds to clinically relevant microorganisms and whether CL-11 induces innate defense mechanisms against these microorganisms. To this end, we studied 6 characterized urine isolates from UTI patients. All these isolates express type 1 fimbriae (or type 1 plus P fimbria), which is a proven virulence factor of UPEC; 3 of these are non-antibiotic-resistant strains, and the other 3 are multiple-antibiotic-resistant strains (Supplementary Tables S1 and S2). Flow cytometry showed that rCL-11 effectively bound to all the isolates, similar to the UPEC model strain (CFT073; Figure 8c). Fluorescence microscopy showed that agglutination was observed clearly in all the isolates following incubation with the rCL-11 (Figure 8d). Phagocytosis assay showed that rCL-11-opsonized isolates (including both the nonresistant and resistant strains) were more efficiently phagocytosed by THP-1 cells than were non-opsonized isolates (Figure 8e). Together, these results demonstrate that CL-11 is present in human urine, and that rCL-11 can bind to clinically relevant microorganisms, including multiple antibiotic-resistant strains, and mediate host defense mechanisms (i.e., agglutination, enhancement of phagocytosis) against urinary microorganisms.

DISCUSSION

CL-11 is a recently described soluble C-type lectin that has been suggested to play roles in host defense against infection. However, the role of CL-11 in kidney infection has not been established yet. There are several compelling reasons for CL-11 to play important roles in kidney infection. First, the urinary tract is constantly exposed to microorganisms. Second, local innate defense mechanisms play important roles in protection against the microorganisms. Third, the kidney is a major organ synthesizing CL-11. In this study, by employing 2 CL-11-deficient mouse strains (global; kidney-specific) and pharmacologic treatment with rCL-11, we demonstrate that CL-11 has a pivotal role in host defense against UPEC, via reduction of susceptibility to and severity of the infection.

In addition to demonstrating that CL-11 plays a protective role in kidney infection, we investigated the underlying mechanisms by which CL-11 confers this protection. Our results show that rCL-11 induced the agglutination in a dose- and time-dependent manner and prevented UPEC adhesion to RTECs *in vitro* (Figure 6c–e). Accordingly, early bacterial colonization in kidney epithelium was significantly increased in CL-11-deficient mice, demonstrating that CL-11 is required for preventing bacterial adhesion and/or colonization (Supplementary Figure S3). Furthermore, our results clearly demonstrate

Figure 7 | (continued) (Ctrl; bovine serum albumin [BSA]) at 24 hours post-infection (hpi). Data were analyzed by Mann-Whitney test ($n = 6$ mice per group). (**b**) Flow cytometry analysis for C3 deposition on uropathogenic *Escherichia coli* (UPEC) following incubating with (5%) different types of sera or CL-11 KO serum plus rCL-11 (600 ng/ml) (at 37 °C for 30 minutes). Left panel: Histogram. Right panel: Quantification of geometric mean fluorescence intensity (MFI) of C3 deposition. (**c,d**) Immunofluorescence for C3 in the (**c**) kidney and (**d**) bladder of wild-type (WT) and CL-11 KO mice at 24 hpi. C3 (red), lens culinaris agglutinin (LCA; for illustrating the kidney and bladder structures; green) and 4′,6-diamidino-2-phenylindole (DAPI; for nuclear staining; blue) are shown. Representative images from 3 mice per group are shown. Bars = (**c**) 50 μm and (**d**) 75 μm. (**e,f**) Colony-forming unit (CFU)–based phagocytosis assay detecting phagocytosis of UPEC (CL-11-opsonized or non-opsonized) in macrophages, in the presence or absence of (1%) different types of sera. (**e**) In the presence or absence of normal serum (ser.; from CL-11 KO mice). (**f**) In the presence of C3 KO or WT serum. Data were analyzed by 1-way analysis of variance with multiple-comparison test ($n = 4$–8 wells per group, from 2–3 individual experiments). L, lumen; SBM, submucosa. To optimize viewing of this image, please see the online version of this article at www.kidney-international.org.

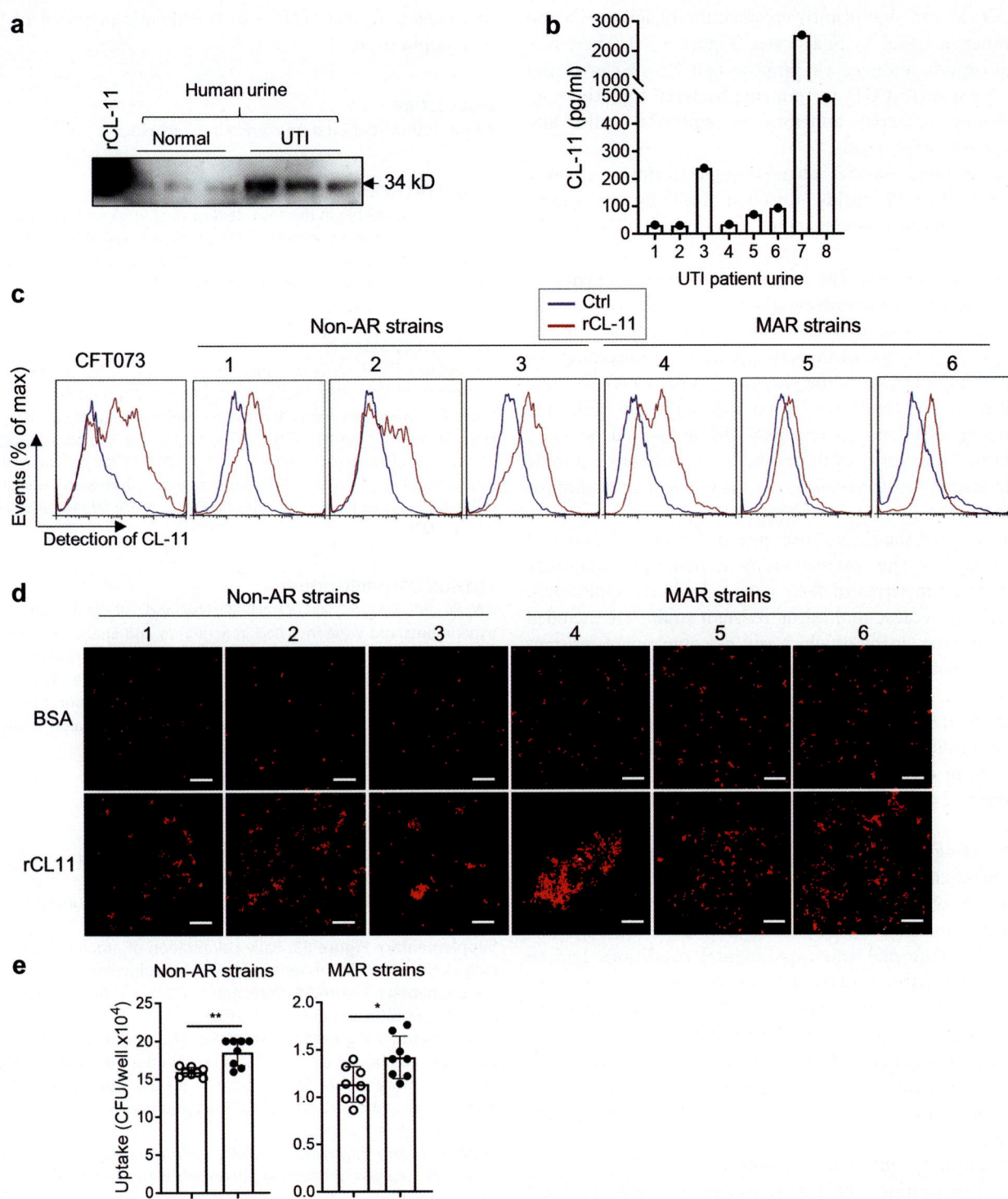

Figure 8 | Clinical relevance of collectin-11 (CL-11) in human urinary tract infection (UTI). (**a**) Western blot for detecting CL-11 in the (10 times concentrated) urine of healthy subjects (normal) and patients with UTI. Each lane represents a urine sample from an individual subject. Recombinant CL-11 (rCL-11; 0.01 ng) was used as a positive control. (**b**) Enzyme-linked immunosorbent assay measuring CL-11 levels in the (nonconcentrated) urine of patients with UTI (diagnosed as acute pyelonephritis). (**c**) Flow cytometry detecting binding of rCL-11 to clinical urinary isolates including 3 non-antibiotic-resistant (Non-AR) strains and 3 multiple-antibiotic-resistant (MAR) strains. (**d**) Microscopy images of bacterial agglutination following incubation of the bacteria with rCL-11 or control (Ctrl; bovine serum albumin [BSA]) at 37 °C for 1 hour. Bar = 25 μm. (**e**) Colony-forming unit (CFU)–based phagocytosis assay detecting phagocytosis of Non-AR strains and MAR strains (CL-11 opsonized, non-opsonized) by THP1 cells. Data were analyzed by unpaired t test ($n = 8$ wells per group, pooled from 2 independent experiments). *$P < 0.05$; **$P < 0.005$. To optimize viewing of this image, please see the online version of this article at www.kidney-international.org.

that CL-11 can significantly enhance the phagocytosis and clearance of UPEC by phagocytes (Figure 6g–i). Therefore, based on our findings, we propose that CL-11 can confer protection against UTI by inducing bacterial agglutination, preventing bacterial adhesion to epithelial cells, and enhancing phagocytosis.

We explored whether pharmacologic treatment of mice with rCL-11 could provide protection in UTI by employing 2 treatment approaches (systemic, intravesical). The results show that both approaches provide protection against kidney and bladder infection. The importance of these findings is 2-fold. First, they support observations made in CL-11-deficient mice, and second, they have strong implications for the therapeutic potential of human application. Concerning the route of administration, the systemic approach may be more effective in systemic or intrarenal infection following ascending infection, whereas local therapy would be more suited to the majority of those who have resistant or chronic lower urinary tract infection, as a supplement to traditional approaches.

We assessed the clinical relevance of CL-11 in the context of human UTI. The observations on human urine isolates are encouraging in terms of their potential clinical application, particularly because multi-drug-resistant strains are included in the analyses, many of which will be complement resistant as well. Another notable point is that the results on agglutination and opsonophagocytosis validate the data in the mouse model, strengthening the case for clinical translation. Patient groups that could benefit are those with recurrent, resistant, or chronic infection of the urinary tract, including catheterized patients, a situation in which current therapy has failed.

Detecting murine serum and urine complement levels presented challenges in our study, owing to the lack of reliable enzyme-linked immunosorbent assay reagents. As a result, our analysis of serum and urine CL-11 levels under both normal and experimental conditions had to rely on estimations derived from Western blot analysis. Although these estimations provided valuable insights, they should be interpreted with caution, as they may not reflect precise CL-11 levels accurately. Future research efforts may benefit from improved methods and reagents for more accurate assessments of CL-11 levels in murine models.

In summary, our results demonstrate that CL-11 is protective in a murine model of ascending UTI, and that local production of CL-11 in the kidney is of fundamental importance for this protection. We propose that CL-11-mediated bacterial agglutination, inhibition of bacterial adhesion and colonization, and promotion of opsonophagocytosis, coupled with downregulation of proinflammatory responses, contribute to the mechanism of protection. We have validated the clinical relevance of these data with patient urine isolates. Taken together, our findings provide evidence for kidney-produced CL-11 as a key defense mechanism against UTI, with therapeutic potential of human application.

DISCLOSURE
All the authors declared no competing interests.

DATA STATEMENT
All data are available in the main text or the Supplementary Material. The custom resources related to the article are available from the corresponding authors upon request. This article does not report large datasets, original code, or reanalyzed data.

ACKNOWLEDGMENTS
The authors thank Mutant Mouse Resource and Research Centers (University of California, Davis, Davis, CA) for providing $Colec11^{-/-}$ mice. This work was supported by the National Natural Science Foundation of China (NSFC 81970596 to KL), the Natural Science Foundation of Shaanxi Province of China (2021JM-287 to XYM and KL; 2023-ZDLSF-10 to YW and KL), and the Medical Research Council UK (MR/L020254/1 to WZ and SS; MR/J006742/1 to SS; MR/M012263/1 to SS and WZ).

AUTHOR CONTRIBUTIONS
KW, BC, WC, WW, SZ, XM, YJ, JH, XD, NW, and YW conducted experiments and were invovled in acquiring and analyzing data. PG provided vital reagents. SHS contributed to designing research studies and provided critical reading and editing of the manuscript. WZ contributed to designing research studies and writing the manuscript. KL supervised the research, designed research studies, and wrote the paper.

SUPPLEMENTARY MATERIAL
Supplementary File (PDF)
Supplementary Figure S1. Generation and characterization of kidney-specific collectin-11 knockout (CL-11 KO) mice.
Supplementary Figure S2. Serum collectin-11 (CL-11) levels in normal and infected mice.
Supplementary Figure S3. Early colonization of uropathogenic *Escherichia coli* (UPEC) in renal and bladder epithelium.
Supplementary Figure S4. Detection of CD45+, Ly6G+, and F4/80+ in wild-type (WT) and *Colec11*−/− mice.
Supplementary Figure S5. Distribution of (intraperitoneal [i.p]) injected recombinant collectin-11 (rCL-11) in the kidney and bladder.
Supplementary Figure S6. Collectin-11 (CL-11) induces uropathogenic *Escherichia coli* (UPEC; CFT073) agglutination in a dose- and time-dependent manner.
Supplementary Figure S7. Stepwise gating strategy used in flow cytometric analysis of bacterial phagocytosis by peritoneal phagocytes.
Supplementary Figure S8. Collectin-11 (CL-11) induces innate defense mechanisms against uropathogenic *Escherichia coli* (UPEC; J96).
Supplementary File (Word)
Supplementary Table S1. Virulent factor expression profiles of urine isolates from UTI patient.
Supplementary Table S2. Antibiotic resistant profiles of urine isolates from UTI patient.
Supplementary Table S3. PCR primer sequences and product sizes.
Supplementary Methods.
Supplementary References.

REFERENCES

1. Zowawi HM, Harris PN, Roberts MJ, et al. The emerging threat of multidrug-resistant Gram-negative bacteria in urology. *Nat Rev Urol*. 2015;12:570–584.
2. Bunduki GK, Heinz E, Phiri VS, et al. Virulence factors and antimicrobial resistance of uropathogenic *Escherichia coli* (UPEC) isolated from urinary tract infections: a systematic review and meta-analysis. *BMC Infect Dis*. 2021;21:753.
3. Ambite I, Butler D, Wan MLY, et al. Molecular determinants of disease severity in urinary tract infection. *Nat Rev Urol*. 2021;18:468–486.
4. Abraham SN, Miao Y. The nature of immune responses to urinary tract infections. *Nat Rev Immunol*. 2015;15:655–663.
5. Ulett GC, Totsika M, Schaale K, et al. Uropathogenic *Escherichia coli* virulence and innate immune responses during urinary tract infection. *Curr Opin Microbiol*. 2013;16:100–107.
6. Butler D, Ambite I, Wan MLY, et al. Immunomodulation therapy offers new molecular strategies to treat UTI. *Nat Rev Urol*. 2022;19:419–437.
7. Gupta G, Surolia A. Collectins: sentinels of innate immunity. *Bioessays*. 2007;29:452–464.
8. Casals C, Garcia-Fojeda B, Minutti CM. Soluble defense collagens: sweeping up immune threats. *Mol Immunol*. 2019;112:291–304.
9. Garred P, Genster N, Pilely K, et al. A journey through the lectin pathway of complement-MBL and beyond. *Immunol Rev*. 2016;274:74–97.
10. Selman L, Hansen S. Structure and function of collectin liver 1 (CL-L1) and collectin 11 (CL-11, CL-K1). *Immunobiology*. 2012;217:851–863.
11. Henriksen ML, Brandt J, Andrieu JP, et al. Heteromeric complexes of native collectin kidney 1 and collectin liver 1 are found in the circulation with MASPs and activate the complement system. *J Immunol*. 2013;191:6117–6127.
12. Keshi H, Sakamoto T, Kawai T, et al. Identification and characterization of a novel human collectin CL-K1. *Microbiol Immunol*. 2006;50:1001–1013.
13. Hansen S, Selman L, Palaniyar N, et al. Collectin 11 (CL-11, CL-K1) is a MASP-1/3-associated plasma collectin with microbial-binding activity. *J Immunol*. 2010;185:6096–6104.
14. Venkatraman Girija U, Furze CM, Gingras AR, et al. Molecular basis of sugar recognition by collectin-K1 and the effects of mutations associated with 3MC syndrome. *BMC Biol*. 2015;13:27.
15. Dong X, Wu W, Ma L, et al. Collectin-11 is an important modulator of retinal pigment epithelial cell phagocytosis and cytokine production. *J Innate Immun*. 2017;9:529–545.
16. O'Hanley P, Lark D, Falkow S, Schoolnik G. Molecular basis of *Escherichia coli* colonization of the upper urinary tract in BALB/c mice. Gal-Gal pili immunization prevents *Escherichia coli* pyelonephritis in the BALB/c mouse model of human pyelonephritis. *J Clin Invest*. 1985;75:347–360.
17. Li K, Wu KY, Wu W, et al. C5aR1 promotes acute pyelonephritis induced by uropathogenic *E. coli*. *JCI insight*. 2017;2:e97626.
18. Wu KY, Cao B, Wang CX, et al. The C5a/C5aR1 axis contributes to the pathogenesis of acute cystitis through enhancement of adhesion and colonization of uropathogenic *E. coli*. *Front Cell Infect Microbiol* 2022;. 2022;12:824505.
19. Mobley HL, Green DM, Trifillis AL, et al. Pyelonephritogenic *Escherichia coli* and killing of cultured human renal proximal tubular epithelial cells: role of hemolysin in some strains. *Infect Immun*. 1990;58:1281–1289.
20. Tang T, Li L, Tang J, et al. A mouse knockout library for secreted and transmembrane proteins. *Nat Biotechnol*. 2010;28:749–755.
21. Hagberg L, Engberg I, Freter R, et al. Ascending, unobstructed urinary tract infection in mice caused by pyelonephritogenic *Escherichia coli* of human origin. *Infect Immun*. 1983;40:273–283.
22. Wei Y, Li K, Wang N, et al. Activation of endogenous anti-inflammatory mediator cyclic AMP attenuates acute pyelonephritis in mice induced by uropathogenic *Escherichia coli*. *Am J Pathol*. 2015;185:472–484.
23. Chernyak S, Salamon C. Intravesical antibiotic administration in the treatment of recurrent urinary tract infections: promising results from a case series. *Female Pelvic Med Reconstr Surg*. 2020;26:152–154.
24. Abrams P, Hashim H, Tomson C, et al. The use of intravesical gentamicin to treat recurrent urinary tract infections in lower urinary tract dysfunction. *Neurourol Urodyn*. 2017;36:2109–2116.
25. Tyagi P, Kashyap M, Hensley H, Yoshimura N. Advances in intravesical therapy for urinary tract disorders. *Expert Opin Drug Deliv*. 2016;13:71–84.
26. Crijnen J, De Reijke TM. Emerging intravesical drugs for the treatment of non muscle-invasive bladder cancer. *Expert Opin Emerg Drugs*. 2018;23:135–147.
27. Ma YJ, Skjoedt MO, Garred P. Collectin-11/MASP complex formation triggers activation of the lectin complement pathway–the fifth lectin pathway initiation complex. *J Innate Immun*. 2013;5:242–250.
28. Taylor PW. Bactericidal and bacteriolytic activity of serum against gram-negative bacteria. *Microbiol Rev*. 1983;47:46–83.
29. Li K, Zhou W, Hong Y, et al. Synergy between type 1 fimbriae expression and C3 opsonisation increases internalisation of *E. coli* by human tubular epithelial cells. *BMC Microbiol*. 2009;9:64.

basic research

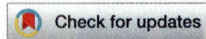

Chronic kidney disease in a murine model of non-alcoholic steatohepatitis (NASH)

Xuezhu Li[1,2,6], Dipankar Bhattacharya[3,6], Yue Yuan[2,6], Chengguo Wei[1], Fang Zhong[1], Feng Ding[2], Vivette D. D'Agati[4], Kyung Lee[1], Scott L. Friedman[3] and John Cijiang He[1,5]

[1]Barbara T. Murphy Division of Nephrology, Department of Medicine, Icahn School of Medicine at Mount Sinai, New York, New York, USA; [2]Division of Nephrology, Shanghai Ninth People's Hospital, Shanghai Jiaotong University, School of Medicine, Shanghai, China; [3]Division of Liver Diseases, Department of Medicine, Icahn School of Medicine at Mount Sinai, New York, New York, USA; [4]Department of Pathology, Columbia University Medical Center, New York, New York, USA; and [5]Renal Program, James J Peters VA Medical Center at Bronx, New York, New York, USA

Clinical studies suggest that non-alcoholic steatohepatitis (NASH) is an independent risk factor for chronic kidney disease (CKD), but causality and mechanisms linking these two major diseases are lacking. To assess whether NASH can induce CKD, we have characterized kidney function, histological features, transcriptomic and lipidomic profiles in a well-validated murine NASH model. Mice with NASH progressively developed significant podocyte foot process effacement, proteinuria, glomerulosclerosis, tubular epithelial cell injury, lipid accumulation, and interstitial fibrosis. The progression of kidney fibrosis paralleled the severity of the histologic NASH-activity score. Significantly, we confirmed the causal link between NASH and CKD by orthotopic liver transplantation, which attenuated proteinuria, kidney dysfunction, and fibrosis compared with control sham operated mice. Transcriptomic analysis of mouse kidney cortices revealed differentially expressed genes that were highly enriched in mitochondrial dysfunction, lipid metabolic process, and insulin signaling pathways in NASH-induced CKD. Lipidomic analysis of kidney cortices further revealed that phospholipids and sphingolipids were the most significantly changed lipid species. Notably, we found similar kidney histological changes in human NASH and CKD. Thus, our results confirm a causative role of NASH in the development of CKD, reveal potential pathophysiologic mechanisms of NASH-induced kidney injury, and established a valuable model to study the pathogenesis of NASH-associated CKD. This is an important feature of fatty liver disease that has been largely overlooked but has clinical and prognostic importance.

Kidney International (2024) 105, 540–561; https://doi.org/10.1016/j.kint.2023.12.009

KEYWORDS: chronic kidney disease; lipidomics analysis; mitochondrial dysfunction; nonalcoholic steatohepatitis; orthotopic liver transplantation; transcriptomes

Published by Elsevier, Inc., on behalf of the International Society of Nephrology.

Translational Statement

Nonalcoholic steatohepatitis (NASH) is the second most common indication for a liver transplant, and it is growing rapidly worldwide, paralleling the obesity epidemic. Although many studies have demonstrated that NASH is an independent risk factor for chronic kidney disease (CKD), models and mechanisms linking these 2 diseases are still lacking. Here, we have characterized renal dysfunction, glomerulosclerosis, tubular injury, interstitial fibrosis, lipid accumulation, and mitochondrial damage in a well-validated murine NASH model. Furthermore, we confirmed the regression of kidney damage and CKD progression in NASH mice following the orthotopic liver transplantation. Transcriptomic and lipidomic analyses revealed the alteration of multiple signaling pathways and lipid species at both intermediate and late stages. Finally, we found similar kidney histologic and ultrastructural changes in human NASH and CKD. These findings confirm a causative role of NASH in the development of CKD and establish a valuable model to study the pathogenesis of NASH-associated CKD, an important feature of fatty liver disease that has been largely overlooked, yet has clinical and prognostic importance.

Correspondence: *John Cijiang He, Division of Nephrology, Department of Medicine, Icahn School of Medicine at Mount Sinai, New York, New York 10029, USA. E-mail: cijiang.he@mssm.edu; or Scott L. Friedman, Division of Liver Disease, Box 1123, Icahn School of Medicine at Mount Sinai, New York, New York 10029, USA. E-mail: scott.friedman@mssm.edu*

[6]XL, DB, and YY contributed equally to the study.

Received 5 August 2023; revised 1 December 2023; accepted 8 December 2023; published online 28 December 2023

Nonalcoholic fatty liver disease (NAFLD) is now the most common chronic liver disease worldwide, associated with the global epidemics of obesity, diabetes, and metabolic syndrome.[1–3] Nonalcoholic steatohepatitis (NASH) is the progressive form of NAFLD, which can lead to cirrhosis, hepatocellular carcinoma, and liver-related mortality, but has limited treatment options. A growing body of clinical evidence established NASH as an independent risk factor for chronic kidney disease (CKD) even after adjustments for traditional risk factors, such as age, sex, body mass index, hypertension, diabetes, smoking, and hyperlipidemia.[4-6] Moreover, the extent of proteinuria and reduction of glomerular filtration rate in individuals with NAFLD/NASH parallel the severity of liver fibrosis.[4,7] Although overlapping mechanisms may underly NASH and CKD pathogenesis, such as insulin resistance, activation of the renin-angiotensin system, oxidative stress, and systemic inflammation,[1,8] whether NASH is involved in CKD development and potential mechanisms linking NASH to CKD are not known.

Previous studies have described kidney injury in NASH animal models induced by a high-fat diet, methionine, and choline-deficient diet,[9] streptozotocin/high-fat diet,[10,11] or genetic modification.[12] However, these models do not replicate the critical metabolic and histologic features of human NASH.[13] In contrast, we previously developed a new mouse model that closely resembles human NASH in histologic features, metabolic abnormalities, and gene expression pathways by administering a Western diet (WD; high-fat, high-fructose, and high-cholesterol diet), combined with a weekly administration of very low-dose carbon tetrachloride (CCl_4).[14] This "FAT-NASH" (**F**ibrosis **a**nd **T**umors) model closely resembles human NASH, including an altered microbiome that parallels those changes seen in humans.[15] This model makes it ideal to investigate whether NASH provokes the development of CKD. In the current study, we have characterized the histologic features and transcriptomic and lipidomic analyses of kidneys in this NASH model to assess the relationship and potential mechanisms linking NASH to CKD. In addition, we have confirmed a causal relationship between NASH and CKD by demonstrating that orthotopic liver transplantation (OLT) leads to attenuation of kidney disease.

METHODS
Animals and treatments
C57BL/6J mice were purchased from Jackson Laboratory. Mice were fed with a WD diet and treated with CCl_4 (0.32 μg/g, i.p., once a week), as previously described.[14] Experimental groups consisted of control mice, treated with chow diet (CD) and vehicle corn oil for 12 or 24 weeks, and NASH mice, treated with WD and CCl_4 for 12 or 24 weeks (n = 10 mice per group, comprising 5 males and 5 females). An additional control group of mice on CD with CCl_4 treatment was included to examine the potential nephrotoxic effects of CCl_4 alone at 12 or 24 weeks after induction (n = 10 mice, 5 males and 5 females; Supplementary Data). All procedures were performed according to protocols approved by the Animal Care and Use Committee of the Icahn School of Medicine at Mount Sinai (IACUC-2015-0112).

Orthotopic liver transplantation
Male WD/CCl_4 mice at 12 weeks, weighing 20 to 25 g, were used for OLT without hepatic artery reconstruction under inhalation anesthesia, according to protocols established by Yokata et al.[16] In brief, a liver graft was procured from 18-week-old wild-type C57BL/6J donor male mice after dissecting vessels, ligaments, and connective tissues around the liver. After clamping the portal vein, intrahepatic inferior vena cava, and suprahepatic inferior vena cava, the recipient liver of NASH mice was removed, and the liver graft was placed orthotopically. Vessels and bile duct were anastomosed through a combined cuff and suture technique. Recipient mice were given CD and corn oil for another 12 weeks after OLT and euthanized at 24 weeks. For control mice, sham operation was performed in parallel, and mice were switched to normal CD and corn oil for another 12 weeks. Three NASH mice completed the procedure with successful OLT and survived.

Liver and kidney histology
Liver and kidney tissues were fixed in 10% neutral-buffered formalin, embedded in paraffin, and sectioned to 3-μm thickness. Liver sections were stained with hematoxylin and eosin for assessment of liver histology. Periodic acid–Schiff staining was used to examine kidney histology. Kidney and liver fibrosis were evaluated by Sirius red staining. Kidney sections were deparaffinized and rehydrated, and then processed with primary antibodies against α-smooth muscle actin (Abcam; ab124964) following an immunohistochemistry standard protocol. Lipid accumulation was determined by oil red O staining. Optimal cutting temperature compound–embedded frozen kidney sections (8 μm thick) were used for oil red O staining, according to the manufacturer's instructions. Frozen kidney sections (3 μm thick) were used for immunofluorescence staining for collagen I (Servicebio; GB11022-3).

Transmission electron microscopy
Mouse kidney tissues were fixed in glutaraldehyde. Sections were mounted on a copper grid, and the ultrastructures were imaged under a Hitachi H-7650 microscope. The thickness of the glomerular basement membrane and widths of the podocyte foot processes were determined as previously described.[17,18]

Morphologic analysis
NASH scores were evaluated from the steatosis grade, inflammation score, and fibrosis stage, according to the NASH Clinical Research Network scoring system.[19] The cross-sectional area of the glomerular tuft and the proportion of the mesangial matrix relative to the glomerular area were measured by using ImageJ software on an equal number of pictures per mouse (20 images) under constant magnification. The severity of tubular vacuolization was assessed by the following grading schema: 0, no vacuolization; 1, <10%; 2, 10% to 25%; 3, 26% to 50%; and 4, >50%. The amount of fibrosis was determined by quantifying the percentage of positive staining areas with Sirius red staining. The proportion of lipid area was quantified by the positive areas with oil red O staining. Semiquantitative histologic analysis was performed by a trained pathologist blinded to the groups (XL), and images were acquired by FZ and YY.

Human kidney biopsy
The human kidney biopsy sample was collected from the Department of Pathology, Columbia University, under Columbia University Medical Center Institutional Review Board number AAAT7999 for archival use of kidney biopsy slides for research purposes. The images provided to investigators were deidentified. No patient consent was required, as per Institutional Review Board protocol.

Urine albumin and creatinine measurements
Urine albumin was measured using a commercial assay enzyme-linked immunosorbent assay kit (E99-134; Bethyl Laboratory). Urine creatinine levels were quantified using a quantiChrom Creatinine Assay Kit (DICT-500; Bioassay Systems). Urine albumin excretion was expressed as the ratio of albumin/creatinine.

Blood urea nitrogen measurement

Blood urea nitrogen (BUN) was measured from mouse sera using a commercial kit (BioAssay Systems), according to the manufacturer's protocol.

mRNA isolation and transcriptome profiling

Total RNA was isolated from kidney cortices by using the RNeasy mini kit (Qiagen; 74104), according to the manufacturer's protocol. mRNA sequencing was performed at the CLC Genomics and Epigenomics Core Facility at Weil Cornell Medical College.

Bioinformatics analysis of mRNA-sequencing data

The RNA-sequencing data were analyzed by following the procedure described below. Briefly, after sequence quality filtering at a cutoff of a minimum quality score Q20 in at least 90% bases for the paired-end 150-bp FASTQ sequencing data, the good-quality reads aligned to reads were processed and aligned to the University of California, Santa Cruz, Mus musculus reference genome and transcriptome (build mm10) using the Burrows-Wheeler Aligner.[20] The reads that are uniquely aligned to the exon and splicing junction sites for each transcript were combined to calculate an expression level for a corresponding transcript and further normalized on the basis of reads per kilobase per million reads[21] to compare transcription levels among samples. The transcripts with a low raw read count of >100 in all the samples were excluded for downstream analysis. Gene expression value was transformed to the log 2 base scale. Principle component analysis was first performed to assess the sample correlations using the expression data of all the genes. The differentially expressed genes in NASH mice compared with control mice were identified by the R package limma test.[22] A specific gene was considered differentially expressed if the P value was ≤ 0.05. The Gene Ontology and pathway analysis for the differentially expressed genes were then performed with a fold change cutoff of ≥ 1.5 using INGENUITY IPA (www.ingenuity.com/products/ipa) and the online tool Enrichr.[23] The read coverage of gene functional elements was also visualized by the Integrative Genome Viewer tool (www.broadinstitute.org/igv/) from the genome alignment file. Heat map analysis was performed for the top 50 differentially expressed genes after the median center was transformed using Multi-Experiment Viewer software.[24]

Tissue lipid extraction

Kidney cortex (10 ± 0.2 mg) tissues were homogenized in 40 μl of cold double-distilled water at 20 Hz. A total of 20 μl of the resulting supernatants was mixed with 225 ul methanol by vortexing. Then, we added 5 ul internal standard and 750 ul methyl tert-butyl ether. Then, the mixture was vibrated for 30 minutes, and 188 μl double-distilled water was added and vortexed to form a 2-phase system. After equilibration for 10 minutes at 4 °C, the mixture was centrifuged at 10,000g for 10 minutes at 4 °C. A total of 700 μl of supernatant was dried under nitrogen. All samples were reconstituted in acetonitrile/isopropyl alcohol/water (65:30:5, v/v/v), and samples were mixed with 20 μl as quality control, and 2 μl was injected into the liquid chromatography–mass spectrometry system.

Lipidomics profiling and bioinformatics analysis

The lipidomic profiling was performed using the Ultra-Performance Liquid Chromatography Mass Spectrometry system (ultra-performance liquid chromatography, Agilent 1290; mass spectrometry, Applied Biosystems SCIEX 6500 + QTRAP) at Core Facility of Basic Medical Sciences, Shanghai Jiaotong University School of Medicine. The samples were separated with reverse-phase chromatography (Kinetex 2.6 μm; C18; 2.1 × 100 mm; Phenomenex). The experiment was performed using multi-reaction monitoring mode, in which each type of lipid was corrected with corresponding lipid isotope standards to ensure the accuracy of the experiment.

LipidSig R package was used to analyze the data.[25] R package, version was 2.11.1, was also used. All samples were normalized using the probabilistic quotient normalization method. Differential analysis was performed using normalized and log-transformed data with the limma package. Lipid with adjusted $P \leq 0.05$ was considered statistically significant.

Statistical analysis

Data are expressed as means ± SEM. Analysis of variance, followed by the Bonferroni correction, was used to analyze means between groups. GraphPad Prism 9 software was used for statistical analyses. $P < 0.05$ was considered statistically significant.

RESULTS

NASH mice develop proteinuria and renal dysfunction

To assess whether NASH can induce CKD, we first assessed their renal function at 12 weeks (intermediate NASH stage) and 24 weeks (late stage) post-NASH induction. At 12 weeks, NASH mice began to show albuminuria development compared with control mice, without significant accumulation of BUN (Figure 1a and b). By 24 weeks, overt albuminuria and BUN accumulation were observed in NASH mice (Figure 1a and b) that were not influenced by sex (Supplementary Figure S1A and B). The renal function decline was not due to a direct kidney injury by CCl_4 administration, as no change in renal function parameters was observed in an independent cohort of control mice after either 12 or 24 weeks post-CCl_4 administration fed with a normal diet that did not develop NASH[14] (Supplementary Figure S2A and B).

NASH promotes glomerulosclerosis and podocyte foot process effacement

Histologic analysis of periodic acid–Schiff–stained kidney sections showed mild to moderate glomerulomegaly (red arrowheads in Figure 2a, top panel) in NASH mice at the intermediate stage, which was marked by increased glomerular cross-sectional area (Figure 2b) and the percentage of mesangial area (Figure 2b). At the late stage, NASH mice developed diffuse moderate to severe mesangial expansion with increased mesangial cell number and accumulation of mesangial matrix and focal segmental glomerular sclerosis, some of which was perihilar focal segmental glomerular sclerosis (Figure 2a, top panel). The glomerular cross-sectional area of the late-stage NASH mice was 78% larger than that of control mice (Figure 2b), and the percentage of mesangial area to the glomerular cross-sectional area of these NASH mice was 2.4-fold higher than that of control mice and 1.25-fold higher than that of the intermediate-stage NASH mice ($P < 0.001$) (Figure 2b). None of the control mice fed with a normal diet developed glomerulosclerosis or tubulointerstitial fibrosis (Figure 2a, top panel).

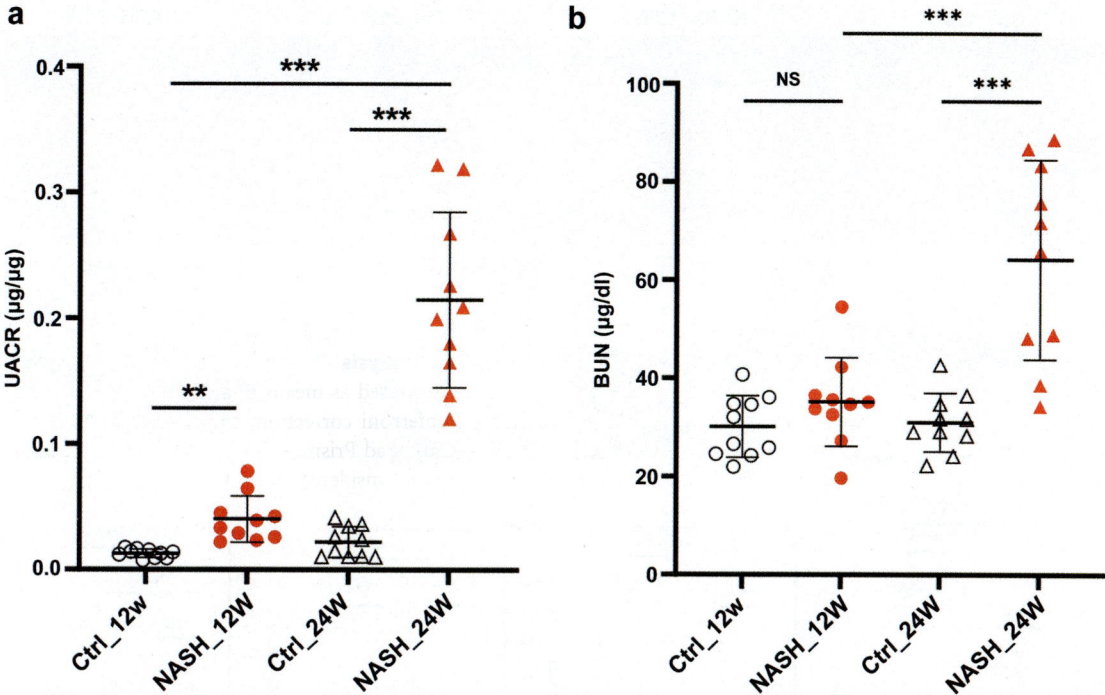

Figure 1 | Nonalcoholic steatohepatitis (NASH) mice develop proteinuria and renal dysfunction. (a) Urinary albumin excretion as quantified by the urinary albumin/creatinine ratio (UACR; μg of albumin/μg of creatinine) at 12 and 24 weeks of Western diet/carbon tetrachloride treatment. UACR at 12 and 24 weeks was significantly higher in the NASH mice than the control (Ctrl) mice. n = 10 in each group. **$P < 0.01$, ***$P < 0.001$. (b) Serum blood urea nitrogen (BUN) at 24 weeks was significantly higher in the NASH mice than in Ctrl mice. n = 10 in each group. ***$P < 0.001$. NS, not significant.

The evaluation of the ultrastructure of podocytes by transmission electron microscopy revealed foot process widening at the intermediate stage and extensive effacement at the late stage of NASH (Figure 2a, bottom panel). The mean foot process width in NASH mice at 12 weeks was 1.25-fold greater than control, and 1.78-fold greater than control mice in late stage of NASH mice (Figure 2b). However, there was no difference in the thickness of the glomerular basement membrane between groups (Figure 2b).

Renal fibrosis parallels the severity of NASH liver damage

Kidney histology also showed significant vacuolation in tubules (asterisks in Figure 2a, top panel) and mild tubulointerstitial fibrosis (Figure 2c, bottom panel) in NASH mice at the intermediate stage. At the late stage, NASH mice had irregular macroscopic scars on the kidney cortical surface (black arrows in Figure 2c, top panel) that represented a large fibrotic area. Microscopically, NASH mice showed a significant increase in tubulointerstitial fibrosis, tubular atrophy, and diffuse infiltrates of inflammatory cells (arrowheads in Figure 2c, middle panel), most of which were macrophages (Supplementary Figure S3). Sirius red histologic staining and immunostaining for collagen and α-smooth muscle actin confirmed a moderate but significantly increased renal fibrosis at the intermediate stage and a more remarkable increase in renal fibrosis by the late stage in NASH kidneys (Figure 2c–e). These results indicate the development of renal fibrosis at the intermediate stage of NASH, which is significantly worsened by the advanced stage of NASH.

Consistent with our original description of the model, CCl_4-treated mice on WD rapidly developed hallmarks of NASH (steatosis, inflammation, hepatocyte ballooning, and fibrosis) within 12 weeks, progressing to hepatocellular carcinoma by 24 weeks (Figure 2f–h). Notably, the extent of renal fibrosis was positively correlated with the NASH activity score and the percentage of liver fibrosis area (Figure 2i and j). These results indicated that renal fibrosis was strongly associated with the histologic severity of NASH, consistent with those reported in human NASH and CKD.[4,7]

OLT attenuates proteinuria, renal dysfunction, and fibrosis in NASH mice

To determine whether liver damage alone contributes to renal dysfunction and fibrosis in NASH mice independent from metabolic dysregulation, we performed OLT of healthy donor livers on NASH recipient mice at the intermediate stage (12 weeks). We compared the effects of OLT or sham operation using the following 3 groups (Figure 3a): (i) control NASH mice on WD for 24 weeks (NASH), (ii) NASH mice receiving sham operation after 12 weeks of induction and switched to CD for 12 weeks (SHAM), and (iii) NASH mice receiving OLT of healthy livers and switched to CD for 12 weeks (OLT). Histologic analysis showed that mice in the OLT group had normal hepatocytes, except mild infiltrating inflammatory cells in periportal and sinusoidal areas (Figure 3b and Supplementary Figure S4), whereas mice in the SHAM group had attenuated liver fibrosis compared with mice in the NASH group. As we expected, mice with OLT had a

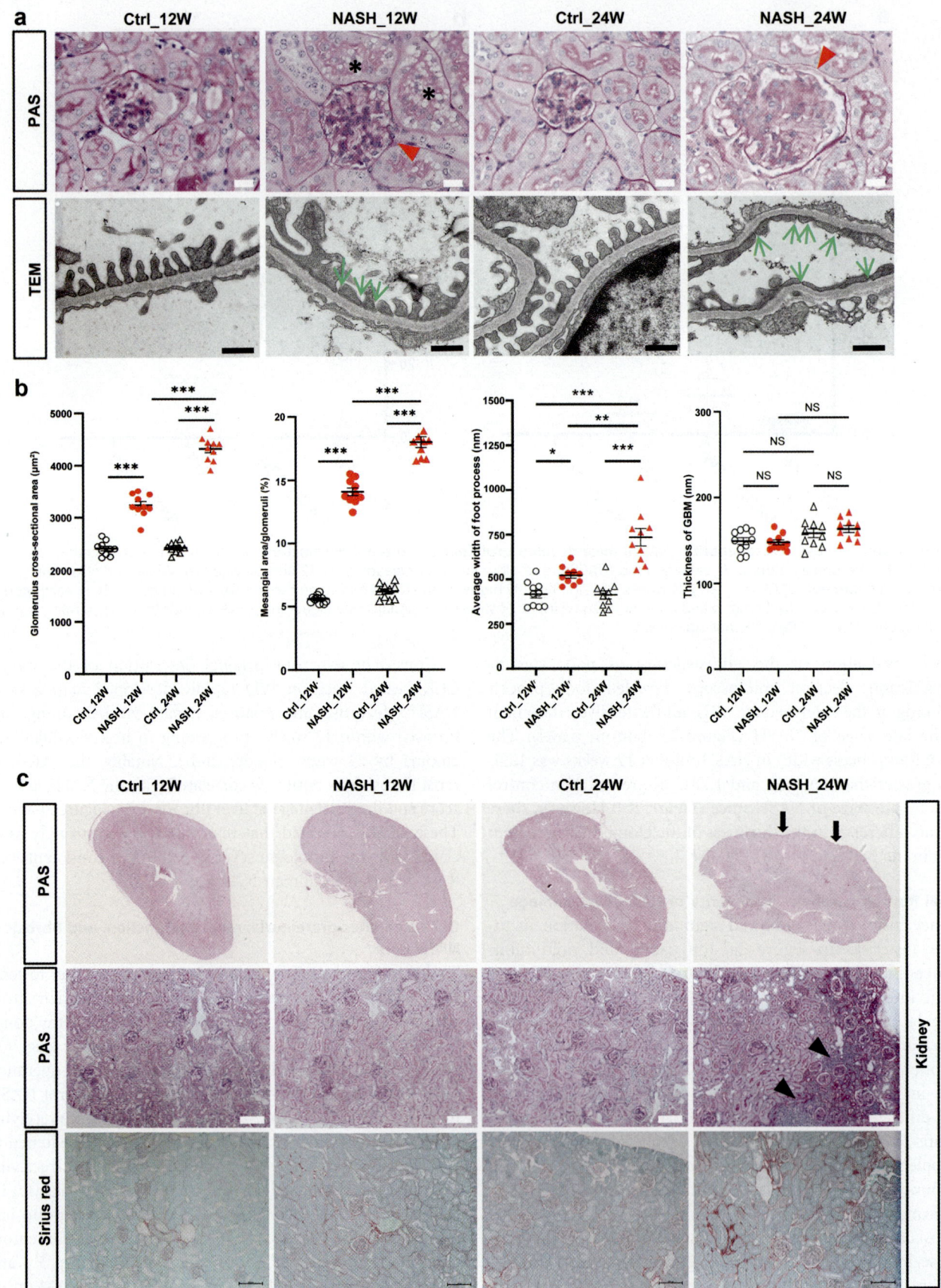

Figure 2 | Nonalcoholic steatohepatitis (NASH) promotes glomerulosclerosis and tubulointerstitial fibrosis. (Continued)

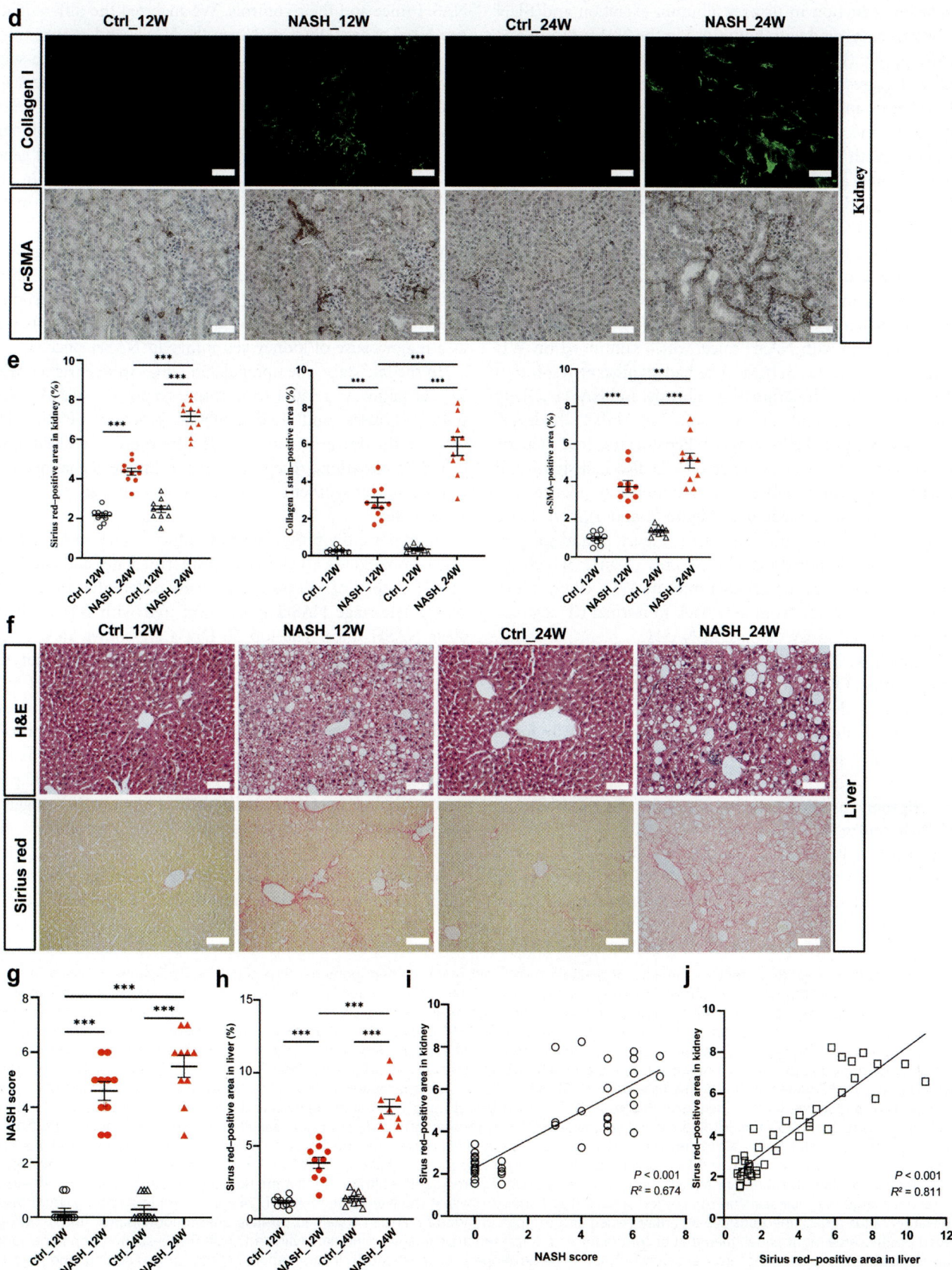

Figure 2 | (Continued)

significant reduction in urinary albumin excretion and BUN level when compared with both mice in the NASH group and SHAM group (Figure 3d and e). Moreover, the OLT mice exhibited regression of glomerulosclerosis and tubulointerstitial fibrosis and significant reduction of glomerular volume (Figure 3f and g) and the percentage of mesangial area, compared with mice in both NASH and SHAM groups (Figure 3f and g). Similarly, the percentages of Sirius red–, collagen I–, and α–smooth muscle actin–positive areas were also significantly decreased in OLT mice compared with the other 2 groups (Figure 3f–i). These results confirm that OLT attenuates kidney injury and fibrosis in NASH mice.

To exclude the influence of a dietary switch, SHAM mice were also switched to normal CD and corn oil for 12 weeks. When compared with NASH mice, which continued on WD for another 12 weeks, SHAM mice had significant resolution of hepatic steatosis, inflammation, fibrosis, and NASH activity score (Figure 3b and c), but still had diffuse hydropic degeneration, mild ballooning of hepatocytes, and hepatic fibrosis (Figure 3b). SHAM mice on CD also had significant reductions in urinary albumin/creatinine ratio (Figure 3d), glomerular cross-sectional area (Figure 3f and g), percentage of mesangial area to glomerular area (Figure 3f and g), percentage of tubulointerstitial fibrosis area (Figure 3f and g), and BUN (Figure 3e) than NASH mice on WD. These results suggest that switching from WD back to normal CD also led to regression of kidney damage in NASH.

Although switching back to a normal diet attenuated kidney injury, OLT mice had additional regression of proteinuria, renal dysfunction, and fibrosis compared with the SHAM group, indicating that NASH alone also contributes to the progression of CKD.

Transcriptomic profile of the kidneys from the NASH mice and their controls

To gain a global, unbiased insight into the mechanisms of kidney injury in the NASH mice, transcriptome analysis using RNA sequencing was performed in the kidney cortices of the NASH mice and their controls. We analyzed the differentially expressed genes (DEGs) between the NASH and control mice. A total of 1680 DEGs were found in the intermediate-stage NASH mice, and 365 DEGs were found in the late-stage NASH mice, compared with their respective control mice. The top 50 DEGs are shown in the heat map (Figure 4a and d). Analysis of the DEGs revealed that the upregulated genes in the 12-week NASH mice were mostly enriched in the pathways of respiratory electron transport chain, lipid metabolic process, adenosine triphosphate synthesis, and oxidation-reduction (Figure 4b), whereas downregulated DEGs were enriched in functions of transcription, phosphorylation, macromolecule catabolic process, and response to stress (Figure 4b), implicating mitochondrial dysfunction as a major cause of kidney cell injury in NASH mice.

In the late stage, the upregulated DEGs were enriched with several pathways related to immune response, mRNA metabolic processes, and lipid catabolic processes (Figure 4e), whereas the downregulated DEGs were mostly involved in fat cell differentiation, receptor tyrosine kinase signaling, carbohydrate biosynthetic process, and response to insulin (Figure 4e).

To explore the progression of kidney injury in NASH, we also compared the DEGs between intermediate- and late-stage NASH. A total of 525 transcripts were differentially expressed in the late-stage NASH mice compared with intermediate-stage NASH mice. The top 50 DEGs are shown in the heat map (Figure 4g). Analysis of the DEGs revealed that the upregulated genes in the 24-week versus 12-week NASH mice were mostly within pathways of fatty acid metabolic process, oxidation-reduction, and retinoid metabolic process (Figure 4h), whereas downregulated genes were enriched in functions of lipid biosynthetic process, sterol metabolic process, and cholesterol metabolic process (Figure 4h), suggesting dysregulation of lipid metabolism promotes the progression of NASH-associated CKD.

Dysregulated signaling pathways were further analyzed by using Ingenuity Pathway Analysis, which identified oxidative

Figure 2 | (Continued) (**a**) Representative images of periodic acid–Schiff (PAS)–stained glomeruli (top panel) and transmission electron microscopy (TEM) (bottom panel) are shown. Bar in PAS stain = 20 μm, bar in TEM = 500 nm. (**b**) Graph of glomerular cross-sectional area, percentage of mesangial area to glomerular area, the podocyte foot process (FP) widths, and width of glomerular basement membrane (GBM) in indicated mice. n = 10 in each group. Values represent mean ± SEM. *$P < 0.05$, **$P < 0.01$, ***$P < 0.001$. NASH mice developed (**a**) significant glomerulomegaly and glomerulosclerosis (top panel, red arrowhead), (**b**) deposition of the mesangial matrix, (**b**) larger glomerular cross-sectional area, and (**b**) the percentage of mesangial area to glomerular area than that of control (Ctrl) mice. (**a**, bottom panels, and **b**) TEM revealed podocyte FP widening in intermediate-stage NASH and extensive FP effacement in late-stage NASH mice. Green arrows: slit diaphragms of podocytes. (**c**) Representative images of PAS-stained kidneys (top and middle panels) and Sirius red–stained kidneys (bottom panel) are shown. Bar = 100 μm. (**d**) Representative images of immunostaining of collagen I (top panel) and α–smooth muscle actin (SMA) (bottom panel) are shown. Bar = 50 μm. (**e**) The average percentage of Sirius red–stained positive area of kidney, and collagen I– and α-SMA–stained positive area per mouse. n = 10 in each group. Values represent mean ± SEM. **$P < 0.01$, ***$P < 0.001$. (**a**) NASH mice developed significant vacuolation on tubules (asterisks, top panel), (**c**) interstitial fibrosis and infiltrate of inflammation cells (middle panel, arrowheads), and (**c**) have large irregular scars on the cortical surface (top panel, arrows) at the late stage of NASH (24 weeks). (**e**) In addition, NASH mice have larger Sirius red–stained positive area (left panel) and the percentage of collagen I–stained positive area (middle panel) and α-SMA–stained positive area (right panel) than that of control mice. (**f**) Representative images of hematoxylin and eosin (H&E)–stained (top panel) and Sirius red–stained (bottom panel) liver are shown. NASH mice developed severe steatosis, inflammation, hepatocyte ballooning, and fibrosis. Bar = 50 μm. (**g,h**) The average percentage of NASH active score and Sirius red–stained positive area of liver per mouse. n = 10 in each group. Values represent mean ± SEM. ***$P < 0.001$. (**i**) Renal fibrosis area was positively correlated with NASH active score. (**j**) Renal fibrosis area was positively correlated with liver fibrosis area. NS, not significant. To optimize viewing of this image, please see the online version of this article at www.kidney-international.org.

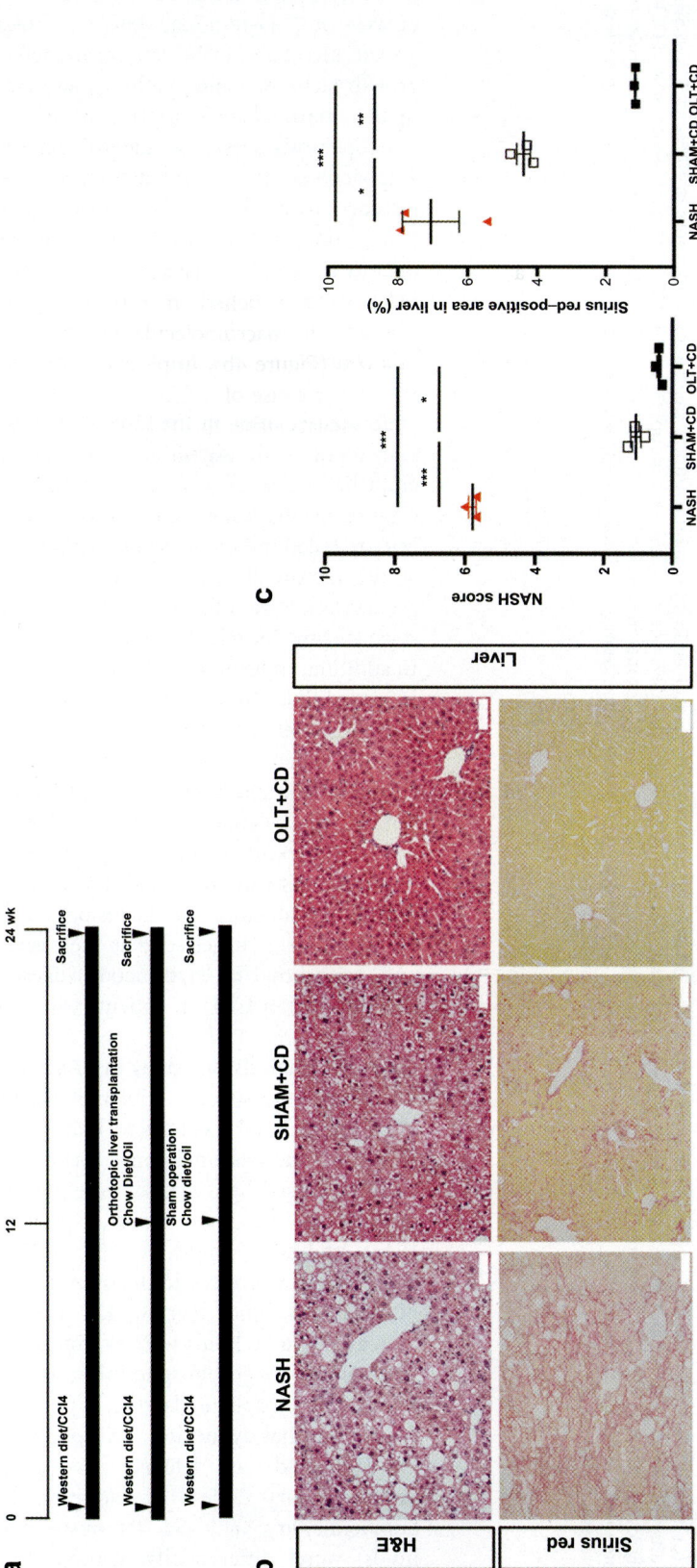

Figure 3 | Orthotopic liver transplantation (OLT) attenuated proteinuria, blood urea nitrogen (BUN), and renal fibrosis in nonalcoholic steatohepatitis (NASH) mice. (a) Schema of study design. OLT was performed 12 weeks after initiation of Western diet and carbon tetrachloride (CCl_4), mice were switched to the normal chow diet (CD) and corn oil, and euthanized at 24 weeks after induction. SHAM operation was performed in parallel, and mice were also switched to a normal CD and corn oil. n = 3 in each group. **(b)** Representative images of hematoxylin and eosin (H&E)–stained livers (top panel) and Sirius red–stained livers (bottom panel) are shown. Bar = 50 μm. **(c)** The average percentage of NASH active score and Sirius red–stained positive area of liver per mouse. n = 3 in each group. Values represent mean ± SEM. $*P < 0.05$, $**P < 0.01$, $***P < 0.001$. Hepatic histology of NASH mice at the late stage (24 weeks) showing severe steatosis, lobular inflammation, ballooning hepatocytes, and severe liver fibrosis. SHAM group mice had regression of steatosis, lobular inflammation, and ballooning hepatocytes after switching to a normal CD and corn oil, but still had diffuse hydropic degeneration, mild ballooning of hepatocytes, and fibrosis. (Continued)

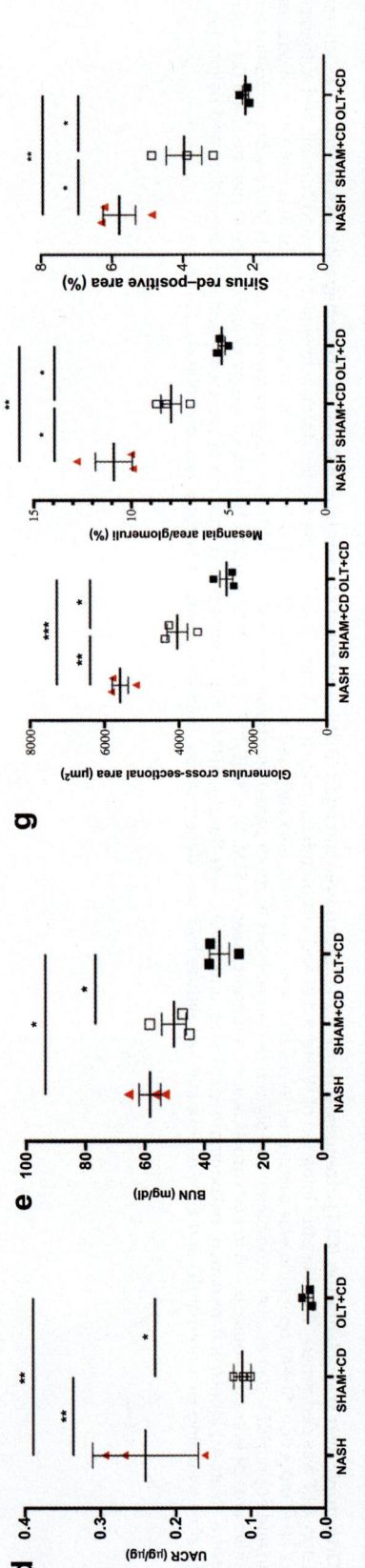

Figure 3 | (Continued) (d) Urinary albumin excretion as quantified by the urinary albumin/creatinine ratio (UACR; μg of albumin/μg of creatinine) at 24 weeks of NASH, OLT, and SHAM operation after 12 weeks. UACR of OLT mice was significantly decreased than that of SHAM mice and NASH mice. n = 3 in each group. *$P < 0.05$, **$P < 0.01$. **(e)** Serum BUN of OLT was significantly lower than that of NASH mice and SHAM mice. n = 3 in each group. *$P < 0.05$, **$P < 0.01$ compared with NASH mice. **(g)** OLT significantly attenuated the glomerular cross-sectional area (left panel), the percentage of mesangial area to glomerular area (middle panel), and the percentage of Sirius red–stained positive area (right panel). n = 3 in each group. Values represent mean ± SEM. *$P < 0.05$, **$P < 0.01$, ***$P < 0.001$. (Continued)

phosphorylation, mitochondrial dysfunction, sirtuin, nuclear factor erythroid 2-related factor 2, stress-activated protein kinase/c-Jun N-terminal kinase, cholesterol biosynthesis, growth arrest and DNA damage-inducible 45 and hepatocyte growth factor signaling pathway, and regulation of cell cycle in the intermediate stage (Figure 4c); glycerol metabolism, atherosclerosis signaling, adenosine monophosphate kinase, adipogenesis, antioxidant action, and Bcl2-associated athanogene 2 pathways in the late stage (Figure 4f); and fatty acid β-oxidation, ketogenesis, mevalonate pathway, and phosphatidylinositol-3′-kinase/protein kinase B pathways in the progression of NASH mice from intermediate to late stage (Figure 4i). Overall, these results reveal DEGs and pathways that contribute to the pathogenesis of NASH-associated CKD.

Lipid accumulation in the kidney of NASH mice
Consistent with significant vacuolations in the tubular epithelial cells (TECs) on periodic acid–Schiff staining (Figure 5a, top panel, and 5i), oil red O staining of NASH mice revealed mild lipid accumulation in TECs and podocytes at the intermediate stage, and significantly increased lipid accumulation was observed in TECs and podocytes at the late stage (Figure 5a, middle panel, Figure 5b, top panel, and 5j). In addition, transmission electron microscopy (TEM) showed increased lipid droplets in the cytoplasm of TECs (Figure 5a, bottom panel, and Figure 5g) and podocytes (Figure 5b, bottom panel), and myelin-like membranous inclusions (Figure 5c, d, and h) in the cytoplasm of TECs. In addition, mitochondria damage, such as swelling and loss of cristae, was also present in TECs (Figure 5e and f). Interestingly, impaired mitochondria and lysosomes were seen around myelin-like membranous inclusions in TECs (Figure 5c and d). These data suggested that increased lipid accumulation and mitochondrial dysfunction likely contribute to the development of CKD in patients with NASH.

Lipidomic analysis of kidney in NASH mice
To identify the specific lipid metabolites that mediate lipotoxicity in NASH-associated kidney injury, we performed lipidomic analysis on kidney cortices. Overall, 5 differentially expressed lipid classes were identified, mainly glycerophospholipids, glycerolipids, sphingolipids, fatty acids (FAs), and sterol lipids. A total of 174 lipid species were differentially expressed in the intermediate stage. Among the discriminant lipid species, 124 lipids were significantly increased and 50 lipids were significantly decreased. Most of them were glycerophospholipids, including phosphatidylglycerol, phosphatidylserine, phosphatidylethanolamine (PE), phosphatidylinositol, phosphatidylcholine, and phosphatidic acid, as detailed in Figure 6a and b and Supplementary Table S1. In addition, Figure 6a and c and Supplementary Table S2 demonstrate that a total of 185 lipids were differentially expressed in the late stage compared with controls. A total of 93 lipids were significantly increased, whereas 92 lipids were significantly decreased. In general, phospholipids showed the most

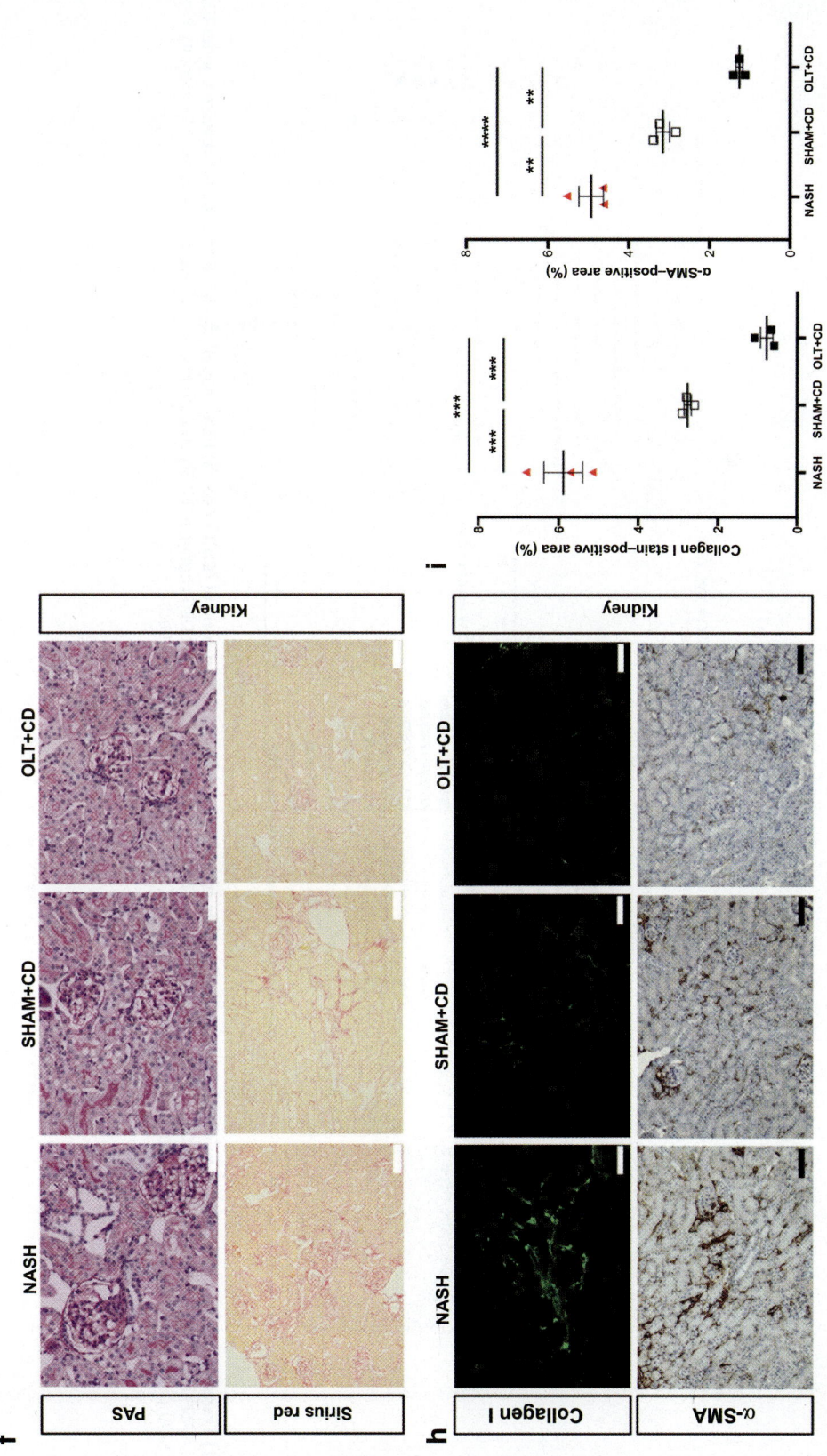

Figure 3 | (Continued) (f) Representative images of periodic acid–Schiff (PAS)–stained kidneys (top panel) and Sirius red–stained kidneys (bottom panel) are shown. Bar = 50 μm. **(h)** Representative images of immunostaining of collagen I (top panel) and α-smooth muscle actin (α-SMA) (bottom panel) are shown. Bar = 50 μm. **(i)** The average percentage of collagen I– and α-SMA–stained positive area per mouse. n = 3 in each group. Values represent mean ± SEM. **$P < 0.01$, ***$P < 0.001$. To optimize viewing of this image, please see the online version of this article at www.kidney-international.org.

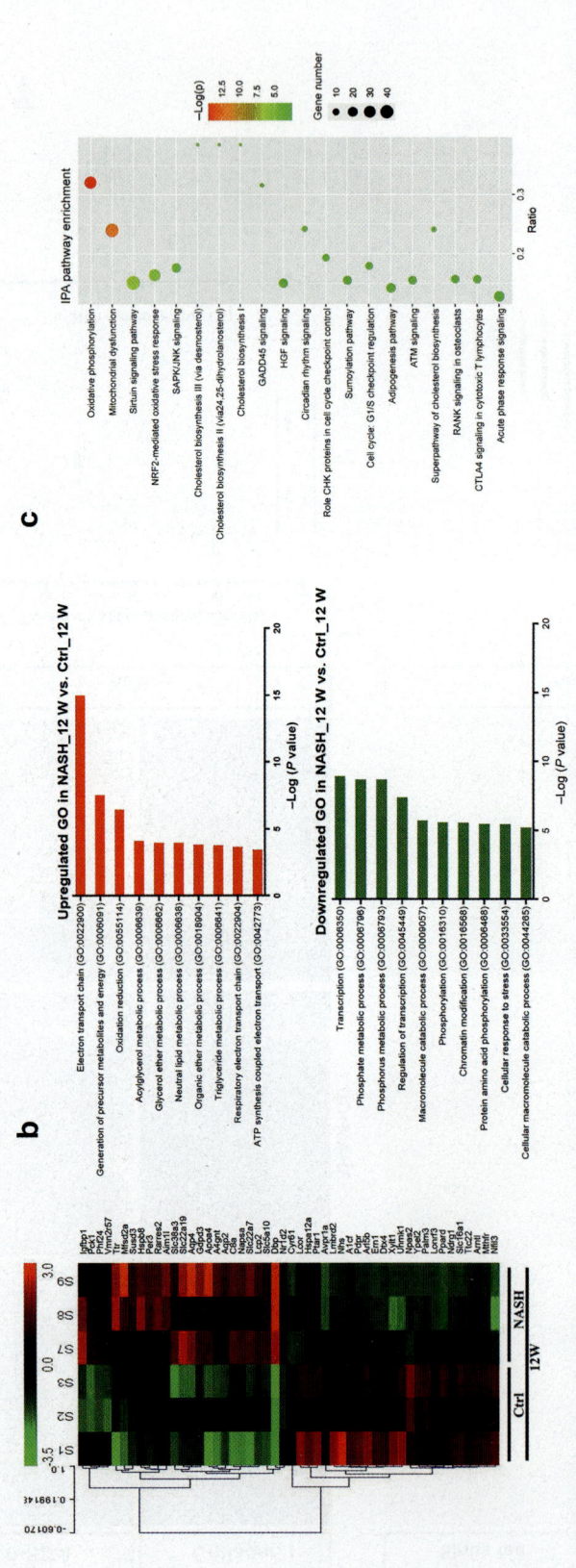

Figure 4 | Transcriptomic profile of kidney cortices from nonalcoholic steatohepatitis (NASH) and control (Ctrl) mice. (a) Heat map of top 50 differentially expressed genes (DEGs) between NASH and Ctrl mice at 12 weeks. (b) Gene Ontology (GO) terms of upregulated or downregulated DEGs between NASH and Ctrl mice at 12 weeks. (c) The top 15 Ingenuity Pathway Analysis (IPA) pathway enrichment analysis for DEGs between NASH and Ctrl mice at 12 weeks. (Continued)

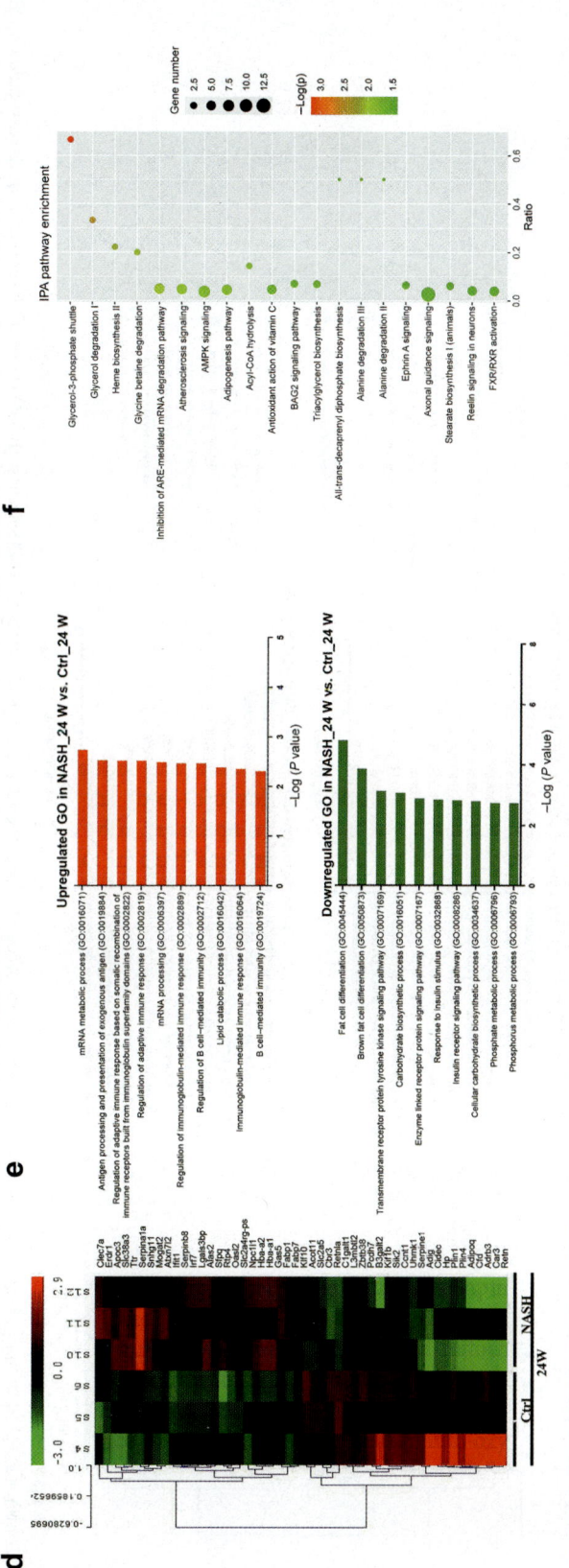

Figure 4 | (Continued) (**d**) Heat map of top 50 DEGs between NASH and Ctrl mice at 24 weeks. (**e**) GO terms of upregulated or downregulated DEGs between NASH and Ctrl mice at 24 weeks. (**f**) The top 15 IPA pathway enrichment analyses for DEGs between NASH and Ctrl mice at 24 weeks. (Continued)

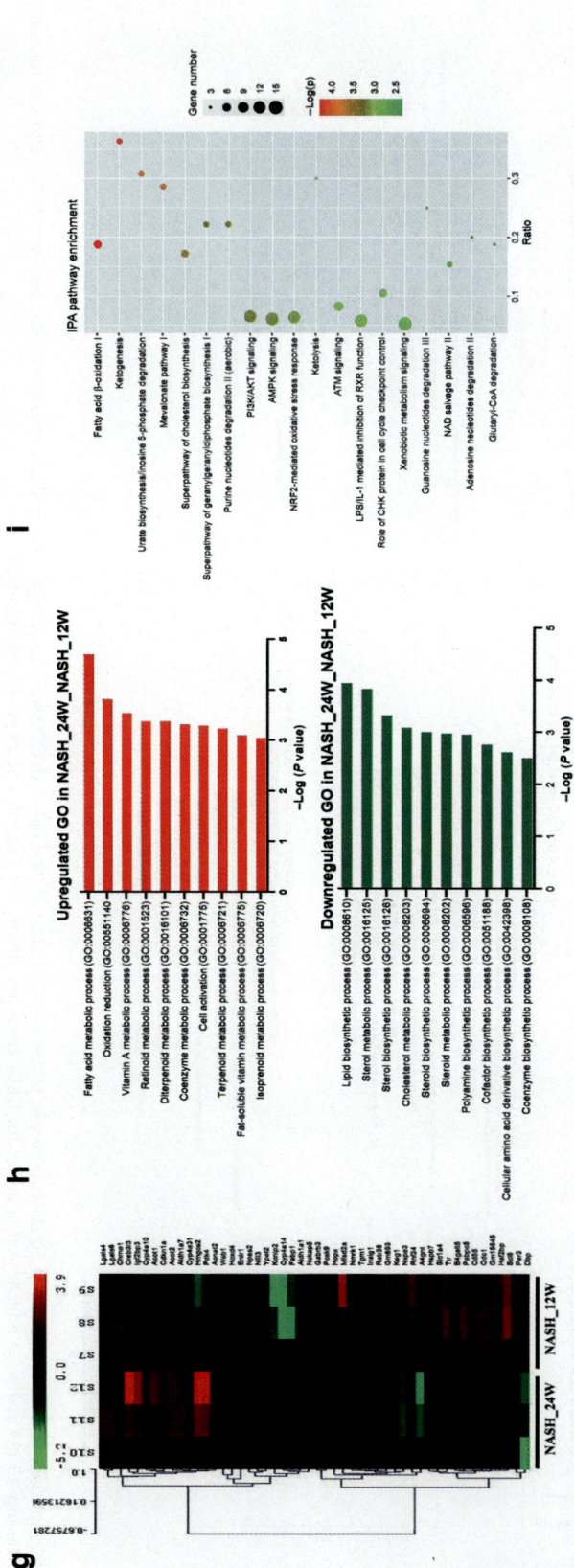

Figure 4 | (Continued) (g) Heat map of top 50 DEGs between intermediate stage (12 weeks) and late stage (24 weeks) of NASH mice. **(h)** GO terms of upregulated or downregulated DEGs between intermediate and late stages of NASH. **(i)** The top 15 IPA pathway enrichment analyses for DEGs between the intermediate and late stage of NASH.

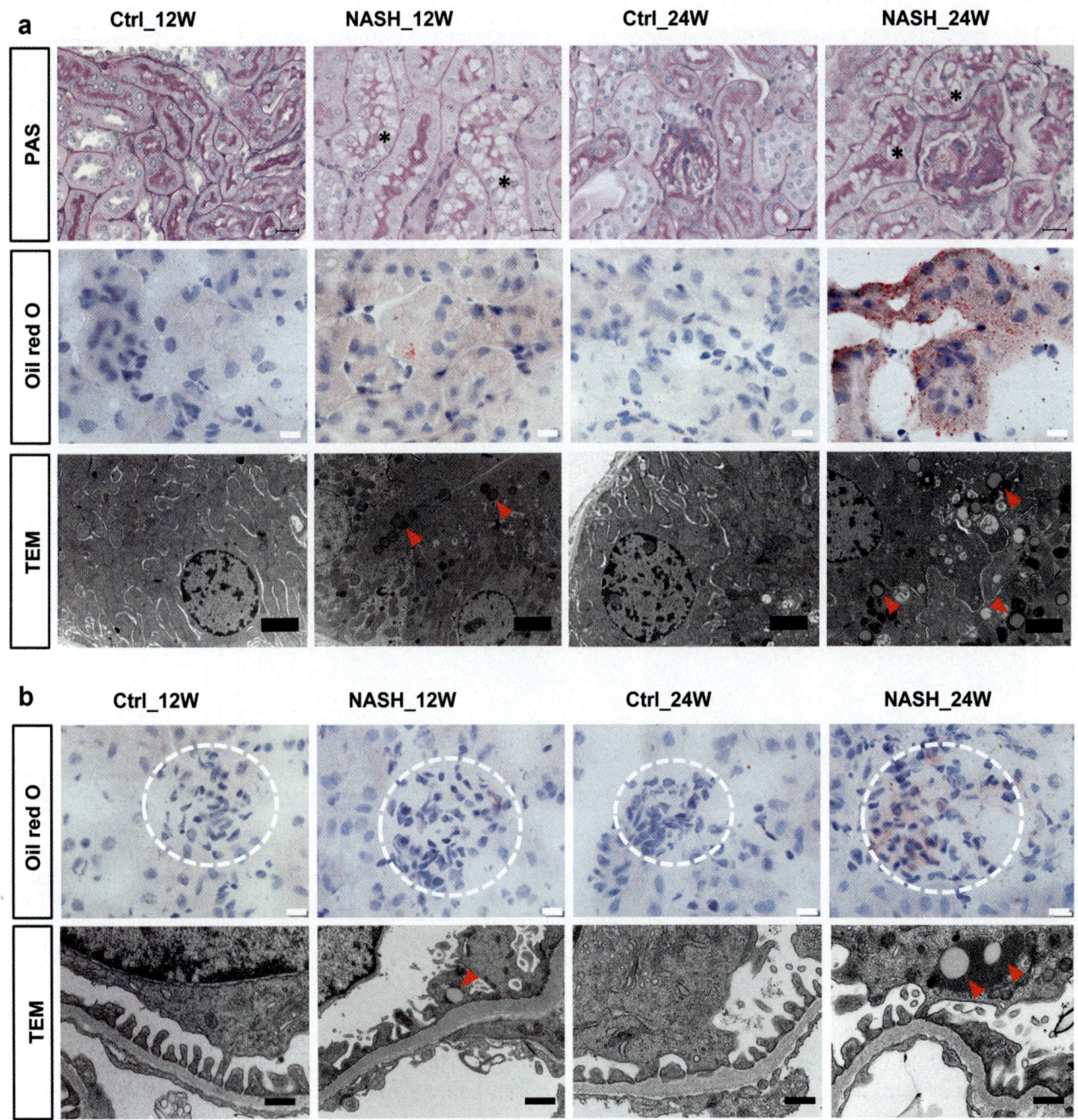

Figure 5 | Lipid accumulation in nonalcoholic steatohepatitis (NASH) mouse kidneys. (a) Representative images of periodic acid–Schiff (PAS)–stained kidneys (top panel, bar = 20 μm.), oil red O–stained kidneys (middle panel, bar = 10 μm), and transmission electric microscopy (TEM) of tubules (bottom panel, bar = 2 μm.) are shown. Compared with control (Ctrl) mice, NASH mice had significant lipid accumulation in tubules (middle panel), consistent with significant vacuolations on tubules (asterisks, top panel) in PAS-stained tissues. Meanwhile, lipid droplets in tubular epithelial cells (TECs) were observed by TEM (bottom panel, red arrowhead). (b) Compared with Ctrl mice, NASH mice had significant lipid accumulation in glomeruli (top panel, bar = 10 μm). Lipid droplets in the cytoplasm of podocytes were observed by TEM (bottom panel, red arrowhead, bar = 500 nm). (Continued)

significant changes in both intermediate and late stages among all lipid classes. Remarkably, 111 lipid species were regulated similarly in intermediate and late stages, including 69 upregulated lipids and 42 downregulated lipids, as detailed in Figure 6e through g and Supplementary Table S3.

Interestingly, the lipid profile also included an increase in sphingolipid families in NASH mice, including sphingomyelin, ceramide, and hexosyl-ceramide. Among them, 3 were upregulated consistently at both intermediate and late stages (namely, sphingomyelin [14:0], sphingomyelin [18:1], and ceramide [14:0]). With regard to glycerolipids, tiracylglycerol-containing polyunsaturated FAs were the most significantly decreased lipid species at both intermediate and late stages of NASH. However, although the trend indicates that tiracyl-glycerol-containing polyunsaturated FAs further decreased in the late stage compared with the intermediate stage, this did

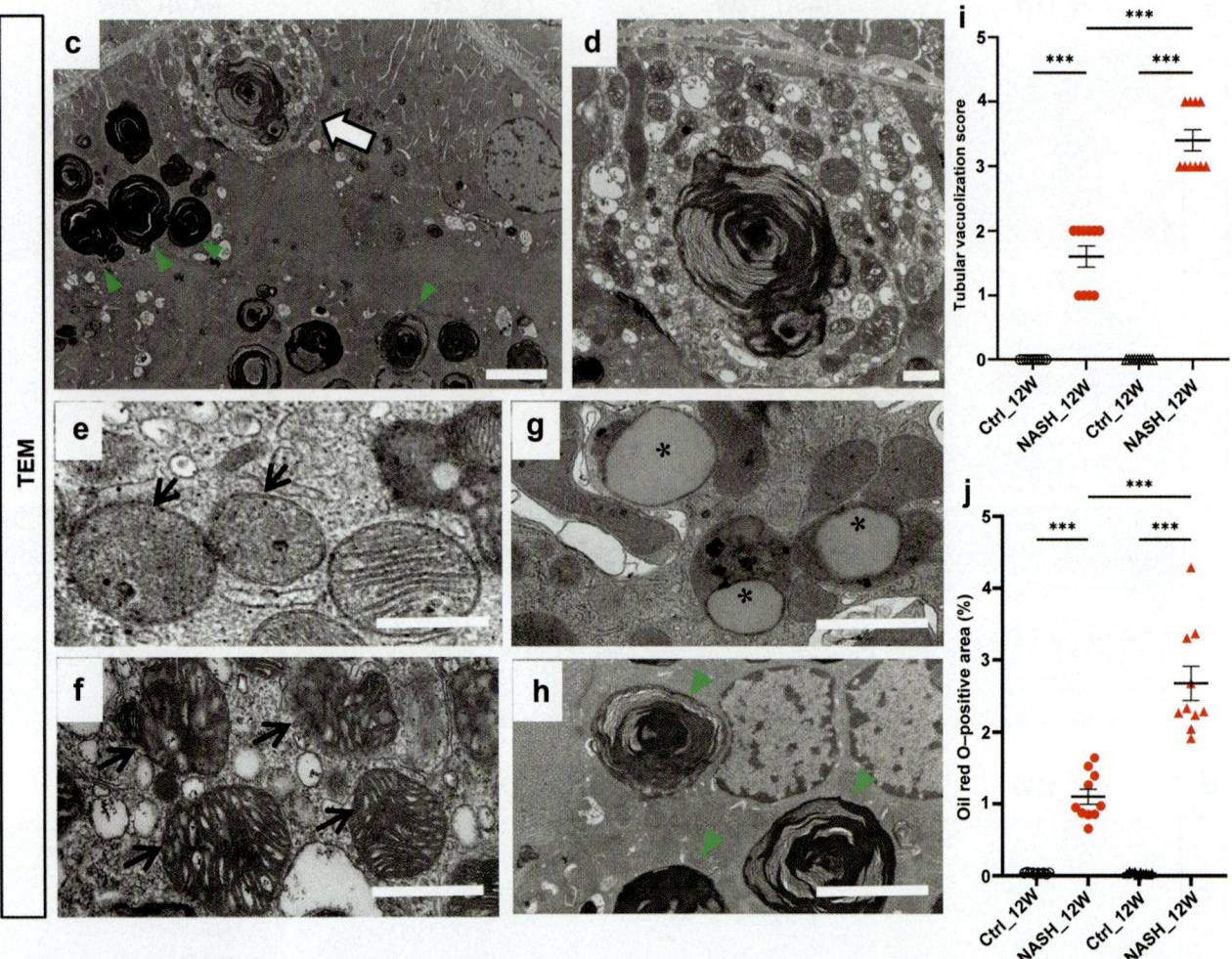

Figure 5 | (Continued) (**c,d**) Impaired mitochondria and lysosomes (white arrow) were seen around myelin-like membranous profile inclusion (green arrowhead) in TECs, bar = 5 μm. (**e,f**) Mitochondria swelling, loss of cristae, black arrows. Bar = 500 nm. (**g**) Lipid droplets in TECs. Bar = 500 nm. (**h**) Myelin-like membranous profile inclusion. Bar = 500 nm. (**i**) The average percentage of tubular vacuolation score per mouse. n = 10 in each group. Values represent mean ± SEM. ***P < 0.001. (**j**) The average percentage of oil red O–stained positive area per mouse. n = 10 in each group. Values represent mean ± SEM. ***P < 0.001. To optimize viewing of this image, please see the online version of this article at www.kidney-international.org.

not reach statistical significance. With regard to other lipid classes, no significant difference was observed between the intermediate and late stages (Figure 6d). Differentially expressed lipids are summarized in the heat map and volcano plots in Figure 6. These studies demonstrate that significant lipid metabolic dysregulation mediates the development of NASH-associated CKD.

Renal histologic changes of NASH mice resemble human NASH and CKD

Kidney biopsy findings from a patient with NASH with elevated transaminases, nephrotic-range proteinuria, and preserved renal function (detailed case presentation is shown in Supplementary Data) showed secondary focal segmental glomerular sclerosis (Figure 7b) with increase of mesangial matrix and glomerulomegaly (Figure 7a) and moderately severe tubulointerstitial fibrosis and inflammation infiltrate (Figure 7b–d) in light microscopy. Some nonatrophic tubules contain intracytoplasmic protein and lipid resorption droplets with focal shedding of lipid-laden epithelial cells into the lumen (Figure 7c and d). TEM revealed mild podocyte foot process effacement with normal glomerular basement membrane thickness (Figure 7e and f). Furthermore, TEM confirmed abundant lipid inclusions in podocytes (Figure 7e, f, and h), mesangial cells (Figure 7g), and TECs (Figure 7h), and myelin figures in TECs (Figure 7h). In addition, TEM also showed mitochondrial abnormalities, such as mitochondrial swelling, loss of cristae, and abnormal patterning of cristae (Figure 7i and j). These histologic findings in human NASH and CKD are reminiscent of the changes illustrated in our animal model.

DISCUSSION

Although prior studies of NASH preclinical models have suggested an association with CKD, the prospect of crosstalk

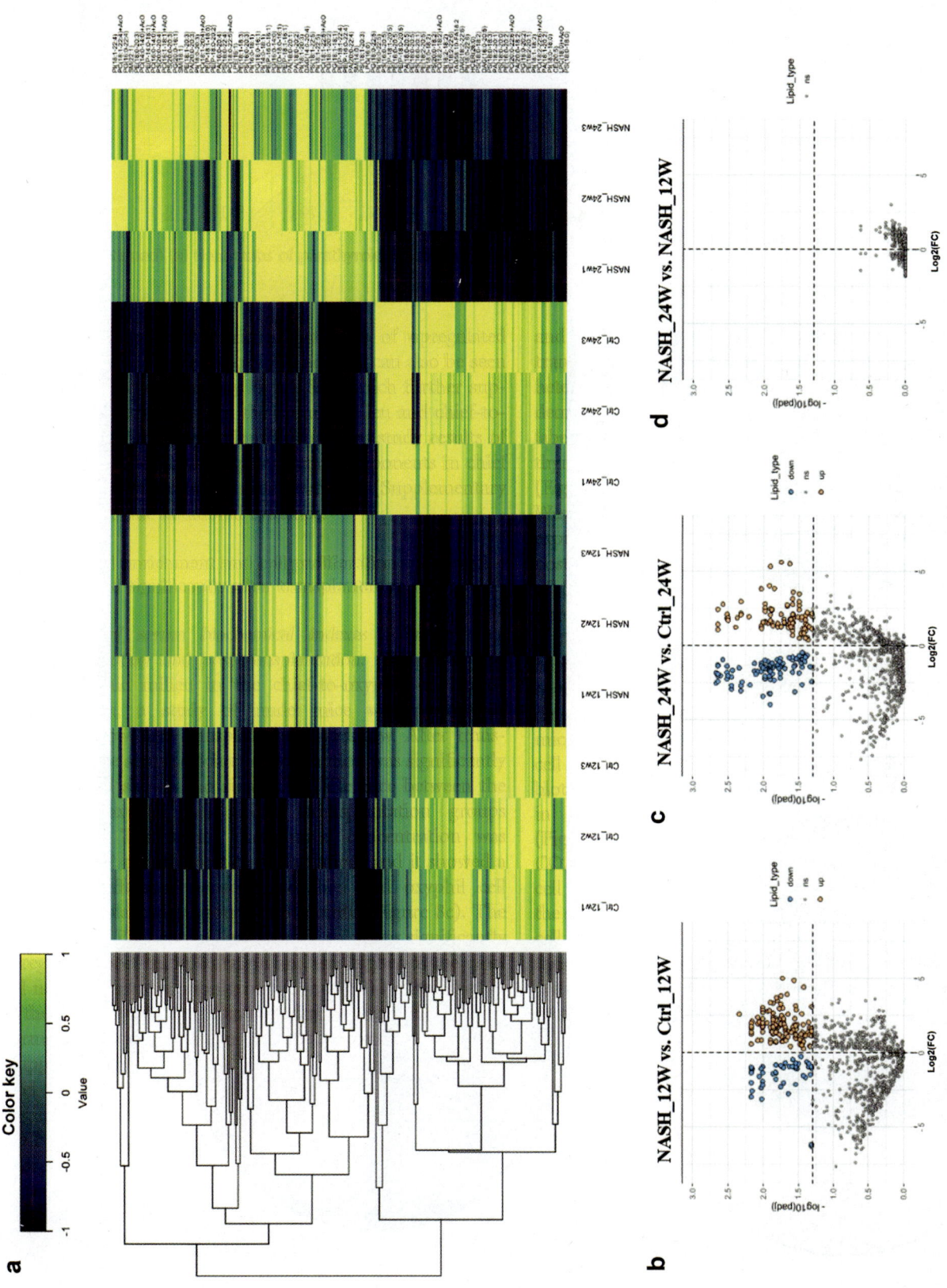

Figure 6 | Lipidomic profile of kidney cortices from nonalcoholic steatohepatitis (NASH) and control (Ctrl) mice. (a) Heat map of discriminant lipid species between NASH and Ctrl mice at intermediate (12 weeks) and late stage (24 weeks). (b) Volcano plots of upregulated and downregulated lipids between NASH and Ctrl mice at intermediate stage (12 weeks). (c) Volcano plots of upregulated and downregulated lipids between NASH and Ctrl mice at late stage (24 weeks). (d) Volcano plots of upregulated and downregulated lipids between intermediate-stage NASH (12 weeks) and late-stage NASH (24 weeks). (Continued)

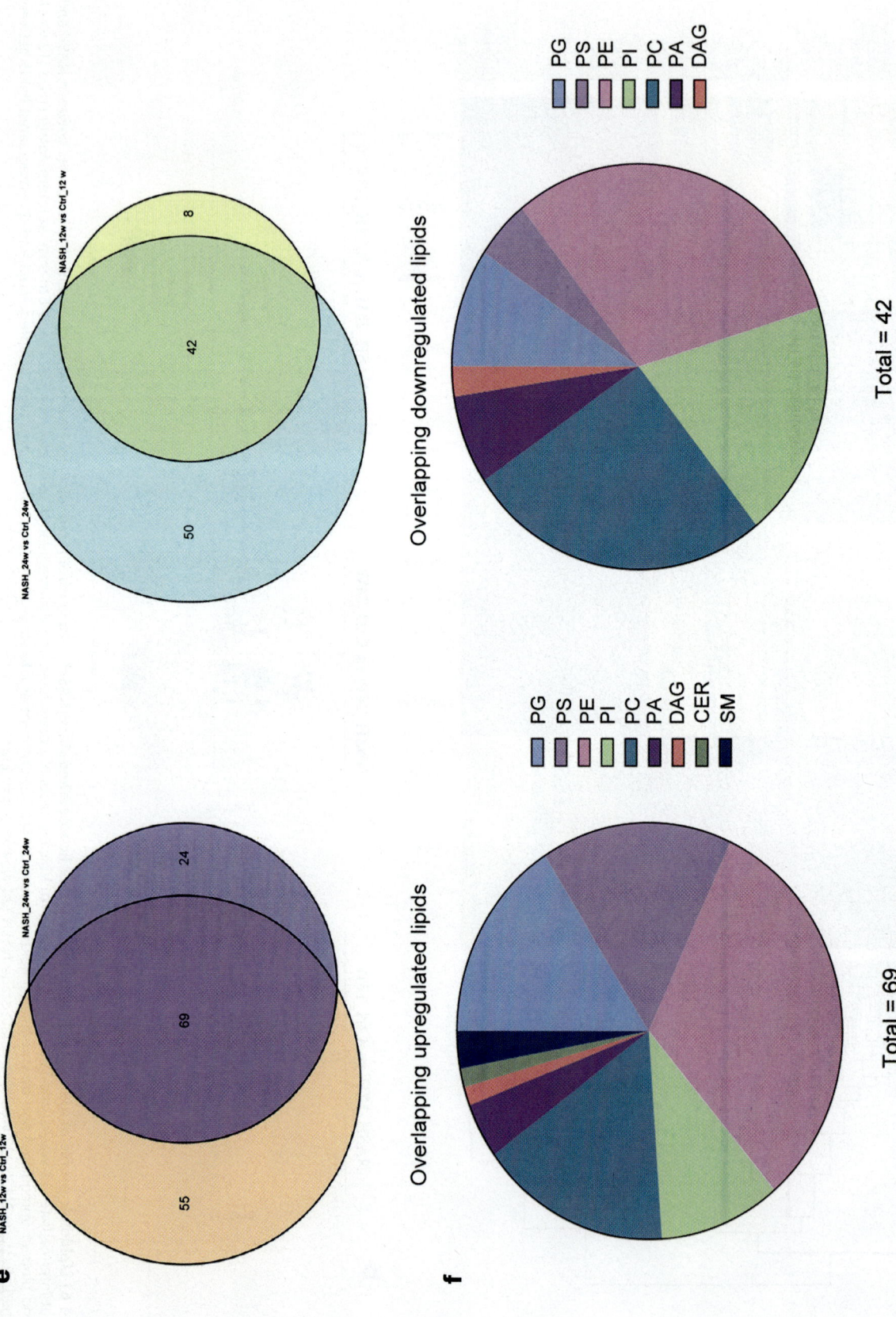

Figure 6 | (Continued) (e) The Venn diagram shows the number of upregulated and downregulated lipids at intermediate-stage NASH (12 weeks) and late-stage NASH (24 weeks) in mice compared with their Ctrls. The number of overlapping lipids is shown in the overlapping regions. (f) The composition of upregulated and downregulated overlapping lipids species at intermediate stage (12 weeks) and late stage (24 weeks) in NASH mice is shown as a pie chart. (Continued)

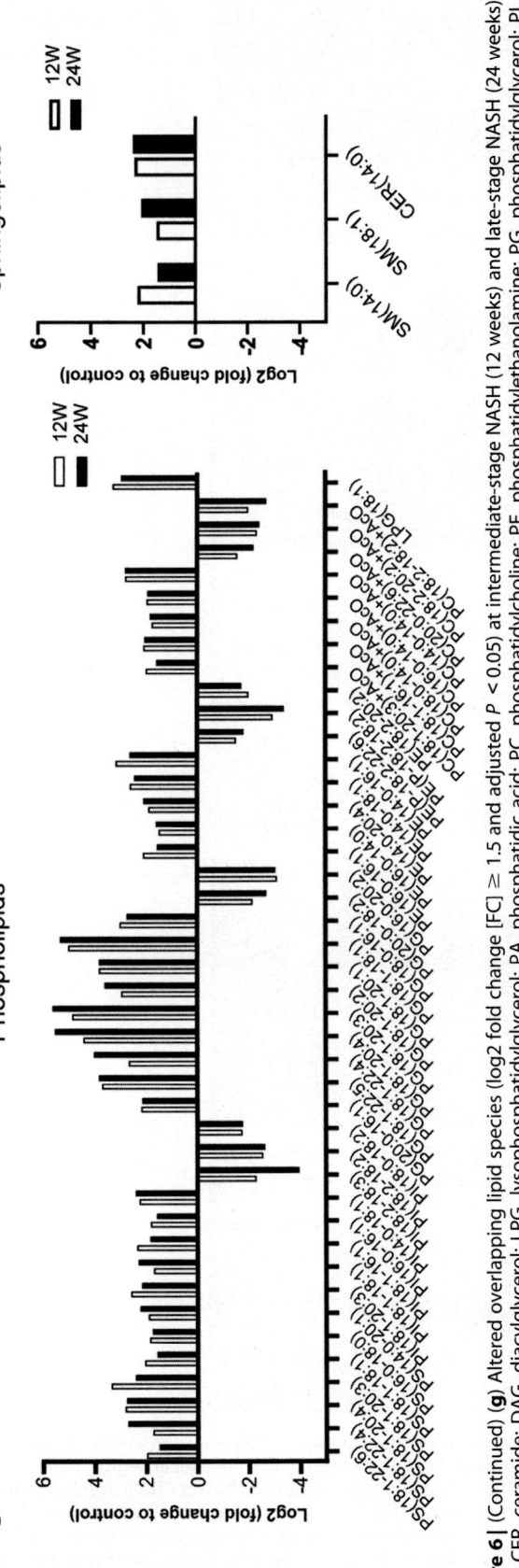

Figure 6 | (Continued) **(g)** Altered overlapping lipid species (log2 fold change [FC] ≥ 1.5 and adjusted $P < 0.05$) at intermediate-stage NASH (12 weeks) and late-stage NASH (24 weeks) in mice. CER, ceramide; DAG, diacylglycerol; LPG, lysophosphatidylglycerol; PA, phosphatidic acid; PC, phosphatidylcholine; PE, phosphatidylethanolamine; PG, phosphatidylglycerol; PI, phosphatidylinositol; PS, phosphatidylserine; SM, sphingomyelin.

between the liver and kidney in NASH remains uncertain. Our murine NASH model, which shows a close resemblance with human NASH, has provided an opportunity to interrogate the link between NASH and kidney disease, with much greater human relevance than the classic dietary and genetic models reported previously.[14,26] In the current study, significant vacuolation of tubular epithelial cells and expansion of mesangial matrix in glomeruli were observed as early as 12 weeks of NASH (intermediate stage). Furthermore, these mice developed significant proteinuria, elevation of BUN, focal segmental glomerular sclerosis, lipid accumulation, and interstitial fibrosis after 24 weeks of feeding WD (late stage). The histologic changes of our NASH model are reminiscent of kidney biopsy findings from a patient with NASH with elevated transaminases and nephrotic-range proteinuria. These findings suggest that the NASH mice develop typical findings of CKD that resemble those observed in humans with NASH.

CCl_4 is reported to induce nephrotoxicity in animals, and a large dose of CCl_4 can reduce glomerular filtration and provoke acute tubular necrosis,[27,28] but the dose of CCl_4 in our study is much lower than doses reported previously (≈8%–10% of the standard dose).[27–29] To confirm that this low dose does not cause toxicity, we treated mice with the same low dose of CCl_4 as used in the NASH model and did not observe any kidney histologic changes, proteinuria, or renal dysfunction in these mice, suggesting that the kidney injury and fibrosis in these NASH mice were not due to CCl_4 nephrotoxicity. C57BL/6 mice fed with a high-fat diet alone usually do not develop significant histologic changes in the kidney.[30] Furthermore, C57BL/6 mice fed with a high-fat and high-fructose diet for 8 months only developed minimal kidney injury without fibrosis and mesangial matrix expansion.[31] Thus, the kidney injury and fibrosis in our NASH model are likely related to NASH or the combination of a high-fat diet and the presence of NASH. Consistent with this, the kidney fibrosis score positively correlated with the NASH activity score.

Switching the diet back to a normal chow diet in NASH mice led to partial resolution of hepatic steatosis and inflammation, along with partial reduction of proteinuria, renal dysfunction, and histologic abnormalities, suggesting the importance of diet on both NASH and CKD. Consistent with this finding, it has been shown that in patients with NASH, lifestyle intervention can lead to improvement of liver fibrosis,[32] and return to normal chow diet leads to regression of hepatic histologic changes.[33] Our results indicate that dietary modifications also have benefits in NASH-associated CKD. However, we could not deduce from these studies whether CKD was caused by WD, NASH, or both.

To confirm the causal effect of NASH on CKD development, we performed OLT. We found that NASH mice receiving OLT had significant improvement in proteinuria, renal dysfunction, glomerulosclerosis, and tubulointerstitial fibrosis compared with the SHAM mice, which were on the same diet. These data suggest that NASH alone contributes to the development of CKD.

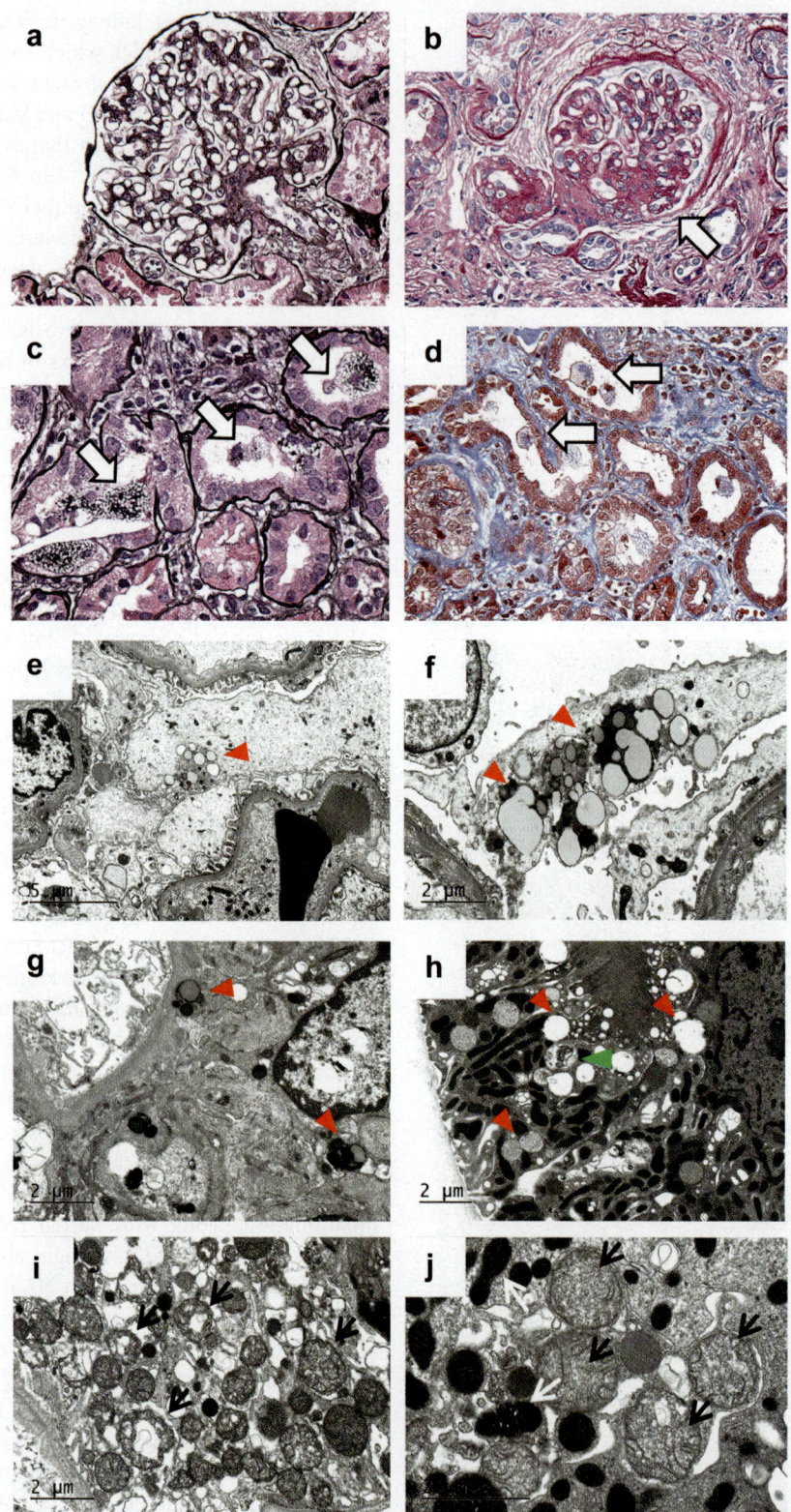

Figure 7 | Kidney biopsy findings in a patient with nonalcoholic steatohepatitis and chronic kidney disease. (**a**) Glomerulomegaly and mild mesangial matrix expansion. Jones methenamine silver (JMS), original magnification ×400. (**b**) Perihilar focal segmental glomerular sclerosis and arteriolosclerosis with hyalinosis. Periodic acid–Schiff, original magnification ×400. (**c**) Cholesterol cleft in tubular lumen and lipid-laden detached tubular epithelial cells. JMS, original magnification ×600. (**d**) Tubular lipid vacuoles and interstitial fibrosis. Masson trichrome, original magnification ×400. (**e**) Lipid vacuoles (red arrowhead) in podocyte cell body and mild podocyte foot process effacement. Electron micrograph, original magnification ×8000. (**f**) Phospholipid (red arrowheads) in the cytoplasm of podocyte primary process. Original magnification ×15,000. (**g**) Mesangial cell lipid inclusions (red arrowheads). Original magnification ×15,000. (**h**) Lipid vacuoles (red arrowheads) and myelin figures (green arrowheads) in proximal tubular (continued)

To gain insight into the pathogenesis of NASH-induced kidney injury, we compared the transcriptomic profiles of kidney cortices between NASH mice and their controls at both intermediate and late stages. Although the DEGs in 2 stages have a temporal pattern, the pathway analysis of DEGs in both stages of NASH indicated that many of the DEGs are involved in lipid metabolism and energetic homeostasis. Consistent with this, there was significant vacuolation and lipid droplets in TECs in the NASH mice. These data suggest that lipid dysregulation in the kidney might be a key event mediating the progression of NASH-associated CKD.

Hepatic steatosis is a consequence of lipid metabolic reprogramming in which lipogenesis surpasses FA oxidation (FAO) in NAFLD.[34] In addition, ectopic lipid accumulation may also affect extrahepatic organs.[35,36] Recent studies suggest that intracellular lipid accumulation in kidney cells, especially TECs, has a key role in the pathogenesis of CKD.[37–39] Excess lipids can damage proximal tubular epithelial cells through various mechanisms, including mitochondrial dysfunction, production of reactive oxygen species and lipid peroxidation, diminished autophagy, and activation of the inflammatory pathway.[40–42] Inhibition of FAO in tubular epithelial cells can also promote renal fibrosis through inflammation and apoptosis of TECs.[40,43] Under NAFLD conditions, the tricarboxylic acid cycle, FAO, and oxidative phosphorylation were accelerated to overcome the free FA burden.[44] Increased mitochondrial activity appears to protect TECs from the deleterious effects of free FAs.[45] Accelerated FAO may be a compensatory response to the lipid accumulation in TECs. However, increased mitochondrial tricarboxylic acid cycle and FAO results in a redundant supply of electrons to the respiratory complexes. This overreduction of the electron transport chain promotes the production of reactive oxygen species, which cause cellular oxidative damage.[46] These findings suggest that ectopic lipid accumulation in the TECs during the progression of NAFLD likely contributes to the development of renal fibrosis in these NASH mice. Thus, the more advanced kidney disease in the late-stage NASH mice could reflect the cumulative effects of liver disease on progressive ectopic lipid accumulation in the kidney.

To further dissect the role of lipid disorder in CKD, we performed lipidomics of the kidneys from these mice. We revealed significant differences in kidney lipid profiles between NASH mice and controls. The dysregulation of many phospholipids, including phosphatidylcholine, phosphatidylserine, PE, phosphatidylglycerol, phosphatidylinositol, and phosphatidic acid, is the most consistent feature in NASH. Phospholipids are major constituents of cellular and subcellular organelle membranes.[47–49] For example, phosphatidylglycerol is a biosynthetic precursor for bis(monoacylglycero) phosphates and cardiolipins,[49] which are essential for normal electron transport and oxidative phosphorylation in the inner mitochondrial membrane.[50] PE is the second most abundant phospholipid in cells and has essential roles in cytochrome c oxidase activity, and PE deficiency reduces the complex IV activity.[51] In addition, PE, along with cardiolipin, phosphatidic acid, and phosphatidylinositol, is an integral member of complex III formation of mitochondria.[52,53] In the current study, TEM revealed mitochondrial damage in TECs of NASH mice, including swelling and loss of cristae. Pathway analysis of DEGs showed that many of the upregulated genes were involved in the electron transport chain and adenosine triphosphate synthesis, and Ingenuity Pathway Analysis also indicates that pathways of mitochondrial dysfunction and oxidative stress were highly enriched. Thus, dysregulation of phospholipids in kidneys of NASH mice likely affects mitochondrial function, such as adenosine triphosphate production, oxidative stress, and crosstalk between organelles,[54] playing a pivotal role in the pathogenesis in NASH-associated CKD.

Sphingolipids are the major components of the lipid raft for membrane protein-protein interaction and are closely associated with insulin resistance and ectopic lipid deposition. Serum and hepatic ceramides elevate in obese patients with NASH with insulin resistance and are associated with systemic and hepatic inflammation and damage of the mitochondrial respiratory chain, resulting in decreased adenosine triphosphate production in patients with NAFLD/NASH.[55]

Ceramide 14:0 and sphingosine were correlated with circulating tumor necrosis factor-α levels in patients with NAFLD.[55] *In vitro*, ceramides can regulate autophagy, reactive oxygen species production, cell proliferation, and apoptosis.[56] Certain serum ceramides, such as dihydroceramide 18:0, may be early biomarkers of diabetes onset in mice and humans.[57] Moreover, accumulation of sphingolipids occurs in kidney tissue in rodent models of type 1 and type 2 diabetes.[58,59] Our results showed that sphingolipid was significantly increased in kidney tissues of NASH mice, and TEM confirmed myelin-like membranous inclusions in TECs, which usually reflect deposition of sphingolipid, and impaired mitochondria and lysosomes were seen around myelin-like membranous inclusion, suggesting a specific role of sphingolipid that has distinct biological functions in NASH-associated CKD. Further studies are required to investigate the role of the sphingolipid–insulin resistance pathway in NASH-associated CKD.

Ingenuity Pathway Analysis also highlights several signaling pathways contributing to the pathogenesis of CKD through the regulation of fibrosis, autophagy, apoptosis, oxidative stress, inflammation, energetic homeostasis, cell growth, differentiation, and stress response.[60–66] Nonetheless,

Figure 7 | (continued) epithelial cells. Original magnification ×12,000. (**i**) Swollen mitochondria with loss of cristae (black arrows) in proximal tubular epithelial cells. Original magnification ×15,000. (**j**) Normal mitochondria (white arrows) adjacent to abnormal swollen mitochondria with loss of cristae (black arrows) in proximal tubular epithelial cells. Original magnification ×25,000. To optimize viewing of this image, please see the online version of this article at www.kidney-international.org.

specific roles of these pathways in the pathogenesis of NASH-associated CKD remain to be confirmed.

Interestingly, we reported here the kidney biopsy findings from a patient with NASH with CKD, which were similar to the findings from our NASH mouse model, further validating the human relevance of our studies. To our knowledge, there are no previous reports on the kidney histology of patients with NASH with CKD. Future studies are required to have more systemic studies of kidney histology in these patients.

In conclusion, we have characterized the kidney phenotype in a novel NASH model that resembles human NASH. NASH mice develop proteinuria, a decline of renal function, glomerulosclerosis, and tubulointerstitial fibrosis, resembling human CKD in patients with NASH. We found that transplantation of normal livers into NASH mice leads to improved renal function and regression of kidney histologic abnormalities, confirming the critical role of NASH in the development and progression of CKD. Our transcriptomic and lipidomic analyses reveal alterations in major signaling pathways and lipid profiles that likely mediate the pathogenesis of NASH-associated CKD. Our study will help better understand the mechanisms of NASH-induced kidney injury and develop potential new therapies for NASH-associated CKD.

DISCLOSURE
All the authors declared no competing interests.

DATA STATEMENT
The authors confirm that the data supporting the findings of this study are available in the article and its supplementary materials. The mRNA-sequencing data set is available at the National Center for Biotechnology Information Gene Expression Omnibus database (www.ncbi.nlm.nih.gov/geo), accession number GSE184256.

FINANCIAL SUPPORT
XL is supported by the National Nature Science Foundation of China (81970622); JCH is supported by National Institutes of Health (NIH)/National Institute of Diabetes and Digestive and Kidney Diseases (NIDDK) R01DK109683, R01DK122980, R01DK129467, and P01DK56492, and VA Merit Award I01BX000345; KL is supported by NIH/NIDDK R01DK117913-01, R01DK129467, and R01DK133912. SLF is supported by grants from the NIH, R01 DK56621 and DK128289.

AUTHOR CONTRIBUTIONS
XL, DB, YY, and FZ performed the experiments and morphologic and other data analysis; CW performed analysis and interpretation of mRNA-sequencing data; XL performed analysis of lipidomic data; VDD acquired and analyzed data of human kidney biopsy; XL wrote the manuscript; and JCH, KL, and SLF designed and supervised the study and revised the manuscript.

SUPPLEMENTARY MATERIAL
Supplementary File (TIF)
Supplementary Figure S1. (**A**) Urinary albumin excretion and (**B**) serum BUN of male (n = 5) and female (n = 5) NASH and control mice at 12 and 24 weeks.
Supplementary Figure S2. (**A**) Urinary albumin excretion, (**B**) serum BUN, and renal histology of CCl_4-treated mice. There was no significant difference between CCl_4-treated mice and control mice at 12 weeks (n = 10) and 24 weeks (n = 10). (**C**) Representative images of PAS-stained paraffin-embedded sections of kidneys in CCl_4 treatment at 12 weeks (n = 10) and 24 weeks (n = 10). Bar = 50 μm (black); 20 μm (red). NS, not significant.
Supplementary Figure S3. Representative images of immunostaining of CD3, CD8, and F4/80 on paraffin sections of NASH kidney at 24 weeks. Bar = 50 μm.
Supplementary Figure S4. Orthotopic liver transplantation in NASH mice. (**A,B**) Recipient operation of OLT. Inset, the harvested fatty liver of recipient mice. (**C**) Histology of recipient mice at the intermediate stage of NASH (12 weeks), showing steatosis, lobular inflammation, and ballooning hepatocytes. Hematoxylin and eosin stain. Bar = 50 μm. (**D**) Histology of liver graft 12 weeks after OLT. There were mild infiltrating inflammatory cells in periportal and sinusoidal areas. Hematoxylin and eosin stain. Bar = 50 μm.
Supplementary File (Word)
Supplementary Renal biopsy case presentation.
Supplementary File (Excel)
Supplementary Table S1. Discriminant lipids between NASH_12W versus Ctrl_12W.
Supplementary Table S2. Discriminant lipids between NASH_24W versus Ctrl_24W.
Supplementary Table S3. Overlap lipids.

REFERENCES
1. Loomba R, Friedman SL, Shulman GI. Mechanisms and disease consequences of nonalcoholic fatty liver disease. *Cell*. 2021;184:2537–2564.
2. Turkish AR. Nonalcoholic fatty liver disease: emerging mechanisms and consequences. *Curr Opin Clin Nutr Metab Care*. 2008;11:128–133.
3. Younossi ZM. Non-alcoholic fatty liver disease - a global public health perspective. *J Hepatol*. 2019;70:531–544.
4. Targher G, Bertolini L, Rodella S, et al. Relationship between kidney function and liver histology in subjects with nonalcoholic steatohepatitis. *Clin J Am Soc Nephrol*. 2010;5:2166–2171.
5. Sinn DH, Kang D, Jang HR, et al. Development of chronic kidney disease in patients with non-alcoholic fatty liver disease: a cohort study. *J Hepatol*. 2017;67:1274–1280.
6. Park H, Dawwas GK, Liu X, et al. Nonalcoholic fatty liver disease increases risk of incident advanced chronic kidney disease: a propensity-matched cohort study. *J Intern Med*. 2019;286:711–722.
7. Mantovani A, Petracca G, Beatrice G, et al. Non-alcoholic fatty liver disease and risk of incident chronic kidney disease: an updated meta-analysis. *Gut*. 2022;71:156–162.
8. Byrne CD, Targher G. NAFLD as a driver of chronic kidney disease. *J Hepatol*. 2020;72:785–801.
9. Kim SH, Lim Y, Park JB, et al. Erratum: comparative study of fatty liver induced by methionine and choline-deficiency in C57BL/6N mice originating from three different sources. *Lab Anim Res*. 2017;33:318.
10. Saito H, Tanaka T, Sugahara M, et al. Inhibition of prolyl hydroxylase domain (PHD) by JTZ-951 reduces obesity-related diseases in the liver, white adipose tissue, and kidney in mice with a high-fat diet. *Lab Invest*. 2019;99:1217–1232.
11. Xie G, Wang X, Liu P, et al. Distinctly altered gut microbiota in the progression of liver disease. *Oncotarget*. 2016;7:19355–19366.
12. Permyakova A, Gammal A, Hinden L, et al. A novel indoline derivative ameliorates diabesity-induced chronic kidney disease by reducing metabolic abnormalities. *Front Endocrinol (Lausanne)*. 2020;11:91.
13. Ibrahim SH, Hirsova P, Malhi H, et al. Animal models of nonalcoholic steatohepatitis: eat, delete, and inflame. *Dig Dis Sci*. 2016;61:1325–1336.
14. Tsuchida T, Lee YA, Fujiwara N, et al. A simple diet- and chemical-induced murine NASH model with rapid progression of steatohepatitis, fibrosis and liver cancer. *J Hepatol*. 2018;69:385–395.
15. Carter JK, Bhattacharya D, Borgerding JN, et al. Modeling dysbiosis of human NASH in mice: loss of gut microbiome diversity and overgrowth of Erysipelotrichales. *PLoS One*. 2021;16:e0244763.
16. Yokota S, Ueki S, Ono Y, et al. Orthotopic mouse liver transplantation to study liver biology and allograft tolerance. *Nat Protoc*. 2016;11:1163–1174.

17. Fujimoto M, Maezawa Y, Yokote K, et al. Mice lacking Smad3 are protected against streptozotocin-induced diabetic glomerulopathy. *Biochem Biophys Res Commun*. 2003;305:1002–1007.
18. Chen A, Feng Y, Lai H, et al. Soluble RARRES1 induces podocyte apoptosis to promote glomerular disease progression. *J Clin Invest*. 2020;130:5523–5535.
19. Kleiner DE, Brunt EM, Van Natta M, et al. Design and validation of a histological scoring system for nonalcoholic fatty liver disease. *Hepatology*. 2005;41:1313–1321.
20. Li H, Durbin R. Fast and accurate short read alignment with Burrows-Wheeler transform. *Bioinformatics*. 2009;25:1754–1760.
21. Mortazavi A, Williams BA, McCue K, et al. Mapping and quantifying mammalian transcriptomes by RNA-Seq. *Nat Methods*. 2008;5:621–628.
22. Ritchie ME, Phipson B, Wu D, et al. limma powers differential expression analyses for RNA-sequencing and microarray studies. *Nucleic Acids Res*. 2015;43:e47.
23. Chen EY, Tan CM, Kou Y, et al. Enrichr: interactive and collaborative HTML5 gene list enrichment analysis tool. *BMC Bioinformatics*. 2013;14:128.
24. Saeed AI, Sharov V, White J, et al. TM4: a free, open-source system for microarray data management and analysis. *Biotechniques*. 2003;34:374–378.
25. Lin WJ, Shen PC, Liu HC, et al. LipidSig: a web-based tool for lipidomic data analysis. *Nucleic Acids Res*. 2021;49:W336–W345.
26. Santhekadur PK, Kumar DP, Sanyal AJ. Preclinical models of non-alcoholic fatty liver disease. *J Hepatol*. 2018;68:230–237.
27. Jaramillo-Juarez F, Rodriguez-Vazquez ML, Rincon-Sanchez AR, et al. Acute renal failure induced by carbon tetrachloride in rats with hepatic cirrhosis. *Ann Hepatol*. 2008;7:331–338.
28. Yilmaz-Ozden T, Can A, Karatug A, et al. Carbon tetrachloride-induced kidney damage and protective effect of Amaranthus lividus L. in rats. *Toxicol Ind Health*. 2016;32:1143–1152.
29. Scholten D, Trebicka J, Liedtke C, et al. The carbon tetrachloride model in mice. *Lab Anim*. 2015;49:4–11.
30. Wicks SE, Nguyen TT, Breaux C, et al. Diet-induced obesity and kidney disease - in search of a susceptible mouse model. *Biochimie*. 2016;124:65–73.
31. Dissard R, Klein J, Caubet C, et al. Long term metabolic syndrome induced by a high fat high fructose diet leads to minimal renal injury in C57BL/6 mice. *PLoS One*. 2013;8:e76703.
32. Promrat K, Kleiner DE, Niemeier HM, et al. Randomized controlled trial testing the effects of weight loss on nonalcoholic steatohepatitis. *Hepatology*. 2010;51:121–129.
33. Ganguly S, Muench GA, Shang L, et al. Nonalcoholic steatohepatitis and HCC in a hyperphagic mouse accelerated by Western diet. *Cell Mol Gastroenterol Hepatol*. 2021;12:891–920.
34. Gluchowski NL, Becuwe M, Walther TC, et al. Lipid droplets and liver disease: from basic biology to clinical implications. *Nat Rev Gastroenterol Hepatol*. 2017;14:343–355.
35. Byrne CD, Targher G. NAFLD: a multisystem disease. *J Hepatol*. 2015;62:S47–S64.
36. Adams LA, Anstee QM, Tilg H, et al. Non-alcoholic fatty liver disease and its relationship with cardiovascular disease and other extrahepatic diseases. *Gut*. 2017;66:1138–1153.
37. Herman-Edelstein M, Scherzer P, Tobar A, et al. Altered renal lipid metabolism and renal lipid accumulation in human diabetic nephropathy. *J Lipid Res*. 2014;55:561–572.
38. Li S, Nagothu KK, Desai V, et al. Transgenic expression of proximal tubule peroxisome proliferator-activated receptor-alpha in mice confers protection during acute kidney injury. *Kidney Int*. 2009;76:1049–1062.
39. Gai Z, Wang T, Visentin M, et al. Lipid accumulation and chronic kidney disease. *Nutrients*. 2019;11:722.
40. Kang HM, Ahn SH, Choi P, et al. Defective fatty acid oxidation in renal tubular epithelial cells has a key role in kidney fibrosis development. *Nat Med*. 2015;21:37–46.
41. Sun H, Sun Z, Varghese Z, et al. Nonesterified free fatty acids enhance the inflammatory response in renal tubules by inducing extracellular ATP release. *Am J Physiol Renal Physiol*. 2020;319:F292–F303.
42. Nosadini R, Tonolo G. Role of oxidized low density lipoproteins and free fatty acids in the pathogenesis of glomerulopathy and tubulointerstitial lesions in type 2 diabetes. *Nutr Metab Cardiovasc Dis*. 2011;21:79–85.
43. Simon N, Hertig A. Alteration of fatty acid oxidation in tubular epithelial cells: from acute kidney injury to renal fibrogenesis. *Front Med (Lausanne)*. 2015;2:52.
44. Alves-Bezerra M, Cohen DE. Triglyceride metabolism in the liver. *Compr Physiol*. 2017;8:1–8.
45. Koliaki C, Szendroedi J, Kaul K, et al. Adaptation of hepatic mitochondrial function in humans with non-alcoholic fatty liver is lost in steatohepatitis. *Cell Metab*. 2015;21:739–746.
46. Irazabal MV, Torres VE. Reactive oxygen species and redox signaling in chronic kidney disease. *Cells*. 2020;9:1342.
47. Acoba MG, Senoo N, Claypool SM. Phospholipid ebb and flow makes mitochondria go. *J Cell Biol*. 2020;219:e202003131.
48. Morita SY, Ikeda Y. Regulation of membrane phospholipid biosynthesis in mammalian cells. *Biochem Pharmacol*. 2022;206:115296.
49. Horvath SE, Daum G. Lipids of mitochondria. *Prog Lipid Res*. 2013;52:590–614.
50. Ren M, Phoon CK, Schlame M. Metabolism and function of mitochondrial cardiolipin. *Prog Lipid Res*. 2014;55:1–16.
51. Hasan SS, Yamashita E, Ryan CM, et al. Conservation of lipid functions in cytochrome bc complexes. *J Mol Biol*. 2011;414:145–162.
52. Ducasa GM, Mitrofanova A, Fornoni A. Crosstalk between lipids and mitochondria in diabetic kidney disease. *Curr Diab Rep*. 2019;19:144.
53. Bottinger L, Horvath SE, Kleinschroth T, et al. Phosphatidylethanolamine and cardiolipin differentially affect the stability of mitochondrial respiratory chain supercomplexes. *J Mol Biol*. 2012;423:677–686.
54. Wang B, Tontonoz P. Phospholipid remodeling in physiology and disease. *Annu Rev Physiol*. 2019;81:165–188.
55. Apostolopoulou M, Gordillo R, Koliaki C, et al. Specific hepatic sphingolipids relate to insulin resistance, oxidative stress, and inflammation in nonalcoholic steatohepatitis. *Diabetes Care*. 2018;41:1235–1243.
56. Siddique MM, Li Y, Chaurasia B, et al. Dihydroceramides: from bit players to lead actors. *J Biol Chem*. 2015;290:15371–15379.
57. Wigger L, Cruciani-Guglielmacci C, Nicolas A, et al. Plasma dihydroceramides are diabetes susceptibility biomarker candidates in mice and humans. *Cell Rep*. 2017;18:2269–2279.
58. Liu G, Han F, Yang Y, et al. Evaluation of sphingolipid metabolism in renal cortex of rats with streptozotocin-induced diabetes and the effects of rapamycin. *Nephrol Dial Transplant*. 2011;26:1493–1502.
59. Matanes F, Twal WO, Hammad SM. Sphingolipids as biomarkers of disease. *Adv Exp Med Biol*. 2019;1159:109–138.
60. Herrero-Fresneda I, Torras J, Franquesa M, et al. HGF gene therapy attenuates renal allograft scarring by preventing the profibrotic inflammatory-induced mechanisms. *Kidney Int*. 2006;70:265–274.
61. Rolo AP, Teodoro JS, Palmeira CM. Role of oxidative stress in the pathogenesis of nonalcoholic steatohepatitis. *Free Radic Biol Med*. 2012;52:59–69.
62. Juszczak F, Caron N, Mathew AV, et al. Critical role for AMPK in metabolic disease-induced chronic kidney disease. *Int J Mol Sci*. 2020;21:7994.
63. Hsu WH, Chen TH, Lee BH, et al. Monascin and ankaflavin act as natural AMPK activators with PPARalpha agonist activity to down-regulate nonalcoholic steatohepatitis in high-fat diet-fed C57BL/6 mice. *Food Chem Toxicol*. 2014;64:94–103.
64. Decleves AE, Zolkipli Z, Satriano J, et al. Regulation of lipid accumulation by AMP-activated kinase [corrected] in high fat diet-induced kidney injury. *Kidney Int*. 2014;85:611–623.
65. Qin L, Guo J, Zheng Q, et al. BAG2 structure, function and involvement in disease. *Cell Mol Biol Lett*. 2016;21:18.
66. Liu Y, Shen P, Zhou Y, et al. c-Jun N-terminal kinase/transforming growth factor-beta/Smad3 pathway: is it associated with endoplasmic reticulum stress-mediated renal interstitial fibrosis? *Mol Med Rep*. 2019;20:755–762.

clinical investigation

www.kidney-international.org

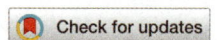

Single-cell RNA sequencing reveals transdifferentiation of parathyroid chief cells into oxyphil cells in patients with uremic secondary hyperparathyroidism

see commentary on page 433

Jianping Mao[1,2], Huaizhou You[1,2], Mengjing Wang[1,2], Yongbing Ba[3], Jing Qian[1], Ping Cheng[1], Chuhan Lu[1] and Jing Chen[1,2]

[1]Division of Nephrology, Huashan Hospital, Fudan University, Shanghai, China; [2]National Clinical Research Center for Aging and Medicine, Huashan Hospital, Fudan University, Shanghai, China; and [3]OE Biotech Co, Ltd, Shanghai, China

The parathyroid gland is one of the main organs that regulate calcium and phosphorus metabolism. It is mainly composed of chief cells and oxyphil cells. Oxyphil cell counts are low in the parathyroid glands of healthy adults but are dramatically increased in patients with uremia and secondary hyperparathyroidism (SHPT). Increased oxyphil cell counts are related to drug treatment resistance, but the origin of oxyphil cells and the mechanism of proliferation remain unknown. Herein, three types of parathyroid nodules (chief cell nodules, oxyphil cell nodules and mixed nodules, respectively) excised from parathyroid glands of uremic SHPT patients were used for single-cell RNA sequencing (scRNA-seq), other molecular biology studies, and transplantation into nude mice. Through scRNA-seq of parathyroid mixed nodules from three patients with uremic SHPT, we established the first transcriptomic map of the human parathyroid and found a chief-to-oxyphil cell transdifferentiation characterized by gradual mitochondrial enrichment associated with the uremic milieu. Notably, the mitochondrial enrichment and cellular proliferation of chief cell and oxyphil cell nodules decreased significantly after leaving the uremic milieu via transplantation into nude mice. Remarkably, the phenotype of oxyphil cell nodules improved significantly in the nude mice as characterized by decreased mitochondrial content and the proportion of oxyphil cells to chief cells. Thus, our study provides a comprehensive single-cell transcriptome atlas of the human parathyroid and elucidates the origin of parathyroid oxyphil cells and their underlying transdifferentiating mechanism. These findings enhance our understanding of parathyroid disease and may open new treatment perspectives for patients with chronic kidney disease.

Kidney International (2024) 105, 562–581; https://doi.org/10.1016/j.kint.2023.11.027

KEYWORDS: cell transdifferentiation; mitochondrion; parathyroid chief cell; parathyroid oxyphil cell; single-cell transcriptomic; uremia

Copyright © 2023, International Society of Nephrology. Published by Elsevier Inc. All rights reserved.

Lay Summary

In patients with uremic secondary hyperparathyroidism (SHPT), increased oxyphil cell counts are related to drug treatment resistance, whereas the origin and proliferation mechanism of oxyphil cells remains unknown. Herein, through single-cell RNA-sequencing analysis and animal study, we found that parathyroid oxyphil cells are derived from chief cells, with mitochondrial enrichment in the uremic milieu as the pathogenic determinant of oxyphil cell transdifferentiation. This finding may stimulate parathyroid research and improve management of patients with SHPT. In addition, these results provide some key clues toward finding more effective therapies for refractory SHPT and have implications for physicians, scientists, and drug developers in the field of SHPT.

The parathyroid gland, which secretes parathyroid hormone (PTH) to increase serum calcium and reduce serum phosphorus levels, is 1 of the main organs that regulate calcium and phosphorus metabolism.[1] Secondary hyperparathyroidism (SHPT), characterized by parathyroid hyperplasia and excessive synthesis and secretion of PTH, is 1 of the most common complications in patients with chronic kidney disease, which can lead to bone metabolism disorders, cardiovascular complications, and increased morbidity and mortality.[2–5] Parathyroid glands of healthy adults are primarily composed of chief cells and few oxyphil cells. However, the parathyroid oxyphil cell content increases dramatically in patients with uremic SHPT, the proportion of which can often exceed 90%.[6–8] Our previous work demonstrated that 84.8% of patients have predominantly oxyphil cells in ≥1 parathyroid glands.[8] Vitamin D receptor (VDR) activators and calcimimetics are the key therapeutic agents in the management of uremic SHPT, but previous studies showed that patients with oxyphil-dominant uremic SHPT are likely

Correspondence: *Jing Chen, Division of Nephrology and National Clinical Research Center for Aging and Medicine, Huashan Hospital, Fudan University, No. 12 Wulumuqi Middle Road, Shanghai 200040, China. E-mail: chenjing1998@fudan.edu.cn*

Received 14 August 2022; revised 28 October 2023; accepted 17 November 2023; published online 21 December 2023

to be refractory to drug treatment.[8–11] These results indicate that oxyphil cell proliferation is the major pathologic process in patients with uremic SHPT and may be a key factor causing treatment failure. Therefore, it is vital to elucidate the origin and proliferation mechanism of oxyphil cells.

The parathyroid gland is composed of 2 major cell types: chief cells and oxyphil cells. Histologically, oxyphil cells are much larger in size than chief cells (12–20 vs. 6–8 μm), and their cytoplasm is more eosinophilic because of a higher mitochondrial content.[7] Oxyphil cells are thought to be derived from chief cells as both express PTH and glial cell missing 2 (GCM2), a parathyroid-specific transcription factor (TF) that is essential for parathyroid cell development.[12,13] The presence of transitional cells that are small, like chief cells, but eosinophilic, like oxyphil cells, provides additional evidence.[7] Another possible mechanism underlying oxyphil cell transdifferentiation was proposed by Müller-Höcker et al., who hypothesized that the defective mitochondrial respiratory chain in chief cells could induce mitochondrial mutations, mitochondrial proliferation could compensate for these mutations, and, consequently, cells could transdifferentiate into oxyphil cells.[14] Although these studies propose chief-to-oxyphil cell transdifferentiation, the origin of oxyphil cells remains unclear because of the lack of conclusive evidence. Single-cell RNA sequencing (scRNA-seq) is an emerging approach that provides transcriptome-wide gene expression information from individual cells.[15] The strongest advantages over traditional bulk sequencing are as follows: (i) the possibility of investigating gene expression patterns for each cell type individually, (ii) the ability to probe heterogeneity within cells of the same type, and (iii) the ability to identify rare cell types within a population.[16,17] Pseudotime analysis is widely used to infer the differentiation trajectory of cell development processes, and it provides a pseudotemporal signature to order cells in developmental time,[18,19] making it suitable for analyzing the origin of oxyphil cells.

In the present study, we conducted scRNA-seq analysis and performed in vitro and in vivo experiments to explore the origin of parathyroid oxyphil cells and elucidate the mechanisms underlying oxyphil cell transdifferentiation as well as to provide a transcriptomic map of parathyroid glands of patients with uremic SHPT.

METHODS
Additional details for all methods are in the Supplementary Methods.

Patients
Parathyroid tissues collected from 20 patients with uremic SHPT were used for scRNA-seq, animal study, and tissue culture in vitro. For details, see the Supplementary Methods.

Tissue culture in vitro
Freshly excised parathyroid chief cell nodules from 3 patients with uremic SHPT were minced and intervened with uremic serum. For details, see the Supplementary Methods.

Animals
Nude BALB/c-nu/nu mice, obtained from Shanghai SLAC Laboratory Animal Co Ltd, were used for transplantation of oxyphil or chief cell nodules. For details, see the Supplementary Methods.

scRNA-seq
Fresh excised parathyroid mixed nodules from 3 patients with uremic SHPT were used for scRNA-seq. For details, see the Supplementary Methods.

RNA sequencing
Chief cell nodules and oxyphil cell nodules pre-transplantation and post-transplantation were collected for RNA sequencing (RNA-seq). For details, see the Supplementary Methods.

Statistical analysis
Data are reported as mean ± SEM. All statistical analyses were performed and graphs were generated in R, version 3.1.0, and GraphPad Prism, version 6.0. $P < 0.05$ was considered statistically significant.

RESULTS
Parathyroid chief cells transdifferentiate into oxyphil cells characterized by gradual mitochondrial enrichment

Characteristics of patients and parathyroid tissues. Table 1 displays the baseline demographic, clinical, and biochemical characteristics of 20 patients with uremic SHPT. Hypercalcemia was noted in 75% of patients, and 85% of patients had hyperphosphatemia. Serum intact PTH, calcium, and phosphorus levels were significantly decreased after surgical therapy. Three pathologic types of parathyroid nodules were identified by hematoxylin and eosin staining among excised parathyroid issues: chief cell nodules (Figure 1a), oxyphil cell nodules (eosinophilic cytoplasm because of a high content of mitochondria) (Figure 1b), and mixed nodules containing both chief and oxyphil cells (Figure 1c). Also, they can be

Table 1 | Clinical and biochemical characteristics of the 20 patients who received PTX with forearm autograft

Characteristic	Value
Age, yr	55 ± 2
Gender, male/female ratio	6:14
HD vintage, mo	138 ± 13
HD frequency, times/wk	3.00 ± 0.00
SpKt/V	1.24 ± 0.04
Pre-PTX serum biochemical indexes	
Corrected Ca, mmol/l	2.67 ± 0.05
Phosphate, mmol/l	2.20 ± 0.13
Intact PTH, pg/ml	1798.00 ± 113.90
Post-PTX serum biochemical indexes	
Corrected Ca, mmol/l	2.11 ± 0.05
Phosphate, mmol/l	1.08 ± 0.08
Intact PTH, pg/ml	37.14 ± 14.80
Parathyroid pathology	
Parathyroid glands, n	3.80 ± 0.12
Maximal parathyroid gland weight, g	2.54 ± 0.73
Total parathyroid gland weight, g	5.02 ± 1.01

Ca, calcium; HD, hemodialysis; PTH, parathyroid hormone; PTX, parathyroidectomy; SpKt/V, single-pool urea clearance index.
Data are given mean ± SEM unless otherwise noted.

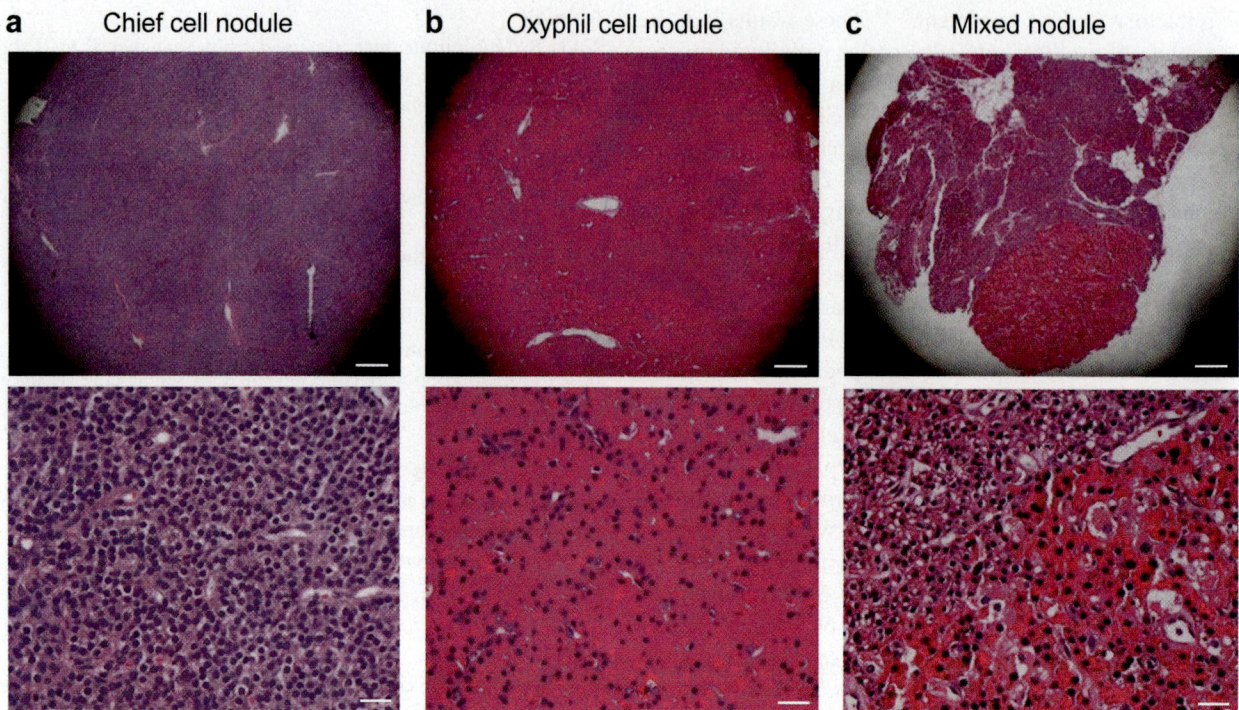

Figure 1 | Pathologic types of excised parathyroid nodules from patients with uremic secondary hyperparathyroidism. Three types of parathyroid nodules were identified by hematoxylin and eosin staining: (a) chief cell nodule, (b) oxyphil cell nodule (eosinophilic cytoplasm because of the high mitochondria content), and (c) mixed nodule containing chief cells and oxyphil cells. Bars = 200 μm (top panels); 20 μm (bottom panels). To optimize viewing of this image, please see the online version of this article at www.kidney-international.org.

identified by the expression of mitochondrial-related indicators and tissue color (Supplementary Figure S1).

Cell diversity in parathyroid cells from patients with uremic SHPT as delineated by single-cell transcriptomic analysis. We set out to obtain single-cell suspensions of parathyroids from 3 patients with uremic SHPT and performed scRNA-seq analysis with a high-throughput droplet-mediated scRNA-seq platform (Figure 2a). Using stringent quality controls, we further analyzed 28,375 cells. Clustering analysis identified 16 distinct cell clusters consisting of as few as 367 cells to as many as 4312 cells per cluster (Figure 2b). To define the identity of each cell cluster, we analyzed cluster-specific marker genes by performing differential gene expression analysis (Figure 2c). In many cases, the unbiased cluster identifier was a known cell type–specific marker, such as *CD68* for macrophages, *COL6A3* for fibroblasts, *CDH5* for endothelial cells, and *CD3E* and *NKG7* for natural killer T cells (Figure 2c and Supplementary Figure S2). Parathyroid-specific factors, namely *PTH* and *GCM2*, were expressed highly in clusters 1, 2, 3, 4, 6, 9, and 13, so these clusters were identified as parathyroid cells.

Trajectory analysis of parathyroid cells. To explore the relationship between chief and oxyphil cells, we used the Monocle 2 toolkit to perform cell trajectory analysis. Figure 3a shows t-distributed stochastic neighbor embedding plots for marker genes (*PTH* and *GCM2*) of parathyroid cells, including clusters 1, 2, 3, 4, 6, 9, and 13. As oxyphil cells were rich in mitochondria, the percentage of mitochondrial transcripts across the 16 main clusters is shown by violin plots (Figure 3b). Furthermore, cluster 1 was divided into 6 subclusters (i.e., subclusters 1-1, 1-2, 1-3, 1-4, 1-5, and 1-6) because of the broad percentage range of mitochondrial transcripts (Figure 3b). Among the clusters of parathyroid cells, clusters 1-4, 1-5, and 9 were likely to be oxyphil cells based on their higher mitochondrial transcript proportion, and clusters 2 and 13 were likely to be chief cells based on their lower mitochondrial transcript proportion, whereas the other clusters may contain chief and oxyphil cells. In addition, oxyphil and chief cell clusters were further identified by comparing the expression of parathyroid function-related genes, which showed lower expression of VDR, calcium-sensing receptor (CASR), and Klotho in oxyphil clusters (1-4, 1-5, and 9) than in chief clusters (2 and 13) (Supplementary Figure S3). The cell trajectory analysis results revealed a differentiation relationship in parathyroid cells (Figure 3c). The mitochondrial transcript proportion in the cell trajectory demonstrated a gradual upward trend (Figure 3d), which suggested that mitochondrial enrichment is the pathogenic determinant of oxyphil cell transdifferentiation. Furthermore, each cluster was displayed separately on the differentiation trajectory to clarify the differentiation relationship. Clusters 2 and 13 were on one end, whereas clusters 1-4, 1-5, and 9 were

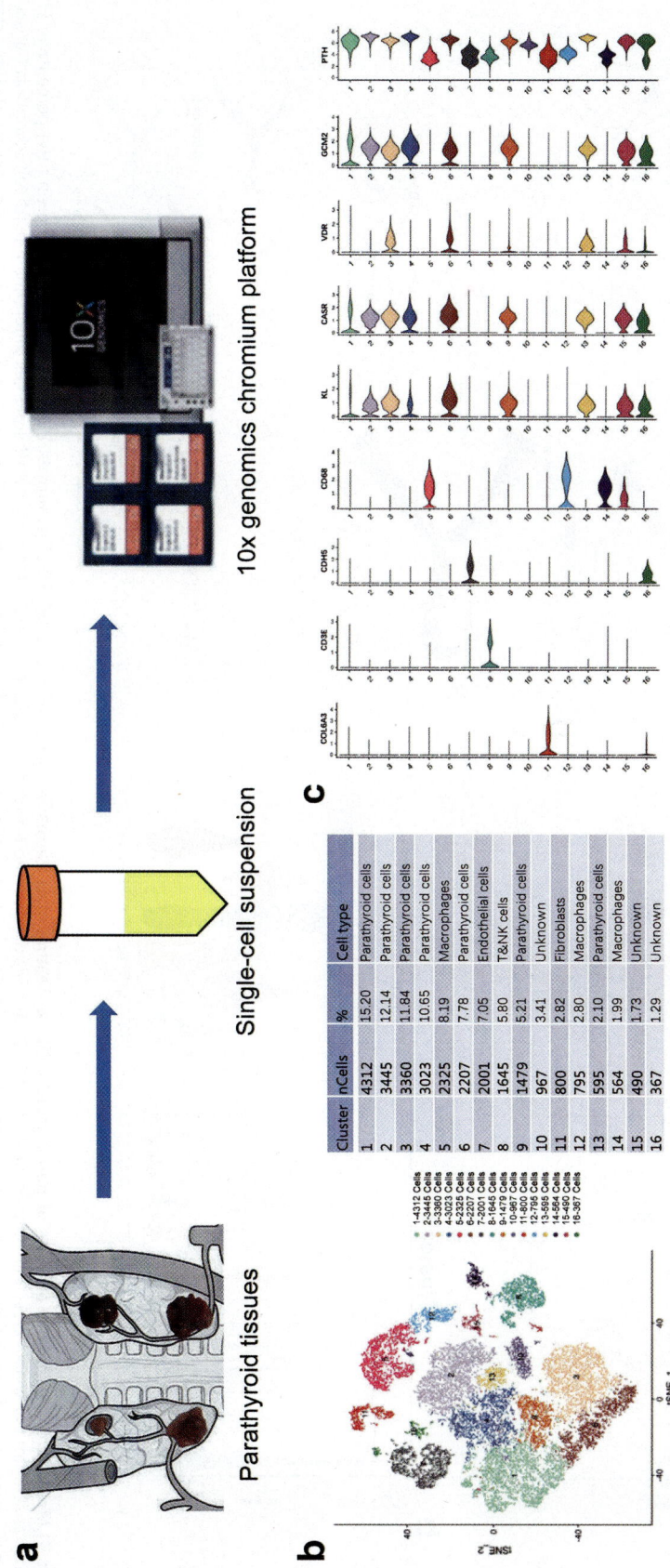

Figure 2 | Cell diversity in parathyroid cells from patients with uremic secondary hyperparathyroidism (SHPT), delineated by single-cell transcriptomic analysis. (a) Overview of the single-cell RNA-sequencing process using parathyroid tissue samples from patients with uremic SHPT. **(b)** Unsupervised clustering demonstrates 16 distinct cell types shown in a t-distributed stochastic neighbor embedding (tSNE) map (left). Percentages of assigned cell types are summarized in the right panel. **(c)** Violin plots showing the expression levels of representative marker genes across the 16 main clusters. The y axis shows the log-scale normalized read count.

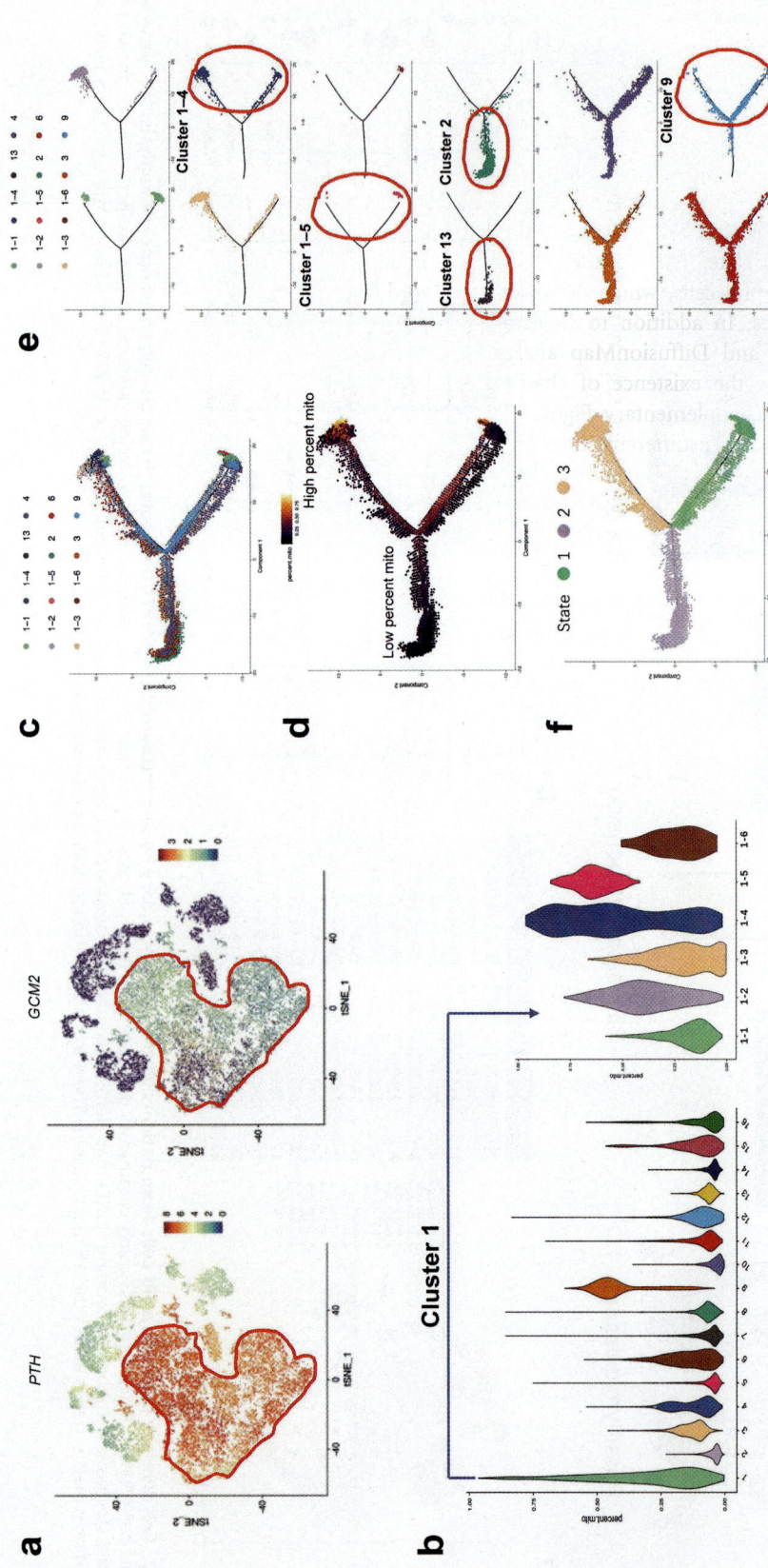

Figure 3 | Monocle cell trajectory analysis of parathyroid cells. (a) Feature plots for marker genes (*PTH* and *GCM2*) of parathyroid cells. (b) Violin plots showing the percentage of mitochondrial (mito) transcript across the 16 main clusters (left). Cluster 1 is divided into 6 subclusters (right). (c) Trajectories for parathyroid cell differentiation. (d) Mitochondrial transcript proportion trajectories of parathyroid cells during differentiation. (e) Cell trajectory map of parathyroid cells, highlighting the contribution of cells coming from each cluster. (f) Three states were identified on the basis of their distribution in the cell trajectory map. Along with trajectory progression, cells experienced 3 states: the starting point of branching (prebranch, state 2) and the 2 other branches (state 1 and state 3). tSNE, t-distributed stochastic neighbor embedding.

on the other end (Figure 3e), which further validated that chief cells and oxyphil cells represent 2 ends of a spectrum of cellular phenotypes and that they may undergo cellular transitions. Considering the pathophysiology background that oxyphil cell content accounts for few in healthy adults but increases dramatically in patients with uremic SHPT,[6–8] we speculated that oxyphil cells were at the late stage and chief cells were at the early stage. As clusters 3, 4, and 6 were distributed on the middle of the differentiation trajectory and closely connected chief and oxyphil cells (Figure 3e), these clusters may be in a transitional state. Therefore, chief cells could transdifferentiate into oxyphil cells, which are associated with mitochondrial changes. In addition to trajectory analysis, RNA velocity analysis and DiffusionMap analysis were also performed to validate the existence of chief-to-oxyphil cell transdifferentiation (Supplementary Figure S4), both of which have confirmed the transdifferentiation direction of parathyroid cells in uremic patients. To further explore the potential mechanisms involved in chief-to-oxyphil cell transdifferentiation, 3 states were identified on the basis of their distribution in the cell trajectory map: the starting point of branching (prebranch, namely state 2) and the 2 other branches (states 1 and 3) (Figure 3f).

Multiple uremia-associated factors participate in chief-to-oxyphil cell transdifferentiation

Evaluation of mitochondrial quality control and metabolic function of parathyroid oxyphil cells. As the chief-to-oxyphil cell transdifferentiation was associated with mitochondrial changes, the mitochondrial characteristics in chief and oxyphil cells were evaluated, such as mitochondrial quality control and metabolic function. The electron microscopy data showed higher mitochondria number and larger mitochondria size in oxyphil cell nodules than chief cell nodules (Figure 4a). The immunohistochemistry and Western blot results demonstrated significant higher expression of mitochondrial biogenesis-related factors (peroxisome proliferator-activated receptor-γ co-activator 1α [PGC1α] and mitochondrial transcription factor A [mtTFA]) (Figure 4b), mitochondrial component-related factors (voltage-dependent anion channel 1 [VDAC1] and mitochondrially encoded cytochrome c oxidase II [MT-CO2]) (Figure 4c), and mitochondrial fusion-related factor optic atrophy 1 (OPA1; Figure 4d) in oxyphil cell nodules. Chief and oxyphil cells were sorted by flow cytometry (Figure 5a) and further validated by hematoxylin and eosin staining (Figure 5b). Subsequently, the oxidative respiration function of mitochondria was evaluated using a Seahorse cell energy metabolism analyzer and showed no significant difference in basal respiration and adenosine triphosphate production-dependent respiration between single chief cell and single oxyphil cell (Figure 5c). Considering the higher mitochondria number in oxyphil cells, it is speculated that the activity of single mitochondria is lower in oxyphil cells. Therefore, compared with chief cells, the mitochondria of oxyphil cells demonstrated many changes, which were manifested in increased mitochondrial biogenesis, components, and fusion, and decreased metabolic function.

Specific transcription factors involved in parathyroid cell differentiation, as determined by SCENIC analysis. To investigate the TFs involved in parathyroid cell differentiation, SCENIC analysis was conducted for TF network inference. The TFs enriched in parathyroid cells were clustered into 4 modules by correlation analysis (Figure 6a). Module 1 is enhanced in states 1 and 3 rather than state 2 (Figure 6b), indicating regulons of module 1 might play an important role in the chief-to-oxyphil cell transdifferentiation. The regulons of module 1 contained *MAFB*, *ATF3*, *FOSB*, *MAFF*, *CEBPD*, *JUND*, *CEBPG*, *DDIT3*, *CEBPB*, *CREM*, *EGR2*, *JUNB*, and *KLF2* (Figure 6a). To clarify the specific TFs driving the chief-to-oxyphil cell transdifferentiation, the regulon activities were analyzed in 3 states (Figure 6c). The regulon activities of *CEBPD*, *JUND*, and *MAFB* were upregulated, whereas the activities of *DDIT3*, *FOSB*, *KLF2*, *JUNB*, and *ATF3* were downregulated, in states 1 and 3 rather than state 2 (Figure 6d), indicating these regulons might participate in the chief-to-oxyphil cell transdifferentiation. More important, these TFs belonged to module 1, which further confirmed the credibility of the results. In addition, the expression profiles of parathyroid function-related genes showed different expression abundance in parathyroid cell clusters (Figure 6e); whether it is related to regulon activities of TFs is worth further research.

KEGG pathway enrichment analysis in parathyroid transcriptomics. To better investigate the underlying molecular mechanisms driving the chief-to-oxyphil cell transdifferentiation, Kyoto Encyclopedia of Genes and Genomes (KEGG) pathway enrichment analysis was performed in parathyroid transcriptomics. In scRNA-seq, differentially expressed genes (DEGs) were displayed in the pseudotime heat map, and KEGG pathway enrichment analysis of DEGs upregulated in states 1 and 3 was performed (Figure 7a). Moreover, we performed KEGG analysis of upregulated DEGs in oxyphil cell nodules using our published RNA-seq data (Figure 7b). Here, 43 pathways in total and 17 common pathways were identified using transcriptomics (Figure 7c). They are listed in Figure 7d[20–36] and could be summarized into the following categories: immunity and inflammation, lipid and energy metabolism, mineral metabolism disorder, endocrine metabolic disorder, kinase signal transduction, cell growth, development and death, and cell adhesion and junction. As most of these pathways are related to the uremic milieu and mitochondrial biogenesis, it was postulated that multiple uremia-associated signaling pathways promote the mitochondria biogenesis of chief cells, resulting in transformation into oxyphil cells. In addition, 2012 DEGs between oxyphil (1-4, 1-5, and 9) and chief clusters (2 and 13) in scRNA-seq and 2686 DEGs between oxyphil and chief nodules in our published RNA-seq were identified, of which 369 DEGs were in common (Supplementary Figure S5A, D, and G). KEGG pathway enrichment analysis of DEGs in scRNA-seq and RNA-seq showed many common pathways, and

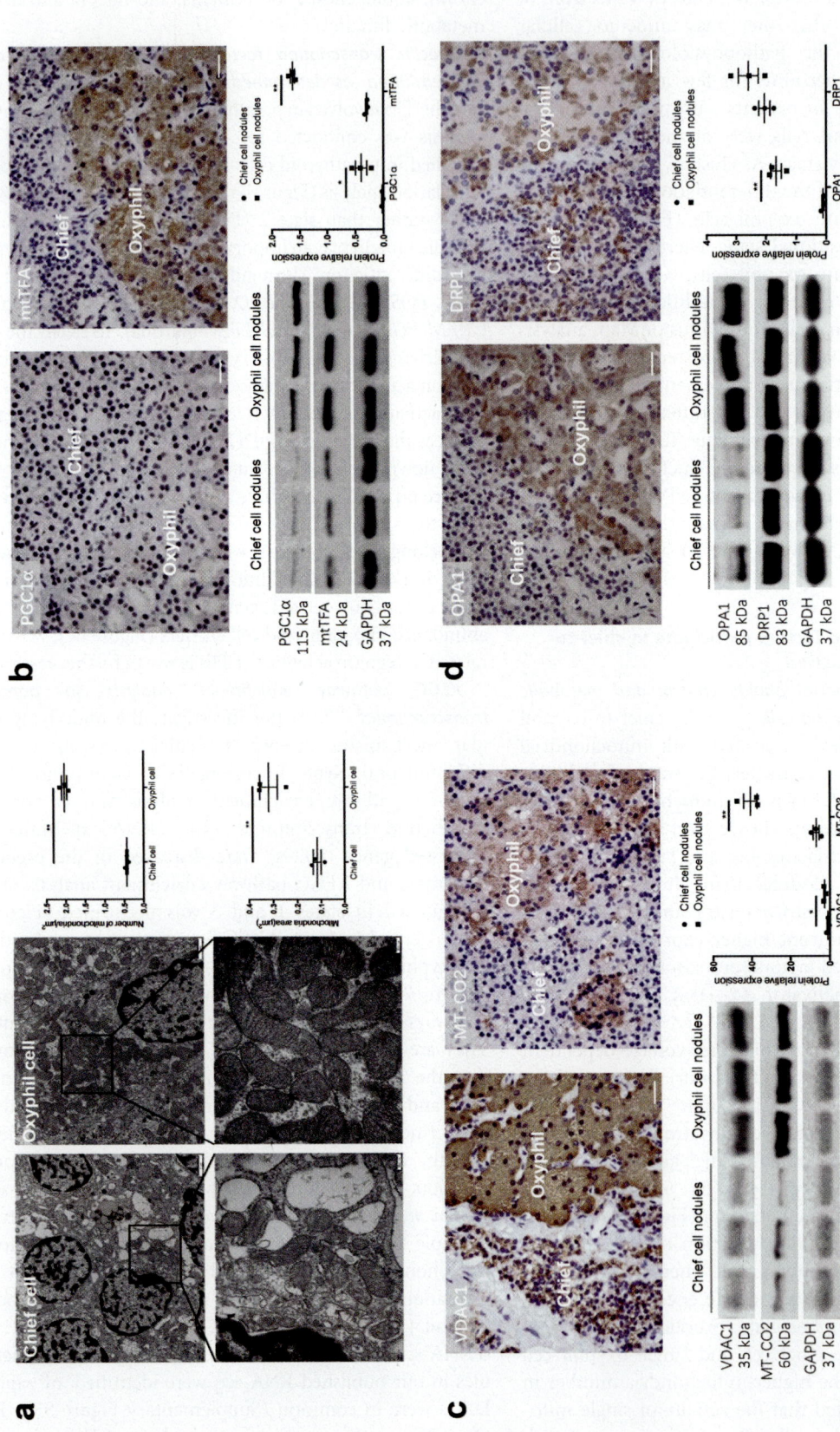

Figure 4 | Increased mitochondrial biogenesis, components, and fusion in oxyphil cell nodules. (a) Representative electron microscopy images of chief and oxyphil cell nodules. The mitochondria were counted and normalized to the area. Bar = 1 μm (top panel); 0.2 μm (bottom panels). **(b–d)** Immunohistochemistry and Western blot showing the expression of **(b)** mitochondrial biogenesis-related factors (peroxisome proliferator-activated receptor-γ co-activator 1α [PGC1α] and mitochondrial transcription factor A [mtTFA]), **(c)** mitochondrial component-related factors (voltage-dependent anion channel 1 [VDAC1] and mitochondrially encoded cytochrome c oxidase II [MT-CO2]), and **(d)** the mitochondrial fusion-related factor optic atrophy 1 (OPA1) and the mitochondrial fission-related factor dynamin-related protein 1 (DRP1) in chief and oxyphil cell nodules. Values are mean ± SEM. $*P < 0.05$, $**P < 0.01$ versus the chief cell group. Bars = 20 μm. GAPDH, glyceraldehyde-3-phosphate dehydrogenase. To optimize viewing of this image, please see the online version of this article at www.kidney-international.org.

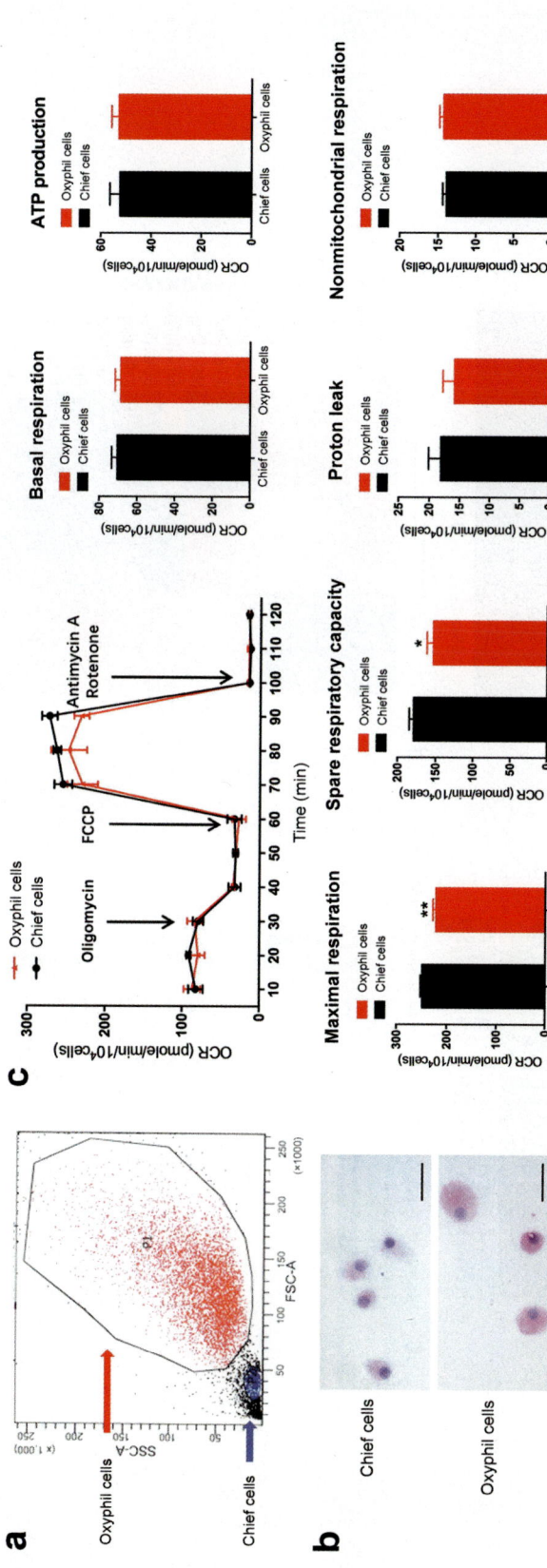

Figure 5 | Mitochondrial respiration in chief and oxyphil cells sorted by flow cytometry. (a) Chief and oxyphil cells were sorted by flow cytometry and (b) further validated by hematoxylin and eosin staining. Oxyphil cells are characterized by large size and eosinophilic staining compared with chief cells. Bars = 20 μm. (c) Oxygen consumption rate (OCR) and quantification of metabolic parameters by Seahorse in chief and oxyphil cells. Values are mean ± SEM. *$P < 0.05$, **$P < 0.01$ versus the chief cell group. ATP, adenosine triphosphate; FCCP, p-trifluoromethoxy carbonyl cyanide phenylhydrazone; FSC, forward scatter; SSC, side scatter.

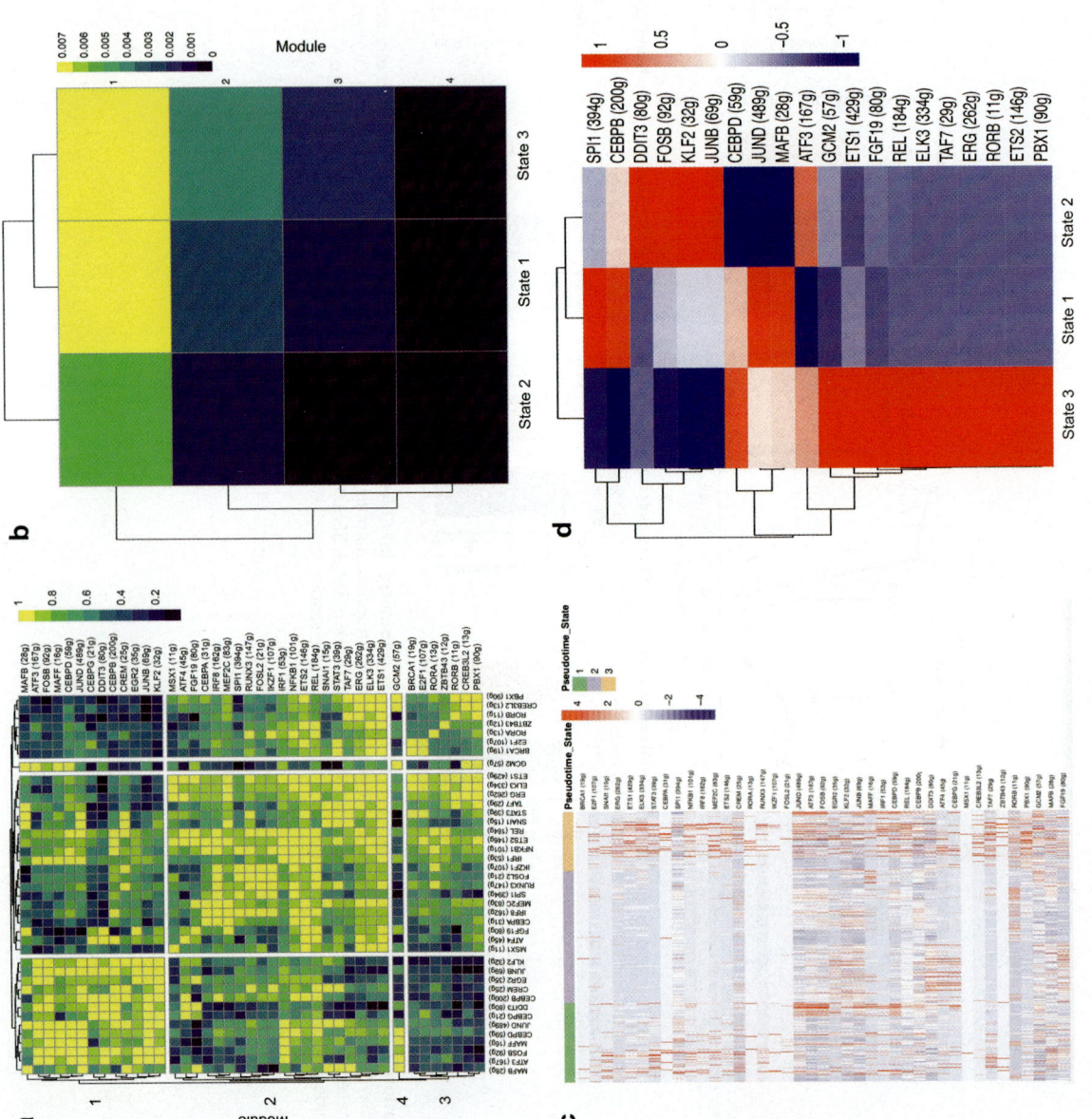

Figure 6 | Specific transcription factors (TFs) involved in parathyroid cell differentiation, as determined by SCENIC analysis. (a) The connection specificity index (CSI) correlation clustering heat map of regulon modules. The rows and columns represent regulons. The color changes from blue to yellow indicate the CSI correlation value changes from low to high. Regulons with high CSI values may have similar cellular functions and jointly regulate downstream genes. (b) Activity heat map of CSI-related modules in 3 states. Rows represent CSI modules manually divided according to the CSI clustering heat map, and columns represent different states. The color changes from blue to yellow indicate the activity of CSI module changes from low to high. The states corresponding to CSI modules with similar activities may have similar gene expression patterns and similar regulatory networks. (c) Heat map of regulon activity analyzed by SCENIC with default thresholds for binarization. The term "regulon" refers to a regulatory network of TFs and their target genes. (d) The heat map displays the average regulon activities of TFs in different states. The color changes from blue to red indicate the relative expression levels changes from low to high. Numbers between parentheses indicate the (extended) regulons for respective TFs. (Continued)

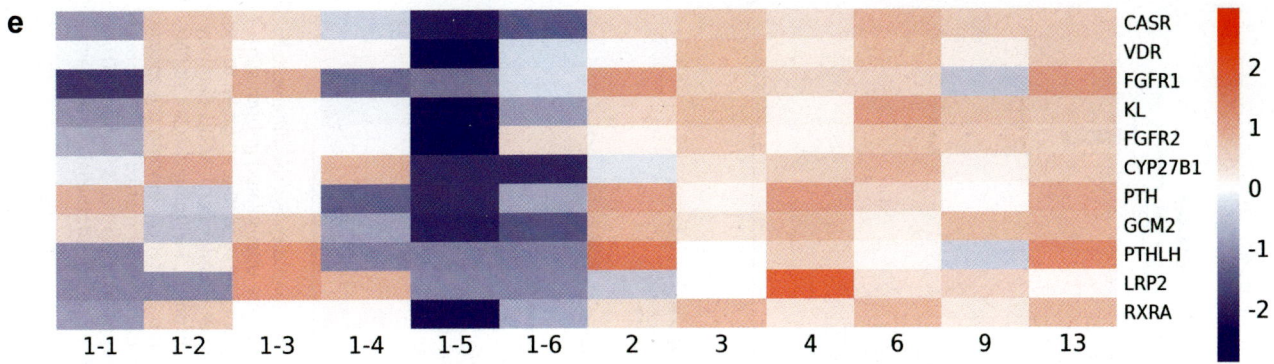

Figure 6 | (Continued) (**e**) Heat maps of parathyroid function-related genes in parathyroid cell clusters.

most of the significant enriched pathways of upregulated DEGs in oxyphil clusters or oxyphil nodules can also be seen in Figure 7d (Supplementary Figure S5), which further support the correlation between the uremic milieu and chief-to-oxyphil cell transdifferentiation. The *in vitro* study results of increased mitochondrial biogenesis and components in chief cell nodules after uremic serum treatment (Supplementary Figure S6) provide additional evidence.

Mitochondrial enrichment and cell proliferation of oxyphil cells improved significantly after transplantation into nude mice

Changes of serum biochemical indexes in nude mice pre-transplantation and post-transplantation. To clarify the role of uremic milieu in the chief-to-oxyphil cell transdifferentiation, a study of nude mice was performed. Figure 8a shows the transplantation workflow. After transplantation, the serum calcium concentration was significantly increased and showed no significant difference between the chief and oxyphil cell nodule transplantation groups (Figure 8b). The serum phosphorus concentration was decreased at 2 months post-transplantation, and it showed a significant difference between the chief and oxyphil cell nodule transplantation groups at 3 months (Figure 8c). The human intact PTH serum level in nude mice was significantly upregulated post-transplantation and was higher in the chief cell nodule transplantation group (Figure 8d) but was higher in the oxyphil cell nodule transplantation group after being normalized by total protein content of transplanted glands (Supplementary Figure S7). The mouse intact PTH serum level showed no significant changes post-transplantation (Figure 8e), but its change trend at different time points can be explained by the change trend of serum calcium and phosphorus levels.

Cell growth and death in parathyroid nodules pre-transplantation and post-transplantation. Hematoxylin and eosin staining showed no significant histologic change in oxyphil and chief cell nodules pre-transplantation and post-transplantation (Figure 9a). Immunohistochemical results revealed that PTH was positively expressed in the oxyphil and chief cell nodules post-transplantation, like pre-transplantation (Figure 9b), which confirmed that resected heterografts were human parathyroid tissues. Terminal deoxynucleotidyl transferase–mediated dUTP nick end-labeling staining showed no obvious apoptosis in parathyroid nodules pre-transplantation and post-transplantation (Figure 9c). The immunohistochemistry (Figure 9d) and Western blot (Figure 9e) results showed significant decreased expression of proliferating cell nuclear antigen in nodules post-transplantation, indicating reduced proliferation ability of both oxyphil and chief cells after transplantation into nonuremic nude mice.

Decreased mitochondrial biogenesis, components, and fusion in oxyphil cell nodules after transplantation into nude mice. Mitochondrial changes of oxyphil cell nodules were further detected after transplantation into nude mice. The electron microscopy data showed smaller mitochondria size in oxyphil cell nodules post-transplantation (Figure 10a). The Western blot results showed significant decreased expression of mtTFA in oxyphil and chief cell nodules post-transplantation (Figure 10b). Moreover, the expression of VDAC1 and MT-CO2 was significantly downregulated in oxyphil and chief cell nodules post-transplantation (Figure 10c). In addition, the expression of OPA1 was significantly decreased in oxyphil cell nodules post-transplantation (Figure 10d). Collectively, these results indicated decreased mitochondrial biogenesis, components, and fusion in oxyphil cell nodules after transplantation into nonuremic nude mice.

Amelioration of phenotype in oxyphil cell nodules after transplantation into nude mice. Chief cell nodules and oxyphil cell nodules pre-transplantation and post-transplantation were collected for RNA-seq to confirm the phenotype amelioration in the nonuremic milieu. DEGs were displayed in heat maps (Figure 11a, d, and g), and KEGG pathway enrichment analysis was performed. Most of the significant enriched pathways were also displayed in Figure 7d. KEGG analysis of upregulated DEGs (pre-transplantation oxyphil vs. pre-transplantation chief) showed that "oxidative phosphorylation," "glycine, serine, and threonine metabolism," "Fc γ R-mediated phagocytosis," "intestinal immune network for

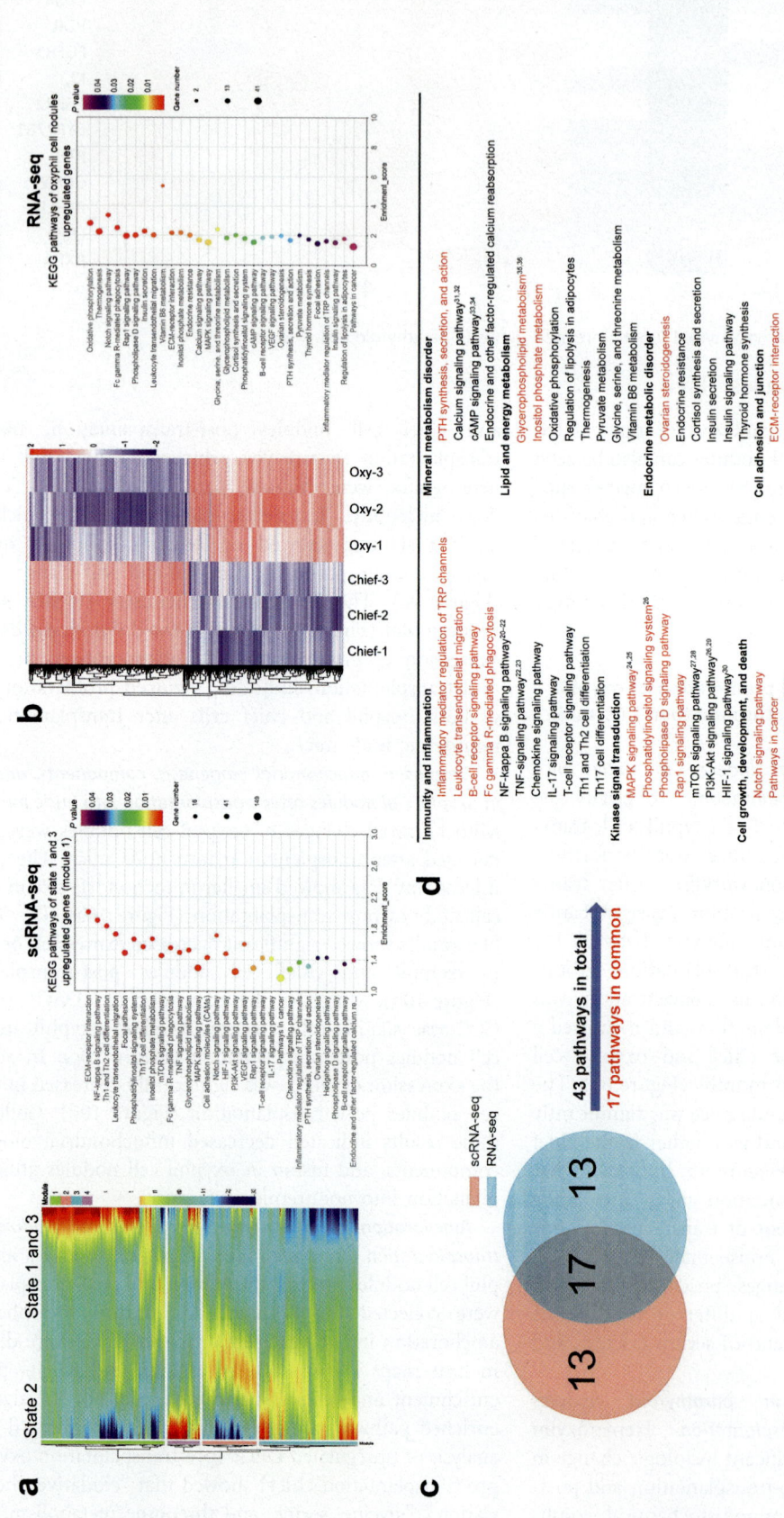

Figure 7 | Kyoto Encyclopedia of Genes and Genomes (KEGG) pathway enrichment analysis in parathyroid transcriptomics. (a) The pseudotime heat map displays the differentially expressed genes (DEGs) during the progression of oxyphil cell transdifferentiation (left). KEGG pathway enrichment analysis of DEGs in module 1, which were upregulated in both state 1 and state 3 (right). The x axis represents the enrichment score; the larger the bubble, the greater the enrichment score; the smaller the enrichment P value, the greater the significance. (b) Heat map of RNA-sequencing (RNA-seq) analysis between chief and oxyphil cell nodules (left). KEGG pathway enrichment analysis of DEGs upregulated in oxyphil cell nodules (right). (c) Venn diagram showing the number of common KEGG pathways in transcriptomics, including single-cell RNA-sequencing (scRNA-seq) and RNA-seq data. (d) A list of total KEGG pathways in transcriptomics; 17 common pathways of transcriptomics are marked in red; references binding the specific pathways to the uremic environment and mitochondrial biogenesis are listed.[20–36] Akt, protein kinase B; cAMP, cyclic adenosine monophosphate; ECM, extracellular matrix; HIF-1, hypoxia-inducible factor 1; IL, interleukin; MAPK, mitogen-activated protein kinase; mTOR, mammalian target of rapamycin; NF-κB, nuclear factor-κB; PI3K, phosphatidylinositol-3′-kinase; PTH, parathyroid hormone; Th1, T helper cell 1; Th2, T helper cell 2; Th17, T helper cell 17; TNF, tumor necrosis factor; TRP, transient receptor potential; VEGF, vascular endothelial growth factor.

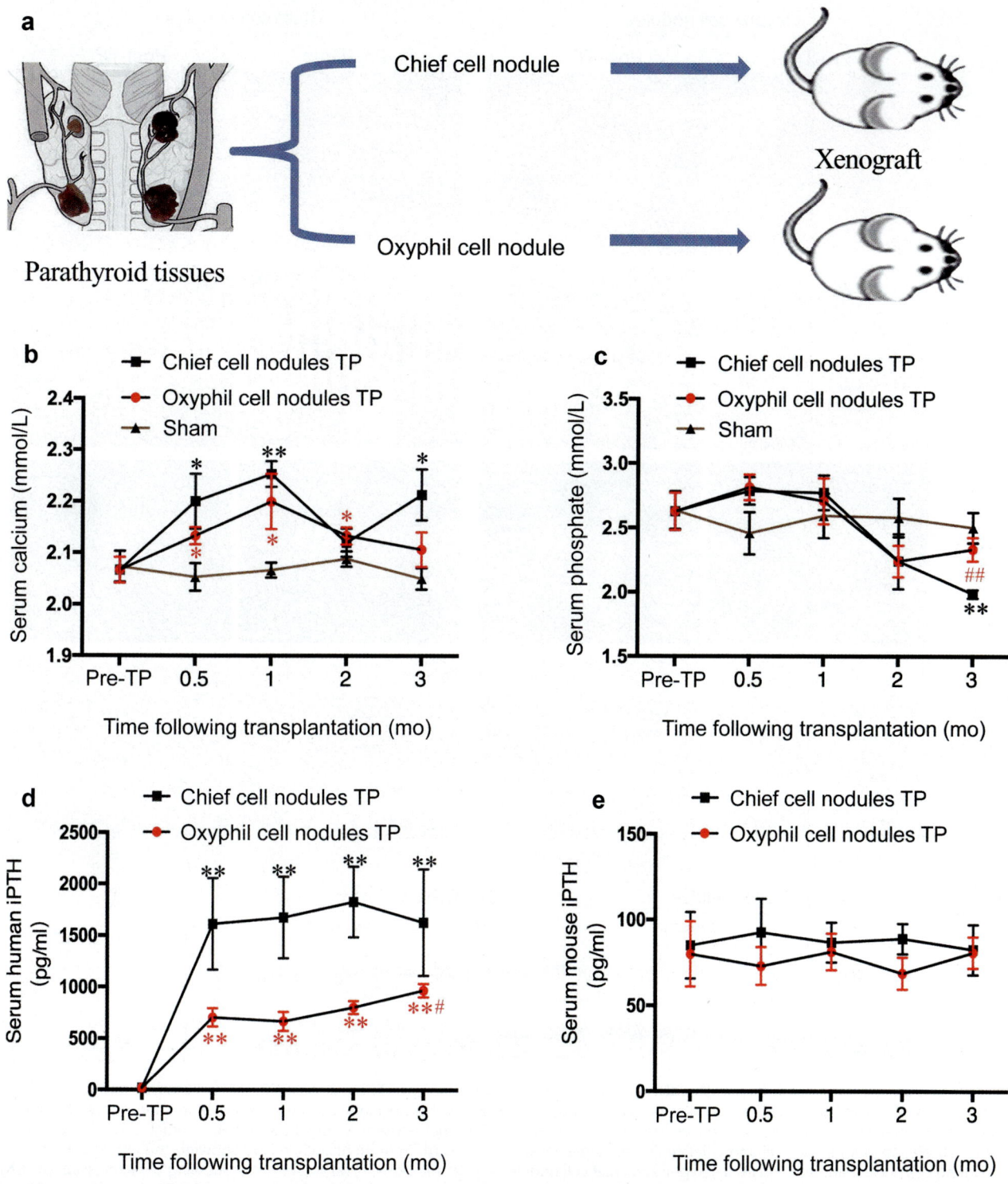

Figure 8 | Changes of serum biochemical indexes in nude mice pre-transplantation (pre-TP) and post-TP. (**a**) Overview of parathyroid nodules from patients with uremic secondary hyperparathyroidism, transplanted into nude mice. (**b**) Serum calcium concentrations at various times following sham surgery and transplantation of the chief and oxyphil cell nodules. (**c**) Serum phosphate concentrations at various times following sham surgery and transplantation of the chief and oxyphil cell nodules. (**d**) Serum human intact parathyroid hormone (iPTH) concentrations at various times following transplantation of the chief and oxyphil cell nodules. (**e**) Serum mouse iPTH concentrations at various times following transplantation of the chief and oxyphil cell nodules. Values are mean ± SEM. *$P < 0.05$, **$P < 0.01$ versus the pre-TP group. #$P < 0.05$, ##$P < 0.01$ versus the chief cell group at the same time point. n = 6 in each group.

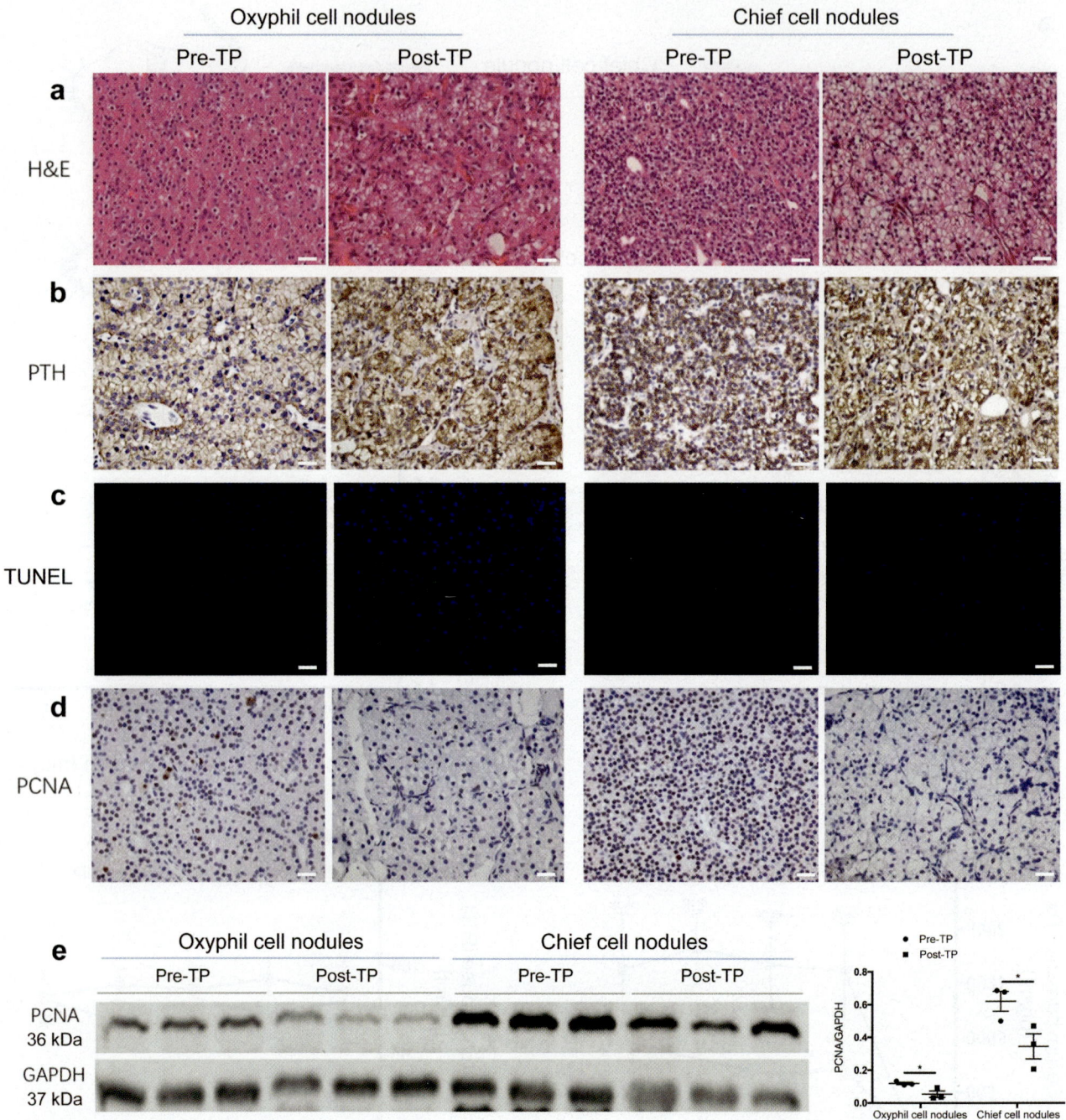

Figure 9 | Cell growth and death in parathyroid nodules pre-transplantation (pre-TP) and post-TP. (**a**) Hematoxylin and eosin (H&E) staining results of oxyphil and chief cell nodules pre-TP and post-TP. (**b**) Immunohistochemistry showing the expression of parathyroid hormone (PTH) in oxyphil and chief cell nodules pre-TP and post-TP. (**c**) Terminal deoxynucleotidyl transferase–mediated dUTP nick end-labeling (TUNEL) staining of oxyphil and chief cell nodules pre-TP and post-TP. (**d**) Immunohistochemistry showing the expression of proliferating cell nuclear antigen (PCNA) in oxyphil and chief cell nodules pre-TP and post-TP. (**e**) Western blot showing the expression of PCNA in oxyphil and chief cell nodules pre-TP and post-TP. Values are mean ± SEM. *$P < 0.05$, **$P < 0.01$ versus the pre-TP group. Bars = 20 μm. GAPDH, glyceraldehyde-3-phosphate dehydrogenase. To optimize viewing of this image, please see the online version of this article at www.kidney-international.org.

IgA production," and "cell adhesion molecules" exhibited significant differences (Figure 11b), and these pathways also exhibited significant differences in KEGG analysis of downregulated DEGs (post-transplantation chief vs. pre-transplantation chief and post-transplantation oxyphil vs. pre-transplantation oxyphil) (Figure 11e and h), indicating

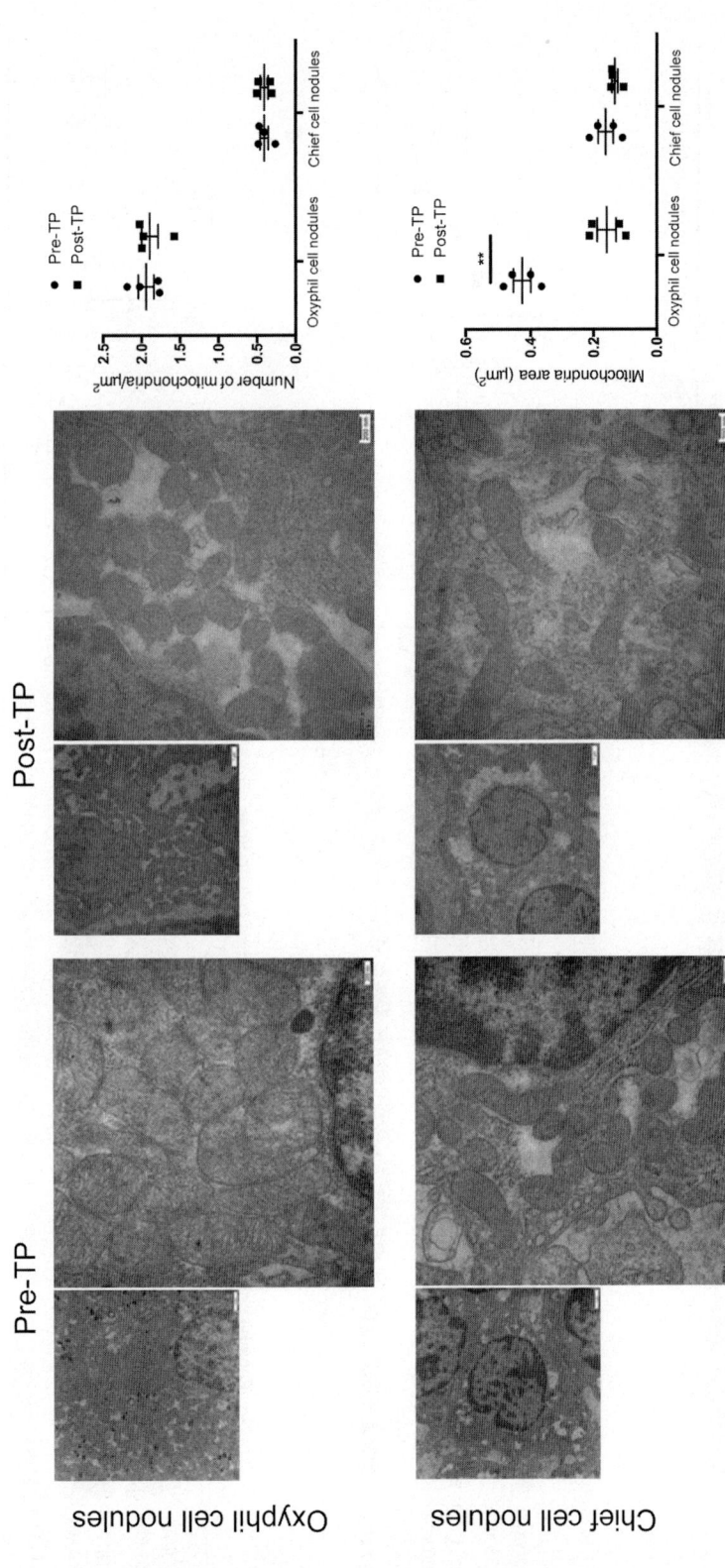

Figure 10 | Decreased mitochondrial biogenesis, components, and fusion in oxyphil cell nodules after transplantation (TP) into nude mice. (a) Representative electron microscopy images of oxyphil and chief cell nodules pre-TP and post-TP. The mitochondria were counted and normalized to the area. Bar = 1 μm (left panels); 0.2 μm (right panels). (Continued)

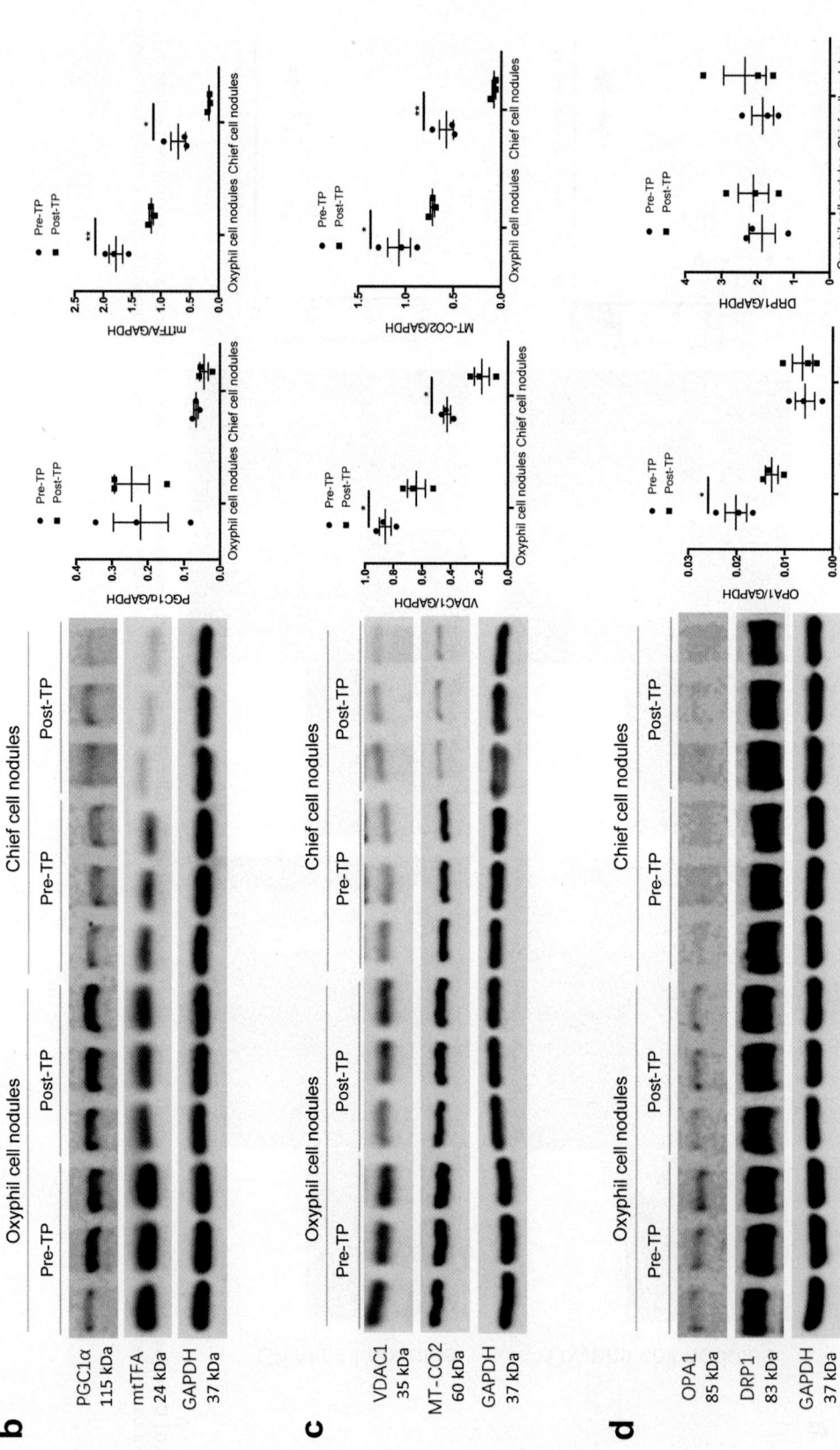

Figure 10 | (Continued) (b–d) Western blot showing the expression of (b) mitochondrial biogenesis-related factors (peroxisome proliferator-activated receptor-γ co-activator 1α [PGC1α] and mitochondrial transcription factor A [mtTFA]), (c) mitochondrial component-related factors (voltage-dependent anion channel 1 [VDAC1] and mitochondrially encoded cytochrome c oxidase II [MT-CO2]), and (d) the mitochondrial fusion-related factor optic atrophy 1 (OPA1) and the mitochondrial fission-related factor dynamin-related protein 1 (DRP1) in oxyphil and chief cell nodules pre-TP and post-TP. Values are mean ± SEM. *$P < 0.05$, **$P < 0.01$ versus the pre-TP group. GAPDH, glyceraldehyde-3-phosphate dehydrogenase. To optimize viewing of this image, please see the online version of this article at www.kidney-international.org.

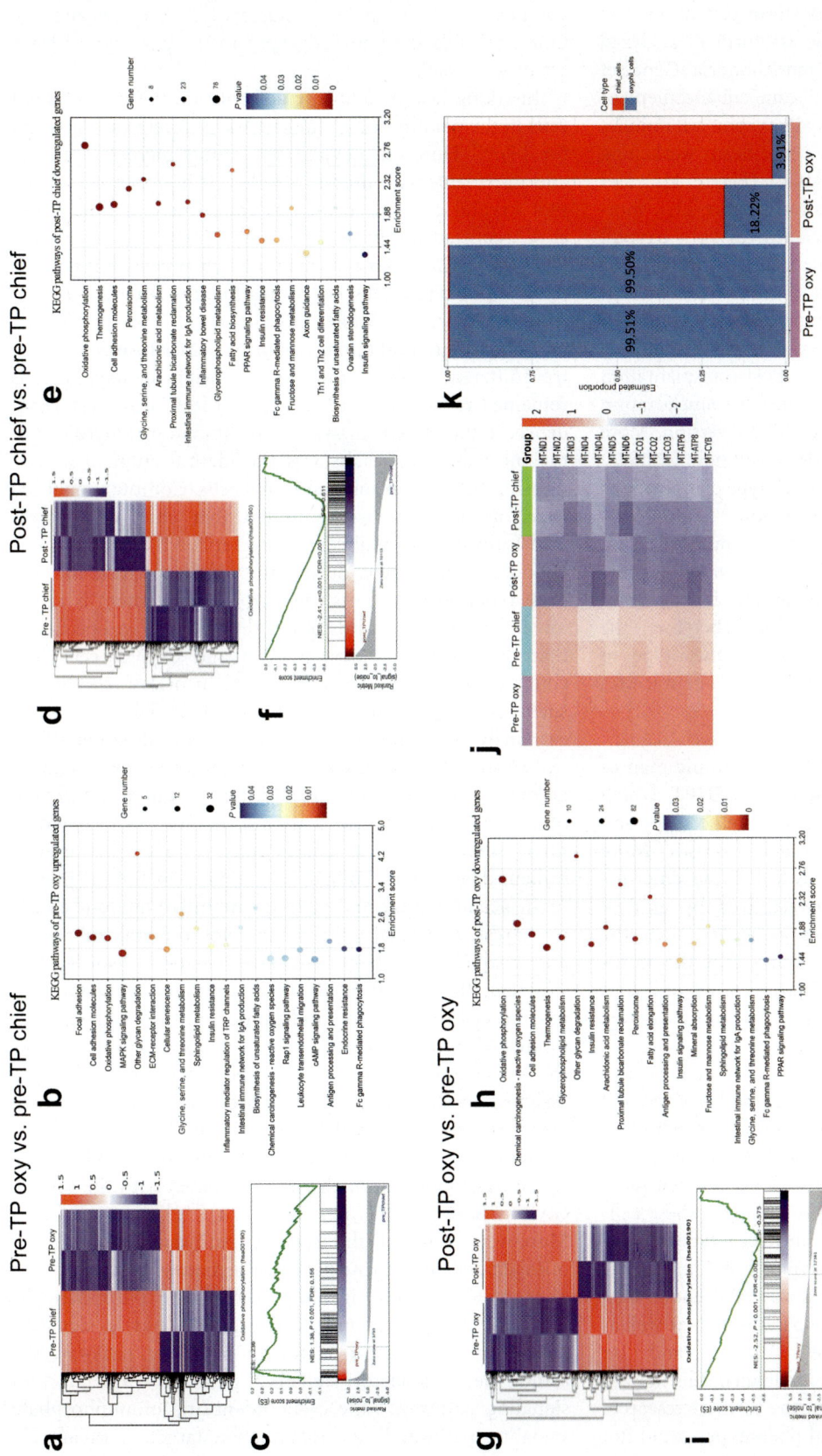

Figure 11 | Transcriptomic analysis of oxyphil and chief cell nodules pre-transplantation (pre-TP) and post-TP in RNA sequencing. (a) Heat map of differentially expressed genes (DEGs) between oxyphil cell nodules pre-TP (pre-TP oxy) and chief cell nodules pre-TP (pre-TP chief). (b) Kyoto Encyclopedia of Genes and Genomes (KEGG) pathway enrichment analysis of DEGs upregulated in pre-TP oxy. (c) Gene set enrichment analysis (GSEA) of oxidative phosphorylation pathway in pre-TP oxy versus pre-TP chief. (d) Heat map of DEGs between chief cell nodules post-TP (post-TP chief) and pre-TP chief. (e) KEGG pathway enrichment analysis of DEGs downregulated in post-TP chief versus pre-TP chief. (f) GSEA of oxidative phosphorylation pathway in post-TP chief versus pre-TP chief. (g) Heat map of DEGs between oxyphil cell nodules post-TP (post-TP oxy) and pre-TP oxy. (h) KEGG pathway enrichment analysis of DEGs downregulated in post-TP oxy. (i) GSEA of oxidative phosphorylation pathway in post-TP oxy versus pre-TP oxy. (j) Heat maps of 13 mitochondrial genes in pre-TP oxy, pre-TP chief, post-TP oxy, and post-TP chief. (k) Multi-subject single-cell deconvolution (MuSiC) to calculate the cell type compositions in oxyphil nodules pre-TP and post-TP. Two independent experiments were sequenced for each group. Genes with a threshold q value < 0.05 and $|\log_2$ (fold change)$| > 1$ between 2 groups were defined as DEGs. cAMP, cyclic adenosine monophosphate; ECM, extracellular matrix; MAPK, mitogen-activated protein kinase; PPAR, peroxisome proliferator–activated receptor; Th1, T helper cell 1; Th2, T helper cell 2; TRP, transient receptor potential.

decreased metabolism ability and immune inflammation of both oxyphil and chief cell nodules post-transplantation. The oxidative phosphorylation pathway is further analyzed because of its important function in mitochondria. Gene set enrichment analysis displayed a significant enhancement of the oxidative phosphorylation pathway in oxyphil cell nodules pre-transplantation (Figure 11c) but a significant weakening in chief cell nodules post-transplantation (Figure 11f) and oxyphil cell nodules post-transplantation (Figure 11i), indicating decreased mitochondria metabolism of both oxyphil and chief cell nodules post-transplantation. Heat maps of 13 mitochondrial genes showed that mitochondrial content was higher in oxyphil cell nodules compared with chief cell nodules pre-transplantation, but decreased significantly in both oxyphil and chief cell nodules post-transplantation (Figure 11j), which furthermore confirmed the amelioration of uremic condition-induced chief-oxyphil conversion. More than that, multi-subject single-cell deconvolution (MuSiC) analysis was performed to calculate the cell type compositions in oxyphil nodules pre-transplantation and post-transplantation, and it clearly showed the proportion of oxyphil cells decreased significantly in oxyphil nodules post-transplantation (Figure 11k), indicating the reduction of oxyphil cells in the nonuremic condition. Therefore, the above data confirmed the amelioration of phenotype in oxyphil cell nodules after transplantation into nude mice.

DISCUSSION

The present study provides the first transcriptomic map of parathyroid cells from patients with uremic SHPT, which improves our understanding of parathyroid cell biology and the relationship between cell types and diseases. More important, our current work first revealed the chief-to-oxyphil cell transdifferentiation characterized by gradual mitochondrial enrichment, which is associated with the uremic milieu. In addition, it was found that the mitochondrial enrichment and cell proliferation of oxyphil cells improved significantly after transplantation into nonuremic nude mice.

Over the past century, it became known that the parathyroid is composed mainly of chief cells and few oxyphil cells.[6] Here, we provide a molecular definition of cell types in human parathyroid obtained by scRNA-seq of 28,375 cells. At this resolution, we distinguished 6 major cell types defined by quantitative gene expression analysis; these cells included almost all previously described cell types (parathyroid cells, including chief and oxyphil cells) and newly described cell types (macrophages, fibroblasts, endothelial cells, and natural killer T cells) in the parathyroid, as well as additional undefined cells (clusters 10, 15, and 16; Figure 2b). It is speculated that these undefined cells may be some new cell types and are worth further research. Although all cell types, subtypes, and phenotypes could not possibly be described here in full, some key observations emerged. Parathyroid cells were more complex and heterogeneous than hitherto appreciated. They were composed of 7 subtypes (i.e., clusters 1, 2, 3, 4, 6, 9, and 13). Our work fills the knowledge gap in the parathyroid transcriptomic map.

In young healthy adults, chief cells are the predominant cells in the parathyroid gland, and oxyphil cells only account for 1%.[6–8] However, oxyphil cell counts increase with age and in patients with uremic SHPT.[6,8] It has been postulated that oxyphil cells are formed by transdifferentiation. Ritter et al. reported the presence of transitional cells expressing PTH and GCM2 that are small, like chief cells, but eosinophilic, like oxyphil cells, suggesting that the latter are derived from chief cells.[7] Müller-Höcker et al. speculated that mitochondrial mutations promote chief-to-oxyphil cell transdifferentiation.[14] However, the origin of oxyphil cells remained to be clarified because of a lack of powerful evidence. In the present analysis of the human parathyroid, 1 of the most striking results was the identification of a relationship between oxyphil and chief cells. Computational cell trajectory analysis first indicated that chief cells might transform into oxyphil cells characterized by gradual mitochondrial enrichment during the process, which has not been reported before. As the oxyphil cell content is rather low in parathyroid glands of healthy humans, we speculated that the transition between chief and oxyphil cells is a constitutive process that is activated in disease conditions, such as uremia, and mitochondrial enrichment is an extremely essential step in oxyphil cell transdifferentiation.

Chronic kidney disease is characterized by reduced glomerular filtration rate, resulting in serum accumulation of toxic substances, called uremic toxins.[37] The environment containing these compounds is called the uremic milieu. The uremic milieu is complex, including uremic toxin accumulation and subsequent inflammation, oxidative stress, abnormal lipid metabolism, mineral imbalance, and water electrolyte acid-base balance disorder.[38–40] Whether the complicated uremic milieu contributes to oxyphil cell proliferation and mitochondrial enrichment is unknown. Our present transcriptomics pathway analysis showed that the pathways enriched in oxyphil cells were assigned to the following categories: mineral metabolism disorder, immunity and inflammation, lipid and energy metabolism, endocrine metabolic disorder, and kinase signal transduction, which were associated with the uremic environment (details in Figure 7d).[20,21,23,24,27,29–31,33,35] Moreover, most of the specific pathways, such as the mitogen-activated protein kinase signaling pathway,[25] the phosphatidylinositol signaling system, the phosphatidylinositol-3′-kinase/protein kinase B (Akt) signaling pathway,[26] the nuclear factor-κB signaling pathway, the tumor necrosis factor signaling pathway,[22] the calcium signaling pathway,[32] the cyclic adenosine monophosphate signaling pathway,[34] the mammalian target of rapamycin signaling pathway,[28] and glycerophospholipid metabolism,[36] have been reported to participate in mitochondrial biogenesis. In addition to the pathways related to the uremic milieu, the *in vitro* study further proved that uremic serum contributed to mitochondrial enrichment. Previous publications reported no such obvious amplification of oxyphil cells in primary hyperparathyroidism because only 11% of nodules were composed of oxyphil cells.[9,41] The aggressive proliferation of parathyroid oxyphil cells is unique to uremic SHPT and participates in drug treatment resistance, which is not associated with primary hyperparathyroidism or aging. Therefore, the chief-to-oxyphil cell transdifferentiation may be the result of multiple factors in the uremic environment.

As an immune-deficient animal model, nude mice are ideal xenotransplantation recipients.[42] To elucidate the role of uremic milieu in chief-to-oxyphil cell transdifferentiation, parathyroid oxyphil cell nodules from patients with uremic SHPT were transplanted into nude mice. Interestingly, our mouse study revealed that not only the mitochondrial content but also the cell proliferation ability of oxyphil cells decreased significantly after leaving the uremic milieu, which further confirmed that the uremic milieu promotes mitochondrial biogenesis in chief cells, stimulating transdifferentiation into oxyphil cells. In addition, oxyphil cell nodules showed higher PTH secretion levels than chief cell nodules in nude mice, which is consistent with our previous *in vitro* research results,[43] suggesting that oxyphil cells contribute to the pathophysiology of uremic SHPT and should be regarded as an independent treatment target. Therefore, these results further proved that the transdifferentiation and proliferation of oxyphil cells may be a special phenomenon in the uremic environment, which participates in the continuous progression of uremic SHPT. Similarly, nodular hyperplasia, characterized by higher PTH expression and proliferative ability as well as lower VDR and CASR expression,[44–47] is a more severe stage than diffuse hyperplasia in uremic SHPT. Studies that will better define the role of the uremic milieu in oxyphil cell transdifferentiation are warranted.

Mitochondria are an important organelle in eukaryotic cells and play a key role in adenosine triphosphate production, regulating various catabolic and anabolic processes and maintaining intracellular calcium and oxidation-reduction homeostasis.[48–50] In the current study, trajectory analysis showed that chief-to-oxyphil cell transdifferentiation was associated with mitochondrial changes. We further found higher mitochondrial biogenesis, components, and fusion and lower metabolic function in oxyphil cells, but whether the dysregulation of oxyphil cells is related to mitochondrial changes merits further investigation. Although mitochondrial changes are the pathogenic determinant of oxyphil cell transdifferentiation, whether it is the cause or the result needs more research. In summary, this study provided the first comprehensive description of mitochondria in parathyroid oxyphil cells, whereas the mechanism and significance of mitochondrial changes in oxyphil cells require further study.

Although the present study revealed that oxyphil cells might be derived from chief cells, the limited number of subjects studied and the limited depth of the experiments impair the ability to draw robust and impactful conclusions. Additional studies are warranted to fully define the exact pathways or factors involved in chief-to-oxyphil cell transdifferentiation. Besides that, 2 branches were formed during the chief-to-oxyphil cell transdifferentiation, and the difference between the 2 branches was not researched. Similarly, the functions of other cell types in parathyroid tissue are also worthy of detailed analysis.

In conclusion, our study provides a comprehensive single-cell transcriptome atlas of parathyroids from patients with uremic SHPT and suggests that oxyphil cells are derived from chief cells, with mitochondrial enrichment in the uremic milieu as the pathogenic determinant of oxyphil cell transdifferentiation, which will facilitate parathyroid research and clinical treatment.

DISCLOSURE
All the authors declared no competing interests.

DATA STATEMENT
Sequencing data reported in this article have been deposited in the Genome Sequence Archive in the National Genomics Data Center (https://www.cncb.ac.cn/) under accession number HRA005855.

ACKNOWLEDGMENTS
This work was supported by Shanghai Sailing Program (grant number 23YF1403900), Key Project of National Natural Science Foundation of China (number 81730017), National Key Research and Development Program of China (2020YFC2005000), Shanghai Medical Leading Talents Fund (number 2019LJ03), and Shanghai Soft Science Research Plan (number 23692113800). We thank Dr. Hongying Wang and Dr. Qiang Zou (Department of General Surgery, Huashan Hospital) for their assistance in the preparation of patient parathyroid tissues.

AUTHOR CONTRIBUTIONS
JM performed experiments; JM analyzed data and prepared figures; HY, MW, JQ, PC, and CL helped with data interpretation; YB helped with bioinformatics analysis; JM wrote and edited the manuscript; and JC designed the research and revised the manuscript. All authors reviewed the manuscript.

SUPPLEMENTARY MATERIAL
Supplementary File (PDF)
Supplementary Methods.
Supplementary Figure S1. Comparison of 3 pathologic types of parathyroid nodules (associated with Figure 1).
Supplementary Figure S2. Cell type identification in parathyroid glands of patients with uremic secondary hyperparathyroidism (SHPT) by known markers (associated with Figure 2).
Supplementary Figure S3. Expression of parathyroid function-related genes in parathyroid cells (associated with Figure 3).
Supplementary Figure S4. RNA velocity analysis and DiffusionMap analysis of parathyroid cells (associated with Figure 3).

Supplementary Figure S5. Transcriptomic analysis of chief and oxyphil cells in single-cell RNA sequencing (scRNA-seq) and published RNA sequencing (RNA-seq).

Supplementary Figure S6. Increased mitochondrial biogenesis and components in chief cell nodules after uremic serum treatment.

Supplementary Figure S7. Changes of serum human intact parathyroid hormone (iPTH) concentrations normalized by total protein content of transplanted glands in nude mice pre-transplantation (pre-TP) and post-transplantation (post-TP) (associated with Figure 8d).

Supplementary References.

REFERENCES

1. Silver J, Naveh-Many T. Phosphate and the parathyroid. *Kidney Int.* 2009;75:898–905.
2. Raggi P, Kleerekoper M. Contribution of bone and mineral abnormalities to cardiovascular disease in patients with chronic kidney disease. *Clin J Am Soc Nephrol.* 2008;3:836–843.
3. Cunningham J, Locatelli F, Rodriguez M. Secondary hyperparathyroidism: pathogenesis, disease progression, and therapeutic options. *Clin J Am Soc Nephrol.* 2011;6:913–921.
4. Go AS, Chertow GM, Fan D, et al. Chronic kidney disease and the risks of death, cardiovascular events, and hospitalization. *N Engl J Med.* 2004;351:1296–1305.
5. Block GA, Klassen PS, Lazarus JM, et al. Mineral metabolism, mortality, and morbidity in maintenance hemodialysis. *J Am Soc Nephrol.* 2004;15:2208–2218.
6. Christie AC. The parathyroid oxyphil cells. *J Clin Pathol.* 1967;20:591–602.
7. Ritter CS, Haughey BH, Miller B, et al. Differential gene expression by oxyphil and chief cells of human parathyroid glands. *J Clin Endocrinol Metab.* 2012;97:E1499–E1505.
8. Li S, Mao J, Wang M, et al. Comparative proteomic analysis of chief and oxyphil cell nodules in refractory uremic hyperparathyroidism by iTRAQ coupled LC-MS/MS. *J Proteomics.* 2018;179:42–52.
9. Lomonte C, Martino R, Selvaggiolo M, et al. Calcitriol pulse therapy and histology of parathyroid glands in hemodialysis patients. *J Nephrol.* 2003;16:716–720.
10. Sumida K, Nakamura M, Ubara Y, et al. Histopathological alterations of the parathyroid glands in haemodialysis patients with secondary hyperparathyroidism refractory to cinacalcet hydrochloride. *J Clin Pathol.* 2011;64:756–760.
11. Lomonte C, Vernaglione L, Chimienti D, et al. Does vitamin D receptor and calcium receptor activation therapy play a role in the histopathologic alterations of parathyroid glands in refractory uremic hyperparathyroidism? *Clin J Am Soc Nephrol.* 2008;3:794–799.
12. Tanaka Y, Funahashi H, Imai T, et al. Oxyphil cell function in secondary parathyroid hyperplasia. *Nephron.* 1996;73:580–586.
13. Nonaka D. Study of parathyroid transcription factor Gcm2 expression in parathyroid lesions. *Am J Surg Pathol.* 2011;35:145–151.
14. Müller-Höcker J, Schäfer S, Krebs S, et al. Oxyphil cell metaplasia in the parathyroids is characterized by somatic mitochondrial DNA mutations in NADH dehydrogenase genes and cytochrome c oxidase activity-impairing genes. *Am J Pathol.* 2014;184:2922–2935.
15. Grün D, van Oudenaarden A. Design and analysis of single-cell sequencing experiments. *Cell.* 2015;163:799–810.
16. Kolodziejczyk AA, Kim JK, Svensson V, et al. The technology and biology of single-cell RNA sequencing. *Mol Cell.* 2015;58:610–620.
17. Grün D, Lyubimova A, Kester L, et al. Single-cell messenger RNA sequencing reveals rare intestinal cell types. *Nature.* 2015;525:251–255.
18. Haghverdi L, Büttner M, Wolf FA, et al. Diffusion pseudotime robustly reconstructs lineage branching. *Nat Methods.* 2016;13:845–848.
19. Weinreb C, Rodriguez-Fraticelli A, Camargo FD, et al. Lineage tracing on transcriptional landscapes links state to fate during differentiation. *Science.* 2020;367:eaaw3381.
20. Mao J, Wang M, Ni L, et al. Local NF-κB activation promotes parathyroid hormone synthesis and secretion in uremic patients. *Endocrinology.* 2021;162:bqab084.
21. Xun T, Lin Z, Wang X, et al. Advanced oxidation protein products downregulate CYP1A2 and CYP3A4 expression and activity via the NF-κB-mediated signaling pathway in vitro and in vivo. *Lab Invest.* 2021;101:1197–1209.
22. Piantadosi CA, Suliman HB. Transcriptional control of mitochondrial biogenesis and its interface with inflammatory processes. *Biochim Biophys Acta.* 2012;1820:532–541.
23. Brito RBO, Rebello JF, Grabulosa CC, et al. 25-Vitamin D reduces inflammation in uremic environment. *Sci Rep.* 2020;10:128.
24. Filiopoulos V, Hadjiyannakos D, Vlassopoulos D. New insights into uric acid effects on the progression and prognosis of chronic kidney disease. *Ren Fail.* 2012;34:510–520.
25. Jornayvaz FR, Shulman GI. Regulation of mitochondrial biogenesis. *Essays Biochem.* 2010;47:69–84.
26. Packer L, Cadenas E. Lipoic acid: energy metabolism and redox regulation of transcription and cell signaling. *J Clin Biochem Nutr.* 2011;48:26–32.
27. Hsu YH, Huang HP, Chang HR. The uremic toxin p-cresol promotes the invasion and migration on carcinoma cells via Ras and mTOR signaling. *Toxicol In Vitro.* 2019;58:126–131.
28. Morita M, Gravel SP, Hulea L, et al. mTOR coordinates protein synthesis, mitochondrial activity and proliferation. *Cell Cycle.* 2015;14:473–480.
29. Chang LC, Sun HL, Tsai CH, et al. 1,25(OH)(2) D(3) attenuates indoxyl sulfate-induced epithelial-to-mesenchymal cell transition via inactivation of PI3K/Akt/β-catenin signaling in renal tubular epithelial cells. *Nutrition.* 2020;69:110554.
30. Nangaku M, Mimura I, Yamaguchi J, et al. Role of uremic toxins in erythropoiesis-stimulating agent resistance in chronic kidney disease and dialysis patients. *J Ren Nutr.* 2015;25:160–163.
31. Torres PA, De Broe M. Calcium-sensing receptor, calcimimetics, and cardiovascular calcifications in chronic kidney disease. *Kidney Int.* 2012;82:19–25.
32. Chin ER. The role of calcium and calcium/calmodulin-dependent kinases in skeletal muscle plasticity and mitochondrial biogenesis. *Proc Nutr Soc.* 2004;63:279–286.
33. Chen WJ, Lai YJ, Lee JL, et al. CREB/ATF3 signaling mediates indoxyl sulfate-induced vascular smooth muscle cell proliferation and neointimal formation in uremia. *Atherosclerosis.* 2020;315:43–54.
34. Matsukawa T, Motojima H, Sato Y, et al. Upregulation of skeletal muscle PGC-1α through the elevation of cyclic AMP levels by cyanidin-3-glucoside enhances exercise performance. *Sci Rep.* 2017;7:44799.
35. Rapa SF, Di Iorio BR, Campiglia P, et al. Inflammation and oxidative stress in chronic kidney disease-potential therapeutic role of minerals, vitamins and plant-derived metabolites. *Int J Mol Sci.* 2019;21:263.
36. Townsend LK, Knuth CM, Wright DC. Cycling our way to fit fat. *Physiol Rep.* 2017;5:e13247.
37. Vanholder RC, Glorieux GL. An overview of uremic toxicity. *Hemodial Int.* 2003;7:156–161.
38. Borges NA, Barros AF, Nakao LS, et al. Protein-bound uremic toxins from gut microbiota and inflammatory markers in chronic kidney disease. *J Ren Nutr.* 2016;26:396–400.
39. Rossi M, Campbell KL, Johnson DW, et al. Protein-bound uremic toxins, inflammation and oxidative stress: a cross-sectional study in stage 3-4 chronic kidney disease. *Arch Med Res.* 2014;45:309–317.
40. Kamiński TW, Pawlak K, Karbowska M, et al. Indoxyl sulfate - the uremic toxin linking hemostatic system disturbances with the prevalence of cardiovascular disease in patients with chronic kidney disease. *BMC Nephrol.* 2017;18:35.
41. DeLellis RA. Parathyroid tumors and related disorders. *Mod Pathol.* 2011;24(suppl 2):S78–S93.
42. Jungheim K, Schumm-Draeger PM, Usadel KH. Graves' disease: xenotransplantation model (athymic nude mice). *J Mol Med (Berl).* 1999;77:185–188.
43. Mao J, You H, Wang M, et al. Integrated transcriptomic and proteomic analyses for the characterization of parathyroid oxyphil cells in uremic patients. *Amino Acids.* 2022;54:749–763.
44. Fukuda N, Tanaka H, Tominaga Y, et al. Decreased 1,25-dihydroxyvitamin D3 receptor density is associated with a more severe form of parathyroid hyperplasia in chronic uremic patients. *J Clin Invest.* 1993;92:1436–1443.
45. Tokumoto M, Tsuruya K, Fukuda K, et al. Reduced p21, p27 and vitamin D receptor in the nodular hyperplasia in patients with advanced secondary hyperparathyroidism. *Kidney Int.* 2002;62:1196–1207.

46. Taniguchi M, Tokumoto M, Matsuo D, et al. Persistent hyperparathyroidism in renal allograft recipients: vitamin D receptor, calcium-sensing receptor, and apoptosis. *Kidney Int.* 2006;70: 363–370.
47. Týcová I, Sulková SD, Štěpánková J, et al. Molecular patterns of diffuse and nodular parathyroid hyperplasia in long-term hemodialysis. *Am J Physiol Endocrinol Metab.* 2016;311: E720–E729.
48. Diogo CV, Yambire KF, Fernández Mosquera L, et al. Mitochondrial adventures at the organelle society. *Biochem Biophys Res Commun.* 2018;500:87–93.
49. Krebs J, Agellon LB, Michalak M. Ca(2+) homeostasis and endoplasmic reticulum (ER) stress: an integrated view of calcium signaling. *Biochem Biophys Res Commun.* 2015;460:114–121.
50. Frezza C. Mitochondrial metabolites: undercover signalling molecules. *Interface Focus.* 2017;7:20160100.

clinical investigation

Evaluation of novel candidate filtration markers from a global metabolomic discovery for glomerular filtration rate estimation

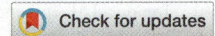

see commentary on page 435

Nora F. Fino[1], Ogechi M. Adingwupu[2], Josef Coresh[3], Tom Greene[1], Ben Haaland[1], Michael G. Shlipak[4], Veronica T. Costa e Silva[5,6], Roberto Kalil[7], Ayse L. Mindikoglu[8,9], Susan L. Furth[10], Jesse C. Seegmiller[11], Andrew S. Levey[2] and Lesley A. Inker[2]

[1]Division of Biostatistics, Department of Population Health Sciences, University of Utah Health, Salt Lake City, Utah, USA; [2]Division of Nephrology, Tufts Medical Center, Boston, Massachusetts, USA; [3]Department of Population Health, NYU Langone, New York, New York, USA; [4]Kidney Health Research Collaborative, San Francisco Veterans Affair Medical Center and University of California, San Francisco, San Francisco, California, USA; [5]Serviço de Nefrologia, Instituto do Câncer do Estado de São Paulo, Faculdade de Medicina, Universidade de São Paulo, São Paulo, Brazil; [6]Laboratório de Investigação Médica 16, Faculdade de Medicina da Universidade de São Paulo, São Paulo, Brazil; [7]Division of Nephrology, Department of Medicine, University of Maryland School of Medicine, Baltimore, Maryland, USA; [8]Margaret M. and Albert B. Alkek Department of Medicine, Section of Gastroenterology and Hepatology, Baylor College of Medicine, Houston, Texas, USA; [9]Michael E. DeBakey Department of Surgery, Division of Abdominal Transplantation, Baylor College of Medicine, Houston, Texas, USA; [10]Department of Pediatrics, Children's Hospital of Philadelphia, and the Perelman School of Medicine at the University of Pennsylvania, Philadelphia, Pennsylvania, USA; and [11]Department of Laboratory Medicine and Pathology, University of Minnesota, Minneapolis, Minnesota, USA

Creatinine and cystatin-C are recommended for estimating glomerular filtration rate (eGFR) but accuracy is suboptimal. Here, using untargeted metabolomics data, we sought to identify candidate filtration markers for a new targeted assay using a novel approach based on their maximal joint association with measured GFR (mGFR) and with flexibility to consider their biological properties. We analyzed metabolites measured in seven diverse studies encompasing 2,851 participants on the Metabolon H4 platform that had Pearson correlations with log mGFR and used a stepwise approach to develop models to estimate mGFR with and without inclusion of creatinine that enabled selection of candidate markers. In total, 456 identified metabolites were present in all studies, and 36 had correlations with mGFR < −0.5. A total of 2,225 models were developed that included these metabolites; all with lower root mean square errors and smaller coefficients for demographic variables compared to estimates using untargeted creatinine. Seventeen metabolites were chosen, including 12 new candidate filtration markers. The selected metabolites had strong associations with mGFR and little dependence on demographic factors. Candidate metabolites were identified with maximal joint association with mGFR and minimal dependence on demographic variables across many varied clinical settings. These metabolites are excreted in urine and represent diverse metabolic pathways and tubular handling. Thus, our data can be used to select metabolites for a multi-analyte eGFR determination assay using mass spectrometry that potentially offers better accuracy and is less prone to non-GFR determinants than the current eGFR biomarkers.

Kidney International (2024) **105**, 582–592; https://doi.org/10.1016/j.kint.2023.11.007

KEYWORDS: filtration markers; glomerular filtration rate; metabolomics

Copyright © 2023, International Society of Nephrology. Published by Elsevier Inc. All rights reserved.

Lay Summary

Creatinine and cystatin C are recommended for estimating glomerular filtration rate (GFR), but accuracy is limited by factors other than GFR that affect both markers, especially in patient populations with acute or chronic illnesses. We used untargeted metabolomics from 7 different studies with a total of 2851 participants to develop a total of 2225 models. Each model had 2 to 15 metabolites. All models provided more accurate predictions of measured GFR than a creatinine-only model and were largely robust across demographic factors. From these models, we identified 17 candidate metabolites for evaluation for their analytical properties by our laboratory. Incorporation of the final selected set of metabolites in a targeted multiplex assay and ultimately development and validation of a panel GFR may provide more accurate GFR estimates across health and disease.

Correspondence: *Lesley A. Inker, Division of Nephrology, Tufts Medical Center, 800 Washington St, Box 391, Boston, Massachusetts 02111, USA. E-mail: linker@tuftsmedicalcenter.org*

Received 24 May 2023; revised 31 October 2023; accepted 10 November 2023; published online 23 November 2023

Glomerular filtration rate (GFR), the key indicator of kidney function in health and disease, is most commonly estimated from creatinine combined with age and sex (eGFRcr).[1,2] (When discussing current and former equations to estimate GFR, we use the term *sex* to align with the terminology used in the orginal papers that developed these equations. In general, we use the term *sex* to describe sex at birth, and *gender* to describe gender identity.) Clinical practice guidelines recommend more accurate tests, such as GFR measured using clearance of exogenous filtration markers (mGFR) or GFR estimated from the combination of creatinine with cystatin-C (eGFRcr-cys) when eGFRcr is thought to be not sufficiently accurate, or when the clinical decision requires a more accurate assessment of GFR.[2] Measurement procedures for mGFR can be difficult to perform and are not widely accessible to many health systems, and even with the more accurate eGFRcr-cys, there is substantial variation between eGFR and mGFR for individual patients,[3] with errors relative to mGFR >30% in 10% to 20% of patients.[4] Notably, higher rates are observed in patients with acute and chronic illness, in whom clinical decisions based on imprecise GFR can have important effects.[4-8] In addition, the inclusion of age and sex in current GFR equations is undesirable as these coefficient reflect the average effect of age and sex in the populations used to develop the equations, contributing to the individual-level errors.

Errors in eGFR are predominantly due to the presence of non-GFR determinants of the serum concentration of endogenous filtration markers (e.g., muscle mass for creatinine).[1,9] In principle, a collection of multiple filtration markers with non-GFR determinants that are largely independent of one another could be used to develop a panel eGFR equation that lowers the importance of any individual marker, consequently reducing the influence of non-GFR determinants on the GFR estimate, improving accuracy for individual patients, and eliminating the need for demographic factors.

Our prior explorations into multimarker panels have not resulted in eGFR that was substantially more accurate than current eGFR.[10-12] We hypothesize that a greater number of metabolites identified from diverse data sets is required for greater accuracy in GFR estimation, especially to be robust to states of health and disease. Untargeted metabolomics assays, where a broad population of metabolites are assessed and compared across a cohort of subjects using relative quantification, can be used for the identification of a set of candidate filtration markers.[13] Selected metabolites can then be used to develop targeted assays that provide absolute quantitative results for widespread clinical applications (Supplementary Figure S1).

In this article, our goal was to select candidate markers using untargeted metabolites from a joint analysis of 7 diverse studies that measured untargeted metabolites using the same platform. We hypothesized that many combinations of metabolites could form the basis of alternative prediction models with similarly high accuracy. We present a systematic process that allows flexibility in choosing among a possible set of metabolites based on relevant biological and chemical characteristics.

METHODS
Data sources
We included the following 7 research studies with existing metabolomics data and available mGFR: African American Study of Kidney,[14] Assessing Long Term Outcomes in Living Kidney Donors (ALTOLD[15]), Onco-GFR Study,[16] Chronic Kidney Disease in Children (CKiD[17]), University of Maryland Baltimore Cirrhosis Cohort,[18,19] Multi-Ethnic Study of Atherosclerosis (MESA[20]), and Modification of Diet in Renal Disease[21] (Supplementary Table S1). GFR was measured using urinary clearance of iothalamate, or plasma clearance of iothalamate, iohexol, or creatinine-EDTA. We increased GFR measured using plasma clearance of iohexol by 5% to calibrate to the other methods, as has been done previously.[4,12,22] All studies were approved by participating institutions' institutional review boards.

Metabolomics
Global, untargeted metabolomics assays were performed at Metabolon on the H4 platform (Durham, NC; Supplementary Table S1). We excluded all exogenous metabolites as well as metabolites and samples with high levels of missingness (>80% and >50% missing, respectively). Remaining missing values were imputed with the lower level of detection. We assessed the appropriateness of this imputation in metabolites with >1% missing by predicting the missing values with a process outlined in the Supplementary Methods. We rescaled all data by the batch-specific median and evaluated within- and between-study batch effects using principal components analysis.[23]

Statistical analysis
Our goal for this analysis was to rigorously select a set of candidate metabolites for exploration by our central laboratory for potential incorporation into a targeted mass spectrometry multiplex assay (Supplementary Figure S1). To allow for the possibility that markers in combination outperformed individual markers with stronger associations with mGFR, we did not restrict this analysis to examination of each metabolite in isolation. In addition, because no single model developed here is likely to be the ultimate panel eGFR, we did not solely focus on the best performing (the statistically optimal model) for a given number of metabolites, but rather a collection of models that perform almost as well as the statistical optimal model (near-optimal models). We expected many collections of metabolites would be highly associated with mGFR, and this flexibility allowed the ultimate selection of metabolites to be guided by assay characteristics, biological characteristics, and predictive accuracy.

We limited our analysis to named metabolites measured in all 7 studies. mGFR was indexed by body surface area and is expressed as ml/min per 1.73 m^2. We log transformed mGFR and each metabolite. Metabolites with an average Pearson correlation with log mGFR across studies <–0.5 were included as candidates, as strong inverse associations are expected for a filtration marker. In sensitivity analysis, we also evaluated metabolites with an average Pearson correlation <–0.3. Separate linear regression models for mGFR were fit for each individual metabolite, along with age, sex, race (Black vs. other), and body mass index (BMI). To account for the lack of cross-study calibration of untargeted assays, which can have arbitrary shifts in location and scale of metabolite distributions, we included terms for study and metabolite-by-study interactions in all modeling.

We developed a novel stepwise (Supplementary Figure S2) approach using linear regression to generate subsets of metabolites for estimating mGFR, detailed in the Supplemental Methods. Prior simulations suggested that a more accurate eGFR would require 8 to 10 metabolites; we performed selection up to 15 metabolites to confirm that additional metabolites did not improve predictive error. Briefly, we began by fitting all models for mGFR using a single metabolite and identifying all models with root mean square error

Table 1 | Summaries of patient characteristics in included atudies

Study	Study description	N	Age, yr	mGFR, ml/min per 1.73 m²	Black	Female	BMI, kg/m²
AASK	RCT of CKD progression	962	54.5 (10.6)	45.8 (13.0)	962 (100.0)	373 (38.8)	30.6 (6.6)
ALTOLD[a]	Cohort study of kidney donor candidates	131	43.7 (11.3)	101.1 (15.3)	3 (2.3)	83 (63.4)	27.0 (4.3)
Onco-GFR	Cohort study of patients with solid tumors in Brazil	100	57.2 (13.3)	80.1 (21.1)	14 (14.0)	51 (51.0)	28.3 (6.1)
CKiD	Cohort study of children with CKD	613	12.1 (4.3)	54.7 (25.5)	88 (14.4)	236 (38.5)	20.6 (5.7)
Cirrhosis	Cohort study of patients with cirrhosis	103	54.5 (8.9)	80.3 (35.3)	26 (25.2)	45 (43.7)	29.5 (6.8)
MDRD	RCT of CKD progression	677	52.9 (12.0)	28.9 (13.1)	51 (7.5)	256 (37.8)	26.8 (4.3)
MESA	General population of older adults	265	70.9 (8.7)	76.3 (20.2)	122 (46.0)	124 (46.8)	29.8 (5.5)

AASK, African American Study of Kidney; ALTOLD, Assessing Long Term Outcomes in Living Kidney Donors; BMI, body mass index; Cirrhosis, University of Maryland Baltimore Cirrhosis Cohort; CKD, chronic kidney disease; CKiD, Chronic Kidney Disease in Children; mGFR, measured glomerular filtration rate; Onco-GFR, Oncology Glomerular Filtration Rate; MDRD, Modification of Diet in Renal Disease; MESA, Multi-Ethnic Study of Atherosclerosis; RCT, randomized controlled trial.
[a]GFR visits in ALTOLD occurred prior to donation.
Data are presented as mean (SD) or as N (percentage).

(RMSE) within 0.005 of the best-fitting single metabolite model. Then, as we incrementally increased the number of metabolites included in the model from 2 to 15, we found the best new metabolite to add to the best-fitting model from the previous model size. Next, we replaced each metabolite in the present model with an alternative metabolite and determined whether the present model RMSE was within a small margin (0.005) of the current best-fitting model for a given model size. Following this approach, we found a collection of near-optimal models across a spectrum of subset sizes. We developed models with and without the inclusion of untargeted creatinine as a candidate predictor. Sets of metabolites that do not include creatinine would be more appropriate as confirmatory tests for eGFRcr and may be optimal in people at the extremes of muscle mass or dietary meat intake, where eGFRcr accuracy is poor.

We assessed the impact of including demographics and clinical factors or age, sex, race, and BMI alone and in combination. We compared all developed models with models fit with demographics and untargeted creatinine as the sole metabolite (hereon referred to as the reference model). We used untargeted creatinine as a reference because we believe it represents a meaningful comparison to untargeted analyses of other metabolites. To examine the degree of overoptimism in our models, we compared the fitted model RMSEs with cross-validated RMSEs. We also evaluated the performance of the models separately by study.

Our final step was to identify the set of metabolites for evaluation by our laboratory for consideration in development of the multiplex assay. Models that did not show evidence of substantial overfitting in cross-validation were retained for further consideration. We removed from consideration models that had at least 1 demographic coefficient (age, sex, race, or BMI) with an absolute value >0.1. After applying the above criteria to the set of models with and without creatinine, we selected metabolites present in at least 20% of all models for consideration of assay development. To better understand the metabolites, we also evaluated the partial correlation of each metabolite with untargeted creatinine after adjusting for mGFR and the association of demographic factors to mGFR after adjusting for each metabolite.

RESULTS
Study populations
Across studies, there were 2851 participants with a wide range of mGFR (6.1–201.8 ml/min per 1.73 m²), age (2.0–91.0 years), BMI (13.1–56.3 kg/m²), and proportion of Black individuals (2.3%–100%; Table 1). More important, we included 3 populations not well represented in studies developing GFR equations: children with chronic kidney disease, patients with cirrhosis, and patients with cancer.

A summary of overlapping metabolites by study is given in Supplementary Table S2. There were 456 named metabolites common to all 7 studies, 36 of which had a pairwise correlation <−0.5 with mGFR (Figure 1). Missing data for the 36 metabolites are summarized in Supplementary Table S3. No evidence of substantial batch effects by study was found using principal components analysis (Supplementary Figure S3). For metabolites with >1% missingness, we found that predicted missing values were generally small in magnitude and similar to predicted values below the fifth percentile of values in a given metabolite. An example of these results using guanidino succinate, which was 12.5% missing, can be found in Supplementary Figure S4; results of other metabolites with missing data were similar (data not shown). Following these results, we concluded that it was reasonable to impute remaining values with the lower limit of detection. The correlations for each of the 36 metabolites with mGFR as well as demographic coefficients for all models fit with each individual metabolite are shown in Supplementary Table S4.

Near-optimal models
Figure 2 shows the RMSE for all near-optimal models by model size. All developed models had lower RMSE compared with the reference model (RMSE, 0.258). When creatinine was included as a candidate marker, we found 1204 models using 36 metabolites. As the number of metabolites included in the model increased, the RMSEs generally decreased: the mean RMSE for 2-metabolite models was 0.210 (range, 0.207–0.211), compared with 0.187 for 15-metabolite models (range, 0.183–0.188). When creatinine was not included, we found 1021 near-optimal models using 35 metabolites. In general, models without creatinine had higher RMSE than those containing creatinine (mean RMSE, 0.193 [range, 0.185–0.212] vs. mean RMSE, 0.191 [range, 0.183–0.211], respectively), although they become more similar as the number of metabolites increased. Cross-validated RMSEs were comparable to original RMSEs when considering models with ≤10 metabolites, whereas cross-validated RMSEs were generally higher for models with >10 metabolites (shaded band in Figure 2).

Impact of demographic factors
Across all models, the magnitude of coefficients for age, sex, race, and BMI was smaller than their size in the reference

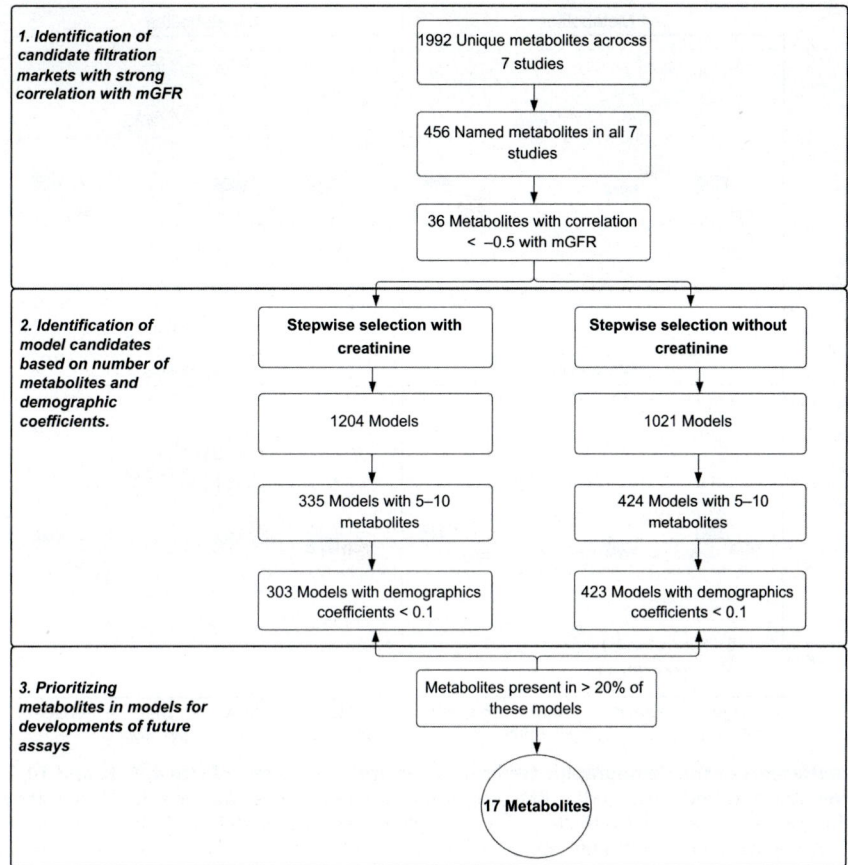

Figure 1 | Flow diagram of metabolite and model selection process. mGFR, measure glomerular filtration rate.

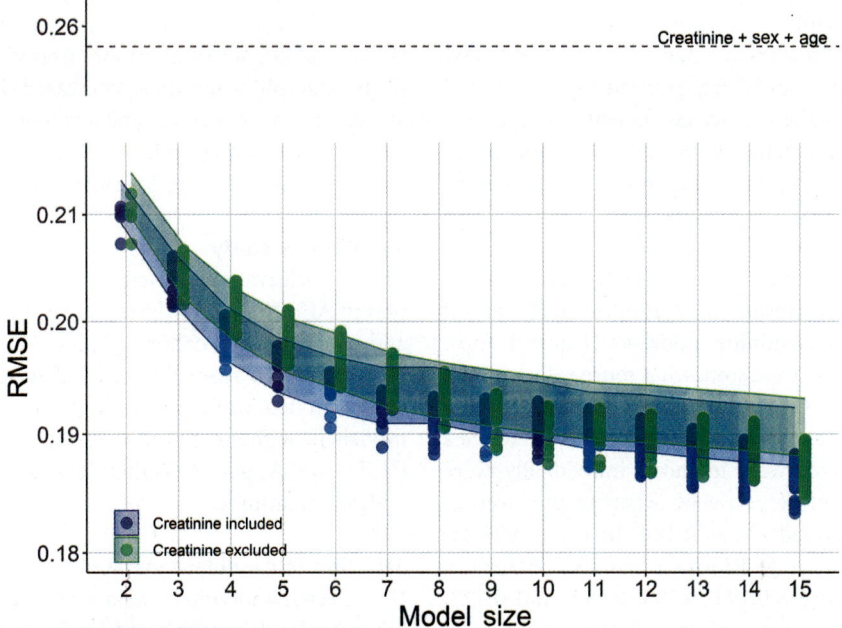

Figure 2 | Comparison of near-optimal models when untargeted creatinine is included as a candidate (Creatinine included) versus when untargeted creatinine is excluded (Creatinine excluded). The colored bands show the range of cross-validated (CV) root mean square errors (RMSEs). Points are non-CV model errors. Cross-validated errors were averaged across 10 random iterations of 5-fold cross-validation. Models are fit with study terms but not with demographic variables.

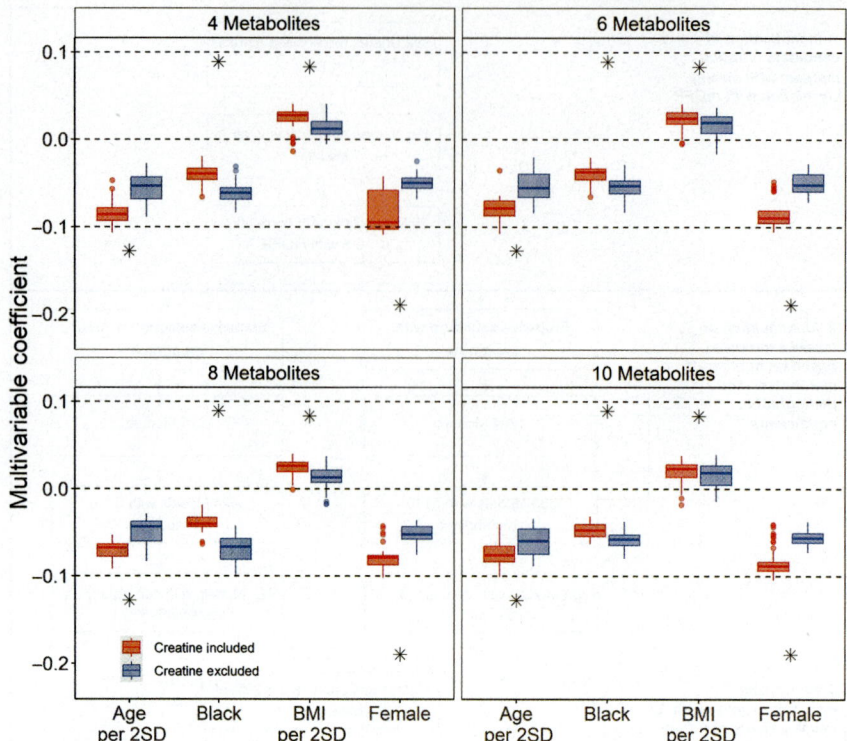

Figure 3 | Multivariable coefficients of the demographic terms for near-optimal models of size 4, 6, 8, and 10, both with and without consideration of creatinine. Age and body mass index (BMI) coefficients are represented as per 2 SDs. Black star points represent the demographic coefficients for the reference model with creatinine only. When selecting models for further consideration in a targeted assay, we excluded models with any demographic coefficients >0.1 in absolute value. Coefficients from other model sizes not shown were similar.

equation (Figure 3). Coefficients from models that did not include creatinine were generally smaller in magnitude than those from models in which creatinine was a candidate predictor. The average coefficients for age, sex, race, and BMI were −0.07, −0.08, −0.05, and 0.02, respectively, in models with creatinine, whereas the average coefficients for age, sex, race, and BMI were −0.05, −0.05, −0.06, and 0.02, respectively, in models without creatinine. Including more metabolites did not appreciably reduce the coefficients' size in either set of models (Supplementary Table S5).

When demographic terms and BMI were included in models individually, the inclusion of sex resulted in the largest decrease in RMSE in the creatinine model set (Figure 4, top). Models without creatinine were somewhat more robust to the addition of demographic variables (Figure 4, bottom). Across all model sizes in the creatinine model set, the average RMSEs when age, BMI, and race were included individually were 0.190, 0.191, and 0.190, respectively, whereas the average RMSE when sex was included was 0.188. In the model set without creatinine, the average RMSEs when age, BMI, race, and sex were included were 0.193, 0.193, 0.193, and 0.192, respectively.

In the creatinine model set, incorporating age and sex together decreased RMSEs compared with the corresponding models without any demographics (average RMSE across all model sizes was 0.191 compared with 0.187 when age and sex are included). In contrast, the incorporation of BMI and race did not substantially decrease RMSEs beyond the age- and sex-adjusted models (average RMSE, 0.186; Supplementary Figure S5, top). In the model set without creatinine, the average RMSE across all model sizes was 0.193. The inclusion of demographics modestly decreased the average RMSE. The average RMSE when age and sex were included together and when all demographics were included was 0.193 (Supplementary Figure S5, bottom).

Variation by study

Model performance varied by study: models performed the best in ALTOLD and MESA and performed the worst in CKiD and the Cirrhosis cohort (Figure 5). Notably, near-optimal models chosen from the entire data set performed similarly to the models optimized to a given study and outperformed models fit with creatinine as the sole metabolite, especially in CKiD, MESA, and ALTOLD. Results were similar in models without creatinine.

Selection of candidate metabolites

We selected individual metabolites for further investigation for assay development based on the performance of the cross-validation and multivariable models (Figure 1). We selected the 17 metabolites present in >20% in either set of models to form our list of top-performing metabolites (Table 2; Supplementary Figure S6). When creatinine was a candidate predictor, it was chosen in 81.5% of models. Two of the most

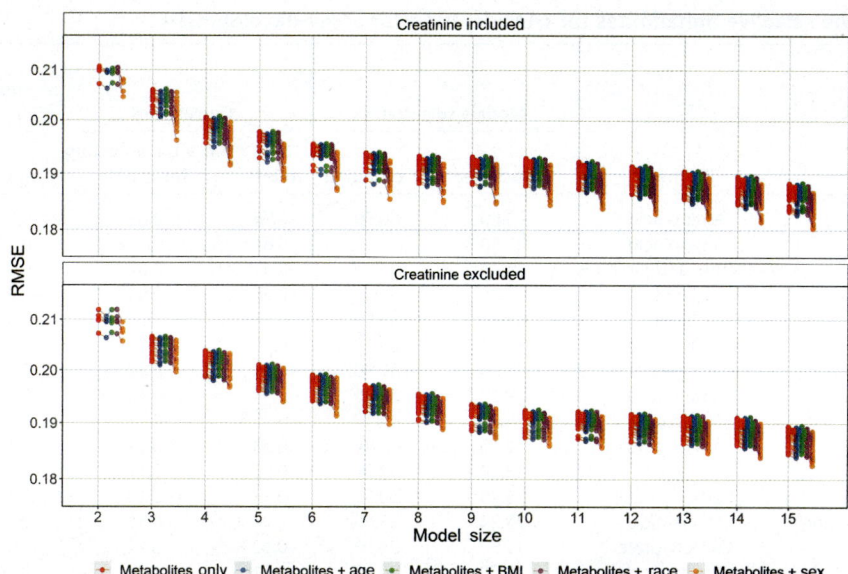

Figure 4 | Comparison of near-optimal models after inclusion of age, body mass index (BMI), and race individually. Top: models with creatinine. Bottom: models without creatinine. Comparison of near-optimal models fit with and without creatinine after individual inclusion of age, BMI, and race terms. Models denoted "Metabolites only" refer to the fact that the near-optimal models with no demographic terms were included. We added each demographic term individually to assess changes in root mean square error (RMSE) after each single demographic term is included. Each near-optimal model is connected by semitransparent lines.

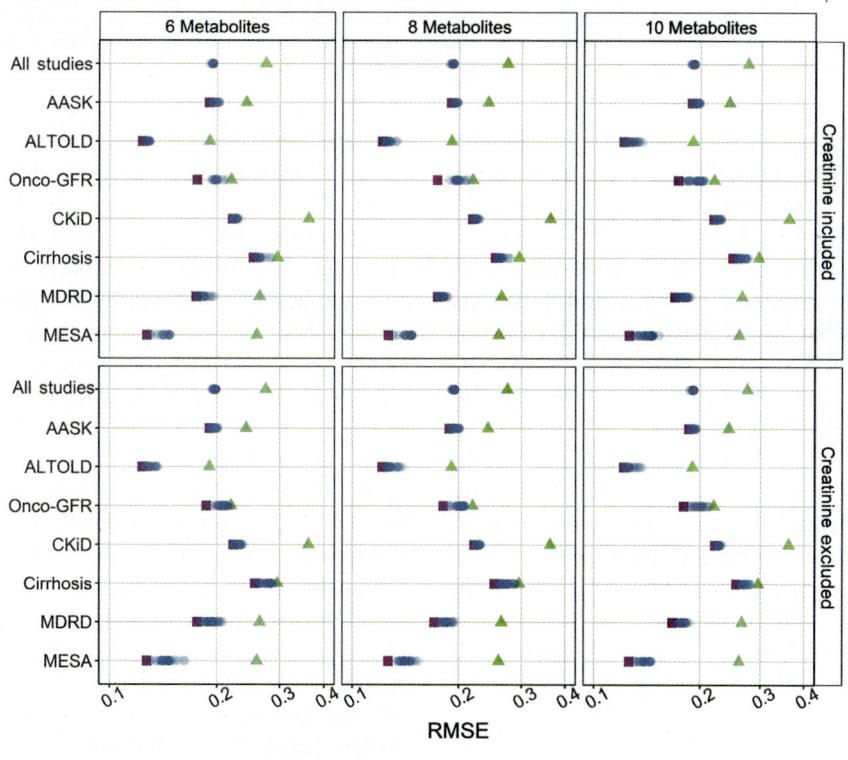

Figure 5 | Root mean square errors (RMSEs) of near-optimal models including all studies and models fit separately by study for model sizes of 6, 8, and 10 metabolites. Top: models could include creatinine. Bottom: models exclude creatinine. Green triangles show the RMSE from the reference model containing creatinine, age, and sex. Purple squares represent the best study-specific model for a given subset size. The axis for RMSE is shown on the log scale. AASK, African American Study of Kidney; ALTOLD, Assessing Long Term Outcomes in Living Kidney Donors; Cirrhosis, University of Maryland Baltimore Cirrhosis Cohort; CKiD, Chronic Kidney Disease in Children; MDRD, Modification of Diet in Renal Disease; MESA, Multi-Ethnic Study of Atherosclerosis; Onco-GFR, Oncology Glomerular Filtration Rate.

Table 2 | Summary of the selective metabolites for consideration for assay development

		Models selected, %		Correlation		Coefficients with demographic and clinical characteristics			
Metabolite	Pathway	Cr included	Cr excluded	mGFR	Cr, after adjusting for mGFR	Age	Female	Black	BMI
C-glycosyltryptophan[a]	Amino acid	90.60	80.60	−0.76	0.08	−0.03	−0.03	−0.08	0.04
Creatinine[b]	Amino acid	81.50	–	−0.64	–	−0.13	−0.19	0.09	0.08
Gulonic acid[a]	Cofactors and vitamins	64.40	45.20	−0.6	0.07	−0.07	−0.05	0.02	0.03
3-Hydroxy-3-methylglutarate[b]	Lipid	63.50	2.90	−0.58	0.05	−0.04	−0.03	−0.01	0.02
Myoinositol[a]	Lipid	61.20	39.60	−0.57	0.1	0.01	−0.06	0.03	0.02
4-Acetamidobutanoate[a]	Amino acid	50.00	63.10	−0.68	0.22	−0.05	−0.05	−0.02	0.01
Erythronate[a]	Carbohydrate	31.30	32.90	−0.7	0.19	−0.07	−0.07	−0.04	0.00
3-Methylglutarylcarnitine (2)[a]	Amino acid	29.40	39.90	−0.53	0.12	−0.07	−0.01	−0.12	0.06
Pseudouridine[a]	Nucleotide	25.50	42.10	−0.77	0.28	−0.06	−0.07	−0.05	0.03
3-Methylglutaconate[b]	Amino acid	25.10	6.10	−0.53	0.14	−0.11	−0.01	−0.06	0.00
Adipoylcarnitine[b]	Lipid	23.60	12.80	−0.52	0.17	−0.07	−0.08	−0.07	0.08
N-acetylneuraminate[a]	Carbohydrate	23.20	30.30	−0.7	0.14	−0.1	−0.03	0.02	−0.02
N6-carbamoylthreonyladenosine[a]	Nucleotide	22.20	33.80	−0.74	0.36	−0.1	−0.09	−0.02	0.06
Arabitol/xylitol[c]	Carbohydrate	11.80	34.00	−0.62	0.12	−0.06	−0.08	−0.06	0.00
Vanillylmandelate[c]	Amino acid	11.70	30.10	−0.61	0.07	0.00	−0.03	−0.06	−0.01
1-Methylimidazoleacetate[c]	Amino acid	9.40	21.90	−0.65	0.22	−0.1	−0.07	−0.07	−0.01
N-acetyl-1-methylhistidine[c]	Amino acid	6.60	42.70	−0.54	0.24	−0.04	−0.06	0.12	0.07

BMI, body mass index; Cr, untargeted creatinine; mGFR, measured glomerular filtration rate.
[a]Metabolites were selected in both scenarios, with and without consideration of creatinine.
[b]Metabolites were selected only when creatinine was considered.
[c]Metabolites were selected only when creatinine was not considered.
Model selection percentages are the fraction of high-performing models across the metabolites that were chosen both when creatinine was included as a candidate predictor and when creatinine was not included as a candidate predictor. Correlations shown are the Pearson correlations of the metabolites with mGFR and the partial correlations of the metabolites with nontargeted creatinine, after adjusting for mGFR. Demographic coefficients are from models fit with a single given metabolite. Models also include study effects. Age and BMI coefficients represent a 2-SD increase. Note these single metabolite coefficients were not used to select metabolites in the final criteria, which used the coefficients from multivariable models. Coefficients in gray are >0.1 in absolute value. Dashes (–) indicate that the cell is not applicable.

common metabolites in models with and without creatinine were C-glycosyltryptophan (selected in 90.6% and 80.6% of models with and without creatinine, respectively) and gulonic acid (selected in 64.4% and 45.2% of models with and without creatinine, respectively). Of the 17 metabolites, 5 had partial correlation with creatinine of >0.2, and 4 had coefficients for demographic factors that were >0.1. Selection percentages for all 36 metabolites are given in Supplementary Table S4. Scatterplots with study-wise locally estimated scatterplot smoothing (LOESS) curves for the 17 selected metabolites and mGFR are given in Supplementary Figure S7.

In sensitivity analysis using a different threshold for initial metabolite inclusion (correlation, < −0.3), model RMSEs were similar (Supplementary Figure S8), and we selected 12 of the same metabolites (Supplementary Table S6). Two of the additional 4 metabolites that might have been included had correlation >−0.5 and were therefore eliminated because of other criteria (Figure 1), and 2 had correlation <−0.3.

DISCUSSION

This article presented analyses of a global untargeted metabolomics platform for selection of candidate novel filtration markers. Our results will be used to develop targeted assays on a subset of markers that will ultimately be used to develop a panel estimated GFR that ideally will provide greater accuracy for individual patients. We found many subsets of metabolites with excellent predictions of mGFR, and models outperformed untargeted creatinine-only–based estimates and were largely robust across demographics. Improved accuracy was observed with more metabolites, but cross-validation results suggested diminishing benefits to adding more metabolites beyond 10. Inclusion of sex did meaningfully improve the accuracy of our models, but age, race, and body size did not. By selecting metabolites common to these high-performing models, we created a list of metabolites with maximal joint association with mGFR and with flexibility in choosing the final metabolites for the panel eGFR based on biological and assay characteristics.

We hypothesized that to improve on existing eGFR, we would first need to identify a large set of candidate markers. We identified 17 metabolites that are candidates for possible inclusion in a panel eGFR. To our knowledge, as many as 12 metabolites may not have been specifically identified as filtration markers in prior work (Supplementary Table S7). We had previously identified 3 of the 17 metabolites: myoinositol, pseudouridine, and arabitol/xylitol, although only pseudouridine had been included in our prior multimarker panel.[10,11] In addition, C-glycosyltryptophan (also known as C-mannosyltryptophan) and erythronate had been identified by other investigators.[24–26] All 17 have promise to be excellent filtration markers. Seven of the 17 metabolites had inverse correlations with mGFR of greater magnitude than that of creatinine. In addition to their low molecular weights, all are eliminated in the urine, consistent with metabolite filtration markers. The 17 represent diverse metabolic pathways and tubular handling, hopefully allowing for selection of nonoverlapping, non–GFR-related properties of metabolites (Supplementary Table S7).

C-glycosyltryptophan was the top most selected metabolite in both model sets. It has a higher correlation to mGFR than does creatinine (–0.76 vs. –0.64) and results from N-glycosylation, a posttranslational modification, of tryptophan.[27] It is not bound to plasma proteins and correlates strongly with measured GFR. However, 1 study showed it did undergo tubular reabsorption.[28] After creatinine, gulonic acid was the next metabolite selected in the highest proportion of models. Gulonic acid appears to be bound to plasma proteins. It is a product of ascorbate and aldarate metabolism, involved in the conversion of D-gluconic acid to the D-xylose as part of the pento phosphate pathway, and in nonhumans to ascorbic acid.[29,30] Further testing in diverse experimental and clinical settings for the included metabolites is necessary to fully characterize these metabolites and assess the potential non-GFR determinants of these markers.

We hypothesized that the use of multiple markers would obviate the need for demographics and would be more robust to body size and composition. Consistent with this hypothesis, the addition of age, race, and BMI did not meaningfully improve the RMSE of the models that included these variables compared with models that did not include these variables. Although race has been excluded from creatinine-based GFR equations, its removal introduced a small but persistent bias observed in several populations.[4,31,32] Thus, our demonstration that inclusion of race did not improve performance is an important finding. In contrast, we found that including sex improved RMSE across all models. Recently, there have been increased questions about using eGFR equations that include sex, given the increase in gender diversity and the use of gender versus biological sex in clinical care,[33–35] and new equations are available that estimate GFR from cystatin-C that do not include sex.[32] Our results suggest 2 important points. First, sets of metabolites that did not include creatinine had smaller female versus male coefficients than sets with creatinine, suggesting that should the ultimately developed panel eGFR not include creatinine, it might be able to exclude sex, whereas a panel eGFR that includes creatinine may need to retain sex. Second, the persistence of the sex coefficient might suggest that biological sex does impact the levels of these markers, and the impact is not related to body size, unlike what has been hypothesized for creatinine. The cause of the sex differences here is not well understood and requires future investigation. Future studies can explore the impact of hormonal and nonhormonal cause on the observed differences, which could have wider implications, such as in the care of individuals in the transgender community or the impact of menopause and hormone replacement therapy on health.

More important, despite substantial variation in relative metabolite quantities by study, the models developed in the pooled data set performed similarly to models optimized for individual studies. This suggests that models developed in the pooled data set are similar to models developed within each study, highlighting the generalizability of our models.

In all studies, our models showed better performance compared with estimates based on GFR estimates from creatinine alone. Despite this consistency, we also noted that the accuracy of the models varied by study. Improvements were particularly notable in CKiD, ALTOLD, and MESA, suggesting that the greatest benefits of a panel eGFR could be seen in children or individuals with relatively healthy kidneys. Future work should investigate causes of these differences.

Our approach had several strengths. First, we identified novel candidate filtration markers using untargeted metabolomics and their relation to mGFR, many of which were not previously noted to be filtration markers.[26] Second, we combined data from 2851 participants in 7 diverse data sources across age, disease, and geography. This diversity allowed us to analyze a wide range of mGFR, from 6 to 202 ml/min per 1.73 m^2, and across health and disease, increasing the likelihood of a novel panel eGFR to be accurate across clinical settings. Third, our approach provided flexibility in selecting metabolites, considering not only predictive accuracy but also biological and assay characteristics. A central challenge was how to estimate the degree of overfitting and optimism when fitting many prediction models. We developed an envelope of cross-validated RMSEs that represented the range of the generalizable predictive accuracy for each model size.

Limitations of this analysis include that the observed results for individual metabolites assayed in the global untargeted platform might not be consistent with targeted assays. However, improved precision is expected with targeted assays.[10] The cross-sectional study design also limits our conclusions. Repeated assessments of the metabolites would allow us to account for possible measurement error in our analysis, as well as allow us to investigate changes in the metabolites over time. In addition, we limited our analysis to metabolites measured in all 7 studies; it is possible that there are important metabolites omitted from our results. In addition, across all studies, there were 68 unknown metabolites (7.4% of the unknown metabolites) with a correlation with mGFR greater than our threshold of >0.5 in absolute value. Future work could include investigating these metabolites in greater detail. Nevertheless, our models were able to predict GFR consistently across numerous collections of metabolites, so it is unlikely that a single omitted metabolite would meaningfully improve accuracy. We were limited to using dichotomous race (Black vs. other) and did not include a more refined assessment of race, ethnicity, and geographic groups. However, previous work showed that using a 4-level race term did not improve prediction beyond that of a dichotomous race term, although this finding may be limited to data from the United States and Europe.[36] In addition, the inclusion of patients with cancer from South America and the consistency of results within this cohort might suggest our results are more robust to geographic region and disease. Last, we did not include cystatin-C in our analysis, which limits our ability to compare to eGFRcr-cys. Our goal was to identify a set of metabolites that could be included in a targeted mass spectrometry multiplex assay; cystatin-C, as a low-molecular-weight protein, would not be included in such an assay as it would only include metabolites that could be assayed together. Future work will incorporate cystatin-C using standard clinical chemistry assays in conjunction with the multiplex metabolite assay. Regardless of the inclusion of cystatin-C in the panel eGFR algorithm, the most relevant future comparison of eGFR panel will be to eGFRcr-cys, the current most accurate eGFR.

In conclusion, these data represent the first step toward our ultimate goal of developing a more accurate panel eGFR across a range of health and disease, with less reliance on demographic terms than the current eGFR. This new panel is intended as an independent complementary test for eGFRcr-cys. Next steps include exploring the physical and biological properties of candidate metabolites for final selection and developing and validating the panel GFR for analytical precision and performance compared with mGFR in various clinical settings.

DISCLOSURE

LAI reports receiving grant and contracts to institution from National Institutes of Health (NIH)/National Institute of Diabetes and Digestive and Kidney Diseases (NIDDK) (1R01DK116790), National Kidney Foundation (NKF), Chinnocks, Omeros, and Reata Pharmaceuticals; consultancy fees from Tricida Inc. and Diamtrix; and participation on medical advisory council for Alport Foundation and scientific advisory board for NKF. SLF reports receiving a grant from the NIH and participation on the advisory board at Genentech. ASL reports receiving a grant to institution from the NKF and NIH and honoraria for academic lectures and participation on advisory board for clinical trials of dapagliflozin at AstraZeneca. MGS reports receiving grants and contracts to institution from Bayer Pharmaceuticals, NIH–National Institute on Aging, NIDDK, and National Heart, Lung, and Blood Institute; consultancy fees from Cricket Health and Intercept Pharmaceuticals; honoraria from Boehringer Ingelheim, AstraZeneca, and Bayer Pharmaceuticals; stock options at TAI Diagnostics; and being chairman of the Board of Directors for NCIRE. TG reports receiving contracts from Boehringer Ingelheim, AstraZeneca, CSL, and Vertex; and consultancy fees from Invokana, Pfizer, Novartis, AstraZeneca, and Janssen Pharmaceuticals. JCS reports receiving subcontracts from the NIH and Centers for Disease Control and Prevention; and participation on data safety and monitoring board for HIV in Nigeria (H3). VTCeS reports funding from FAPESP (Fundação de Amparo à Pesquisa do Estado de São Paulo, project number 2014/19286-4), a local public research agency from São Paulo, Brazil. ALM reports funding from NIH-NIDDK (5 K23 DK089008-05) and the University of Maryland School of Medicine, Department of Medicine funds, University of Maryland Clinical Translational Science Institute, University of Maryland General Clinical Research Center, and NIH Public Health Service grant P30DK056338. All the other authors declared no competing interests.

DATA STATEMENT

Data of African American Study of Kidney, Assessing Long Term Outcomes in Living Kidney Donors Study, and Modification of Diet in Renal Disease Study are available at NIH Common Fund's National Metabolomics Data Repository website, the Metabolomics Workbench, https://www.metabolomicsworkbench.org, where they have has been assigned project identifier PR001762 and DOI: https://doi.org/10.21228/M8ZB1D. Data of Multi-Ethnic Study of Atherosclerosis can be requested through the study website, https://www.mesa-nhlbi.org/MesaInternal/Publications.aspx. Data of Chronic Kidney Disease in Children can be requested through the study website, https://statepi.jhsph.edu/ckid/investigator-resources/. Data of Oncology Glomerular Filtration Rate (Onco-GFR) Study and University of Maryland Baltimore Cirrhosis Cohort can be requested directly from study investigators (ALM [University of Maryland Baltimore] and VTCeS [Onco-GFR]). R code for the stepwise procedure is included in the Supplementary Material.

ACKNOWLEDGMENTS

We would like to acknowledge collaborators of participating studies: Assessing Long Term Outcomes in Living Kidney Donors: Bertram Kasiske, Matthew Weir, and Todd Pesavento; Multi-Ethnic Study of Atherosclerosis: Tariq Shafi, Wendy Post, and Peter Rossing; Onco-GFR Study: Emmanuel de Almeida Burdmann and Renato Antunes Caires; Chronic Kidney Disease in Children: Bradley Warady, Alvaro Munoz, Derek Ng, and George Schwartz; University of Maryland Baltimore Cirrhosis Cohort: Laurence S. Magder, Thomas C. Dowling, Matthew R. Weir, and Robert H. Christenson.

FUNDING

The measurements and analyses were supported by the National Institute of Diabetes and Digestive and Kidney Diseases (NIDDK) grant 1R01DK116790 to Tufts Medical Center.

African American Study of Kidney (AASK) received support from NIDDK U01 DK045388 and the NCMHHD M01 RR00071. The Assessing Long Term Outcomes in Living Kidney Donors (ALTOLD) study was funded by the National Institutes of Health (NIH) under the cooperative agreement U01 DK066013. The NIH participated in the interpretation of data, writing the report, and the decision to submit the report for publication. This study was also supported by the Minneapolis Medical Research Foundation, Minneapolis, MN, which did not participate in any aspect of the study. The Multi-Ethnic Study of Atherosclerosis (MESA) research was supported by contracts 75N92020D00001, HHSN268201500003I, N01-HC-95159, 75N92020D00005, N01-HC-95160, 75N92020D00002, N01-HC-95161, 75N92020D00003, N01-HC-95162, 75N92020D00006, N01-HC-95163, 75N92020D00004, N01-HC-95164, 75N92020D00007, N01-HC-95165, N01-HC-95166, N01-HC-95167, N01-HC-95168, and N01-HC-95169 from the National Heart, Lung, and Blood Institute, and by grants UL1-TR-000040, UL1-TR-001079, and UL1-TR-001420 from the National Center for Advancing Translational Sciences (NCATS). The authors thank the other investigators, the staff, and the participants of the MESA study for their valuable contributions. A full list of participating MESA investigators and institutions can be found at http://www.mesa-nhlbi.org. The Chronic Kidney Disease in Children (CKiD) study was supported by NIDDK grants U01DK106982, U01DK085689, U01DK103225, and K23DK093556. The Modification of Diet in Renal Disease (MDRD) study received support from NIDDK U01 DK35073. The University of Maryland Baltimore Cirrhosis Cohort project was supported in part by award 5 K23 DK089008-05 from the NIH NIDDK (to ALM), and its contents are solely the responsibility of the authors and do not necessarily represent the official views of the NIDDK or the NIH. The project was also supported in part by the University of Maryland School of Medicine, Department of Medicine funds, University of Maryland Clinical Translational Science Institute, University of Maryland General Clinical Research Center, and NIH Public Health Service grant P30DK056338, which funds the Texas Medical Center Digestive Diseases Center, and its contents are solely the responsibility of the authors and do not necessarily represent the official views of the NIDDK or the NIH.

AUTHOR CONTRIBUTIONS

NFF performed formal analysis, methods, writing (original draft), and writing (review and editing); OMA performed project administration, methods, writing (original draft), and writing (review and editing); JC performed investigation, methods, writing (original draft), and writing (review and editing); TG performed data curation, methods, formal analysis, writing (original draft), and writing (review and editing); BH performed formal analysis, methods, writing (original draft), and writing (review and editing); MGS performed data curation and writing (review and editing); VTCeS performed data curation and writing (review and editing); RK performed data curation and writing (review and editing); ALM performed data curation and writing (review and editing); SLF performed data curation and writing (review and editing); JS performed methods and writing (review and editing); ASL performed data curation, investigation, methods, writing (original draft), and writing (review and editing); LAI performed conceptualization, data curation, funding acquisition, supervision, investigation, methods, writing (original draft), and writing (review and editing).

SUPPLEMENTARY MATERIAL

Supplementary File (Word)
Funding for studies.
Supplementary Methods.
Supplementary Table S1. Descriptions of study populations.
Supplementary Figure S1. Overall process to ultimately develop targeted assay for panel estimated glomerular filtration rate (GFR).
Supplementary Figure S2. Summary of the stepwise procedure to find near-optimal models.
Supplementary Table S2. Summary of overlapping named metabolites in each study.
Supplementary Table S3. Summary of missing metabolite data.
Supplementary Figure S3. Pairwise scatterplots of the 4 components from principal components analysis to evaluate batch effect.
Supplementary Figure S4. Exploration of the imputation of guanidino succinate.
Supplementary Table S4. Summary of all metabolites under consideration and model selection results. All metabolites with correlation <−0.5 with measured glomerular filtration rate (mGFR) are included.
Supplementary Table S5. Multivariable coefficients of the demographic terms for all near-optimal models by metabolite subset size for models with and without untargeted creatinine.
Supplementary Figure S5. Comparison of near-optimal models after inclusion of sex and age only and after inclusion of race, sex, age, and body mass index (BMI).
Supplementary Figure S6. Scatterplots for the 17 selected metabolites and measured glomerular filtration rate (mGFR).
Supplementary Figure S7. Scatterplots with study-wise LOESS curves for the 17 selected metabolites and measured glomerular filtration rate (mGFR).
Supplementary Table S6. Summary of metabolite selection when varying the correlation threshold for metabolite inclusion.
Supplementary Table S7. Characteristics of top metabolites in high-performing models.
Supplementary Figure S8. Root mean square errors (RMSEs) of near-optimal models when varying the correlation threshold for metabolite inclusion.

Supplementary References.
Supplementary File (R Code)
KINT_stepwise_model_code.R

REFERENCES

1. Levey AS, Coresh J, Tighiouart H, et al. Measured and estimated glomerular filtration rate: current status and future directions. *Nat Rev Nephrol*. 2020;16:51–64.
2. Kidney Disease: Improving Global Outcomes (KDIGO) CKD Work Group. KDIGO 2012 clinical practice guideline for the evaluation and management of chronic kidney disease. *Kidney Int Suppl*. 2013;3:1–150.
3. Shafi T, Zhu X, Lirette ST, et al. Quantifying individual-level inaccuracy in glomerular filtration rate estimation: a cross-sectional study. *Ann Intern Med*. 2022;175:1073–1082.
4. Inker LA, Eneanya ND, Coresh J, et al. New creatinine- and cystatin C-based equations to estimate GFR without race. *N Engl J Med*. 2021;385:1737–1749.
5. Levey AS, Stevens LA, Schmid CH, et al. A new equation to estimate glomerular filtration rate. *Ann Intern Med*. 2009;150:604–612.
6. Levey AS, Becker C, Inker LA. Glomerular filtration rate and albuminuria for detection and staging of acute and chronic kidney disease in adults: a systematic review. *JAMA*. 2015;313:837–846.
7. Kervella D, Lemoine S, Sens F, et al. Cystatin C versus creatinine for GFR estimation in CKD due to heart failure. *Am J Kidney Dis*. 2017;69:321–323.
8. Torre A, Aguirre-Valadez JM, Arreola-Guerra JM, et al. Creatinine versus cystatin C for estimating GFR in patients with liver cirrhosis. *Am J Kidney Dis*. 2016;67:342–344.
9. Levey AS, Bosch JP, Lewis JB, et al. A more accurate method to estimate glomerular filtration rate from serum creatinine: a new prediction equation. *Ann Intern Med*. 1999;130:461–470.
10. Coresh J, Inker LA, Sang Y, et al. Metabolomic profiling to improve glomerular filtration rate estimation: a proof-of-concept study. *Nephrol Dial Transplant*. 2019;34:825–833.
11. Freed TA, Coresh J, Inker LA, et al. Validation of a metabolite panel for a more accurate estimation of glomerular filtration rate using quantitative LC-MS/MS. *Clin Chem*. 2019;65:406–418.
12. Inker LA, Couture SJ, Tighiouart H, et al. A new panel-estimated GFR, including beta2-microglobulin and beta-trace protein and not including race, developed in a diverse population. *Am J Kidney Dis*. 2021;77:673–683.e1.
13. Roberts LD, Souza AL, Gerszten RE, Clish CB. Targeted metabolomics. *Curr Protoc Mol Biol*. 2012;98:30.2.1–30.2.24.
14. Wright JT Jr, Bakris G, Greene T, et al. Effect of blood pressure lowering and antihypertensive drug class on progression of hypertensive kidney disease: results from the AASK trial. *JAMA*. 2002;288:2421–2431.
15. Kasiske BL, Anderson-Haag T, Israni AK, et al. A prospective controlled study of living kidney donors: three-year follow-up. *Am J Kidney Dis*. 2015;66:114–124.
16. Costa E Silva VT, Gil LA Jr, Inker LA, et al. A prospective cross-sectional study estimated glomerular filtration rate from creatinine and cystatin C in adults with solid tumors. *Kidney Int*. 2022;101:607–614.
17. Schwartz GJ, Furth SL. Glomerular filtration rate measurement and estimation in chronic kidney disease. *Pediatr Nephrol*. 2007;22:1839–1848.
18. Mindikoglu AL, Opekun AR, Putluri N, et al. Unique metabolomic signature associated with hepatorenal dysfunction and mortality in cirrhosis. *Transl Res*. 2018;195:25–47.
19. Mindikoglu AL, Dowling TC, Magder LS, et al. Estimation of glomerular filtration rate in patients with cirrhosis by using new and conventional filtration markers and dimethylarginines. *Clin Gastroenterol Hepatol*. 2016;14:624–632.e2.
20. Inker LA, Shafi T, Okparavero A, et al. Effects of race and sex on measured GFR: the Multi-Ethnic Study of Atherosclerosis. *Am J Kidney Dis*. 2016;68:743–751.
21. Klahr S, Levey AS, Beck GJ, et al. Modification of Diet in Renal Disease Study Group. The effects of dietary protein restriction and blood-pressure control on the progression of chronic renal disease. *N Engl J Med*. 1994;330:877–884.
22. Inker LA, Levey AS, Tighiouart H, et al. Performance of glomerular filtration rate estimating equations in a community-based sample of Blacks and Whites: the Multiethnic Study of Atherosclerosis. *Nephrol Dial Transplant*. 2018;33:417–425.

23. Han W, Li L. Evaluating and minimizing batch effects in metabolomics. *Mass Spectrom Rev*. 2022;41:421–442.
24. Sekula P, Goek O-N, Quaye L, et al. A metabolome-wide association study of kidney function and disease in the general population. *J Am Soc Nephrol*. 2016;27:1175–1188.
25. Takahira R, Yonemura K, Yonekawa O, et al. Tryptophan glycoconjugate as a novel marker of renal function. *Am J Med*. 2001;110:192–197.
26. Cheng Y, Li Y, Benkowitz P, et al. The relationship between blood metabolites of the tryptophan pathway and kidney function: a bidirectional Mendelian randomization analysis. *Sci Rep*. 2020;10:12675.
27. Gutsche B, Grun C, Scheutzow D, Herderich M. Tryptophan glycoconjugates in food and human urine. *Biochem J*. 1999;343(pt 1):11–19.
28. Sekula P, Dettmer K, Vogl FC, et al. From discovery to translation: characterization of C-mannosyltryptophan and pseudouridine as markers of kidney function. *Sci Rep*. 2017;7:17400.
29. Linster CL, Van Schaftingen E. Vitamin C: biosynthesis, recycling and degradation in mammals. *FEBS J*. 2007;274:1–22.
30. DBGET integrated database retrieval system. KEGG COMPOUND: C00800. Accessed August 3, 2023. https://www.kegg.jp/entry/C00800
31. Hsu C-Y, Yang W, Parikh RV, et al. Race, genetic ancestry, and estimating kidney function in CKD. *N Engl J Med*. 2021;385:1750–1760.
32. Pottel H, Björk J, Rule AD, et al. Cystatin C–based equation to estimate GFR without the inclusion of race and sex. *N Engl J Med*. 2023;388:333–343.
33. Collister D, Saad N, Christie E, Ahmed S. Providing care for transgender persons with kidney disease: a narrative review. *Can J Kidney Health Dis*. 2021;8:2054358120985379.
34. Gandhi P, Medeiros W, Shah AD. Physiology or pathology? elevated serum creatinine in a female-to-male transgender patient. *Am J Kidney Dis*. 2020;75:A13–A14.
35. Whitley CT, Greene DN. Transgender man being evaluated for a kidney transplant. *Clin Chem*. 2017;63:1680–1683.
36. Stevens LA, Claybon MA, Schmid CH, et al. Evaluation of the CKD-EPI equation in multiple races and ethnicities. *Kidney Int*. 2011;79:555.

clinical investigation

Idiopathic collapsing glomerulopathy is associated with *APOL1* high-risk genotypes or Mendelian variants in most affected individuals in a highly admixed population

see commentary on page 437

Precil D. Neves[1,2,3], Andreia Watanabe[2,4], Elieser H. Watanabe[1,2], Amanda M. Narcizo[5], Kelly Nunes[6], Antonio M. Lerario[7], Frederico M. Ferreira[8], Lívia B. Cavalcante[8], Janewit Wongboonsin[9,10], Denise M. Malheiros[8], Lectícia B. Jorge[1], Matthew G. Sampson[9], Irene L. Noronha[1] and Luiz F. Onuchic[1,2]

[1]Division of Nephrology, University of São Paulo School of Medicine, São Paulo, Brazil; [2]Division of Molecular Medicine, University of São Paulo School of Medicine, São Paulo, Brazil; [3]Nephrology and Dialysis Center, Oswaldo Cruz German Hospital, São Paulo, Brazil; [4]Division of Pediatric Nephrology, University of São Paulo School of Medicine, São Paulo, Brazil; [5]Large-Scale Sequencing Laboratory, University of São Paulo School of Medicine, São Paulo, Brazil; [6]Human Genome Center, Institute of Biosciences/University of São Paulo, São Paulo, Brazil; [7]Division of Endocrinology, University of Michigan, Ann Arbor, Michigan, USA; [8]Department of Pathology, University of São Paulo School of Medicine, São Paulo, Brazil; [9]Division of Pediatric Nephrology, Boston Children's Hospital, Boston, Massachusetts, USA; and [10]Division of Nephrology, Department of Medicine, Faculty of Medicine Siriraj Hospital, Mahidol University, Bangkok, Thailand

Collapsing glomerulopathy (CG) is most often associated with fast progression to kidney failure with an incidence apparently higher in Brazil than in other countries. However, the reason for this occurrence is unknown. To better understand this, we performed an integrated analysis of clinical, histological, therapeutic, causative genetic and genetic ancestry data in a highly genetically admixed cohort of 70 children and adult patients with idiopathic CG (ICG). The disease onset occurred at 23 (interquartile range: 17-31) years and approximately half of patients progressed to chronic kidney disease requiring kidney replacement therapy (CKD-KRT) 36 months after diagnosis. Causative genetic bases, assessed by targeted-gene panel or whole-exome sequencing, were identified in 58.6% of patients. Among these cases, 80.5% harbored *APOL1* high-risk genotypes (HRG) and 19.5% causative Mendelian variants (MV). Self-reported non-White patients more frequently had HRG. MV was an independent risk factor for progression to CKD-KRT by 36 months and the end of follow-up, while remission was an independent protective factor. All patients with HRG manifested CG at 9-44 years of age, whereas in those with *APOL1* low-risk genotype, the disease arose throughout life. HRGs were associated with higher proportion of African genetic ancestry. Novel causative MVs were identified in *COL4A5*, *COQ2* and *PLCE1* and previously described causative MVs were identified in *MYH9*, *TRPC6*, *COQ2*, *COL4A3* and *TTC21B*. Three patients displayed HRG combined with a variant of uncertain significance (*ITGB4*, *LAMA5* or *PTPRO*). MVs were associated with worse kidney prognosis. Thus, our data reveal that the genetic status plays a major role in ICG pathogenesis, accounting for more than half of cases in a highly admixed Brazilian population.

Kidney International (2024) **105,** 593–607; https://doi.org/10.1016/j.kint.2023.11.028

KEYWORDS: *APOL1*; collapsing glomerulopathy; genetically admixed population; genetic ancestry; Mendelian variants; nephrotic syndrome

Copyright © 2023, International Society of Nephrology. Published by Elsevier Inc. All rights reserved.

Lay Summary

Collapsing glomerulopathy is a severe kidney disease that often leads to chronic dialysis or kidney transplantation. To expand its understanding, we performed a broad clinical and genetic analysis of a highly admixed patient population with idiopathic collapsing glomerulopathy. Interestingly, we identified a genetic cause in more than half of the 70 evaluated patients. Moreover, in a significant majority of the cases with a genetic form, the disease was associated with the presence of risk variants in both alleles of the *APOL1* gene, which are genetic variants associated with African ethnicity. These patients, in fact, displayed a higher proportion of African genetic ancestry. The other genetic cases occurred due to causative variants in other genes, being classified as Mendelian forms. Mendelian cases had a higher risk of progression to kidney failure, and all patients with 2 *APOL1* risk alleles manifested collapsing glomerulopathy between 9 and 44 years of age.

Correspondence: *Luiz F. Onuchic, Department of Medicine, Divisions of Nephrology and Molecular Medicine, University of São Paulo School of Medicine, Avenida Doutor Arnaldo, 455—Sala 4304, São Paulo SP, 01246-903, Brazil. E-mail: lonuchic@usp.br*

Received 19 April 2023; revised 4 September 2023; accepted 16 November 2023; published online 22 December 2023

Collapsing glomerulopathy (CG) is an entity first described by Weiss *et al.*[1] in 6 patients who presented with nephrotic syndrome (NS) and underwent fast chronic kidney disease progression with requirement of kidney replacement therapy (CKD-KRT). As per the Columbia classification, CG is classified as a histologic subtype of focal segmental glomerulosclerosis (FSGS), whereas other authors recommend it to be classified separately from FSGS, using the term CG.[2,3] A recent study sought to investigate protein signatures through proteomic analysis of the glomerular extracellular matrix that could potentially differentiate CG from other FSGS forms.[4] In support to the concept of a distinct entity, different expression profiles of cathepsins B and C were identified in CG compared with other FSGS subtypes. The available studies addressing CG prevalence, however, were performed in the setting of CG as an FSGS subtype.[5] Interestingly, although most of these studies reported CG as accounting for 4% to 12% of FSGS cases,[5–7] this rate reached up to 36.6% in a Brazilian FSGS population.[8] The most frequent presentation of CG is isolated NS, although in some cases, it may be associated with hematuria and hypertension. Of note, many patients already exhibit significant loss of kidney function upon admission and progress rapidly to CKD-KRT,[9,10] facing a scenario of limited response to immunosuppression.[11–13]

CG is diagnosed through kidney biopsy by identifying at least 1 glomerulus with loop collapse associated with hypertrophy/hyperplasia of podocytes covering the glomerular capillary loops.[2,10,14] In addition, podocytes express dedifferentiation markers in CG compared with FSGS, including Ki-67 and PAX2, and fail to express podocyte maturity markers such as podocin, synaptopodin, and WT1.[10,15] CG has been associated with infections (HIV, HCV, parvovirus B19, COVID-19, *Mycobacterium tuberculosis*, and *Schistosoma mansoni*),[16–18] vaccines (COVID-19),[17] systemic and autoimmune diseases (systemic lupus erythematosus, hematologic malignancies, diabetes mellitus, and sickle cell disease),[19,20] drug use (interferon, anabolic steroids, and bisphosphonates),[21,22] and micro- or macrovascular kidney ischemia.[23] When such secondary causes are not identified upon investigation, CG is defined as idiopathic (ICG).

The predominance of African/African descendant patients in a previous series of CG cases[9] suggested that genetic factors linked to ethnicity might predispose individuals to this nephropathy. In this sense, *APOL1* high-risk genotypes (HRGs) have been recognized as the most prevalent susceptibility factor for the development of CG in African individuals or descendants.[24–26] It is currently proposed that the *APOL1*-HRG–mediated pathogenesis involves a 2-hit mechanism, where *APOL1* HRG functions as the first event, whereas a second hit of a different nature (potentially including infections or/and inflammatory disorders) triggers the kidney disease process.[10,27–30] CG can also occur in patients with pathogenic variants in genes whose products are directly involved in mitochondrial function, such as *COQ2*,[31] *COQ6*,[31] *COQ8B*,[31] and *PDSS2*.[32] These genes encode proteins that belong to the coenzyme Q10 biogenesis pathway, whose deficiency leads to the development of CG. Mutations in the *MYH9*,[33] *TRPC6*,[34,35] *INF2*,[34,36] *NUP93*,[37] *NUP107*,[34] *RNASEH2B*,[38] *TMEM173*,[39] *SCARB2*,[40] and *MSH6*[41] genes have also been associated with CG.

The assessment of CG pathogenesis, clinical features, and treatment, however, has currently been limited by the lack of studies including large numbers of CG cases as well as addressing specific CG issues. A number of questions, therefore, remain unclear. It is currently unknown how frequently CG is associated with *APOL1* HRG and Mendelian pathogenic variants and how it is distributed throughout life. Along this line, it is unclear how *APOL1*-associated and Mendelian forms of CG are distributed throughout different age ranges. Moreover, we do not know if and how a non-African genetic background impacts the *APOL1* HRG effect. To address these fundamental points, we performed the current study to evaluate molecular-genetic, clinical, and histologic parameters in a large, highly admixed Brazilian population of adult and pediatric patients diagnosed with ICG.

METHODS
Study design and approval
Adult and pediatric patients with histologic diagnosis of CG established by kidney biopsy were initially selected and screened for potential secondary causes of this disorder based on clinical evaluation and complementary tests. Those with negative assessment were classified as ICG cases and initially included in this retrospective cohort. These patients were then submitted to comprehensive demographic, clinical, laboratory, and therapeutic responsiveness characterization. Therapeutic response was assessed based on the course of proteinuria and estimated glomerular filtration rate (eGFR). As per the 2021 Kidney Disease: Improving Global Outcomes (KDIGO) on glomerular diseases,[42] a reduction in proteinuria by 50% or more from baseline, however without reaching normal levels, was considered partial remission, whereas full return to the normal range was deemed as complete remission. Progression to CKD-KRT was the primary analyzed outcome, whereas the secondary outcomes comprised time to reach CKD-KRT, response to therapy—categorized into partial remission, complete remission, or no response—and development of CG in the graft. All kidney biopsies were evaluated by specialized renal pathologists.

The study was approved by the ethics committee of Hospital das Clínicas da Faculdade de Medicina da Universidade de São Paulo under the numbers CAAE 17279219.8.0000.0068 for the adult patients and CAAE 70756317.7.0000.0068 for the pediatric patients.

Molecular genetics evaluation
DNA was extracted from peripheral blood using the QIAamp DNA Blood Mini Kit (Qiagen). Samples were submitted to target sequencing using 2 customized gene panels or to whole-exome sequencing (WES). The first customized gene panel was assembled to capture 845 target regions including all exons of 42 genes associated with NS (*ACTN4, ADCK4, ARHGDIA, NPHS2, CD2AP, COQ2, CRB2, CUBN, DGKE, EMP2, EYA1, COQ6, FAT1, INF2, ITGA3, ITGB4, KANK1, KANK2, KANK4, LAMB2, LMX1B, MYO1E, NPHS1, PAX2, PDSS2, PLCE1, PODXL, PTPRO, SCARB2, SMARCAL1, TRPC6, TTC21B, WDR73, WT1, XPO5, APOL1, ARHGAP24, MEFV, NXF5, NUP107, NUP205,* and *NUP93*), with a mean coverage >99%. DNA libraries were prepared applying the Nextera Rapid Capture enrichment protocol (Illumina) following the manufacturer's instructions.

The second customized gene panel was designed to generate 579 target regions of 20 genes related to glomerulopathies and/or NS (*NEIL1, COL4A3, COL4A4, COL4A5, CFH, CFI, CD46, C3, CFHR5, ADAMTS13, FN1, MCP1, ANLN, MYH9, MAGI2, TNS2, DLC1, CDK20, ITSN1,* and *ITSN2*), also with a mean coverage >99%. In this case, DNA libraries were prepared using the Ampliseq protocol (Illumina) according to the manufacturer's orientations. The MiSeq platform (Illumina) was used to sequence the targeted regions. This task was carried out using the MiSeq Reagent Kit v2 as dual index and paired-end runs (2 × 150 cycles for Nextera Rapid Capture enrichment and 2 × 250 cycles for Ampliseq).

WES was performed using 2 protocols. In the first one, DNA libraries were prepared on the Nextera Exome Rapid Capture enrichment protocol (Illumina). In this case, sequencing was performed in the NextSeq500 platform (Illumina) as dual index and paired-end runs (2 × 150 cycles) using the NextSeq High-Output Kit. In the second protocol, DNA libraries were prepared with a customized Illumina kit (Illumina) developed for the Mendelics Genomic Analysis facility (Mendelics). This approach included approximately 33 MB of targeted regions, coverage of at least 95% of targeted regions with ≥10 reads of horizontal coverage, and 100× mean depth. Each allele of the target regions located in autosomes in all patients and in X chromosomes in women was therefore represented in approximately 50% of the reads. Nova Seq 6000 (Illumina) was used for targeted gene enrichment and sequencing.

The generated sequencing reads were aligned to the human reference genome GRCh37/hg19 using the Burrows-Wheeler Aligner (BWA-MEM aligner, GNU General Public License version 0.7.17; MIT License) and screened for duplicate reads with the Biobambam tool. Variant calling was performed with FreeBayes and the resulting variant call formats were annotated with the ANNOVAR software package (http://annovar.openbioinformatics.org).[43] To warrant similar variant analysis in all cases, the patients submitted to WES were analyzed for the same genes included in the 2 customized gene panels.

Assessment of variant pathogenicity

The resulting data were filtered targeting variants with at least 10 reads and with low frequency (≤0.1% according to the American College of Medical Genetics and Genomics [ACMG] guidelines) in control populations (gnomAD [https://gnomad.broadinstitute.org/], AbraOM [https://abraom.ib.usp.br/], and SELAdb [http://intranet.fm.usp.br/sela/]). It must be noted that AbraOM and SELAdb are Brazilian databases generated for populations of the São Paulo state, Brazil, which represent the background population of the current study. All but 2 patients, in fact, live/lived in the São Paulo state. The variants were ranked thereafter according to their pathogenicity potential. Stop-gain, splice-site disrupting, and frameshift variants were initially considered, since they are related to potential loss of function. Prediction of pathogenicity of missense variants was based on multiple *in silico* programs, including PolyPhen2, Mutation Assessor, SIFT, and PROVEAN. The assessed variants had their sequencing reads visually inspected using Integrative Genomics Viewer. Sanger sequencing was performed to confirm the potential causative variants, to proceed with segregation analysis when parental DNA was available, and to confirm *APOL1* G1 and/or G2 variants.

Pathogenicity of potentially causative variants was assessed applying the ACMG criteria.[44] Variants of uncertain significance (VUSs) in *COQ2* (coenzyme Q2), associated with high pathogenicity scores predicted by *in silico* programs and phenotypes strongly correlated with the mutated gene, were submitted to additional molecular mechanics evaluation to significantly strengthen the assessment of pathogenicity. This analysis was included in a recently submitted manuscript from our group, which strongly supported pathogenicity for both VUSs.[45]

ACMG-based pathogenic and likely pathogenic variants as well as the *COQ2* VUSs were considered causative for the disease. Segregation was analyzed in all pedigrees with available structure and information. All monogenic variants and *APOL1*-HRG genotyping were confirmed by Sanger sequencing.

Evaluation of genetic ancestry

All patients were genotyped with a specifically designed high-density single nucleotide polymorphism (SNP) array (Infinium Global Screening Array version 3.0; Illumina) to ascertain the individual genetic ancestry. The data were cleaned and filtered according to the manufacturer's recommendations using the GWASTools pipeline.[46] Relatedness analyses of the genetic data were performed using the methodology contained in the R SNPRelate package.[47] Runs of homozygosity were performed with PLINK[48] using a sliding window with 50 SNPs. A maximum of 1 heterozygous genotype and 5 missing calls were allowed per window, whereas a series of overlapping windows were used to form a homozygous genomic segment of 5%. A density of at least 1 SNP per 50 kb was employed, with a maximum gap of 100 kb between consecutive SNPs. Homozygosity-based inbreeding coefficient (FROH) was inferred according to the approach by McQuillan *et al.*[49] Analyses of genomic ancestry average were performed using the ADMIXTURE program version 1.3[50] through supervised analysis with K = 4 and 2000 bootstrap replicates, windows of 50 kb and step size of 10 kb, and LD r2 threshold of 0.1. We used Africans, Europeans, East Asians, and Native Americans as parental populations, anchored on samples from the Human Genome Diversity Panel–Centre d'Étude du Polymorphisme Humain.[51] Of note, only parental samples with more than 95% ancestry of their population group were included in this genome diversity panel.

Statistical analyses

We used the D'Agostino-Pearson Omnibus and Shapiro-Wilk tests to evaluate variable distribution. Because almost all variables presented nonparametric distribution, continuous variables are expressed as median (interquartile range). Parametric data were compared using the Student *t* test when in 2 groups and analysis of variance when in 3 or more groups. When variances (analyzed by the Levene test) were significantly different between the groups, the Welch correction was applied. Post-test analyses were performed using the Tukey HSD (honestly significant difference) test. Nonparametric data were compared using the Mann-Whitney *U* test for 2 groups and the Kruskal-Wallis test for 3 or more groups. Post-test analyses were carried out using the Dunn test. Comparisons involving nominal variables were performed using the Fisher exact test for variables with 2 categories or the χ^2 test when 1 or more of the variables had more than 2 categories. For these cases, the standardized and adjusted residuals were calculated for each cell, and "p" was obtained and then corrected with the Benjamini-Hochberg method. The Pearson test for parametric data and the Spearman test for nonparametric data were used for correlation analyses. Comparative analyses of kidney survival over time were performed using Kaplan-Meyer curves, log-rank test for univariable analysis, and Cox regression for multivariable analyses. *P* values < 0.05 were considered statistically significant, and in the case of multiple comparisons,

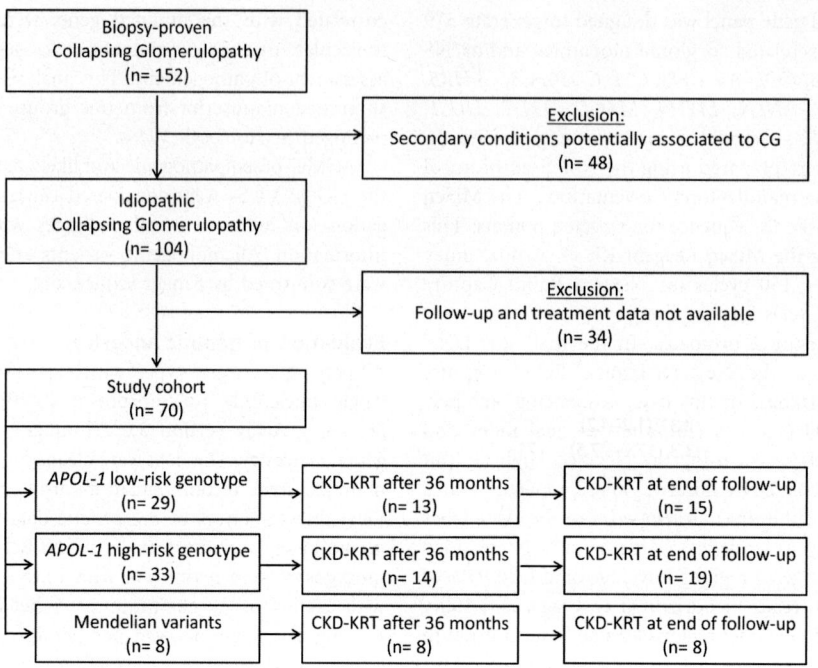

Figure 1 | Study flowchart. A total of 70 patients diagnosed with idiopathic collapsing glomerulopathy were eligible for the study and were submitted to molecular genetic analysis. CG, collapsing glomerulopathy; CKD-KRT, chronic kidney disease with need of kidney replacement therapy.

$q < 0.05$. All analyses were performed using GraphPad Prism version 8.00 (GraphPad Software) and SPSS 25.0 (SPSS Inc.).

RESULTS

Demographic, clinical, laboratorial, and histologic characterization of the patient population

From a total of 152 patients with histologic diagnosis of CG, 70 classified as ICG were eligible after applying the exclusion criteria (Figure 1). The most recent case manifested the disease in January 2019, indicating that the analyzed cohort predated the COVID-19 pandemic. This observation allows the exclusion of SARS-CoV-2 as the etiology of CG in our cohort, strengthening the diagnoses as idiopathic. The median follow-up time was 27.0 (11.5–36.5) months. Sex distribution was essentially even (52.9% male); the median age at disease onset was 23 (17–31) years, with higher prevalence in adults (74.3%); most patients self-reported as White (64.3%); family history of kidney disease was reported by 22.9% of patients (16 of 70, Supplementary Table S1) and consanguinity by 5.7%. The patients already had kidney dysfunction on kidney biopsy, characterized by an eGFR of 56.1 (31.2–108.4) ml/min per 1.73 m^2, in addition to high proteinuria (6.85 [4.22–10.69] g/24 h) and hypoalbuminemia (2.10 [1.50–3.10] g/dl; Table 1). Most patients were treated with glucocorticoids (90%) and calcineurin inhibitors (62.9%), whereas steroid resistance was observed in 85.7%. The median eGFR decline was 28.4 (7.3–56.8) ml/min per 1.73 m^2/yr, and remission was absent in 57% of the cases. Approximately half (51.4%) of patients progressed to CKD-KRT by 36 months after diagnosis, and 71.4% by the end of follow-up.

Close to 40% received a kidney transplant, and 15.4% of them developed CG in the kidney graft.

Patients who progressed to CKD-KRT within 36 months of diagnosis were younger than patients who did not (21.0 [16.2–26.0] vs. 27.0 [18.8–37.8] years, $P = 0.021$) and had higher serum creatinine ($P = 0.006$) at diagnosis, reflected by lower eGFR (43.3 [17.9–77.5] vs. 71.7 [51.5–120.7] ml/min per 1.73 m^2, $P = 0.005$; Table 1). Along these lines, they also showed a higher percentage of glomeruli with synechiae (25% [11%–50%] vs. 10% [0%–25%], $P = 0.045$) and sclerotic glomeruli (17.6% [0.0%–42.2%] vs. 0.0% [0.0%–11.5%], $P = 0.023$) on kidney biopsy. Interestingly, calcineurin inhibitor was less often used in patients who progressed to CKD-KRT by 36 months (44.0% vs. 82.4%, $P = 0.001$) and these patients were less likely to achieve partial remission (13.9% vs. 52.9%, $P = 0.001$).

Progression to CKD-KRT by the end of follow-up occurred more often among patients with worse kidney function at diagnosis (eGFR of 47.4 [25.4–83.9] vs. 85.4 [52.6–112.1] ml/min per 1.73 m^2, $P = 0.022$; Table 1). As expected, patients who progressed to KRT tended to have more extensive tubulointerstitial fibrosis/tubular atrophy. Such patients also used less angiotensin-converting enzyme inhibitors/angiotensin receptor blockers (74% vs. 100%, $P = 0.014$). Moreover, having any type of remission was associated with a lower risk of progression to CKD-KRT ($P < 0.001$).

Most patients with ICG have an identifiable genetic basis and approximately half of them harbor an *APOL1* HRG

Mendelian or susceptibility genotypes associated with CG were identified in 41 patients (58.6%): HRG in 33 (80.5% of

Table 1 | Clinical, laboratory, and histologic profiles of patients with ICG who progressed or not progressed to CKD-KRT up to 36 months after biopsy and to the end of follow-up; patients who progressed to CKD-KRT within 36 months of diagnosis were younger than those who did not

	36 months after biopsy			End of follow-up			
	CKD-KRT (n = 36)	No CKD-KRT (n = 34)	P value	CKD-KRT (n = 50)	No CKD-KRT (n = 20)	P value	Total (n = 70)
Age, yr	21 (16.2–26.0)	27 (18.8–37.8)	**0.021**	23 (17–31)	27 (19–34)	0.214	23 (17–31)
Male, n (%)	22 (61.1)	15 (44.1)	0.231	28 (56)	9 (45)	0.438	37 (52.9)
Self-declared ethnicity, n (%)			0.326			1.000	
White	21 (58.3)	24 (70.6)		32 (64)	13 (65)		45 (64.3)
Non-White	15 (41.7)	10 (29.4)		18 (36)	7 (35)		25 (35.7)
Family history of kidney disease, n (%)	9 (25.0)	7 (20.6)	0.778	13 (26)	3 (15)	0.529	16 (22.9)
Consanguinity, n (%)	1 (2.8)	3 (8.8)	0.350	4 (8)	0 (0)	0.319	4 (5.7)
Laboratory tests at kidney biopsy							
Creatinine, mg/dl	2.31 (1.2–4.2)	1.22 (0.78–1.55)	**0.006**	1.57 (1.20–3.00)	1.10 (0.77–1.37)	**0.018**	1.39 (0.80–2.60)
eGFR, ml/min per 1.73 m^2	43.3 (17.9–77.5)	71.7 (51.5–120.7)	**0.005**	47.4 (25.4–83.9)	85.4 (52.6–112.1)	**0.022**	56.1 (31.2–108.4)
Albumin, g/dl	2.05 (1.57–3.12)	2.30 (1.50–3.02)	0.931	2.10 (1.50–3.00)	2.30 (1.55–3.25)	0.518	2.10 (1.50–3.10)
Proteinuria, g/d	7.2 (4.6–11.5)	6.6 (4.2–10.7)	0.621	6.50 (4.40–16.41)	7.13 (4.1–10.7)	0.904	6.85 (4.22–10.69)
Hematuria, n (%)	19 (54.3)	12 (37.5)	0.222	24 (48)	7 (35)	0.289	31 (44.3)
Hypertension, n (%)	26 (74.3)	23 (71.9)	1.000	35 (70)	14 (70)	1.000	49 (70)
Kidney biopsy findings							
Glomerular compartment							
Mesangial hypercellularity, n (%)	20 (55.5)	13 (38.2)	0.145	24 (48)	9 (45)	0.793	33 (48.5)
Mesangial matrix expansion, n (%)	27 (75)	26 (76.5)	1.000	37 (74)	17 (85)	0.532	54 (79.4)
Segmental sclerosis with synechiae, %	25 (11–50)	10 (0–25)	**0.045**	25 (10–35)	10 (0–28.3)	0.242	13 (0–29.6)
Global sclerosis, %	17.6 (0–42.2)	0 (0–11.5)	**0.023**	8.35 (0–32.5)	2.5 (0–17.3)	0.221	5 (0–20.7)
Tubulointerstitial compartment, n (%)							
Interstitial fibrosis/tubular atrophy			0.271			0.050	
Absent	3 (8.3)	6 (17.6)		5 (10)	5 (25)		10 (14.3)
<25%	14 (38.8)	17 (50)		19 (38)	12 (60)		31 (44.3)
25%–50%	9 (25)	7 (20.6)		13 (26)	2 (10)		15 (21.4)
>50%	10 (27.9)	4 (11.8)		13 (26)	1 (5)		14 (20)
Microcystic tubular dilatation	28 (77.7)	23 (67.6)	0.262	36 (72)	15 (75)	0.992	51 (72.8)
Vascular compartment, n (%)							
Arteriolar hyalinosis	7 (19.4)	9 (26.5)	0.576	10 (20)	6 (30)	0.532	16 (22.8)
Intimal thickening	14 (38.9)	12 (35.3)	0.803	16 (32)	10 (50)	0.274	26 (37.1)
Arteriolosclerosis	5 (13.8)	2 (5.9)	0.411	4 (8)	3 (15)	0.411	7 (10)
Treatment, n (%)							
ACEi/ARB	26 (72.2)	31 (91.2)	0.064	37 (74)	20 (100)	**0.014**	57 (81.4)
Glucocorticoids	30 (85.7)	33 (97.1)	0.198	44 (88)	19 (95)	0.664	63 (90)
Calcineurin inhibitor	16 (44.4)	28 (82.4)	**0.001**	29 (58)	15 (75)	0.274	44 (62.9)
Cyclophosphamide	2 (5.9)	5 (13.9)	0.430	5 (10)	2 (10)	1.000	7 (10)
Mycophenolate mofetil	7 (19.4)	6 (17.6)	1.000	10 (20)	3 (15)	0.744	13 (18.6)
Rituximab	2 (5.6)	3 (8.8)	0.669	3 (6)	2 (10)	0.619	5 (7.1)
Steroid resistance, n/N (%)	28/30 (93.3)	26/33 (78.8)	0.152	40/44 (90.9)	14/19 (73.7)	0.114	54/63 (85.7)
Remission, n (%)							
Any	7 (20)	24 (70.5)	**<0.001**	14 (28)	17 (85)	**<0.001**	8 (11.4)
Complete	2 (5.6)	6 (17.6)	0.145	2 (4)	6 (30)	**0.005**	23 (32.9)
Partial	5 (13.9)	18 (52.9)	**0.001**	12 (24)	11 (55)	**0.023**	39 (55.7)
ΔeGFR-CKD-EPI/yr, ml/min per 1.73 m^2	−28.44 (−56.81; −7.30)	−20.8 (−55.1; −7.1)	0.145	−22.6 (−76.7; −7.3)	−34.7 (−56.9; 13.5)	0.681	−28.44 (−56.8; −7.30)

ACEi, angiotensin-converting enzyme inhibitors; ARB, angiotensin receptor blockers; CKD-KRT, chronic kidney disease with need of kidney replacement therapy; eGFR-CKD-EPI, estimated glomerular filtration rate by Chronic Kidney Disease-Epidemiology Collaboration equation; ICG, idiopathic collapsing glomerulopathy.
Continuous data are expressed as median (interquartile range). Bold data indicate statistical significance ($P < 0.05$).

these cases) and causative Mendelian variants (MVs) in 8 (19.5%; Figure 2a). Among the 33 patients with HRG, 18 displayed the G1/G1 genotype (54.5%), 13 G1/G2 (39.4%), and 2 G2/G2 (6.1%). Nine patients harbored only 1 *APOL1* risk allele (12.9% of all patients), whereas 19 presented the G0/G0 genotype (27.1%), which together constituted the *APOL1* low-risk genotype (LRG) group.

Patients with HRG self-declared non-White and reported family history of kidney disease more often than LRG individuals (57.6% vs. 17.2%, $P = 0.002$, and 36.4% vs. 10.6%, $P = 0.02$, respectively; Supplementary Table S2). No significant differences in laboratory tests were detected, whereas intimal thickening was lower in HRG compared with LRG (25.8% vs. 55.2%, $P = 0.034$). Patients with HRG were less often treated with

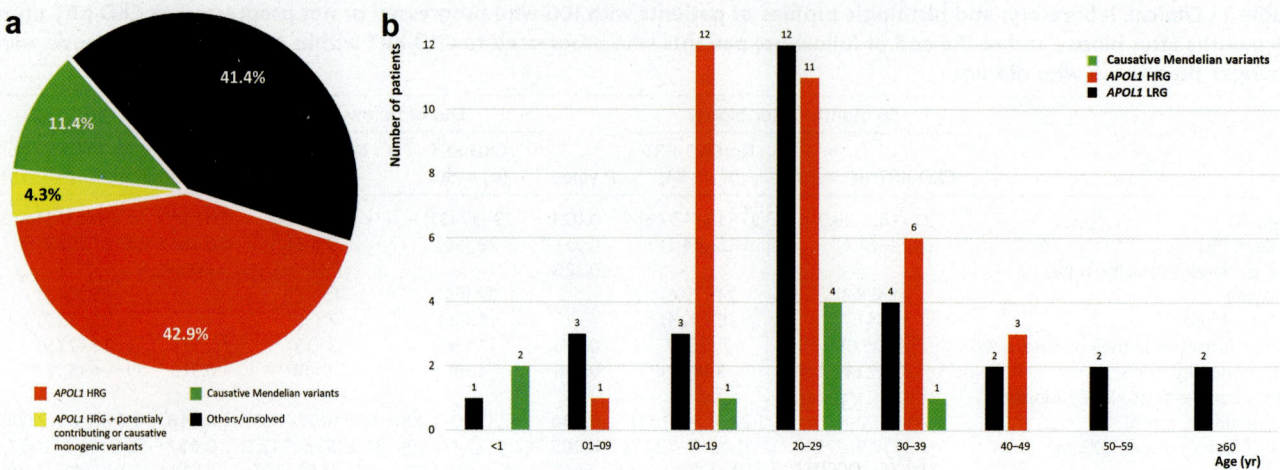

Figure 2 | Most patients of the ICG cohort displayed causative genetic findings. (**a**) Percent distribution of genetic findings. (**b**) Age distribution of patients with *APOL1* HRG, Mendelian variants, or *APOL1* LRG. HRG, high-risk genotype; ICG, idiopathic collapsing glomerulopathy; LRG, low-risk genotype.

cyclophosphamide (3.0% vs. 20.7%, $P = 0.044$) and rituximab (0% vs. 17.2%, $P = 0.018$), whereas the HRG and LRG groups did not differ with respect to therapeutic response, progression to CKD-KRT, and post-transplant development of CG.

A remarkable finding was that although individuals with LRG manifested the disease across all ages, all patients with HRG had the CG onset within the 9 to 44–year range (Figure 2b). Although the age of patients with HRG was expressed as median (interquartile range) because a nonparametric test was used for comparison with other groups with nonparametric age distributions, in the HRG group, age displayed a parametric distribution, yielding a 2-SD interval of 4.3–43.5 years. This profile contrasts with the age distribution of the LRG group, which is not normal and includes a substantial number of patients in the age extremes. Our data support, therefore, that HRG-associated CG rarely occurs in younger children and older adults and leads to an odds ratio: 14.4 (95% confidence interval [CI]: 1.69–122.41; $P = 0.003$) of a patient with HRG with CG to manifest the disease between the second decade and the middle of the fifth decade compared with a patient with LRG.

APOL1 HRG is found in different ancestry backgrounds in Brazilian patients with ICG

The high genetic admixture of the Brazilian population allowed us to investigate the genetic backgrounds in which HRGs occurred in patients with ICG. Although our systematic assessment revealed an overall mean African genetic ancestry of 35%, 54% European, 10% Native American, and 1% Eastern Asian, the proportions of each of the first 3 components displayed a wide variation among the patients (Figure 3). Interestingly, the correlation of the proportions of European and African genetic ancestries between self-reported White and non-White patients was weak ($r^2 = 0.16$).

Notably, the fraction of African genetic ancestry in our cohort was higher than the ones described in previous studies performed in populations from other Brazilian regions, except for those identified in remaining Brazilian hinterland settlements founded by people of African origin (quilombo) groups and in the city of Salvador (Supplementary Table S3). As expected, the HRG subgroup had a higher proportion of African ancestry than the G0/G0 subgroup (Supplementary Figure S1A). Comparisons between G1/G1 versus G0/any

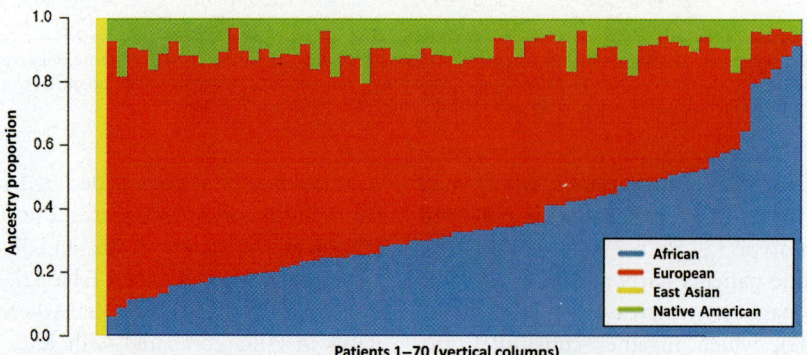

Figure 3 | The ICG cohort patient population is highly genetically admixed. Bar plot of genetic ancestry inference for each patient of the cohort. ICG, idiopathic collapsing glomerulopathy.

risk allele and between G2/G2 versus G0/any risk allele also revealed different proportions (Supplementary Figure S1B).

The relative frequency of CG Mendelian forms was similar among adults and children
Despite the high frequency of adults in our ICG cohort (74.3%), causative MVs were identified in 8 patients (11.4%), 6 of them being adult (11.5% of all adult cases) and 2 pediatric (11.1% of all pediatric cases). Most of these patients self-declared as White (7 of 8, 87.5%). Six of the 7 cases treated with glucocorticoids were steroid-resistant (85.7%), 4 of whom did not show any remission (57.1%). All 8 patients with causative MVs progressed to CKD-KRT by the end of follow-up (Tables 2 and 3).

The most frequent causative MVs occurred in genes encoding collagen IV chains: 2 variants in *COL4A5* accounting for 2 cases and 2 variants in *COL4A3* accounting for 1 case (Tables 2 and 3). Causative MVs were also identified in *TRPC6* (heterozygosity), *MYH9* (heterozygosity), *TTC21B* (homozygosity), *COQ2* (compound heterozygosity), and *PLCE1* (homozygosity; Tables 2 and 3). Of note, pathogenic variants in the *MYH9*, *TRPC6*, and *COQ2* have already been associated with CG.[33,52] Two of the causative MVs are novel (both in *COL4A5*), while pathogenicity analyses—including *in silico* molecular mechanics assessment—of the 2 variants in *COQ2* and the variant in *PLCE1*, recently reported in a submitted manuscript of our group,[45] strongly supported pathogenicity for these 3 VUSs. The c.1147T>C:p.Phe383Leu variant in *COQ2* has been previously reported.[53] Allele segregation analyses were performed for patients with variants in *COL4A5*, *COQ2*, *MYH9*, and *PLCE1*. A comprehensive characterization of the identified causative variants, including frequencies, pathogenicity analyses, and available information, is depicted in Tables 2 and 3.

Harboring a Mendelian variant increased while achieving remission reduced the risk of progression to CKD-KRT
Patients self-reported as non-White more often harbored HRG (57.6% vs. 17.2% in LRG vs. 12.5% in MV, $P = 0.001$) and reported more frequently family history of kidney disease (36.4% vs. 10.3% vs. 12.5%, respectively; $P = 0.039$; Table 4). The 3 groups did not differ regarding laboratory tests at diagnosis. Patients with LRG were more often treated with cyclophosphamide and rituximab than individuals with HRG and MV ($P = 0.042$ and $P = 0.022$, respectively). Of note, a higher percentage of patients with LRG presented intimal proliferation as a histologic finding than the HRG and MV groups (55.2% vs. 25.8% vs. 25.0%, respectively; $P = 0.046$).

Three patients with HRG also harbored VUSs in *ITGB4* (homozygosity), *LAMA5* (compound heterozygosity), or *PTPRO* (compound heterozygosity; Tables 5 and 6). To rule out potential interference of such VUSs in the analyses performed for the HRG group, we also ran the analyses excluding the 3 HRG+VUS cases from the HRG group (30 patients). One patient with LRG also harbored a VUS in the *MAGI2* gene (Tables 5 and 6). Although a possible causative role for this VUS cannot be excluded, the ACMG-based prediction was not sufficiently strong to suggest a pathogenic effect. A comprehensive characterization of the *ITGB4*, *LAMA5*, *PTPRO*, and *MAGI2* variants, including frequencies, pathogenicity analyses, segregation analyses, and additional information, is presented in Tables 5 and 6. To also rule out a potential influence of this VUS in the analyses conducted with the LRG group, we removed this patient from the LRG group (28 patients) when we compared it with the HRG group without the HRG+VUS cases. Analyses including the HRG and LRG groups without associated VUS led to similar results, confirming a higher prevalence of HRG in self-declared non-White than White patients (53.3% vs. 17.9%, $P = 0.007$) and a higher rate of reported family history of kidney disease in patients with HRG compared with those with LRG (36.7% vs. 10.6%, $P = 0.031$). When comparing the 3 groups in this context, patients self-reported as non-White remained more often harboring HRG (53.3% vs. 17.9% in LRG vs. 12.5% in MV, $P = 0.007$) and more frequently reporting family history of kidney disease (36.7% vs. 10.7% vs. 12.5%, respectively; $P = 0.047$). The 3 groups remained not differing regarding laboratory tests at diagnosis. Two patients with LRG and 2 patients with MV developed CG in the kidney graft, of whom 3 had the respective donors genotyped for *APOL1*. In all 3 cases, 1 patient with LRG and 2 patients with MV, the donors harbored the G0/G0 genotype.

Multivariable analysis using Cox regression revealed that older age (hazard ratio [HR]: 0.961, 95% CI: 0.927–0.996; $P = 0.029$) and achieving any type of remission (HR: 0.230, 95% CI: 0.085–0.623, $P = 0.004$) were protective factors against progression to CKD-KRT by 36 months after diagnosis, whereas having an MV increased the risk of progression to CKD-KRT (HR: 2.583, 95% CI: 1.151–7.076; $P = 0.024$). When this analysis was performed for the entire follow-up, achieving any type of remission was also identified as a protective factor against progression to CKD-KRT (HR: 0.155, 95% CI: 0.069–0.351; $P \leq 0.001$), whereas harboring an MV was also a risk factor for reaching CKD-KRT (HR: 2.355, 95% CI: 1.018–5.447; $P = 0.045$; Table 7). Similar conclusions were obtained when using the HRG and LRG groups without an associated VUS. A negative impact of MVs on renal survival can also be observed by using the generated Kaplan-Meier curve and analysis ($P = 0.042$, log-rank test; Figure 4). Interestingly, the Cox regression analyses by 36 months and by the end of the follow-up showed statistically nonsignificant lower risks of patients with HRG to reach CKD-KRT compared with patients with LRG (Table 7). This apparent contrast with a lower renal survival observed for patients with HRG in the Kaplan-Meier plot at the end of the follow-up was caused by a higher proportional loss of follow-up of CKD-KRT–free patients in the HRG compared with the LRG group.

Table 2 | Characterization of causative Mendelian variants according to the ACMG criteria for pathogenicity

Pt	Gene	Inheritance pattern	Variant	Chromosomal position (hg38)	Zygosity	Segregation analysis	gnomAD frequency	ACMG pathogenicity criteria for classification of genetic variants	Variant classification according to the ACMG criteria	APOL1 genotype
1[a]	COL4A5 (NM_033380.3)	X-linked	c.4359delT:p.(Pro1453fs)	X:108687543	Hetero	Mother Het/father neg	—	PVS1, PM2, PP4	Pathogenic	G0/G0
2	COL4A5 (NM_033380.3)	X-linked	c.1033-2A>G	X:108586613	Hemi	Mother neg/father neg	—	PSV1, PM2, PM6, PP3	Pathogenic	G0/G0
3	COL4A3 (NM_000091.5)	AD/AR	c.4421T>C:p.(Leu1474Pro) c.1354G>A:p.(Gly452Arg)	2:227307878 2:227266455	Hetero Hetero	Not performed Not performed	0.27%	PM1, PM2, PP2, PP3, PP5 PM1, PP2, PP3	Likely pathogenic VUS	G0/G0
4	TRPC6 (NM_004621.6)	AD	c.643C>T:p.(Arg215Trp)	11:101504326	Hetero	Not performed	0.002%	PM2, PM5, PP3, PP5	Likely pathogenic	G0/G0
5	MYH9 (NM_002473.6)	AD	c.287C>T:p.(Ser96Leu)	22:36348950	Hetero	Mother neg/father neg	—	PM2, PM6, PP3, PP4, PP5	Likely pathogenic	G0/G0
6[a]	TTC21B (NM_024753.5)	AR	c.626C>T:p.(Pro209Leu)	2:165941111	Homo	Not performed	0.01%	PS3, PM2, PP3, PP5	Likely pathogenic	G0/G0
7	COQ2 (NM_001358921.2)	AR	c.424C>G:p.(Pro142Ala) c.1147T>C:p.(Phe383Leu)	4:83279094 4:83264318	Hetero Hetero	Mother Het/father NA Mother neg/father NA	— 0.009%	PM2, PP3, PP4 PM2, PP3, PP4	VUS VUS	G0/G0
8	PLCE1 (NM_016341.4)	AR	c.3698T>C:p.(Leu1233Pro)	10:94259034	Homo	Mother Het/father Het	—	PM2, PP3, PP4	VUS	G0/G0

ACMG, American College of Medical Genetics and Genomics; AD, autosomal dominant; AR, autosomal recessive; Hetero, heterozygosis; Hemi, hemizygosis; Homo, homozygosis; ICG, idiopathic collapsing glomerulopathy; NA, not analyzed; neg, negative; Pt, patient; VUS, variant of uncertain significance.
[a]Patients who also presented the heterozygous p.Arg229Gln variant in NPHS2.
The identified Mendelian forms of ICG included AD, AR, and X-linked inheritance patterns.

Table 3 | Clinical profile and treatment response of patients with ICG who harbored causative Mendelian variants

Pt	Gene	Inheritance pattern	Variant	Zygosity	Age at diagnosis	Self-declared ethnicity	Response to glucocorticoids	Remission	Progression to CKD-KRT	Time to CKD-KRT, mo	APOL1 genotype
1[a]	COL4A5 (NM_033380.3)	X-linked	c.4359delT:p.(Pro1453fs)	Hetero	29 yr	White	Resistant	Partial	Yes	34	G0/G0
2	COL4A5 (NM_033380.3)	X-linked	c.1033-2A>G	Hemi	21 yr	Non-White	Resistant	Absent	Yes	27	G0/G0
3	COL4A3 (NM_000091.5)	AD/AR	c.4421T>C:p.(Leu1474Pro) c.1354G>A:p.(Gly452Arg)	Hetero Hetero	23 yr	White	Not treated	Not treated	Yes	3	G0/G0
4	TRPC6 (NM_004621.6)	AD	c.643C>T:p.(Arg215Trp)	Hetero	33 yr	White	Resistant	Partial	Yes	31	G0/G0
5	MYH9 (NM_002473.6)	AD	c.287C>T:p.(Ser96Leu)	Hetero	19 yr	White	Resistant	Absent	Yes	33	G0/G0
6[a]	TTC21B (NM_024753.5)	AR	c.626C>T:p.(Pro209Leu)	Homo	24 yr	White	Resistant	Absent	Yes	3	G0/G0
7	COQ2 (NM_001358921.2)	AR	c.424C>G:p.(Pro142Ala) c.1147T>C:p.(Phe383Leu)	Hetero Hetero	3 mo	White	Resistant	Absent	Yes	18	G0/G0
8	PLCE1 (NM_016341.4)	AR	c.3698T>C:p.(Leu1233Pro)	Homo	5 mo	White	Resistant	Absent	Yes	3	G0/G0

AD, autosomal dominant; AR, autosomal recessive; CKD-KRT, chronic kidney disease with need of kidney replacement therapy; Hemi, hemizygosis; Hetero, heterozygosis; Homo, homozygosis; ICG, idiopathic collapsing glomerulopathy; Pt, patient.
All patients progressed to CKD-KRT by the end of the follow-up.
[a]Patients who also presented the heterozygous p.Arg229Gln variant in NPHS2.

DISCUSSION

The pathogenesis of CG is yet largely unclear, although isolated or combined pathogenic contributions of genetic, immunologic, mitochondrial, and exogenous-drug nature have been well described.[9,10,18] Although the kidney histologic and cellular patterns of this podocytopathy have also been well defined, including significant hypertrophy, proliferation and dedifferentiation of podocytes, and loss of cell maturation markers,[9,10,14] associated genetic findings have been reported only in subanalyses of small-sample studies or case reports. In fact, to date, no study has focused on correlation analyses among genetic, clinical, histologic, and therapeutic response findings in CG based on appropriately sample-sized studies.

The reason why the relative frequency of CG in Brazil, and likely its prevalence, is apparently strikingly higher than the rates observed in studies from other countries, employing the Columbia classification,[2] is yet unknown. An attractive hypothesis relies on the 2-hit hypothesis for APOL1, where Brazilian individuals, living in a tropical country, would be more often exposed to potential second-hits, particularly to infectious triggers such as arboviruses and protozoa.[54,55] This hypothesis is specially strengthened by the fact that the Brazilian population has a high African global ancestry and is highly genetically admixed,[56,57] which in principle leads to a considerable rate of APOL1 HRG also in admixed genetic backgrounds. The finding of almost half of the cohort harboring an HRG supports the aforementioned hypothesis, as well as the remarkably high global and individual genetic admixture confirmed by our genetic ancestry analysis. The observation that the patients with HRG manifested the disease essentially between the second and the half of the fifth decade of life, while part of a cohort of patients with patients that manifested the disease along the full age spectrum, is also consistent with the raised hypothesis, because the 10- to 45-year range is expected to be associated with a mature immunologic response[58] and high exposure to infectious agents[59], such as viruses, as well as emergence of autoimmune diseases,[60] also a potential trigger. It must be noted, however, that our cohort included only patients with ICG; thus, the known secondary causes of CG were *a priori* excluded. Therefore, if the infection-based 2-hit hypothesis is indeed the basis of our high HRG frequency in our ICG cohort and the high rate of relative frequency of CG in Brazil, additional yet nonidentified agents are likely to act as second hits. Interestingly, it is indeed possible that the Brazilian population is exposed to a diversity of second hits, represented by a myriad of viral infections, a feature of a mostly tropical country.[61] Future studies, therefore, should address this capital issue. It is interesting to note that preliminary data from our group suggest that the relative prevalence of HRG in patients with secondary causes of CG may be just mildly above what we found in our patients with ICG.

Although the relatively narrow age window in which patients with HRG developed CG is a new description, it is in agreement with previous studies that did not report individuals younger than 10 years old in FSGS cases harboring an HRG[62]

Table 4 | Clinical, laboratory, and histologic profiles of patients with ICG according to the genetic findings

	APOL1 LRG (n = 29)	APOL1 HRG (n = 33)	Mendelian variants (n = 8)	P value
Age, yr	25.5 (20–35)	23 (17–33)	22 (5–27)	0.362
Male, n (%)	11 (37.9)	18 (54.5)	4 (50.0)	0.419
Self-declared ethnicity, n (%)				**0.001**
White	24 (82.8)[a,m]	14 (42.4)[b,m]	7 (87.5)[c]	
Non-White	5 (17.2)[a,m]	19 (57.6)[b,m]	1 (12.5)[c]	
Family history of renal disease, n (%)	3 (10.3)[d]	12 (36.4)[e,m]	1 (12.5)[f]	**0.039**
Consanguinity, n (%)	2 (6.9)	1 (3.0)	2 (12.5)	0.549
Laboratory tests at renal biopsy				
Creatinine, mg/dl	1.41 (1.1–2.9)	1.37 (0.8–2.3)	1.71 (0.5–4.0)	0.718
eGFR, ml/min per 1.73 m^2	51.9 (23.5–113)	62 (35.3–103.7)	45 (17–119)	0.599
Albumin, g/dl	2.20 (1.50–3.15)	2.00 (1.57–2.70)	3.25 (1.72–4.00)	0.062
Proteinuria, g/d	5.61 (4.2–9.9)	8.0 (4.5–12.6)	5.0 (2.6–8.2)	0.165
Hematuria, n (%)	16 (55.2)	11 (36.7)	4 (50.0)	0.353
Hypertension, n (%)	22 (75.9)	20 (66.7)	7 (87.5)	0.452
Renal biopsy findings				
Glomerular compartment				
Mesangial hypercellularity, n (%)	15 (51.7)	12 (38.7)	6 (75.0)	0.169
Mesangial matrix expansion, n (%)	25 (86.2)	23 (74.2)	6 (75.0)	0.489
Segmental sclerosis with synechia, %	12 (0–34)	20 (10–30)	10 (0–26)	0.619
Global glomerular sclerosis, %	0 (0–20.8)	5 (0–22.1)	13 (0–45)	0.669
Tubulointerstitial compartment				
Interstitial fibrosis/tubular atrophy, n (%)				0.145
Absent	8 (27.6)	2 (6.5)	1 (12.5)	
<25%	19 (65.6)	17 (54.8)	4 (50.0)	
25%–50%	1 (3.4)	5 (16.1)	1 (12.5)	
>50%	1 (3.4)	7 (22.6)	2 (25.0)	
Microcystic tubular dilatation	22 (75.9)	24 (77.4)	5 (62.5)	0.679
Vascular compartment, n (%)				
Arteriolar hyalinosis	9 (31.0)	5 (16.1)	2 (25.0)	0.394
Intimal thickening	16 (55.2)	8 (25.8)	2 (25.0)	**0.046**
Arteriolosclerosis	4 (13.8)	2 (6.5)	1 (12.5)	0.631
Treatment, n (%)				
ACEi/ARB	23 (79.3)	28 (84.8)	6 (75.0)	0.756
Glucocorticoids	25 (86.2)	30 (90.9)	6 (75.0)	0.474
Calcineurin inhibitor	16 (55.2)	23 (69.7)	5 (62.5)	0.498
Cyclophosphamide	6 (20.7)	1 (3.0)	0 (0)	**0.042**
Mycophenolate mofetil	5 (17.2)	5 (15.2)	3 (37.5)	0.335
Rituximab	5 (17.2)	0 (0)	0 (0)	**0.022**
Steroid resistance, n (%)	21 (87.5)	27 (84.4)	6 (85.7)	0.947
Remission, n (%)				
Any	14 (48.3)	14 (42.4)	3 (37.5)	0.826
Complete	5 (17.2)	2 (6.1)	1 (12.5)	0.384
Partial	9 (31.0)	12 (36.4)	2 (25)	0.798
Outcome, n (%)				
CKD-KRT 36 months after biopsy	13 (46.4)[g]	14 (42.4)[h]	8 (100)[i,m]	**0.012**
CKD-KRT at the end of follow-up	15 (53.6)[j]	19 (57.6)[k]	8 (100)[l]	0.109
Kidney transplant, n (%)	8 (27.6)	14 (42.4)	6 (75.0)	**0.049**
Development of CG in the graft, n (%)	2 (25)	0 (0)	2 (33.3)	0.088

ACEi, angiotensin-converting enzyme inhibitors; ARB, angiotensin receptor blockers; CKD-KRT, chronic kidney disease with need of kidney replacement therapy; eGFR-CKD-EPI, estimated glomerular filtration rate by the Chronic Kidney Disease-Epidemiology Collaboration equation; HRG, high-risk genotype; ICG, idiopathic collapsing glomerulopathy. Patients with APOL1 HRG more frequently self-declared as non-White and reported family history of kidney disease.
Post hoc analysis of χ^2: [a]P = **0.02**; [b]P = **0.0009**; [c]P = 0.43; [d]P = 0.10; [e]P = **0.03**; [f]P = 1.00; [g]P = 1.00; [h]P = 0.46; [i]P = **0.01**; [j]P = 0.49; [k]P = 1.00; [l]P = 0.17; [m]P < 0.05.
Continuous data are expressed as median (interquartile range). Bold data indicate statistical significance (P < 0.05).

and, when assessing pediatric or adult patients, reported most FSGS/CG cases with HRG occurring between 20 and 40 years of age.[24,62–65] On the basis of a significant number of patients, we could also show that HRG and LRG CG patients did not present different rates of kidney disease progression. This is an important finding, because in a broader range of nephropathies including FSGS, the results are controversial, with some studies reporting worse progression in pediatric and adult patients with HRG[62,66,67] and others not doing so.[65,68]

Notably, the proportion of African genetic ancestry in our patients was higher than those found in other Brazilian regions, except for the ones identified in quilombo remnant groups and in the city of Salvador.[57,69,70] This finding is likely explained by the enrichment of African genetic ancestry in our cohort, because, as expected, the HRG subgroup had a higher proportion of African ancestry than the LRG subgroup, and the HRG frequency was significantly higher in our cohort than in the general population.

Table 5 | Characterization of potentially contributing or causative monogenic variants according to the ACMG criteria for pathogenicity

Pt.	Gene	Inheritance pattern	Variant	Chromosomal position (hg38)	Zygosity	Segregation analysis	gnomAD frequency	ACMG pathogenicity criteria for classification of genetic variants	Variant classification according to the ACMG criteria	APOL1 genotype
1	ITGB4 (NM_000213.5)	AR	c.469+5G>A	17:75727860	Homo	Not performed	0.08%	PM2, PP3	VUS	G1/G1
2	LAMA5 (NM_005560.4)	AR	c.4007A>G:p.(His1336Arg)	20:62329889	Hetero	Mother neg/father Het	0.03%	PM2, BP1, BP4	VUS	G1/G1
			c.1421C>T:p.(Thr474Met)	20:62345874	Hetero	Mother Het/father neg	0.009%	PM2, PP3, BP1	VUS	
3	PTPRO (NM_030667.3)	AR	c.2473G>A:p.(Val825Met)	12:15551586	Hetero	Mother Het/father neg	0.003%	PM2	VUS	G1/G1
			c.3478A>G:p.(Ile1160Val)	12:15594952	Hetero	Mother neg/father Het	0.003%	PM2, PP3	VUS	
4[a]	MAGI2 (NM_012301.4)	AR	c.210C>G:p.(Asn70Lys)	7:79453111	Homo	Mother neg/father neg	–	PM2, PP3	VUS	G0/G0

ACMG, American College of Medical Genetics and Genomics; AD, autosomal dominant; AR, autosomal recessive; Hemi, hemizygosis; Hetero, heterozygosis; Homo, homozygosis; neg, negative; NA, not analyzed; Pt, patient; VUS, variant of uncertain significance.
All variant patterns were consistent with AR inheritance.
[a]Patient who also presented the heterozygous p.Arg229Gln variant in NPHS2.

Table 6 | Clinical profile and treatment response of patients with ICG with potentially contributing or causative monogenic variants associated or not with APOL1 HRG

Pt.	Gene	Inheritance pattern	Variant	Zygosity	Age at diagnosis, yr	Self-declared ethnicity	Response to glucocorticoids	Remission	Progression to CKD-KRT	Time to CKD-KRT, mo	APOL1 genotype
1	ITGB4 (NM_000213.5)	AR	c.469+5G>A	Homo	34	Non-White	Resistant	Partial	No	–	G1/G1
2	LAMA5 (NM_005560.4)	AR	c.4007A>G:p.(His1336Arg)	Hetero	17	Non-White	Sensitive	Complete	No	–	G1/G1
			c.1421C>T:p.(Thr474Met)	Hetero							
3	PTPRO (NM_030667.3)	AR	c.2473G>A:p.(Val825Met)	Hetero	26	Non-White	Resistant	Partial	Yes	11	G1/G1
			c.3478A>G:p.(Ile1160Val)	Hetero							
4[a]	MAGI2 (NM_012301.4)	AR	c.210C>G:p.(Asn70Lys)	Homo	23	White	Resistant	Partial	No	–	G0/G0

AR, Autosomal recessive; CKD-KRT, chronic kidney disease with need of kidney replacement therapy; Hemi, hemizygosis; Hetero, heterozygosis; Homo, homozygosis; HRG, high-risk genotype; ICG, idiopathic collapsing glomerulopathy; Pt, patient.
Only 1 patient progressed to CKD-KRT by the end of the follow-up.
[a]Patient who also presented the heterozygous p.Arg229Gln variant in NPHS2.

Table 7 | Cox regression analysis of potential risk factors associated with progression to CKD-KRT 36 months after biopsy and by the end of the follow-up

Variable	HR	95% confidence interval	P value
36 months after biopsy			
APOL1 LRG	1.000		
Older age at kidney biopsy, yr	0.961	0.927–0.996	**0.029**
eGFR at kidney biopsy, ml/min per 1.73 m²	0.992	0.984–1.001	0.094
CNI	0.443	0.184–1.069	0.070
Any remission	0.230	0.085–0.623	**0.004**
APOL1 HRG	0.529	0.240–1.116	0.114
Mendelian variant	2.853	1.151–7.076	**0.024**
End of follow-up			
APOL1 LRG	1.000		
Older age at kidney biopsy, yr	0.982	0.949–1.016	0.303
eGFR at kidney biopsy, ml/min per 1.73 m²	0.996	0.990–1.003	0.261
ACE/ARB	1.288	0.550–3.014	0.560
Any remission	0.155	0.069–0.351	**<0.001**
APOL1 HRG	0.591	0.302–1.157	0.125
Mendelian variant	2.355	1.018–5.447	**0.045**

ACEi, angiotensin-converting enzyme inhibitor; ARB, angiotensin receptor blockers; CKD-KRT, chronic kidney disease with need of kidney replacement therapy; CNI, calcineurin inhibitor; eGFR-CKD-EPI, estimated glomerular filtration rate by the Chronic Kidney Disease-Epidemiology Collaboration equation; HR, hazard ratio.
Older age at kidney biopsy was a protective factor against progression to CKD-KRT by 36 months, remission was a protective factor by 36 months and the end of follow-up, and Mendelian variant was a risk factor by 36 months and the end of follow-up.
Bold data indicate statistical significance ($P < 0.05$).

To date, no studies have systematically evaluated the association between MVs and ICG. This is the first report to quantify the frequency of such causative variants in an ICG population. In contrast to a previous observation in an FSGS cohort,[63] in our CG population, the majority of MV-related cases were identified in adults. The currently available data on MV and CG are derived from subpopulations of studies where CG has been classified as a subtype of FSGS. Gribouval et al.[63] performed WES in 135 adult European patients with sporadic FSGS or steroid-resistant NS, which identified MV or HRG in 30 of them; 16 harbored monogenic variants, whereas 14 presented HRG. Only 2 of such patients were diagnosed with CG, one with a variant in *INF2* and the other with HRG. Another North American study[71] assessed the potential presence of variants in *NPHS2*, *TRPC6*, *ACTN4*, *INF2*, and *PLCE1*, as well as HRG, in 65 patients diagnosed with sporadic FSGS (28 children and 37 adults). Among these patients, 15 had a histologic diagnosis of CG (8 children and 7 adults). No single-gene variants were identified in patients with CG, and 9 of 10 African American patients had at least 1 *APOL1* risk allele, with no reference on how many of them harbored HRG.

It has been previously shown that most monogenic forms of FSGS are associated with MVs in genes encoding collagen IV chains.[63,72–74] Although such reported cases do not include ICG, our findings followed a similar trend, with collagen IV–related variants affecting 3 of our patients with CG. We also detected causative variants in genes that encode a cation channel permeable to calcium (*TRPC6*), a mitochondrial enzyme (*COQ2*), a component of the intraflagellar transport complex in the primary apical cilium (*TTC21B*), a protein that acts in cytoskeleton stabilization (*MYH9*), and a protein involved in cytoskeleton regulation and migration in podocytes (*PLCE1*). The patient with variants in *COQ2* was started on CoQ10 3 months after the onset of symptoms—1 month after kidney biopsy, still with normal eGFR. However, despite being supported by previous evidence of benefit of CoQ10 supplementation[75] and receiving treatment with glucocorticoids, calcineurin inhibitor, and CoQ10 replacement, he quickly progressed to CKD-KRT 8 months after being

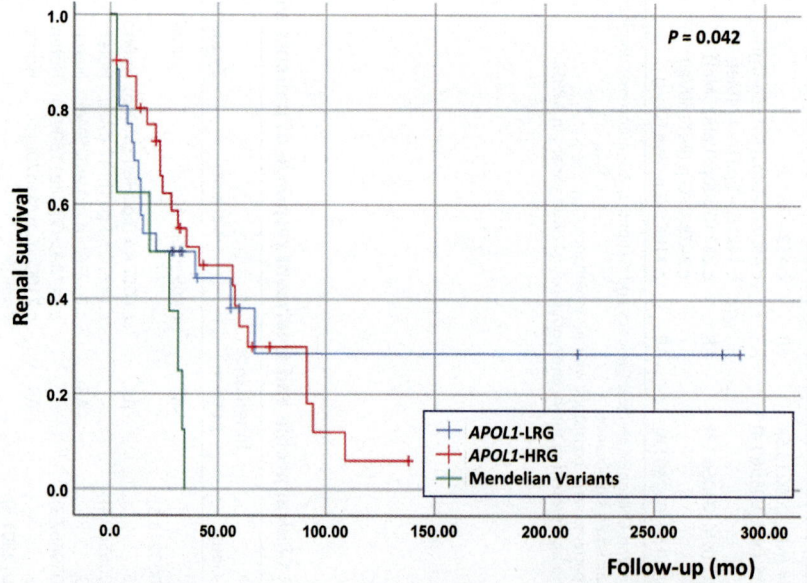

Figure 4 | Mendelian variants are associated with worse kidney prognosis. Renal survival of patients with ICG according to their genetic findings. Univariable *P* value was obtained applying the log-rank test. HRG, high-risk genotype; ICG, idiopathic collapsing glomerulopathy; LRG, low-risk genotype.

started on CoQ10. This clinical course supports that this replacement must be initiated early in the course of CG associated with this etiology to significantly increase the probability of improvement in kidney prognosis. Of note, we not only identified causative variants in genes not previously associated with ICG (*COL4A3*, *COL4A5*, and *TTC21B*) but also novel causative variants in genes previously associated and not with ICG.

An unexpected finding of our study was the identification of VUSs in *ITGB4*, *LAMA5*, or *PTPRO* in 3 patients with HRG. Given the previously established association between *APOL1* HRG and CG, the high prevalence of HRG in our CG cohort, and the insufficient ACMG criteria to strongly predict pathogenicity for the identified VUSs, the likeliest molecular basis for the development of CG in these patients is the *APOL1* HRG–driven mechanism. However, because the HRG-mediated mechanism is based on susceptibility, the VUS status does not rule out potential pathogenicity, in the 3 cases the variants obey the expected Mendelian segregation, and the HRG-VUS combination was observed in 3 cases, one cannot completely rule out the possibility that such VUSs may have a contributing or pathogenic effect on determining the CG phenotype. Interestingly, association of monogenic pathogenic variants with *APOL1* HRG has been previously described in a child with congenital NS with the G1/G1 genotype and 2 variants in compound heterozygosity in the *NPHS1* [c.106delG: p.(Ala36Profs*6) and c.2728T>C:p.(Ser910Pro)].[64] Although the *NPHS1* variants on their own can explain the development of CNS in this case, the HRG status may have contributed to the severity of the phenotype. It is important to mention, however, that the exclusion of these 3 cases from the HRG group did not impact the conclusions related to the HRG patient population. The inclusion of the patient with the *MAGI2* VUS did not impact the conclusions regarding the LRG group either.

Our study has some limitations. First, it is a single-center study; however, because our medical center is the largest in Latin America and is located in São Paulo, a huge metropolitan area with migrants from all regions of the country and very high genetic admixture, we could gather a high number of CG cases highly representative of genetic diversity and admixture. This reality significantly minimizes the single-center effect. Second, electron microscopy was not systematically employed in the kidney histologic assessment. Finally, genetic analyses were performed using 2 approaches, targeted-gene panel or WES, due to cost limitations in the beginning of the study. Although this reality limited our analyses to the genes contained in the gene panels, the comprehensiveness of our panels warranted that this effect should be very minor on the obtained results.

In conclusion, this is the first study to perform an integrated analysis of clinical, histologic, therapeutic, causative genetic, and genetic ancestry data in a CG population with a high number of patients, encompassing children and adults. Our data revealed that ICG is more common in young patients, has low therapeutic responses to immunosuppressive treatment, and quickly progresses to CKD-KRT. We detected a causative genetic basis in approximately 59% of the cases, the majority harboring HRG, but causative variants were present in approximately 20% of the identified genetic cases. Patients with HRG were all aged between 9 and 44 years and more often self-declared non-White. Of note, harboring MVs was associated with worse kidney prognosis. This study reveals that the genetic status plays a major role in the pathogenesis of ICG, accounting for more than 50% of cases in a representative Brazilian population, and provides strategic information for future studies on this disease.

DISCLOSURE
All the authors declared no competing interests.

DATA STATEMENT
The data of whole-exome sequencing supporting the findings of this study are openly available in the repository European Genome-phenome Archive (EGA) at accession number EGAD50000000091 (https://ega-archive.org/datasets/EGAD50000000091). Additional clinical data are available on request to the corresponding author.

ACKNOWLEDGMENTS
We thank Fernanda M. Franzin, PhD, and Vivian C.D. Pinto for support in molecular genetics analyses.

FUNDING STATEMENT
This work was supported by Fundação de Amparo à Pesquisa do Estado de São Paulo, Brazil (grants 2013/02162-8 and 2020/02988-7 to LFO), Coordenação de Aperfeiçoamento de Pessoal de Nível Superior, Brazil (fellowship 88887.352526/2019-00 to PDN), and Hospital das Clínicas da Faculdade de Medicina da USP.

SUPPLEMENTARY MATERIAL
Supplementary File (Word)
Supplementary Table S1. Patients of the cohort with referred family history of kidney disease.
Supplementary Table S2. Clinical, laboratory, and histologic profiles of patients with *APOL1* high-risk genotype (HRG) and low-risk genotype (LRG). Patients with HRG self-declared as non-White more often than those with LRG.
Supplementary Table S3. The proportion of African genetic ancestry in our cohort was higher than in most previously assessed Brazilian populations. The proportion of African, European, Native American, and East Asian genetic ancestries in populations from different regions of Brazil and in our cohort are depicted.
Supplementary References.
Supplementary Figure S1. Comparative analysis of genetic ancestry proportions among subgroups with different genotypes for *APOL1*. The *APOL1* high-risk genotype group had a higher proportion of African ancestry. (**A**) Distribution of genetic ancestry proportions within each subgroup. (**B**) Statistical significance for comparisons of genetic ancestry proportions between the subgroups.

REFERENCES
1. Weiss MA, Daquioag E, Margolin EG, Pollak VE. Nephrotic syndrome, progressive irreversible renal failure, and glomerular "collapse": a new clinicopathologic entity? *Am J Kidney Dis*. 1986;7:20–28.

2. D'Agati VD, Fogo AB, Bruijn JA, Jennette JC. Pathologic classification of focal segmental glomerulosclerosis: a working proposal. *Am J Kidney Dis.* 2004;43:368–382.
3. Schwimmer JA, Markowitz GS, Valeri A, Appel GB. Collapsing glomerulopathy. *Semin Nephrol.* 2003;23:209–218.
4. Merchant ML, Barati MT, Caster DJ, et al. Proteomic analysis identifies distinct glomerular extracellular matrix in collapsing focal segmental glomerulosclerosis. *J Am Soc Nephrol.* 2020;31:1883–1904.
5. D'Agati VD, Alster JM, Jennette JC, et al. Association of histologic variants in FSGS clinical trial with presenting features and outcomes. *Clin J Am Soc Nephrol.* 2013;8:399–406.
6. Deegens JKJ, Steenbergen EJ, Borm GF, Wetzels JFM. Pathological variants of focal segmental glomerulosclerosis in an adult Dutch population—epidemiology and outcome. *Nephrol Dial Transplant.* 2008;23:186–192.
7. Raja R, Nada R, Yadav AK, et al. A prospective study of collapsing focal segmental glomerulosclerosis. *Ren Fail.* 2016;38:894–898.
8. Testagrossa L, Azevedo Neto R, Resende A, et al. Immunohistochemical expression of podocyte markers in the variants of focal segmental glomerulosclerosis. *Nephrol Dial Transplant.* 2013;28:91–98.
9. Albaqumi M, Soos TJ, Barisoni L, Nelson PJ. Collapsing glomerulopathy. *J Am Soc Nephrol.* 2006;17:2854–2863.
10. Cutrim ÉMM, Neves PDM de M, Campos MAG, et al. Collapsing glomerulopathy: a review by the Collapsing Brazilian Consortium. *Front Med (Lausanne).* 2022;9:846173.
11. Valeri A, Barisoni L, Appel GB, et al. Idiopathic collapsing focal segmental glomerulosclerosis: a clinicopathologic study. *Kidney Int.* 1996;50:1734–1746.
12. Laurinavicius A, Hurwitz S, Rennke HG. Collapsing glomerulopathy in HIV and non-HIV patients: a clinicopathological and follow-up study. *Kidney Int.* 1999;56:2203–2213.
13. Laurin LP, Gasim AM, Derebail VK, et al. Renal survival in patients with collapsing compared with not otherwise specified FSGS. *Clin J Am Soc Nephrol.* 2016;11:1752–1759.
14. Fogo AB, Lusco MA, Najafian B, Alpers CE. AJKD Atlas of Renal Pathology: collapsing glomerulopathy. *Am J Kidney Dis.* 2015;66:e3–e4.
15. Barisoni L, Kriz W, Mundel P, D'agati V. The dysregulated podocyte phenotype: a novel concept in the pathogenesis of collapsing idiopathic focal segmental glomerulosclerosis and HIV-associated nephropathy. *J Am Soc Nephrol.* 1999;10:51–61.
16. Teixeira Júnior AAL, Neves PDM de M, Lages JS, et al. Brazilian consortium for the study on renal diseases associated with COVID-19: a multicentric effort to understand SARS-CoV-2-related nephropathy. *Front Med (Lausanne).* 2020;7:584235.
17. Neves PD, Caires RA, Guimarães MP, et al. Collapsing glomerulopathy following SARS-CoV-2 adenovirus-vector–based vaccine: report of 2 cases. *Kidney Int.* 2022;101:637–639.
18. Muehlig AK, Gies S, Huber TB, Braun F. Collapsing focal segmental glomerulosclerosis in viral infections. *Front Immunol.* 2022;12:800074.
19. Salvatore SP, Barisoni LMC, Herzenberg AM, et al. Collapsing glomerulopathy in 19 patients with systemic lupus erythematosus or lupus-like disease. *Clin J Am Soc Nephrol.* 2012;7:914–925.
20. Salvatore SP, Reddi AS, Chandran CB, et al. Collapsing glomerulopathy superimposed on diabetic nephropathy: insights into etiology of an under-recognized, severe pattern of glomerular injury. *Nephrol Dial Transplant.* 2014;29:392–399.
21. Markowitz GS, Nasr SH, Stokes MB, D'Agati VD. Treatment with IFN-α, -β, or -γ is associated with collapsing focal segmental glomerulosclerosis. *Clin J Am Soc Nephrol.* 2010;5:607–615.
22. Barri YM, Munshi NC, Sukumalchantra S, et al. Podocyte injury associated glomerulopathies induced by pamidronate. *Kidney Int.* 2004;65:634–641.
23. Buob D, Decambron M, Gnemmi V, et al. Collapsing glomerulopathy is common in the setting of thrombotic microangiopathy of the native kidney. *Kidney Int.* 2016;90:1321–1331.
24. Kopp JB, Winkler CA, Zhao X, et al. Clinical features and histology of apolipoprotein L1-associated nephropathy in the FSGS clinical trial. *J Am Soc Nephrol.* 2015;26:1443–1448.
25. Freedman BI, Limou S, Ma L, Kopp JB. APOL1-associated nephropathy: a key contributor to racial disparities in CKD. *Am J Kidney Dis.* 2018;72: S8–S16.
26. Genovese G, Friedman DJ, Ross MD, et al. Association of trypanolytic ApoL1 variants with kidney disease in African Americans. *Science.* 2010;329:841–845.
27. McNicholas BA, Nelson PJ. Immunity unmasks APOL1 in collapsing glomerulopathy. *Kidney Int.* 2015;87:270–272.
28. Yusuf AA, Govender MA, Brandenburg JT, Winkler CA. Kidney disease and APOL1. *Hum Mol Genet.* 2021;30:R129–R137.
29. Friedman DJ, Pollak MR. APOL1 nephropathy: from genetics to clinical applications. *Clin J Am Soc Nephrol.* 2021;16:294–303.
30. Daneshpajouhnejad P, Kopp JB, Winkler CA, Rosenberg AZ. The evolving story of apolipoprotein L1 nephropathy: the end of the beginning. *Nat Rev Nephrol.* 2022;18:307–320.
31. Drovandi S, Lipska-Ziętkiewicz BS, Ozaltin F, et al. Variation of the clinical spectrum and genotype-phenotype associations in coenzyme Q10 deficiency associated glomerulopathy. *Kidney Int.* 2022;102:592–603.
32. Gasser DL, Winkler CA, Peng M, et al. Focal segmental glomerulosclerosis is associated with a PDSS2 haplotype and, independently, with a decreased content of coenzyme Q 10. *Am J Physiol Renal Physiol.* 2013;305:F1228–F1238.
33. Reeves-Daniel AM, Iskandar SS, Bowden DW, et al. Is collapsing C1q nephropathy another MYH9-associated kidney disease? A case report. *Am J Kidney Dis.* 2010;55:e21–e24.
34. Nagano C, Hara S, Yoshikawa N, et al. Clinical, pathological, and genetic characteristics in patients with focal segmental glomerulosclerosis. *Kidney360.* 2022;3:1384–1393.
35. Gigante M, Caridi G, Montemurno E, et al. *TRPC6* mutations in children with steroid-resistant nephrotic syndrome and atypical phenotype. *Clin J Am Soc Nephrol.* 2011;6:1626–1634.
36. Morales-Alvarez MC, Knob A, Rennke HG, Pollak MR, Denker BM. Clinical and pathological heterogeneity in FSGS due to INF2 mutations. *Kidney Int Rep.* 2022;7:2741–2745.
37. Cason RK, Williams A, Chryst-Stangl M, et al. Collapsing focal segmental glomerulosclerosis in siblings with compound heterozygous variants in NUP93 expand the spectrum of kidney phenotypes associated with nucleoporin gene mutations. *Front Pediatr.* 2022;10:915174.
38. Fenaroli P, Rossi GM, Angelotti ML, et al. Collapsing glomerulopathy as a complication of type I interferon–mediated glomerulopathy in a patient with RNASEH2B-related Aicardi-Goutières syndrome. *Am J Kidney Dis.* 2021;78:750–754.
39. Abid Q, Best Rocha A, Larsen CP, et al. APOL1-associated collapsing focal segmental glomerulosclerosis in a patient with stimulator of interferon genes (STING)-associated vasculopathy with onset in infancy (SAVI). *Am J Kidney Dis.* 2020;75:287–290.
40. Berkovic SF, Dibbens LM, Oshlack A, et al. Array-based gene discovery with three unrelated subjects shows SCARB2/LIMP-2 deficiency causes myoclonus epilepsy and glomerulosclerosis. *Am J Hum Genet.* 2008;82: 673–684.
41. Jain NG, Ahram DF, Marasa M, et al. Clinical real-time genome sequencing to solve the complex and confounded presentation of a child with focal segmental glomerulosclerosis and multiple malignancies. *Kidney Int Rep.* 2022;7:2312–2316.
42. Rovin BH, Adler SG, Barratt J, et al. KDIGO 2021 clinical practice guideline for the management of glomerular diseases. *Kidney Int.* 2021;100(4S):S1–S276.
43. Wang K, Li M, Hakonarson H. ANNOVAR: functional annotation of genetic variants from high-throughput sequencing data. *Nucleic Acids Res.* 2010;38:e164.
44. Richards S, Aziz N, Bale S, et al. Standards and guidelines for the interpretation of sequence variants: a joint consensus recommendation of the American College of Medical Genetics and Genomics and the Association for Molecular Pathology. *Genet Med.* 2015;17:405–424.
45. Watanabe A. *Patogênese Genética-Molecular da Síndrome Nefrótica Córtico-Resistente, Síndrome Nefrótica Congênita e Glomeruloesclerose Segmentar e Focal: Realidade e Contribuições da Análise de Uma População Pediátrica Brasileira.* Doctoral thesis. University of São Paulo School of Medicine; 2023.
46. Gogarten SM, Bhangale T, Conomos MP, et al. GWASTools: an R/Bioconductor package for quality control and analysis of genome-wide association studies. *Bioinformatics.* 2012;28:3329–3331.
47. Zheng X, Levine D, Shen J, et al. A high-performance computing toolset for relatedness and principal component analysis of SNP data. *Bioinformatics.* 2012;28:3326–3328.
48. Chang CC, Chow CC, Tellier LC, et al. Second-generation PLINK: rising to the challenge of larger and richer datasets. *Gigascience.* 2015;4:7.
49. McQuillan R, Leutenegger AL, Abdel-Rahman R, et al. Runs of homozygosity in European populations. *Am J Hum Genet.* 2008;83: 359–372.

50. Alexander DH, Novembre J, Lange K. Fast model-based estimation of ancestry in unrelated individuals. *Genome Res.* 2009;19:1655–1664.
51. Almarri MA, Bergström A, Prado-Martinez J, et al. Population structure, stratification, and introgression of human structural variation. *Cell.* 2020;182:189–199.e15.
52. Starr MC, Chang IJ, Finn LS, et al. COQ2 nephropathy: a treatable cause of nephrotic syndrome in children. *Pediatr Nephrol.* 2018;33:1257–1261.
53. Feltran LS, Varela P, Silva ED, et al. Targeted next-generation sequencing in Brazilian children with nephrotic syndrome submitted to renal transplant. *Transplantation.* 2017;101:2905–2912.
54. Araújo SDA, Macedo E, Cordeiro T, Belisário AR, et al. First report of collapsing variant of focal segmental glomerulosclerosis triggered by arbovirus: dengue and Zika virus infection. *Clin Kidney J.* 2019;12:355–361.
55. Neves PD, Bridi RA, Ramalho JA, et al. Schistosoma mansoni infection as a trigger to collapsing glomerulopathy in a patient with high-risk APOL1 genotype. *PLoS Negl Trop Dis.* 2020;14:e0008582.
56. Pena SDJ, Santos FR, Tarazona-Santos E. Genetic admixture in Brazil. *Am J Med Genet C Semin Med Genet.* 2020;184:928–938.
57. Kehdy FSG, Gouveia MH, Machado M, et al. Origin and dynamics of admixture in Brazilians and its effect on the pattern of deleterious mutations. *Proc Natl Acad Sci U S A.* 2015;112:8696–8701.
58. Simon AK, Hollander GA, McMichael A. Evolution of the immune system in humans from infancy to old age. *Proc Biol Sci.* 2015;282:20143085.
59. Gavazzi G, Herrmann F, Krause KH. Aging and infectious diseases in the developing world. *Clin Infect Dis.* 2004;39:83–91.
60. Cooper GS, Stroehla BC. The epidemiology of autoimmune diseases. *Autoimmun Rev.* 2003;2:119–125.
61. Campos FS, de Arruda LB, da Fonseca FG. Special issue "viral infections in developing countries.". *Viruses.* 2022;14:405.
62. Kopp JB, Nelson GW, Sampath K, et al. APOL1 genetic variants in focal segmental glomerulosclerosis and HIV-associated nephropathy. *J Am Soc Nephrol.* 2011;22:2129–2137.
63. Gribouval O, Boyer O, Hummel A, et al. Identification of genetic causes for sporadic steroid-resistant nephrotic syndrome in adults. *Kidney Int.* 2018;94:1013–1022.
64. Gribouval O, Boyer O, Knebelmann B, et al. APOL1 risk genotype in European steroid-resistant nephrotic syndrome and/or focal segmental glomerulosclerosis patients of different African ancestries. *Nephrol Dial Transplant.* 2019;34:1885–1893.
65. Atta MG, Estrella MM, Kuperman M, et al. HIV-associated nephropathy patients with and without apolipoprotein L1 gene variants have similar clinical and pathological characteristics. *Kidney Int.* 2012;82:338–343.
66. Kasembeli AN, Duarte R, Ramsay M, et al. APOL1 risk variants are strongly associated with HIV-associated nephropathy in black South Africans. *J Am Soc Nephrol.* 2015;26:2882–2890.
67. Hung RKY, Binns-Roemer E, Booth JW, et al. Genetic variants of APOL1 are major determinants of kidney failure in people of African ancestry with HIV. *Kidney Int Rep.* 2022;7:786–796.
68. Waziri B, Raji YE, Ekrikpo UE, Naicker S. Apolipoprotein L1 gene variants and kidney disease in patients with HIV: a systematic review and meta-analysis. *J Nephrol.* 2023;36:1119–1134.
69. Kimura L, Ribeiro-Rodrigues EM, de Mello Auricchio MTB, et al. Genomic ancestry of rural African-derived populations from Southeastern Brazil. *Am J Hum Biol.* 2013;25:35–41.
70. de Souza AM, Resende SS, de Sousa TN, de Brito CFA. A systematic scoping review of the genetic ancestry of the Brazilian population. *Genet Mol Biol.* 2019;42:495–508.
71. Laurin LP, Lu M, Mottl AK, et al. Podocyte-associated gene mutation screening in a heterogeneous cohort of patients with sporadic focal segmental glomerulosclerosis. *Nephrol Dial Transplant.* 2014;29:2062–2069.
72. Malone AF, Phelan PJ, Hall G, et al. Rare hereditary COL4A3/COL4A4 variants may be mistaken for familial focal segmental glomerulosclerosis. *Kidney Int.* 2014;86:1253–1259.
73. Yao T, Udwan K, John R, et al. Integration of genetic testing and pathology for the diagnosis of adults with FSGS. *Clin J Am Soc Nephrol.* 2019;14:213–223.
74. Groopman EE, Marasa M, Cameron-Christie S, et al. Diagnostic utility of exome sequencing for kidney disease. *N Engl J Med.* 2019;380:142–151.
75. Drovandi S, Lipska-Ziętkiewicz BS, Ozaltin F, et al. Oral coenzyme Q10 supplementation leads to better preservation of kidney function in steroid-resistant nephrotic syndrome due to primary coenzyme Q10 deficiency. *Kidney Int.* 2022;102:604–612.

clinical investigation

A multi-institutional study found a possible role of anti-nephrin antibodies in post-transplant focal segmental glomerulosclerosis recurrence

see commentary on page 440

Yoko Shirai[1], Kenichiro Miura[1], Kiyonobu Ishizuka[1], Taro Ando[1], Shoichiro Kanda[2], Junya Hashimoto[3], Yuko Hamasaki[3], Kiyohiko Hotta[4], Naoko Ito[5], Kazuho Honda[6], Kenji Tanabe[7], Tomoko Takano[8] and Motoshi Hattori[1]

[1]Department of Pediatric Nephrology, Tokyo Women's Medical University, Tokyo, Japan; [2]Department of Pediatrics, Tokyo University, Tokyo, Japan; [3]Department of Nephrology, Toho University Faculty of Medicine, Tokyo, Japan; [4]Department of Urology, Hokkaido University, Graduate School of Medicine, Hokkaido, Japan; [5]Department of Surgical Pathology, Tokyo Women's Medical University, Tokyo, Japan; [6]Department of Anatomy, Showa University School of Medicine, Tokyo, Japan; [7]Medical Research Institute, Tokyo Women's Medical University, Tokyo, Japan; and [8]Division of Nephrology, McGill University Health Centre, Montreal, Québec, Canada

Possible roles of anti-nephrin antibodies in post-transplant recurrent focal segmental glomerulosclerosis (FSGS) have been reported recently. To confirm these preliminary results, we performed a multi-institutional study of 22 Japanese pediatric kidney transplant recipients with FSGS including eight genetic FSGS and 14 non-genetic (presumed primary) FSGS. Eleven of the 14 non-genetic FSGS patients had post-transplant recurrent FSGS. Median (interquartile range) plasma levels of anti-nephrin antibodies in post-transplant recurrent FSGS measured using ELISA were markedly high at 899 (831, 1292) U/mL (cutoff 231 U/mL) before transplantation or during recurrence. Graft biopsies during recurrence showed punctate IgG deposition co-localized with nephrin that had altered localization with increased nephrin tyrosine phosphorylation and Src homology and collagen homology A expressions. Graft biopsies after remission showed no signals for IgG and a normal expression pattern of nephrin. Anti-nephrin antibody levels decreased to 155 (53, 367) U/mL in five patients with samples available after remission. In patients with genetic FSGS as in those with non-genetic FSGS without recurrence, anti-nephrin antibody levels were comparable to those of 30 control individuals, and graft biopsies had no signals for IgG and a normal expression pattern of nephrin. Thus, our results suggest that circulating anti-nephrin antibodies are a possible candidate for circulating factors involved in the pathogenesis of post-transplant recurrent FSGS and that this may be mediated by nephrin phosphorylation. Larger studies including other ethnicities are required to confirm this finding.

Kidney International (2024) **105**, 608–617; https://doi.org/10.1016/j.kint.2023.11.022

KEYWORDS: focal segmental glomerulosclerosis; kidney transplantation; nephrin

Copyright © 2023, International Society of Nephrology. Published by Elsevier Inc. All rights reserved.

Lay Summary

Possible roles of anti-nephrin antibodies in post-transplant recurrent focal segmental glomerulosclerosis (FSGS) have been reported recently. To confirm these preliminary results, we performed a multi-institutional study. Plasma anti-nephrin antibodies in 11 patients with post-transplant recurrent FSGS were high before transplantation or during recurrence. Graft biopsies during recurrence showed punctate IgG deposition colocalized with nephrin that had altered localization with increased nephrin tyrosine phosphorylation and Src homology and collagen homology A expression. Plasma anti-nephrin antibody levels decreased after remission, and graft biopsies after remission showed no signals for IgG and a normal expression pattern of nephrin. In patients with genetic FSGS and nongenetic FSGS without recurrence, anti-nephrin antibody levels were comparable with those in controls consisting of healthy individuals and disease controls. These results suggest that circulating anti-nephrin antibodies are a possible candidate for circulating factors involved in the pathogenesis of post-transplant recurrent FSGS.

Correspondence: Motoshi Hattori, Department of Pediatric Nephrology, Tokyo Women's Medical University, 8-1, Kawada-cho, Shinjuku-ku, Tokyo 162-8666, Japan. E-mail: hattori@twmu.ac.jp

Received 31 August 2023; revised 7 November 2023; accepted 10 November 2023; published online 16 December 2023

P ost-transplant recurrence of primary focal segmental glomerulosclerosis (FSGS) is a major challenge in kidney transplantation. Kidney transplant recipients with primary FSGS face a high risk of post-transplant recurrence in the form of nephrotic range proteinuria (>2.0 g/g creatinine), which leads to allograft damage.[1] The role of circulating factors has long been presumed in the pathogenesis of primary FSGS, but the definitive identity of such factors remains unknown. Previous studies reported that an i.v. injection of monoclonal anti-nephrin antibodies in rats induced massive proteinuria in <24 hours[2,3] and led to a decrease in nephrin expression in 1 hour.[4] In addition, anti-nephrin antibodies, when injected in rodents, changed the nephrin staining pattern from linear to coarse granular and induced nephrin tyrosine phosphorylation, likely via Src family kinase activation.[5,6] Furthermore, nephrin mRNA was decreased in the nephropathy induced by anti-nephrin antibodies.[4]

Recently, a patient who presented with early post-transplant massive proteinuria recurrence was reported to have pretransplant anti-nephrin antibodies.[7] We also reported a case of post-transplant recurrent FSGS (rFSGS) where circulating anti-nephrin antibodies were detected in the plasma before transplantation.[8] In the 1-hour post-implantation biopsy of this patient, IgG deposition, nephrin tyrosine phosphorylation, upregulation of Src homology and collagen homology A (ShcA), and altered nephrin distribution were observed together with foot process effacement (FPE).[8] ShcA is involved in nephrin endocytosis and signaling cascades that contribute to actin polymerization, cell survival, and barrier turnover.[9]

To confirm these findings from a single patient, we conducted a multi-institutional study examining patients with FSGS who underwent kidney transplantation between 1986 and 2022, including those without post-transplant recurrence. We confirmed that anti-nephrin antibodies and associated changes in graft biopsy (IgG deposition, nephrin tyrosine phosphorylation, ShcA upregulation, altered nephrin distribution, and FPE) were observed only in rFSGS but not in non-rFSGS and genetic FSGS. In addition, in patients with rFSGS who achieved remission, anti-nephrin antibody levels were significantly decreased and graft biopsies showed the disappearance of IgG, nephrin tyrosine phosphorylation, and ShcA staining and recovered a normal expression pattern of nephrin and no FPE. Our results suggest that anti-nephrin antibodies may be causally linked to the post-transplant recurrence of FSGS.

METHODS

The clinical and research activities reported here are consistent with the Principles of the Declaration of Istanbul as outlined in the "Declaration of Istanbul on Organ Trafficking and Transplant Tourism," the ethical principles in the 1964 Declaration of Helsinki (2013 update), and the ethical guidelines for epidemiological studies issued by the Ministry of Health, Labour and Welfare, Japan. This study was approved by the Research Ethics Board of Tokyo Women's Medical University (approval number 2021-0184). All participants and/or their guardians provided informed consent to be enrolled in the study.

Patient cohort

Overall, 109 Japanese patients with childhood-onset FSGS underwent their first kidney transplantation from 1986 to 2022 at the Department of Pediatric Nephrology, Tokyo Women's Medical University; Department of Nephrology, Toho University Faculty of Medicine; and Department of Urology, Hokkaido University, Graduate School of Medicine. Patients with congenital nephrotic syndrome (onset within 3 months of birth) and repeat kidney transplantation were not included in this study. Of 109 recipients, 8 patients with secondary FSGS and 56 recipients with FSGS who did not undergo genetic testing were excluded (Figure 1). Of these, 45 patients underwent whole exome sequencing, which identified disease-causing variants in 65 genes associated with FSGS/steroid-resistant nephrotic syndrome in 28 patients (genetic FSGS) (Supplementary Tables S1 and S2).[10] The remaining 17 patients had no pathogenic variants in genes associated with FSGS/steroid-resistant nephrotic syndrome (nongenetic, presumed primary FSGS). Of 17 patients with nongenetic (presumed primary) FSGS, 12 had rFSGS and 5 did not (non-rFSGS).[11–13] Furthermore, 10 of 12 patients with rFSGS achieved remission (responders). The remaining 2 did not achieve remission and had a progression to graft failure (non-responders). Patients without stored frozen plasma samples and graft biopsy specimens were excluded. Consequently, 8 patients with genetic FSGS and 14 patients with nongenetic (presumed primary) FSGS including 11 with rFSGS and 3 with non-rFSGS were analyzed in this study (Figure 1).

Measurement of circulating anti-nephrin autoantibodies by enzyme-linked immunosorbent assay

Circulating anti-nephrin antibodies were quantified by enzyme-linked immunosorbent assay as previously described,[7] except that the recombinant extracellular domain of human nephrin was obtained commercially (R&D Systems, Inc). Briefly, Nunc MaxiSorp enzyme-linked immunosorbent assay plates (Thermo Fisher Scientific) were coated with 100 ng/well of the recombinant extracellular domain of human nephrin (R&D Systems, Inc.) and incubated overnight at 4 °C. Uncoated control wells were used to determine nonspecific binding (in the absence of antigen) for each patient sample, and this allowed for background subtraction. After washing, plates were blocked with 300 μl of SuperBlock (Thermo Fisher Scientific) for 1 hour at room temperature and then incubated overnight with patient samples diluted at 1:400. Plates were incubated with biotin-conjugated goat anti-human IgG Fc, highly cross-absorbed antibody (Thermo Fisher Scientific), followed by incubation with horseradish peroxidase–conjugated avidin (BioLegend). Then, 3,3',5,5'-tetramethylbenzidine substrate was added, followed by stop solution 10 minutes later, and the absorbance at 450 nm was measured. Anti-nephrin antibody titers were determined using a standard curve derived from serial 2-fold dilutions of the index patient's sample (Supplementary Table S2, patient rFSGS1), whose titer was arbitrarily defined as 1000 U/ml. The *cutoff for positivity* was defined as the maximum antibody titer in controls consisting of healthy individuals ($n = 13$) and disease controls including membranous nephropathy ($n = 13$) and lupus nephritis ($n = 4$). Serum samples were obtained from patients with membranous nephropathy and lupus nephritis when they presented with proteinuria, with a median urinary protein excretion of 0.9 (interquartile range [IQR] 0.4–1.8) and 2.9 (IQR 2.3–5.1) g/g creatinine, respectively. Anti-nephrin antibodies were also measured using serum samples from 13 patients with minimal change disease (MCD), who had serial serum samples at relapse and remission. Of 13 patients at relapse, 8 had nephrotic range proteinuria (>2.0 g/g creatinine) and 5 showed proteinuria less than 2 g/g creatinine at the time of serum sampling during relapse.

Immunofluorescence staining

Dual immunofluorescence (IF) staining for IgG and nephrin was performed using frozen specimens of graft and native kidney biopsies as in our previous report.[8] Frozen specimens contained 3 to 5

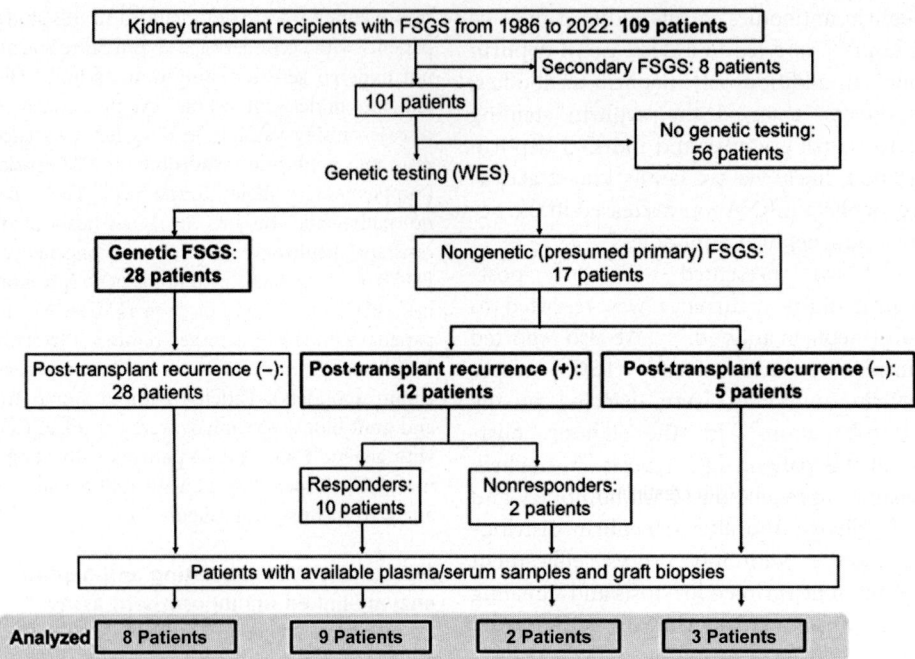

Figure 1 | Flowchart of patient selection. Overall, 109 Japanese patients with childhood-onset focal segmental glomerulosclerosis (FSGS) underwent their first kidney transplantation from 1986 to 2022 at the Department of Pediatric Nephrology, Tokyo Women's Medical University; Department of Nephrology, Toho University Faculty of Medicine; and Department of Urology, Hokkaido University, Graduate School of Medicine. Of 109 recipients, 8 with secondary FSGS and 56 with FSGS who did not undergo genetic testing were excluded. Of these, 45 patients underwent whole exome sequencing (WES), which identified disease-causing variants in genes associated with FSGS/steroid-resistant nephrotic syndrome (SRNS) in 28 patients (genetic FSGS). The remaining 17 patients had no pathogenic variants in the genes associated with FSGS/SRNS (nongenetic, presumed primary FSGS). Of 17 patients with nongenetic (presumed primary) FSGS, 12 had recurrent FSGS (rFSGS) and 5 did not (non-rFSGS), and 10 of 12 patients with rFSGS achieved remission (responders). The remaining 2 did not achieve remission and had a progression to graft failure (non-responders). Consequently, 8 patients with genetic FSGS and 14 patients with nongenetic (presumed primary) FSGS including 11 with rFSGS and 3 with non-rFSGS were analyzed in this study.

glomeruli, and all glomeruli in the specimens were evaluated. IgG depositions colocalized with nephrin in 3 glomeruli per biopsy sample were evaluated by 2 experienced pathologists blinded to the groups with scores ranging from 0 to 3, with 0 representing "no IgG deposition colocalized with nephrin," 1 "IgG deposition colocalized with a small portion (<10%) of nephrin," 2 "IgG deposition colocalized with 10%–50% of nephrin," and 3 "IgG deposition colocalized with >50% of nephrin." The representative images of each score of IgG deposition are shown in Supplementary Figure S1. Dual IF staining for nephrin and IgG subclasses (IgG1–IgG4, 1:50, Sigma-Aldrich) and fluorescein isothiocyanate–conjugated polyclonal antibodies against IgM, C3, and C1q (Dako) with anti-nephrin was also performed using frozen specimens. Dual IF staining for IgG and nephrin tyrosine phosphorylation in all specimens was performed using a rabbit polyclonal anti–Phospho-Nephrin (Tyr1176) antibody (PA5-105709, Thermo Fisher Scientific) at a dilution of 1:50,[8] a rabbit polyclonal anti–Phospho-Nephrin (Tyr1193) antibody (PA5-72369, Thermo Fisher Scientific) at a dilution of 1:50, and a rabbit monoclonal anti–Phospho-Nephrin (Tyr1217) antibody (ab80298, Abcam) at a dilution of 1:50. Dual IF staining for nephrin and ShcA was performed as in our previous report.[8]

All IF images were obtained by the 2-dimensional structured illumination microscopy mode with a Nikon microscope (N-SIM, Nikon), and image reconstruction was carried out using NIS-Elements software (Nikon) on the basis of a previous report with kind support from Dr. Noriko Tokai of the Imaging Core Laboratory (Institute of Medical Science, The University of Tokyo).[8,14]

Foot process width in graft biopsies
The average foot process width (FPW) in electron microscope images was calculated using the Deegens method,[15] as previously reported.[16]

Definitions
Post-transplant FSGS recurrence was defined as (i) the occurrence of nephrotic-range proteinuria (urine protein-creatinine ratio > 2 g/g creatinine) after kidney transplantation and/or (ii) diffuse FPE in graft biopsy on electron microscopy.[10] *Remission* was defined as urine protein excretion < 0.3 g/d.[17]

Statistical analysis
Continuous variables of the patients' clinical characteristics are presented as median (IQR). Anti-nephrin antibody levels were compared using the Wilcoxon rank-sum test. Statistical evaluations were performed using JMP Pro 14.0.0 (SAS Institute).

RESULTS
Patients' clinical characteristics
Patients' clinical characteristics are listed in Table 1 and Supplementary Table S2. The median (IQR) age of all 22 patients at kidney transplantation was 9.5 (8.1–15.2) years. Of 11 patients with rFSGS, prophylactic plasma exchange (PE) was performed in 7 patients, of whom 3 received rituximab before transplantation (Supplementary Table S2).[17] All patients with

Table 1 | Patients' clinical characteristics

Characteristic	Genetic FSGS	Nongenetic FSGS rFSGS	Nongenetic FSGS Non-rFSGS
No. of patients	8	11	3
Ethnicity: Japanese	8 (100)	11 (100)	3 (100)
Male	4 (50)	7 (64)	3 (100)
Age at the onset of NS, yr	3.2 (2.8–4.4)	2.1 (1.5–4.8)	5.5 (4.8–6.4)
Age at kidney failure, yr	10.2 (5.2–14.1)	5.2 (2.4–12.2)	7.1 (6.0–8.2)
Age at transplantation, yr	12.3 (9.2–15.5)	8.1 (6.9–15.0)	12.4 (10.8–12.8)
Donor type: living donor	7 (88)	7 (64)	3 (100)
Prophylactic maneuver	3 (38)[a]	7 (64)[b]	3 (100)
Induction and immunosuppressant regimen			
Basiliximab, Tac, MMF, MP	7 (88)	11 (100)	3 (100)
Basiliximab, CsA, MMF, MP	1 (12)	0 (0)	0 (0)
1 h graft biopsy	1 (12)	6 (55)[c]	3 (100)
Graft biopsies	8 (100)	9 (82)[d]	3 (100)
Days from transplantation to recurrence	N/A	1 (1–1)	N/A
Maximum proteinuria after transplantation, g/g creatinine	N/A	17.9 (7.6–102.3)	N/A
Treatment for recurrence			
Plasma exchange	N/A	9 (82)[e]	N/A
Rituximab	N/A	3 (27)[f]	N/A
Days from transplantation to graft biopsy during recurrence	N/A	22 (20–55)[g]	N/A
Treatment response			
Responder	N/A	9 (82)	N/A
Non-responder	N/A	2 (18)	N/A

CsA, cyclosporine A; FSGS, focal segmental glomerulosclerosis; MMF, mycophenolate mofetil; MP, methylprednisolone; N/A, not applicable; non-rFSGS, nonrecurrent focal segmental glomerulosclerosis; NS, nephrotic syndrome; rFSGS, recurrent focal segmental glomerulosclerosis; SRNS, steroid-resistant nephrotic syndrome; Tac, tacrolimus.
Data are expressed as median (interquartile range) or n (%).
[a]Three of 8 recipients with genetic FSGS underwent a prophylactic maneuver because they did not undergo genetic analysis before transplantation.
[b]Three of 11 patients with rFSGS did not receive a prophylactic maneuver because they underwent deceased donor kidney transplantation. A patient with rFSGS had no pathogenic variants in genes associated with FSGS/SRNS, but his brother also presented with FSGS, so the patient was considered to have variants in undiscovered causative genes associated with FSGS/SRNS and did not undergo a pretransplant prophylactic maneuver.
[c]Graft biopsies: we did not perform 1 h biopsy for a certain period.
[d]Graft biopsies during recurrence were not performed in 2 patients with rFSGS, but 1 h biopsies were analyzed in these 2 patients.
[e]Spontaneous remission was achieved in 1 patient, and MP pulse monotherapy induced remission in 1 patient.
[f]Pretransplant prophylactic rituximab infusion was not used before 2008.
[g]Graft biopsy during recurrence was performed in 9 cases.

rFSGS were anuric-treated with dialysis therapy before transplantation. Post-transplant FSGS recurrence occurred immediately after transplantation in all 11 patients with rFSGS, with the median (IQR) onset of proteinuria at postoperative day 1 (1–1) (Table 1; Supplementary Table S2). The median (IQR) maximum proteinuria after transplantation was 17.9 (7.6–102.3) g/g creatinine in patients with rFSGS (Table 1; Supplementary Table S2). Of 11 patients with rFSGS, 9 achieved remission with and without treatment for recurrence including PE and rituximab (responders) whereas 2 had no response to PE and rituximab and had a progression to graft failure (non-responders) (Table 1; Supplementary Table S2). No patients with genetic FSGS had post-transplant FSGS recurrence (Table 1; Supplementary Table S2).

Circulating anti-nephrin antibodies

Anti-nephrin antibody levels in membranous nephropathy ($n = 13$) and lupus nephritis ($n = 4$) were comparable with those in healthy individuals ($n = 13$). Therefore, these 3 groups were collectively considered controls ($n = 30$) and the *cutoff for anti-nephrin antibody positivity* (231 U/ml) was defined as the maximum antibody level observed in controls. In 11 patients with rFSGS, the median (IQR) anti-nephrin antibody levels before prophylactic PE or during post-transplant recurrence were markedly high at 899 (831–1292) U/ml, with large variability among patients (Figure 2). The median (IQR) anti-nephrin antibody levels before transplantation in patients with non-rFSGS and those with genetic FSGS were 165 (153–244) and 113 (33–172) U/ml, respectively, which were comparable with those in controls (Figure 2).

In MCD, anti-nephrin antibody levels in 5 of 13 patients at relapse (38%) were higher than the cutoff, with a significant reduction at remission (Supplementary Figure S2), which was consistent with a previous report.[7]

Dual IF staining for nephrin and IgG or IgM

Nephrin had a normal linear staining pattern along the glomerular capillary wall in pre-perfusion graft biopsies but had a granular staining pattern in 1-hour postperfusion biopsies obtained from 6 patients with rFSGS with available samples (Table 2 and Figure 3[8]). All six 1-hour biopsies showed punctate deposition of IgG colocalized with nephrin (Table 2 and Figure 3; Supplementary Table S3 and Supplementary Figure S3). These findings were consistent with our previous report.[8] Similar punctate IgG colocalized

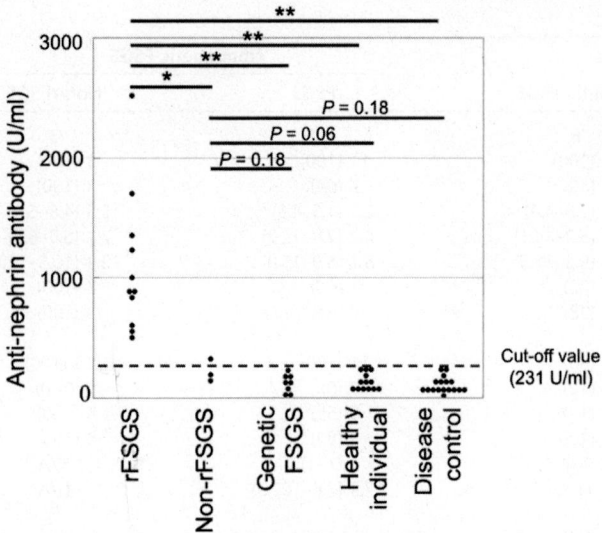

Figure 2 | Anti-nephrin antibody levels during post-transplant focal segmental glomerulosclerosis (FSGS) recurrence. The cutoff (231 U/ml, dotted line) was defined as the maximum antibody level observed in controls consisting of healthy individuals ($n = 13$) and disease controls including membranous nephropathy ($n = 13$) and lupus nephritis ($n = 4$). Patients with recurrent FSGS (rFSGS) had significantly higher plasma anti-nephrin antibody levels than did patients with nonrecurrent FSGS (non-rFSGS), genetic FSGS, healthy individuals, and disease controls. *$P = 0.01$, **$P < 0.01$.

with nephrin was observed in the subsequent biopsies obtained from all recurrent patients during recurrence (Table 2 and Figure 3; Supplementary Table S3 and Supplementary Figure S3). IgG depositions were located at the slit diaphragm and podocyte intracellular areas in 1-hour biopsies, and podocyte intracellular depositions were more frequently observed during recurrence (Figure 3; Supplementary Table S3 and Supplementary Figure S3). IgG depositions that did not colocalize with nephrin were observed in 7 patients (Supplementary Table S3 and Supplementary Figure S4). Trace IgM depositions were observed in some biopsies obtained during post-transplant recurrence, but these IgM depositions did not colocalize with nephrin (Supplementary Figure S5). The graft biopsies obtained from patients with non-rFSGS and genetic FSGS did not show IgG deposition (Table 3; Supplementary Figure S6).

Among patients with MCD, kidney biopsy specimens at relapse in 2 of 5 patients with positive circulating anti-nephrin antibodies showed similar punctate IgG deposition colocalized with nephrin (Supplementary Figure S7), which was consistent with a previous report.[7]

Dual IF staining for nephrin and IgG subclasses

All patients with rFSGS showed depositions of ≥1 IgG subclasses colocalized with nephrin. They showed various patterns of IgG subclass depositions (Supplementary Table S4 and Supplementary Figure S8).

Dual IF staining for nephrin and C3 or C1q

All 1-hour biopsies showed no C3 depositions. Some biopsies during post-transplant recurrence showed trace C3 depositions, which did not colocalize with nephrin (Supplementary Figure S9). C1q was negative in all specimens obtained from patients with rFSGS (Supplementary Figure S10).

Table 2 | Serial changes in circulating anti-nephrin antibody levels and pathological findings in responders and non-responders

Variable	Responders[a] ($n = 9$)	Non-responders ($n = 2$)
Anti-nephrin antibody levels (U/ml)		
Before KTx or during recurrence	860 (829–1231)	1000, 2516
After remission	155 (53–367)[b]	N/A
IgG deposition colocalizing with nephrin		
1 h graft biopsy	4/4 (100)[c]	2/2 (100)
Graft biopsy during recurrence	7/7 (100)[d]	2/2 (100)
Graft biopsy after remission	0/8 (0)	N/A
Increased expression of pY1176/pY1193/pY1217 nephrin		
1 h graft biopsy	3/3 (100)[c]	2/2 (100)
Graft biopsy during recurrence	7/7 (100)[d]	2/2 (100)
Graft biopsy after remission	0/8 (0%)[e]	N/A
Increased ShcA expression		
1 h graft biopsy	3/3 (100)[c]	2/2 (100)
Graft biopsy during recurrence	7/7 (100)[d]	0/2 (0)[f]
Graft biopsy after remission	0/8 (0)[e]	N/A
FPW		
1 h graft biopsy, nm	2184 (2050–2449)[c]	2272, 2204
Graft biopsy during recurrence, nm	4190 (3571–4442)[d]	3854, 7665
Graft biopsy after remission, nm	1683 (1294–2081)[e]	N/A

FPW, foot process width; KTx, kidney transplantation; N/A, not applicable; pY, phosphotyrosine; ShcA, Src homology and collagen homology A.
Data are expressed as median (interquartile range) or n/total n (%). In non-responders, data of the 2 were given.
[a]Remission was defined as urine protein excretion < 0.3 g/d.
[b]Serum samples were available in 5 of 9 patients after remission.
[c]1 h graft biopsies were performed in 3 of 9 responders.
[d]Graft biopsies during recurrence were performed in 7 of 9 responders.
[e]Graft biopsies after remission were available in 8 of 9 responders.
[f]Non-responders showed glomerulosclerosis and decreased expression of nephrin, which might affect the expression of ShcA.

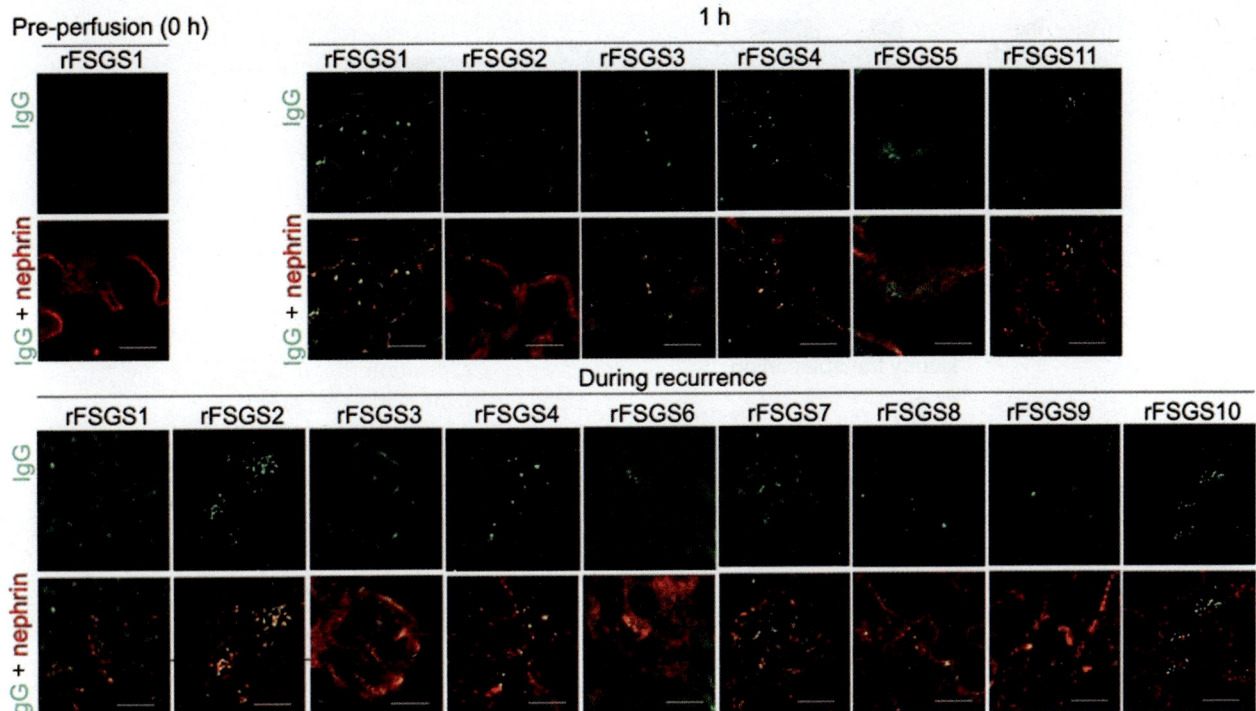

Figure 3 | Dual immunofluorescence staining for IgG and nephrin in graft biopsies at 1 hour postperfusion and during recurrence under structured illumination microscopy observations. Pre-perfusion graft biopsy had no IgG deposition and normal linear staining of nephrin (0 hour). One-hour postperfusion biopsies obtained from 6 patients with recurrent focal segmental glomerulosclerosis (rFSGS) and graft biopsy specimens during recurrence obtained from 9 patients with rFSGS[8] showed punctate IgG deposition colocalized with nephrin. Nephrin expression was decreased in specimens obtained from 2 patients with non-responders (rFSGS1 and rFSGS2) during recurrence. Postoperative days at graft biopsies during recurrence are provided in Supplementary Table S2. Patient rFSGS1 was previously reported.[8] Larger images are shown in Supplementary Figure S3. Bar = 5 μm. To optimize viewing of this image, please see the online version of this article at www.kidney-international.org.

IF staining for phospho-Y1176/Y1193/Y1217

Tyrosine phosphorylation of nephrin at Y1176, Y1193, and Y1217 is important for interacting with its partner proteins including the noncatalytic region of tyrosine kinase and ShcA and can be detected by phospho-specific antibodies.[18] One or more of phosphotyrosine (pY) residues on nephrin, pY1176/pY1193/pY1217, were increased in all 1-hour biopsies and graft biopsies during recurrence in patients with rFSGS (Table 2; Supplementary Figure S11). The graft specimens obtained from patients with non-rFSGS and genetic FSGS did not show an increase in any pY nephrin (Table 3).

IF staining for nephrin and ShcA

Expression of ShcA was increased in all 1-hour biopsies obtained from 5 patients with rFSGS with available samples, which was consistent with our previous report[8] (Table 2). In biopsies obtained during post-transplant recurrence, responders had increased expression of ShcA but non-responders had no expression of ShcA (Table 2); however, non-responders had glomerulosclerosis and decreased expression of nephrin, which may have affected the expression of ShcA. ShcA expression did not increase in protocol biopsies obtained from patients with non-rFSGS and genetic FSGS (Table 3).

FPW

In patients with non-rFSGS, the median (IQR) FPW in protocol graft biopsies was 1473 (1436–1510) nm, which was comparable with those with genetic FSGS (Table 3). All 1-hour graft biopsies obtained from 5 patients with rFSGS had no FSGS lesions on light microscopy, and the median (IQR) FPW was 2204 (2184–2272) nm, reflecting segmental

Table 3 | Results of immunofluorescence studies and FPW of graft biopsies in all patients

Variable	rFSGS (n = 11)	Non-rFSGS (n = 3)	Genetic FSGS (n = 8)
IgG deposition colocalized with nephrin	11 (100)	0 (0)	0 (0)
Increased expression of pY1176/pY1193/pY1217 nephrin	11 (100)	0 (0)	0 (0)
Increased ShcA expression	11 (100)	0 (0)	0 (0)
FPW (nm)	4313 (3873–4515)[a]	1436 (998–1473)	1627 (1618–1637)

FPW, foot process width; FSGS, focal segmental glomerulosclerosis; Non-rFSGS, nonrecurrent focal segmental glomerulosclerosis; pY, phosphotyrosine; rFSGS, post-transplant recurrence of focal segmental glomerulosclerosis; ShcA, Src homology and collagen homology A.
Data are expressed as median (interquartile range) or n/total n (%).
Graft biopsies obtained at 1 h postperfusion or during recurrence were analyzed in rFSGS, and protocol biopsies were analyzed in non-rFSGS and genetic FSGS.
[a]FPW was evaluated in 9 patients with rFSGS with available graft biopsies during recurrence.

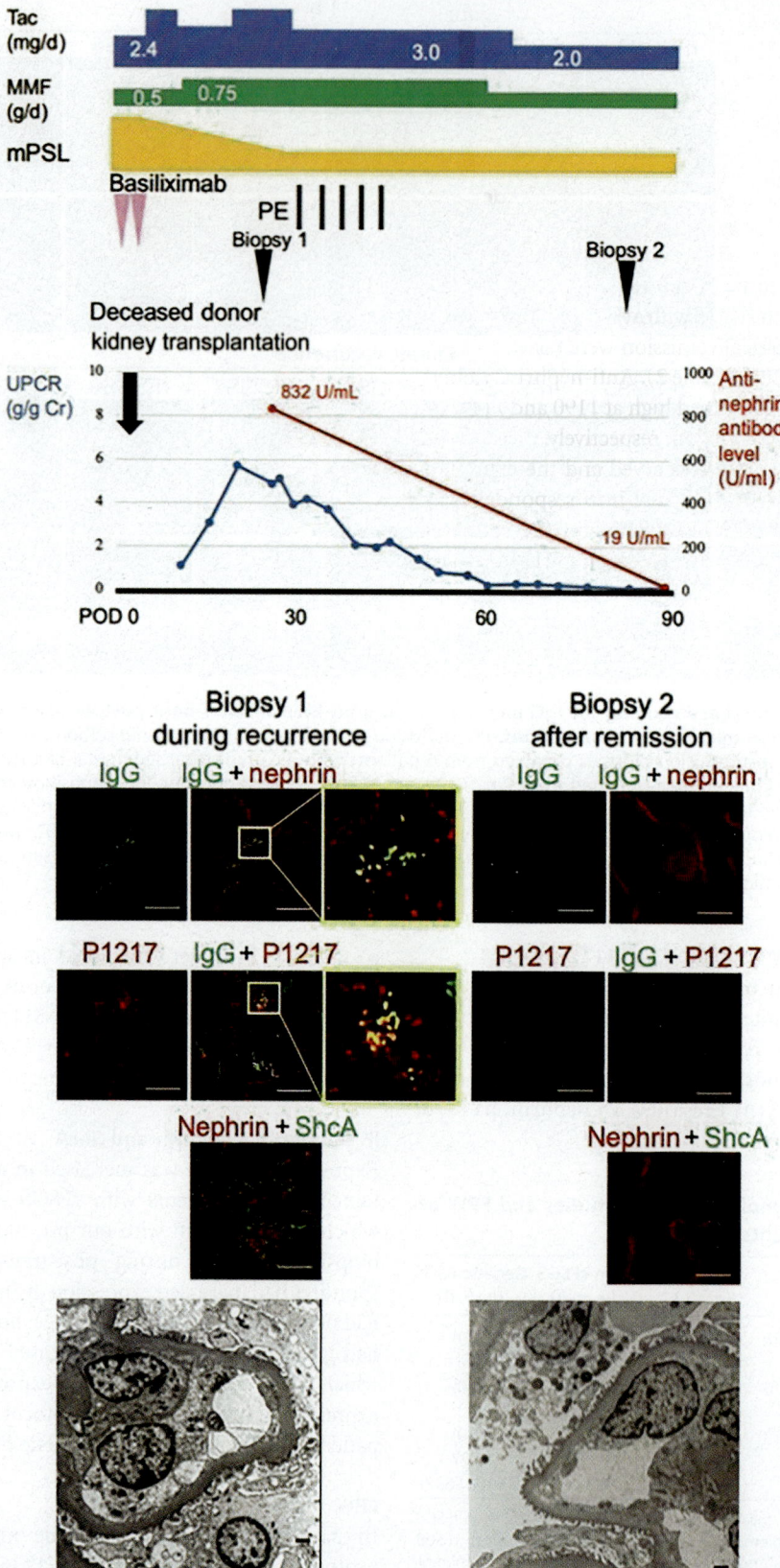

Figure 4 | Representative images of immunostaining for IgG, nephrin, nephrin tyrosine phosphorylation, and Src homology and collagen homology A (ShcA) and electron microscopy during recurrence and after remission. Patient recurrent focal segmental glomerulosclerosis 10 (rFSGS10), who achieved remission after treatment for recurrence including plasma exchange (PE), had a high level of anti-nephrin antibody (832 U/ml) during recurrence, which subsequently decreased to 19 U/ml after remission. Punctate IgG (continued)

FPE. Subsequent graft biopsies obtained from 10 patients with rFSGS during recurrence showed that the median (IQR) FPW was high at 4313 (3873–4515) nm, reflecting diffuse FPE (Table 3), which was consistent with our previous report.[16]

Serial changes in anti-nephrin antibody levels and pathological findings in responders and non-responders with rFSGS

The median (IQR) anti-nephrin antibody levels of responders were significantly decreased from 860 (829–1231) to 155 (53–367) U/ml in 5 patients with rFSGS with available serum samples after remission. The samples at remission were collected at ≥1 year after achieving remission (Table 2). Anti-nephrin antibody levels in 2 non-responders remained high at 1190 and 714 U/ml at 4 and 6 years after transplantation, respectively.

Notably, no IgG staining was observed and the expression pattern of nephrin returned to normal in 8 responders with available graft biopsy samples after remission (Table 2). No staining of pY nephrin (pY1176/pY1193/pY1217) or ShcA was observed after remission (Table 2). In addition, graft biopsies at remission showed no FPE and the median (IQR) FPW was 1683 (1294–2081) nm in responders, which was comparable with genetic FSGS (Table 2). The representative images of IF staining and electron microscopy during recurrence and after remission are shown in Figure 4 and Supplementary Figure S12.

Relationships between anti-nephrin antibody levels and clinical manifestations

Anti-nephrin antibody levels tended to correlate with maximum proteinuria after transplantation in patients with rFSGS ($P = 0.09$; Supplementary Figure S13A), but did not correlate with days from recurrence to remission in 9 responders ($P = 0.32$; Supplementary Figure S13B).

DISCUSSION

The present study confirmed the results of our previous case report[8] and showed that in rFSGS, anti-nephrin antibody levels are elevated, and graft biopsies show IgG deposition colocalized with nephrin, increased pY nephrin/ShcA, altered nephrin distribution, and diffuse FPE. The localization of IgG depositions shifted with disease progression from the slit diaphragm to intracellular areas of podocytes in accordance with altered nephrin expression possibly mediated by endocytosis. Importantly, we demonstrated that anti-nephrin antibodies and associated changes in graft biopsy are absent in non-rFSGS and genetic FSGS cases. Furthermore, in patients with rFSGS who achieved remission, anti-nephrin antibody levels were significantly decreased and graft biopsies showed the disappearance of IgG, pY nephrin, and ShcA staining and recovered a normal expression pattern of nephrin as well as no FPE after remission.

Primary FSGS is thought to be caused by circulating factors that injure podocytes, but the identity of these factors remains elusive despite intensive efforts for many decades.[19,20] Our results indicate an association between circulating anti-nephrin antibodies, the phosphorylation/localization of nephrin in the glomerulus, and disease activity. Strikingly, elevated anti-nephrin antibodies were observed only in rFSGS but not in non-rFSGS or genetic FSGS cases. These findings indicate that anti-nephrin antibodies are an attractive candidate circulating factor responsible for rFSGS. Consistent with this notion, anti-nephrin antibody levels in patients with rFSGS tended to correlate with maximum proteinuria after transplantation.

Anti-nephrin antibody levels before prophylactic PE or during post-transplant recurrence were not significantly different between responders and non-responders, in spite of similar treatment regimens including PE and rituximab after recurrence. Although the precise reason for the different treatment responses is unclear, pathogenic processes of B cell dysregulation may be different between them.[21] The exact mechanisms underlying the pathogenic role of B cells in patients with rFSGS after transplantation should be elucidated in future studies.

All patients with rFSGS showed depositions of ≥1 IgG subclasses including IgG3 and IgG4 colocalized with nephrin. Dominant IgG subclass depositions were varied among patients in our study. Watts et al. described that IgG1 or IgG2 depositions were dominant in patients with MCD.[7] The significance of IgG subclass depositions and the difference in dominant subclasses between MCD and rFSGS after transplantation should be analyzed in future studies.

In the present study, IF staining showed that C3 depositions did not colocalize with nephrin and that C1q was negative in all specimens obtained from patients with rFSGS. Therefore, complement activation may not be critically involved in the pathogenesis of anti-nephrin antibody–mediated FSGS recurrence, which is consistent with the previous study of rat models of MCD induced by mouse monoclonal antibody 5-1-6 against rat nephrin.[2] In patients with rFSGS, slit diaphragms might be injured directly by autoantibodies without fixing complement nor mediating inflammation as identified in the pathogenesis of pemphigus.[22]

Our study was limited by small numbers of patients, especially those with non-rFSGS ($n = 3$). However, given the

Figure 4 | (continued) deposition colocalized with nephrin that had altered localization was observed in graft biopsy during recurrence. Expression of nephrin tyrosine phosphorylation Y1217 and ShcA was increased during recurrence, and their signals were not detected after remission. Notably, no signals for IgG were observed and nephrin had a normal distribution after remission. No staining of nephrin tyrosine phosphorylation or ShcA was observed after remission. Electron microscopy showed diffuse foot process effacement (foot process width 4448 nm) during recurrence and no foot process effacement (foot process width 862 nm) after remission. Larger images are shown in Supplementary Figure S12. Bar = 5 μm. Cr, creatinine; MMF, mycophenolate mofetil; mPSL, methylprednisolone; POD, postoperative day; Tac, tacrolimus; UPCR, urine protein-creatinine ratio. To optimize viewing of this image, please see the online version of this article at www.kidney-international.org.

rarity of primary FSGS and the low rate (20%) of nonrecurrence after transplantation in presumed primary FSGS,[23] collecting a larger number of patients with non-rFSGS is difficult. Further studies are needed to precisely evaluate the relationships between anti-nephrin antibody levels and clinical characteristics of rFSGS and to evaluate whether anti-nephrin antibody levels can be used to predict the post-transplant recurrence of FSGS. In addition, anti-nephrin antibody titers after remission remained above the cutoff level in some patients with rFSGS and MCD (Table 2; Supplementary Figure S2). The significance of slightly elevated anti-nephrin antibody titers in the absence of proteinuria in rFSGS and MCD should be determined in future studies.

Circulating autoantibodies other than anti-nephrin antibody have been implicated in the pathogenesis of post-transplant FSGS recurrence.[24,25] Delville et al. developed a 7-antibody panel, including anti-CD40 antibodies, to predict post-transplant FSGS recurrence.[26] In the present study, IgG depositions that did not colocalize with nephrin were observed in some patients with rFSGS. Therefore, antibodies targeting various podocyte-associated molecules need to be analyzed in future studies.

Of interest, Watts et al. reported that anti-nephrin antibodies were detected in 29% of patients with MCD, with a significant decrease at remission.[7] They also described that 5 of 7 Asian patients with MCD had anti-nephrin antibodies.[7] Consistent with that study,[7] we detected anti-nephrin antibodies in 38% of patients with MCD at relapse, with a significant reduction at remission.

In conclusion, given these results, we propose that circulating nephrin antibodies are a possible candidate for circulating factors involved in the pathogenesis of rFSGS. Larger studies including other ethnicities are required to confirm these findings. In addition, future studies should address how anti-nephrin antibodies affect podocyte functions via nephrin tyrosine phosphorylation.

DISCLOSURE
YS reports grant funding for the Development of Human Resources in Science and Technology "Initiative for Realizing Diversity in the Research Environment" from the Ministry of Education, Culture, Sports, Science and Technology of Japan. MH reports grant funding from Grants-in-Aid for Scientific Research (C) (JP18K07857) from the Ministry of Education, Culture, Sports, Science and Technology of Japan. KM reports grant funding from Grants-in-Aid for Scientific Research (C) (JP21K07829) from the Ministry of Education, Culture, Sports, Science and Technology of Japan. KI reports grant funding from Grants-in-Aid for Scientific Research (C) (JP23K07276) from the Ministry of Education, Culture, Sports, Science and Technology of Japan. TT has declared receiving consultant fees from Otsuka (Canada) and SGK (Canada) and honorarium from Kyowa Kirin (Japan). All the other authors declared no competing interests.

DATA STATEMENT
The data underlying this article will not be made publicly available because of the privacy of the study participants. These data will be shared on reasonable request to the corresponding author.

ACKNOWLEDGMENTS
This work was supported by the Medical Research Institute, Tokyo Women's Medical University (TWMU), and in part by a research grant from the TWMU Career Development Center for Medical Professionals. This work was supported by JSPS Grants-in-Aid for Scientific Research grant numbers JP18K07857, JP21K07829, and JP23K07276. We thank J. Ludovic Croxford, PhD, from Edanz (https://jp.edanz.com/ac) for editing a draft of this manuscript.

SUPPLEMENTARY MATERIAL
Supplementary File (Word)
Supplementary Table S1. List of 65 genes associated with focal segmental glomerulosclerosis/steroid-resistant nephrotic syndrome used for whole exome sequencing.
Supplementary Table S2. Detailed clinical characteristics of kidney transplant recipients with recurrent focal segmental glomerulosclerosis (rFSGS), non-rFSGS, and genetic FSGS.
Supplementary Table S3. Summary of the results of immunofluorescence staining for IgG and nephrin in biopsy specimens obtained at 1 hour and during recurrence in patients with recurrent focal segmental glomerulosclerosis (FSGS).
Supplementary Table S4. Summary of the results of immunofluorescence staining for IgG subclass and nephrin in biopsy specimens obtained during recurrence in patients with recurrent focal segmental glomerulosclerosis (FSGS).
Supplementary Reference.
Supplementary Figure S1. Representative images of each score of IgG deposition colocalized with nephrin.
Supplementary Figure S2. Anti-nephrin antibodies in minimal change disease (MCD) at relapse and remission.
Supplementary Figure S3. Immunofluorescence staining for IgG and nephrin in graft biopsy specimens from patients with recurrent focal segmental glomerulosclerosis (rFSGS) under structured illumination microscopy observations (larger images of Figure 3).
Supplementary Figure S4. IgG depositions that did not colocalize with nephrin in graft biopsy specimens from patients with recurrent focal segmental glomerulosclerosis (rFSGS).
Supplementary Figure S5. Immunofluorescence staining for IgM and nephrin in graft biopsy specimens from patients with recurrent focal segmental glomerulosclerosis (rFSGS) under structured illumination microscopy observations.
Supplementary Figure S6. Immunofluorescence staining for IgG and nephrin in graft biopsy specimens from patients with nonrecurrent focal segmental glomerulosclerosis (non-rFSGS) and genetic FSGS.
Supplementary Figure S7. Immunofluorescence staining for IgG and nephrin in native kidney biopsy specimens from patients with minimal change disease (MCD).
Supplementary Figure S8. Immunofluorescence staining for IgG subclass and nephrin in graft biopsy specimens from patients with recurrent focal segmental glomerulosclerosis (rFSGS) under structured illumination microscopy observations.
Supplementary Figure S9. Immunofluorescence staining for C3 and nephrin in graft biopsy specimens from patients with recurrent focal segmental glomerulosclerosis (rFSGS) under structured illumination microscopy observations.
Supplementary Figure S10. Immunofluorescence staining for C1q and nephrin in graft biopsy specimens from patients with recurrent focal segmental glomerulosclerosis (rFSGS) under structured illumination microscopy observations.
Supplementary Figure S11. Immunofluorescence staining for IgG and phospho-nephrin in graft biopsies during recurrence in patients with recurrent focal segmental glomerulosclerosis (rFSGS).

Supplementary Figure S12. Representative images of immunosaining for IgG, nephrin, nephrin tyrosine phosphorylation, and Src homology and collagen homology A (ShcA) (larger images of Figure 4).

Supplementary Figure S13. Relationships between anti-nephrin antibody levels and maximum proteinuria after transplantation or days from recurrence to remission.

REFERENCES

1. Cravedi P, Kopp JB, Remuzzi G. Recent progress in the pathophysiology and treatment of FSGS recurrence. *Am J Transplant*. 2013;13:266–274.
2. Orikasa M, Matsui K, Oite T, et al. Massive proteinuria induced in rats by a single intravenous injection of a monoclonal antibody. *J Immunol*. 1988;141:807–814.
3. Topham PS, Kawachi H, Haydar SA, et al. Nephritogenic mAb 5-1-6 is directed at the extracellular domain of rat nephrin. *J Clin Invest*. 1999;104:1559–1566.
4. Kawachi H, Koike H, Kurihara H, et al. Cloning of rat nephrin: expression in developing glomeruli and in proteinuric states. *Kidney Int*. 2000;57:1949–1961.
5. Takeuchi K, Naito S, Kawashima N, et al. New anti-nephrin antibody mediated podocyte injury model using a C57BL/6 mouse strain. *Nephron*. 2018;138:71–87.
6. Lahdenperä J, Kilpeläinen P, Liu XL, et al. Clustering-induced tyrosine phosphorylation of nephrin by Src family kinases. *Kidney Int*. 2003;64:404–413.
7. Watts AJB, Keller KH, Lerner GL, et al. Discovery of autoantibodies targeting nephrin in minimal change disease support a novel autoimmune etiology. *J Am Soc Nephrol*. 2022;33:238–252.
8. Hattori M, Shirai Y, Kanda S, et al. Circulating nephrin autoantibodies and posttransplant recurrence of primary focal segmental glomerulosclerosis. *Am J Transplant*. 2022;22:2478–2480.
9. Martin CE, Jones N. ShcA expression in podocytes is dispensable for glomerular development but its upregulation is associated with kidney disease. *Am J Transl Res*. 2021;13:9874–9882.
10. Miura K, Kaneko N, Hashimoto T, et al. Precise clinicopathologic findings for application of genetic testing in pediatric kidney transplant recipients with focal segmental glomerulosclerosis/steroid-resistant nephrotic syndrome. *Pediatr Nephrol*. 2023;38:417–429.
11. Ohta T, Kawaguchi H, Hattori M, et al. Effect of pre- and postoperative plasmapheresis on posttransplant recurrence of focal segmental glomerulosclerosis in children. *Transplantation*. 2001;71:628–633.
12. Hattori M, Akioka Y, Chikamoto H, et al. Increase of integrin-linked kinase activity in cultured podocytes upon stimulation with plasma from patients with recurrent FSGS. *Am J Transplant*. 2008;8:1550–1556.
13. Harita Y, Ishizuka K, Tanego A, et al. Decreased glomerular filtration as the primary factor of elevated circulating suPAR levels in focal segmental glomerulosclerosis. *Pediatr Nephrol*. 2014;29:1553–1560.
14. Gustafsson MG. Surpassing the lateral resolution limit by a factor of two using structured illumination microscopy. *J Microsc*. 2000;198:82–87.
15. Deegens JK, Dijkman HB, Borm GF, et al. Podocyte foot process effacement as a diagnostic tool in focal segmental glomerulosclerosis. *Kidney Int*. 2008;74:1568–1576.
16. Ishizuka K, Miura K, Hashimoto T, et al. Degree of foot process effacement in patients with genetic focal segmental glomerulosclerosis: a single-center analysis and review of the literature. *Sci Rep*. 2021 8;11:12008.
17. Ban H, Miura K, Kaneko N, et al. Amount and selectivity of proteinuria may predict the treatment response in post-transplant recurrence of focal segmental glomerulosclerosis: a single-center retrospective study. *Pediatr Nephrol*. 2021;36:2433–2442.
18. Jones N, Blasutig IM, Eremina V, et al. Nck adaptor proteins link nephrin to the actin cytoskeleton of kidney podocytes. *Nature*. 2006;440:818–823.
19. Candelier JJ, Lorenzo HK. Idiopathic nephrotic syndrome and serum permeability factors: a molecular jigsaw puzzle. *Cell Tissue Res*. 2020;379:231–243.
20. McCarthy ET, Sharma M, Savin VJ. Circulating permeability factors in idiopathic nephrotic syndrome and focal segmental glomerulosclerosis. *Clin J Am Soc Nephrol*. 2010;5:2115–2121.
21. Colucci M, Oniszczuk J, Vivarelli M, Audard V. B-cell dysregulation in idiopathic nephrotic syndrome: what we know and what we need to discover. *Front Immunol*. 2022;13:823204.
22. Hammers CM, Stanley JR. Mechanisms of disease: pemphigus and bullous pemphigoid. *Annu Rev Pathol*. 2016;11:175–197.
23. Bierzynska A, McCarthy HJ, Soderquest K, et al. Genomic and clinical profiling of a national nephrotic syndrome cohort advocates a precision medicine approach to disease management. *Kidney Int*. 2017;91:937–947.
24. Musante L, Candiano G, Bruschi M, et al. Circulating anti-actin and anti-ATP synthase antibodies identify a subset of patients with idiopathic nephrotic syndrome. *Clin Exp Immunol*. 2005;141:491–499.
25. Alachkar N, Gupta G, Montgomery RA. Angiotensin antibodies and focal segmental glomerulosclerosis. *N Engl J Med*. 2013;368:971–973.
26. Delville M, Sigdel TK, Wei C, et al. A circulating antibody panel for pretransplant prediction of FSGS recurrence after kidney transplantation. *Sci Transl Med*. 2014;6:256ra136.

clinical investigation

A population-based cohort defined risk of hyperkalemia after initiating SGLT-2 inhibitors, GLP1 receptor agonists or DPP-4 inhibitors to patients with chronic kidney disease and type 2 diabetes

see commentary on page 442

Edouard L. Fu[1], Julianna Mastrorilli[1], Katsiaryna Bykov[1], Deborah J. Wexler[2], Alexander Cervone[1], Kueiyu Joshua Lin[1,3], Elisabetta Patorno[1] and Julie M. Paik[1,4,5]

[1]Division of Pharmacoepidemiology and Pharmacoeconomics, Department of Medicine, Brigham and Women's Hospital and Harvard Medical School, Boston, Massachusetts, USA; [2]Diabetes Center, Massachusetts General Hospital and Harvard Medical School, Boston, Massachusetts, USA; [3]Department of Medicine, Massachusetts General Hospital and Harvard Medical School, Boston, Massachusetts, USA; [4]Division of Renal (Kidney) Medicine, Department of Medicine, Brigham and Women's Hospital, Boston, Massachusetts, USA; and [5]New England Geriatric Research Education and Clinical Center, VA Boston Healthcare System, Boston, Massachusetts, USA

Hyperkalemia is a common adverse event in patients with chronic kidney disease (CKD) and type 2 diabetes and limits the use of guideline-recommended therapies such as renin-angiotensin system inhibitors. Here, we evaluated the comparative effects of sodium-glucose cotransporter-2 inhibitors (SGLT-2i), glucagon-like peptide-1 receptor agonists (GLP-1RA) and dipeptidyl peptidase-4 inhibitors (DPP-4i) on the risk of hyperkalemia. We conducted a population-based active-comparator, new-user cohort study using claims data from Medicare and two large United States commercial insurance databases (April 2013-April 2022). People with CKD stages 3-4 and type 2 diabetes who newly initiated SGLT-2i vs. DPP-4i (141671 patients), GLP-1RA vs. DPP-4i (159545 patients) and SGLT-2i vs. GLP-1RA (93033 patients) were included. The primary outcome was hyperkalemia diagnosed in inpatient or outpatient settings. Secondary outcomes included hyperkalemia diagnosed in inpatient or emergency department setting, and serum potassium levels of 5.5 mmol/L or more. Pooled hazard ratios and rate differences were estimated after propensity score matching to adjust for over 140 potential confounders. Initiation of SGLT-2i was associated with a lower risk of hyperkalemia compared with DPP-4i (hazard ratio 0.74; 95% confidence interval 0.68-0.80) and contrasted to GLP-1RA (0.92; 0.86-0.99). Compared with DPP-4i, GLP-1RA were also associated with a lower risk of hyperkalemia (0.80; 0.75-0.86). Corresponding absolute rate differences/1000 person-years were -24.8 (95% confidence interval -31.8 to -17.7), -5.0 (-10.9 to 0.8), and -17.7 (-23.4 to -12.1), respectively. Similar findings were observed for the secondary outcomes, among subgroups, and across single agents within the SGLT-2i and GLP-1RA classes. Thus, SGLT-2i and GLP-1RA are associated with a lower risk of hyperkalemia than DPP-4i in patients with CKD and type 2 diabetes, further supporting the use of these drugs in this population.

Kidney International (2024) 105, 618–628; https://doi.org/10.1016/j.kint.2023.11.025

KEYWORDS: chronic kidney disease; dipeptidyl peptidase-4 inhibitors; glucagon-like peptide-1 receptor agonists; hyperkalemia; sodium-glucose cotransporter-2 inhibitors; type 2 diabetes

Copyright © 2023, International Society of Nephrology. Published by Elsevier Inc. All rights reserved.

Lay Summary

Hyperkalemia means that the potassium level in the blood is too high. It commonly occurs in people who have type 2 diabetes and kidney disease. Hyperkalemia often leads physicians to stop medications that protect the kidney, such as angiotensin-converting enzyme inhibitors, because these medications also increase potassium levels in the blood. It is therefore important to find treatments that can prevent hyperkalemia. Sodium-glucose cotransporter-2 inhibitors (SGLT-2i), glucagon-like peptide-1 receptor agonists (GLP-1RAs), and dipeptidyl peptidase-4 inhibitors (DPP-4i) are commonly used medications to lower blood glucose in patients with type 2 diabetes. We were interested in investigating whether these medications could prevent hyperkalemia. In this study, we found that people with type 2 diabetes and kidney disease who used SGLT-2i and GLP-1RAs had a lower risk of developing hyperkalemia than people who started DPP-4i. Our study, therefore, supports the use of these medications in people with type 2 diabetes and kidney disease.

Correspondence: *Julie Paik, Division of Pharmacoepidemiology and Pharmacoeconomics, Brigham and Women's Hospital, 1620 Tremont St, BC-3012C, Boston, Massachusetts 02120, USA. E-mail: jmpaik@bwh.harvard.edu*

Received 24 May 2023; revised 2 November 2023; accepted 10 November 2023; published online 13 December 2023

Hyperkalemia is a common problem among people with chronic kidney disease (CKD) and type 2 diabetes (T2D).[1] Lower kidney function and T2D are independent risk factors for developing hyperkalemia.[2,3] Furthermore, various common medication classes that are used to improve clinical outcomes in these patients, such as renin-angiotensin system inhibitors (RASi)[4] and mineralocorticoid receptor antagonists (MRAs), increase the risk of hyperkalemia.[5–9] In addition to the risk of life-threatening arrhythmias, the occurrence of hyperkalemia negatively affects clinical outcomes in patients with CKD and T2D because of the necessity of discontinuing or reducing the dose of guideline-recommended medications, such as RASi.[10,11]

In recent years, sodium-glucose cotransporter-2 inhibitors (SGLT-2i), glucagon-like peptide-1 receptor agonists (GLP-1RAs), and dipeptidyl peptidase-4 inhibitors (DPP-4i) have become common drugs for treating T2D[12,13] in clinical practice, with the former 2 drug classes showing cardiovascular and kidney benefits.[14–16] Moreover, SGLT-2i have been shown to reduce the risk of hyperkalemia compared with placebo in randomized trials.[17,18] However, several key knowledge gaps remain: first, it is unknown whether the beneficial effects of SGLT-2i for reducing hyperkalemia that were observed in highly controlled trial conditions are similarly observed in real-world settings. Second, head-to-head comparisons between SGLT-2i, GLP-1RAs, and DPP-4i are currently lacking. Last, there are small-scale randomized trials that suggest GLP-1RAs influence tubular handling of electrolytes and increase potassium excretion,[19,20] although it is unknown whether this increase in potassium excretion also leads to a reduced risk of hyperkalemia in clinical settings.

The aim of this study was, therefore, to investigate the comparative effectiveness of SGLT-2i, GLP-1RAs, and DPP-4i in lowering the risk of hyperkalemia among patients with CKD and T2D in a real-world setting.

METHODS
Data source
We used data from 3 large US administrative claims databases: Optum's deidentified Clinformatics Data Mart Database (CDM), IBM MarketScan, and Medicare fee-for-service Parts A, B, and D. CDM and IBM MarketScan include a national commercially insured US population. Medicare is a federal health insurance program providing health care coverage for US residents aged ≥65 years or <65 years with disabilities. All databases contain deidentified longitudinal information, including patient demographics, health care use, inpatient and outpatient medical diagnoses and procedures, outpatient laboratory results (≈45% of patients in CDM and 5%–10% of patients in IBM MarketScan), and prescription dispensing records. The study was approved by the Mass General Brigham Institutional Review Board with waiver of informed consent, and signed data license agreements were in place for all data sources.

Study design and study population
We constructed 3 active-comparator, new-user cohorts[21–23] of patients who newly initiated SGLT-2i versus DPP-4i (cohort 1), GLP-1RA versus DPP-4i (cohort 2), and SGLT-2i versus GLP-1RA (cohort 3) between April 2013 and the end of available data (April 2022 in CDM, December 2020 in IBM MarketScan, and December 2019 in Medicare) (Supplementary Figure S1). New initiation was defined as a filled prescription for 1 of the 2 drug classes in each pairwise comparison, with no dispensing of either drug in the previous 365 days. Eligible patients were required to be aged ≥18 years (aged ≥65 years for Medicare), have at least 12 months of continuous insurance enrollment before drug initiation, and have diagnoses for CKD and T2D. We defined CKD as at least 1 inpatient or 2 outpatient diagnosis codes for CKD stage 3 to 4[24] (Supplementary Table S1). This definition was based on a previously validated algorithm, which showed sufficient accuracy to identify a CKD population (positive predictive value, >80%).[25] Exclusion criteria were a history of type 1 diabetes, secondary or gestational diabetes, CKD stage 5/end-stage kidney disease, nursing home admission, organ transplant, pancreatitis, cirrhosis, acute hepatitis, or multiple endocrine neoplasia type 2 (Supplementary Table S1). Furthermore, we excluded individuals who had a hyperkalemia diagnosis or used potassium binders in the 90 days preceding cohort entry to decrease the possibility that early outcomes during follow-up would be related to a previous hyperkalemia diagnosis (i.e., reverse causation bias) or that the drugs under comparison were started differentially based on history of hyperkalemia (i.e., confounding).

Treatment strategies and follow-up
Our treatment strategies of interest were initiation of SGLT-2i, GLP-1RA, or DPP-4i. Follow-up began on the day after cohort entry and continued in an "as-treated" approach until treatment discontinuation or switch to a drug in the comparator class, outcome occurrence, death, end of continuous health plan enrollment, or end of available data, whichever occurred first. Discontinuation was defined as no prescription refill for the index exposure within the 30 days after the most recent prescription had ended, based on days' supply. We chose an as-treated follow-up approach as our primary analysis to address the high rate of treatment discontinuation in routine care[26] and reduce exposure misclassification.[22]

Study outcomes
The primary outcome was a diagnosis code for hyperkalemia in the inpatient or outpatient setting (definitions provided in Supplementary Table S2). Secondary outcomes included a hyperkalemia diagnosis in the inpatient or emergency department setting, and a composite of serum potassium level ≥5.5 mmol/L in the outpatient setting or hyperkalemia diagnosis in the inpatient setting. The latter outcome was only assessed in CDM among the individuals who had at least 1 serum potassium level measured in the 365 days before cohort entry, as IBM MarketScan and Medicare contain few or no laboratory measurements.

We also performed an internal validation study in CDM to test the specificity and sensitivity of the claims-based hyperkalemia definitions. We included all adult individuals who had a serum potassium measurement (LOINC [Logical Observation Identifier Names and Codes] 6298-4, 77142-8, 12812-4, 12813-2, and 42569-4) and assessed whether there was a hyperkalemia diagnosis in the 90-day window after the serum potassium measurement. Among 12.3 million individuals, we found a specificity of 99.5% and a sensitivity of 22.3% for the primary outcome definition when serum potassium level ≥5.5 mmol/L was used to define hyperkalemia, and specificity of 99.3% and sensitivity of 37.1% when serum potassium level ≥6.0 mmol/L was used to define hyperkalemia. Because specificity is high and misclassification is likely nondifferential, even when sensitivity is low, the relative risk estimates will be unbiased.[27] However, when sensitivity is low, absolute rate differences will be biased toward the null. Hence, the observed associations on the absolute scale for the primary outcome will represent an underestimate of the true absolute rate difference.

Covariates

Patient baseline characteristics were measured during the 365 days before cohort entry date. On the basis of subject matter knowledge and previous studies evaluating outcomes of medication use in people with CKD and T2D,[28] we chose covariates that were associated with the outcome or were confounders or confounder proxies. Ascertainment of comorbid conditions was based on *International Classification of Diseases, Ninth Revision*, and *International Statistical Classification of Diseases and Related Health Problems, Tenth Revision*, diagnosis and procedure codes, and ascertainment of drug use was based on generic drug names, in the 365 days before and including the cohort entry date. Covariates of interest included the following: (i) demographics, including age, sex, and race (race was only available in CDM and Medicare); (ii) comorbid conditions; (iii) diabetes-specific complications; (iv) use of cardiovascular and diabetes drugs; (v) use of other comedications; (vi) measures of health care use, including number of hospitalizations, emergency department visits, cardiologist and nephrologist visits, and number of laboratory tests; (vii) healthy behavior markers, including vaccinations and screening; and (viii) calendar year. To address potential confounding by frailty, we also used a claims-based frailty index.[29] Race was self-reported in the claims data sources. There were no missing data for the other covariates, as the absence of a diagnosis or procedure code was interpreted as the absence of a particular condition.

Statistical analysis

To adjust for baseline confounders, we used 1:1 propensity score matching using the nearest neighbor method and a caliper of 0.01 of the propensity score.[30] We estimated the probability of receiving SGLT-2i versus DPP-4i (cohort 1), GLP-1RA versus DPP-4i (cohort 2), and SGLT-2i versus GLP-1RA (cohort 3) as a function of >140 preexposure covariates using multivariable logistic regression. We included all covariates from Supplementary Table S3 in the propensity score model, except for laboratory results, which were only available in a subset of patients ($\approx$22% of the overall population). Covariate balance before and after matching was assessed using standardized mean differences.[31,32] We also assessed balance in laboratory results to assess potential residual confounding by unmeasured factors, because these were not included in the propensity score. For each outcome, we calculated numbers of events, incidence rates, incidence rate differences, and hazard ratios (HRs) in the propensity score–matched cohorts. The HRs and incidence rate differences with their 95% confidence intervals (CIs) were estimated in each data source and then pooled using a fixed-effects meta-analysis. HRs were estimated using Cox regression, and incidence rate differences were determined using generalized linear regression with identity link function and normal error distribution.[33] We constructed survival plots with the Aalen-Johansen estimator, which does not overestimate risks in the presence of the competing risk of death.[34] Analyses were performed using R, version 3.6.2, and the Aetion Evidence Platform, version 4.53.[35]

Subgroup analyses and effectiveness of individual agents

We performed subgroup analyses in the following prespecified subgroups: age (<75 vs. ≥75 years), sex, race (White vs. Black), baseline cardiovascular disease, heart failure, and use of RASi, MRA, and loop diuretics (definitions for cardiovascular disease and heart failure are provided in Supplemental Table S3). Subgroup analyses according to race were only performed in the Medicare group. Cardiovascular disease was defined as a composite of myocardial infarction, stable angina, acute coronary syndrome, coronary atherosclerosis, history of coronary procedure, heart failure, ischemic stroke, and peripheral vascular disease. For subgroup analyses, propensity score estimation and matching were reperformed for each subgroup. In secondary analyses, to investigate potential differences between agents within the SGLT-2i and GLP-1RA classes, we assessed the associations between empagliflozin, canagliflozin, dapagliflozin, liraglutide, dulaglutide, exenatide, and semaglutide versus DPP-4i.

Sensitivity analyses

We performed the following sensitivity analyses: first, we defined treatment discontinuation as no prescription refill within 60 days (instead of 30 days); second, to investigate the influence of informative censoring, we applied an intention-to-treat follow-up approach, where follow-up was continued for a maximum of 180 and 365 days regardless of treatment discontinuation or switch; third, we excluded all patients who had a history of hyperkalemia or potassium binder use in the prior 365 days, and used a broad outcome defined as hyperkalemia diagnosis in the inpatient or outpatient setting or initiation of potassium binders during follow-up.

RESULTS

Baseline characteristics of study populations

Flowcharts for study inclusion are shown in Supplementary Figure S2. After 1:1 propensity score matching, the SGLT-2i versus DPP-4i cohort included 21,196 propensity score–matched pairs, the GLP-1RA versus DPP-4i cohort included 33,402 pairs, and the SGLT-2i versus GLP-1RA cohort included 27,997 propensity score–matched pairs. After matching, baseline characteristics in the 3 cohorts were well balanced, with standardized mean difference <0.10 (Table 1 and Supplementary Tables S4–S6). In the SGLT-2i versus DPP-4i cohort, mean age was 72 years, 56% were men, 90% had CKD stage 3, 59% had cardiovascular disease, and 26% had heart failure. Among those with available laboratory measurements (22% of the overall population), mean estimated glomerular filtration rate was 43 ml/min per 1.73 m^2 and mean serum potassium level was 4.5 mmol/L. Furthermore, 81% used angiotensin-converting enzyme inhibitor or angiotensin II receptor blocker, 10% used MRA, 35% used loop diuretics, and 36% used insulin during the baseline period. Baseline characteristics were similar across the 3 cohorts, although insulin use was higher for the GLP-1RA versus DPP-4i cohort (46% vs. 34%–36%). In the SGLT-2i versus DPP-4i cohort, the most commonly used SGLT-2i were empagliflozin (52.5%), followed by canagliflozin (32.9%) and dapagliflozin (14.4%). In the GLP-1RA versus DPP-4i cohort, the most commonly used GLP-1RAs were liraglutide (38.5%), dulaglutide (36.0%), exenatide (13.1%), and semaglutide (10.3%) (Supplementary Table S7).

Hyperkalemia risk associated with SGLT-2i, GLP-1RA, and DPP-4i

After propensity score matching, the mean follow-up for the primary outcome was 7.8 months in the SGLT-2i versus DPP-4i cohort, 8.0 months in the GLP-1RA versus DPP-4i cohort, and 7.6 months in the SGLT-2i versus GLP-1RA cohort (Supplementary Table S8). Initiation of SGLT-2i was

Table 1 | Selected baseline characteristics of patients with chronic kidney disease and type 2 diabetes initiating SGLT-2i versus DPP-4i, GLP-1RA versus DPP-4i, and SGLT-2i versus GLP1-1RA after 1:1 propensity score matching

Characteristic	SGLT-2i vs. DPP-4i		GLP-1RA vs. DPP-4i		SGLT-2i vs. GLP-1RA	
	SGLT-2i	DPP-4i	GLP-1RA	DPP-4i	SGLT-2i	GLP-1RA
Total	21,196	21,196	33,402	33,402	27,997	27,997
Demographics						
Age, mean (SD), yr	72.2 (7.4)	72.2 (7.4)	71.8 (7.1)	71.7 (7.1)	72.3 (7.4)	72.3 (7.4)
Male sex, n (%)	11,918 (56.2)	11,832 (55.8)	16,607 (49.7)	16,634 (49.8)	15,466 (55.2)	15,496 (55.3)
Race/ethnicity, n (%)[a]						
White	13,804 (65.1)	13,810 (65.2)	22,228 (66.5)	22,305 (66.8)	17,917 (64.0)	17,915 (64.0)
Black	2179 (10.3)	2152 (10.2)	3672 (11.0)	3630 (10.9)	2846 (10.2)	2822 (10.1)
Other	3030 (14.3)	3051 (14.4)	4036 (12.1)	4001 (12.0)	4157 (14.8)	4183 (14.9)
Burden of comorbidities, mean (SD)						
Combined comorbidity score	4.1 (2.5)	4.1 (2.4)	4.1 (2.4)	4.1 (2.4)	4.0 (2.4)	4.0 (2.4)
Frailty score	0.21 (0.06)	0.21 (0.06)	0.21 (0.06)	0.21 (0.06)	0.20 (0.06)	0.21 (0.06)
Comorbidities, n (%)						
CKD stage 3	19,064 (89.9)	19,031 (89.8)	28,113 (84.2)	28,060 (84.0)	25,011 (89.3)	24,946 (89.1)
CKD stage 4	2132 (10.1)	2165 (10.2)	5289 (15.8)	5342 (16.0)	2986 (10.7)	3051 (10.9)
Hyperkalemia	1138 (5.4)	1130 (5.3)	1989 (6.0)	1965 (5.9)	1571 (5.6)	1614 (5.8)
Hypokalemia	1054 (5.0)	1081 (5.1)	1803 (5.4)	1750 (5.2)	1329 (4.7)	1367 (4.9)
Acute kidney injury	3536 (16.7)	3554 (16.8)	6247 (18.7)	6187 (18.5)	4528 (16.2)	4535 (16.2)
Hypertension	20,413 (96.3)	20,397 (96.2)	32,229 (96.5)	32,224 (96.5)	26,949 (96.3)	26,959 (96.3)
Hyperlipidemia	18,845 (88.9)	18,835 (88.9)	29,606 (88.6)	29,538 (88.4)	24,931 (89.0)	24,924 (89.0)
Cardiovascular disease[b]	12,588 (59.4)	12,497 (59.0)	19,184 (57.4)	19,310 (57.8)	16,346 (58.4)	16,216 (57.9)
Acute myocardial infarction	1008 (4.8)	997 (4.7)	1306 (3.9)	1280 (3.8)	1187 (4.2)	1187 (4.2)
Heart failure	5543 (26.2)	5589 (26.4)	8516 (25.5)	8421 (25.2)	6971 (24.9)	6931 (24.8)
Atrial fibrillation	3960 (18.7)	3936 (18.6)	5891 (17.6)	5855 (17.5)	5006 (17.9)	4993 (17.8)
Ischemic stroke	3098 (14.6)	3070 (14.5)	4817 (14.4)	4856 (14.5)	4005 (14.3)	4004 (14.3)
Peripheral arterial disease	3918 (18.5)	3890 (18.4)	6188 (18.5)	6194 (18.5)	5159 (18.4)	5188 (18.5)
Diabetes-related conditions, n (%)						
Diabetic nephropathy	14,493 (68.4)	14,495 (68.4)	22,821 (68.3)	22,823 (68.3)	18,975 (67.8)	18,940 (67.7)
Diabetic retinopathy	3836 (18.1)	3773 (17.8)	6496 (19.4)	6559 (19.6)	5044 (18.0)	5033 (18.0)
Diabetic neuropathy	7631 (36.0)	7654 (36.1)	12,694 (38.0)	12,647 (37.9)	9995 (35.7)	9973 (35.6)
Hypoglycemia	3857 (18.2)	3871 (18.3)	6005 (18.0)	6022 (18.0)	4941 (17.6)	4988 (17.8)
No. of distinct medications, mean (SD)	15.4 (6.4)	15.5 (6.5)	15.7 (6.3)	15.8 (6.5)	15.6 (6.5)	15.7 (6.4)
Diabetes medications on day of entry to cohort, n (%)						
No. of diabetes drugs, mean (SD)	2.20 (0.85)	2.21 (0.83)	2.15 (0.84)	2.16 (0.84)	2.44 (0.95)	2.45 (0.96)
Metformin	12,365 (58.3)	12,438 (58.7)	16,144 (48.3)	16,281 (48.7)	16,013 (57.2)	16,053 (57.3)
Sulfonylureas	9640 (45.5)	9760 (46.0)	14,924 (44.7)	15,180 (45.4)	13,944 (49.8)	14,003 (50.0)
DPP-4i	N/A	N/A	N/A	N/A	10,902 (38.9)	10,930 (39.0)
SGLT-2i	N/A	N/A	2619 (7.8)	2600 (7.8)	N/A	N/A
GLP-1RA	3452 (16.3)	3416 (16.1)	N/A	N/A	N/A	N/A
Insulin	7643 (36.1)	7770 (36.7)	15,258 (45.7)	15,149 (45.4)	9588 (34.2)	9568 (34.2)
Other medication use, n (%)						
ACEi or ARB	17,203 (81.2)	17,201 (81.2)	26,588 (79.6)	26,572 (79.6)	22,813 (81.5)	22,864 (81.7)
ARNI	326 (1.5)	337 (1.6)	288 (0.9)	298 (0.9)	365 (1.3)	364 (1.3)
Mineralocorticoid receptor antagonists	2080 (9.8)	2079 (9.8)	3215 (9.6)	3178 (9.5)	2605 (9.3)	2621 (9.4)
β-Blockers	12,828 (60.5)	12,874 (60.7)	20,382 (61.0)	20,386 (61.0)	16,912 (60.4)	16,868 (60.2)
Calcium channel blockers	9330 (44.0)	9245 (43.6)	15,064 (45.1)	15,051 (45.1)	12,612 (45.0)	12,649 (45.2)
Loop diuretics	7314 (34.5)	7285 (34.4)	12,929 (38.7)	12,865 (38.5)	9496 (33.9)	9545 (34.1)
Statins	17,815 (84.0)	17,738 (83.7)	27,679 (82.9)	27,649 (82.8)	23,666 (84.5)	23,537 (84.1)
Antiplatelet agents	3940 (18.6)	3988 (18.8)	5799 (17.4)	5863 (17.6)	5167 (18.5)	5160 (18.4)
Anticoagulants	3368 (15.9)	3294 (15.5)	5119 (15.3)	5117 (15.3)	4270 (15.3)	4272 (15.3)
Potassium binders	94 (0.4)	89 (0.4)	216 (0.6)	221 (0.7)	162 (0.6)	173 (0.6)
Potassium supplements	3133 (14.8)	3207 (15.1)	5129 (15.4)	5133 (15.4)	4040 (14.4)	3992 (14.3)
Health care utilization markers						
No. of hospitalizations, mean (SD)	0.3 (0.78)	0.3 (0.79)	0.3 (0.8)	0.3 (0.8)	0.3 (0.8)	0.3 (0.8)
No. of emergency department visits, mean (SD)	0.8 (1.95)	0.9 (1.82)	0.9 (2.1)	0.9 (1.9)	0.8 (1.9)	0.8 (2.0)
No. of internist visits, mean (SD)	22.5 (27.85)	22.7 (27.69)	21.3 (25.9)	21.3 (25.9)	22.3 (27.4)	22.4 (27.0)
No. of cardiologist visits, mean (SD)	5.7 (10.8)	5.6 (10.9)	5.1 (9.7)	5.1 (9.7)	5.4 (10.1)	5.4 (10.2)
No. of endocrinologist visits, mean (SD)	1.9 (7.17)	1.8 (6.81)	2.1 (7.2)	2.0 (7.0)	1.7 (6.5)	1.8 (6.7)
No. of nephrologist visits, mean (SD)	1.9 (5.56)	1.8 (5.24)	2.3 (5.9)	2.3 (5.8)	1.9 (5.6)	1.9 (5.6)
Potassium test order, n (%)	928 (4.4)	944 (4.5)	1554 (4.7)	1572 (4.7)	1152 (4.1)	1210 (4.3)

(Continued on following page)

Table 1 | (Continued) Selected baseline characteristics of patients with chronic kidney disease and type 2 diabetes initiating SGLT-2i versus DPP-4i, GLP-1RA versus DPP-4i, and SGLT-2i versus GLP1-1RA after 1:1 propensity score matching

Characteristic	SGLT-2i vs. DPP-4i		GLP-1RA vs. DPP-4i		SGLT-2i vs. GLP-1RA	
	SGLT-2i	DPP-4i	GLP-1RA	DPP-4i	SGLT-2i	GLP-1RA
Laboratory measurements, mean (SD)						
eGFR, ml/min per 1.73 m^2[c]	45 (16)	42 (15)	42 (15)	42 (15)	45 (16)	42 (15)
Serum potassium, mmol/L[c]	4.5 (0.4)	4.5 (0.5)	4.5 (0.4)	4.5 (0.5)	4.5 (0.4)	4.5 (0.4)

ACEi, angiotensin-converting enzyme inhibitor; ARB, angiotensin II receptor blocker; ARNI, angiotensin receptor/neprilysin inhibitor; CKD, chronic kidney disease; DPP-4i, dipeptidyl peptidase-4 inhibitor; eGFR, estimated glomerular filtration rate; GLP-1RA, glucagon-like peptide-1 receptor agonist; N/A, not applicable; SGLT-2i, sodium-glucose cotransporter-2 inhibitor.
[a]Pooled across Clinformatics Data Mart Database and Medicare database only, and therefore does not add up to 100%.
[b]Cardiovascular disease was defined as a composite of myocardial infarction, stable angina, acute coronary syndrome, coronary atherosclerosis, history of coronary procedure, heart failure, ischemic stroke, and peripheral vascular disease.
[c]After propensity score matching, eGFR was available for 21.5% of participants in the SGLT-2i versus DPP-4i cohort, 17.6% for the GLP-1RA versus DPP-4i cohort, and 20.0% for the SGLT-2i versus GLP-RA cohort. Serum potassium level was available in 21.3%, 17.4%, and 19.8%, respectively.

associated with a lower risk of hyperkalemia compared with DPP-4i, with an adjusted HR of 0.74 (95% CI, 0.68–0.80) and incidence rate difference of −24.8 (95% CI, −31.8 to −17.7) per 1000 person-years (Table 2). Furthermore, GLP-1RAs were associated with a lower risk of hyperkalemia compared with DPP-4i, with an adjusted HR of 0.80 (95% CI, 0.75–0.86) and incidence rate difference of −17.7 (95% CI, −23.4 to −12.1) per 1000 person-years. The adjusted HR for SGLT-2i versus GLP-1RA was 0.92 (95% CI, 0.86–0.99), with an incidence rate difference of −5.0 (95% CI, −10.9 to 0.8). The lower risk of hyperkalemia for SGLT-2i and GLP-1RA compared with DPP-4i was observed within the first 6 months of follow-up (Figure 1). When comparing SGLT-2i versus GLP-1RA, the cumulative incidence curves for hyperkalemia overlapped for the first 9 months of follow-up and started to diverge thereafter. Absolute risks and absolute risk differences at 6-month intervals are reported in Supplementary Table S9. At 2 years of follow-up, the absolute risk was 4.3% (95% CI, 2.8%–5.7%) lower for SGLT-2i versus DPP-4i and 2.3% (95% CI, 1.2%–3.5%) lower for GLP-1RA versus DPP-4i.

When the outcome definition was changed to hyperkalemia diagnosis in the inpatient or emergency department setting, the results were consistent for SGLT-2i versus DPP-4i and GLP-1RA versus DPP-4i comparisons, with HRs of 0.76 (95% CI, 0.58–0.99) and 0.66 (95% CI, 0.54–0.80), respectively. Furthermore, the HR for SGLT-2i versus GLP-1RA was 1.06 (95% CI, 0.82–1.38) (Supplementary Table S10). Similar

Table 2 | Comparative effectiveness of SGLT-2i versus DPP-4i, GLP-1RA versus DPP-4i, and SGLT-2i versus GLP-1RA on risk of hyperkalemia diagnosis in inpatient or outpatient setting before and after 1:1 propensity score matching

SGLT-2i vs. DPP-4i	Before 1:1 propensity score matching		After 1:1 propensity score matching	
	SGLT-2i	DPP-4i	SGLT-2i	DPP-4i
Sample size, n	25,257	116,414	21,196	21,196
Total events, n	1160	9682	960	1441
Follow-up, PY	15,085	92,642	12,758	14,408
Incidence rate/1000 PY (95% CI)	76.9 (72.5 to 81.5)	104.5 (102.4 to 106.6)	75.3 (70.6 to 80.2)	100.0 (94.9 to 105.3)
Rate difference/1000 PY (95% CI)	**−27.6 (−32.5 to −22.7)**	Ref	**−24.8 (−31.8 to −17.7)**	Ref
Hazard ratio (95% CI)	**0.69 (0.65 to 0.74)**	Ref	**0.74 (0.68 to 0.80)**	Ref

GLP-1RA vs. DPP-4i	Before 1:1 propensity score matching		After 1:1 propensity score matching	
	GLP-1RA	DPP-4i	GLP-1RA	DPP-4i
Sample size, n	44,208	115,337	33,402	33,402
Total events, n	2257	9507	1723	2401
Follow-up, PY	27,195	91,990	20,763	23,839
Incidence rate/1000 PY (95% CI)	83.0 (79.6 to 86.5)	103.3 (101.3 to 105.5)	83.0 (79.1 to 87.0)	100.7 (96.7 to 104.8)
Rate difference/1000 PY (95% CI)	**−20.5 (−24.4 to −16.4)**	Ref	**−17.7 (−23.4 to −12.1)**	Ref
Hazard ratio (95% CI)	**0.76 (0.73 to 0.80)**	Ref	**0.80 (0.75 to 0.86)**	Ref

SGLT-2i vs. GLP-1RA	Before 1:1 propensity score matching		After 1:1 propensity score matching	
	SGLT-2i	GLP-1RA	SGLT-2i	GLP-1RA
Sample size, n	31,708	61,325	27,997	27,997
Total events, n	1480	3401	1300	1462
Follow-up, PY	19,310	39,918	17,059	17,994
Incidence rate/1000 PY (95% CI)	76.6 (72.8 to 80.7)	85.2 (82.4 to 88.1)	76.2 (72.1 to 80.5)	81.3 (77.1 to 85.5)
Rate difference/1000 PY (95% CI)	**−8.6 (−13.4 to −3.7)**	Ref	**−5.0 (−10.9 to 0.8)**	Ref
Hazard ratio (95% CI)	**0.88 (0.83 to 0.94)**	Ref	**0.92 (0.86 to 0.99)**	Ref

CI, confidence interval; DPP-4i, dipeptidyl peptidase-4 inhibitor; GLP-1RA, glucagon-like peptide-1 receptor agonist; HR, hazard ratio; PY, person-years; Ref, reference; SGLT-2i, sodium-glucose cotransporter-2 inhibitor.
Data in bold are the rate difference/1000 person-years (95% CI) and HR (95% CI).

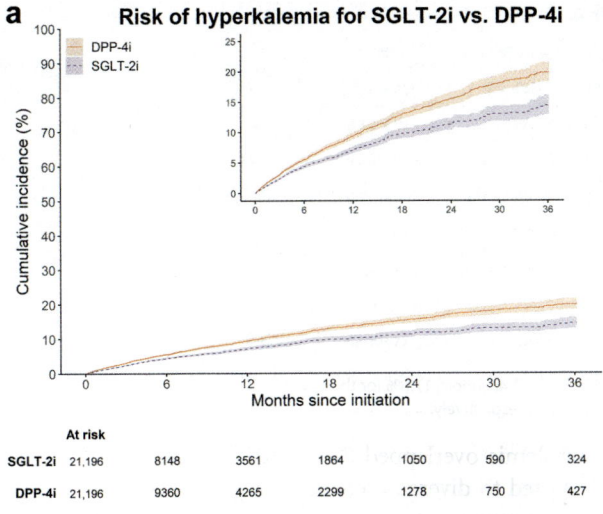
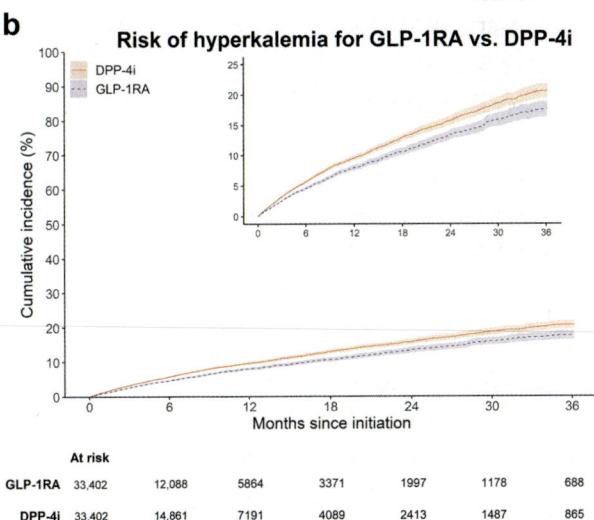
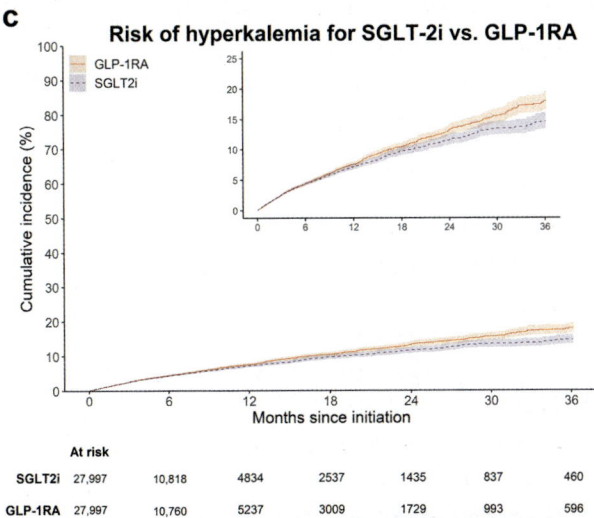

Figure 1 | Cumulative incidence curves for (a) sodium-glucose cotransporter-2 inhibitors (SGLT-2i) versus dipeptidyl peptidase-4 inhibitors (DPP-4i), (b) glucagon-like peptide-1 receptor agonists (GLP-1RAs) versus DPP-4i, and (c) SGLT-2i versus GLP-1RAs on risk of hyperkalemia diagnosis in inpatient or outpatient setting after 1:1 propensity score matching.

findings were observed when using a laboratory-based outcome definition (serum potassium level, ≥5.5 mmol/L) in the subset of patients who had serum potassium measurements available in the CDM data set, although CIs were wide (Supplementary Table S11): HRs were 0.88 (95% CI, 0.69–1.13) for SGLT-2i versus DPP-4i, 0.86 (95% CI, 0.69–1.06) for GLP-1RA versus DPP-4i, and 1.14 (95% CI, 0.91–1.43) for SGLT-2i versus GLP-1RA.

Subgroup analyses, effectiveness of individual agents, and sensitivity analyses

Findings were consistent across all subgroups for all 3 cohorts (Figure 2), including in patients with history of heart failure and cardiovascular disease, as well as patients on medications that influence potassium levels (i.e., RASi, MRAs, and loop diuretics). The lower risk of hyperkalemia was consistent among individual agents within the SGLT-2i class (HRs between 0.72 and 0.77) and GLP-1RA classes (HRs between 0.75 and 0.86) (Supplementary Table S12). Findings were also consistent among all sensitivity analyses (Supplementary Table S13).

DISCUSSION

In this large, nationwide, US cohort study of persons with CKD and T2D, we found that both SGLT-2i and GLP-1RAs were associated with a lower risk of hyperkalemia compared with DPP-4i. Furthermore, we observed consistent findings across subgroups of demographics, comorbid conditions, and medications known to influence potassium levels, and in multiple sensitivity analyses, as well as across individual agents within the SGLT-2i and GLP-1RA classes.

Our findings have important clinical implications. Hyperkalemia occurs frequently among patients with CKD and T2D, particularly those with low kidney function.[1] These patients are also at the highest risk for adverse cardiovascular and renal events. Our findings suggest that both SGLT-2i and GLP-1RAs are associated with a lower risk of hyperkalemia. Initiating these medications may therefore enable patients to use other guideline-recommended therapies that are associated with an increased risk of hyperkalemia, such as inhibitors of the renin-angiotensin-aldosterone system (angiotensin-converting enzyme inhibitor/angiotensin II receptor blocker, MRA, and angiotensin receptor/neprilysin inhibitor). Indeed, hyperkalemia often leads to dose reduction or discontinuation of these therapies, which has been associated with worse clinical outcomes.[10,11]

Our study has several novel findings. A previous meta-analysis of 6 randomized trials found that SGLT-2i lowered the risk of hyperkalemia compared with placebo in people with T2D.[17] Our results extend the protective effects of SGLT-2i on hyperkalemia observed in controlled trial settings to the broad group of patients with CKD and T2D seen in routine clinical practice. There are several differences between the trials and our observational study worth highlighting. First, our study population was on average 10 years older, included a larger proportion of women, and included a larger proportion of patients with heart failure. Second,

a

SGLT-2i vs. DPP-4i

	No. (%) of patients	SGLT-2i No. events	DPP-4i No. events	SGLT-2i IR/1000 PY	DPP-4i IR/1000 PY	Rate difference (95% CI)	HR (95% CI)
Overall	21,196 (100.0%)	960	1141	75.2	100.0	-24.8 (-31.8 to -17.7)	0.74 (0.68 to 0.80)
Age ≥75 yr	7884 (37.5%)	356	520	81.3	99.4	-18.2 (-30.2 to -6.2)	0.77 (0.70 to 0.85)
Age <75 yr	13,143 (62.5%)	606	888	72.9	96.3	-23.4 (-32.0 to -14.8)	0.66 (0.59 to 0.74)
Male	11,779 (55.9%)	574	824	78.6	102.3	-23.7 (-33.2 to -14.2)	0.76 (0.69 to 0.84)
Female	9277 (44.1%)	378	604	70.2	96.4	-26.2 (-36.7 to -15.8)	0.71 (0.62 to 0.80)
White[a]	9842 (90.6%)	411	636	74.2	98.2	-24.0 (-34.4 to -13.5)	0.74 (0.65 to 0.84)
Black[a]	1017 (9.4%)	32	58	63.2	85.0	-21.8 (-52.8 to 9.2)	0.70 (0.46 to 1.09)
Heart failure	5390 (25.7%)	319	420	108.9	126.1	-17.2 (-34.2 to -0.2)	0.84 (0.72 to 0.97)
No heart failure	15,621 (74.3%)	635	948	65.5	84.9	-19.5 (-26.9 to -12.0)	0.75 (0.68 to 0.83)
CVD	12,477 (59.3%)	639	932	88.8	114.3	-25.5 (-35.6 to -15.5)	0.76 (0.68 to 0.84)
No CVD	8571 (40.7%)	319	504	58.6	79.4	-20.9 (-30.3 to -11.4)	0.72 (0.63 to 0.83)
ACEi/ARB/ARNI	14,210 (67.5%)	659	977	74.5	97.2	-22.7 (-31.0 to -14.3)	0.75 (0.68 to 0.83)
No ACEi/ARB/ARNI	6843 (32.5%)	287	434	75.0	101.0	-26.1 (-38.9 to -13.2)	0.73 (0.63 to 0.85)
MRA	1253 (6.0%)	99	123	137.7	155.3	-17.6 (-56.2 to 21.0)	0.88 (0.67 to 1.14)
No MRA	19,571 (94.0%)	850	1264	71.2	93.1	-21.9 (-28.9 to -14.8)	0.75 (0.69 to 0.82)
Loop diuretic	4969 (23.7%)	297	432	104.4	132.6	-28.2 (-45.4 to -11.0)	0.76 (0.66 to 0.89)
No loop diuretic	16,013 (76.3%)	663	960	67.7	86.8	-19.1 (-26.6 to -11.6)	0.77 (0.70 to 0.85)
RAASi (ACE/ARB/ARNI/MRA)	14,728 (70.0%)	701	1012	77.0	98.3	-21.3 (-29.7 to -13.0)	0.77 (0.70 to 0.84)
No RAASi	6315 (30.0%)	264	400	74.3	99.8	-25.5 (-38.7 to -12.2)	0.74 (0.63 to 0.86)

Favors SGLT-2i ← HR → Favors DPP-4i

b

GLP-1RA vs. DPP-4i

	No. (%) of patients	GLP-1RA No. events	DPP-4i No. events	GLP-1RA IR/1000 PY	DPP-4i IR/1000 PY	Rate difference (95% CI)	HR (95% CI)
Overall	33,402 (100.0%)	1723	2401	83.0	100.7	-17.7 (-23.4 to -12.1)	0.80 (0.75 to 0.86)
Age ≥75 yr	16,060 (48.3%)	815	1137	82.2	98.3	-16.1 (-24.2 to -8.1)	0.81 (0.73 to 0.90)
Age <75 yr	17,181 (51.7%)	775	1058	71.7	86.6	-14.9 (-22.2 to -7.7)	0.82 (0.75 to 0.89)
Male	16,334 (49.2%)	949	1243	94.6	107.4	-12.8 (-21.3 to -4.4)	0.86 (0.79 to 0.94)
Female	16,866 (50.8%)	771	1112	72.8	91.7	-18.9 (-26.4 to -11.5)	0.78 (0.71 to 0.85)
White[a]	16,979 (88.9%)	845	1232	84.1	104.2	-20.1 (-28.3 to -12.0)	0.79 (0.72 to 0.86)
Black[a]	2127 (11.1%)	89	152	76.3	98.2	-21.9 (-44.2 to 0.3)	0.73 (0.56 to 0.95)
Heart failure	6052 (24.7%)	355	486	105.3	127.9	-22.6 (-38.4 to -6.8)	0.80 (0.70 to 0.92)
No heart failure	18,455 (75.3%)	828	1182	70.4	89.2	-18.8 (-25.8 to -11.8)	0.78 (0.71 to 0.85)
CVD	7439 (47.1%)	469	586	97.0	111.4	-14.5 (-27.1 to -1.9)	0.87 (0.77 to 0.97)
No CVD	8340 (52.9%)	376	517	65.3	81.6	-16.2 (-25.9 to -6.6)	0.79 (0.69 to 0.90)
ACEi/ARB/ARNI	21,445 (64.6%)	1136	1626	82.5	103.7	-21.2 (-28.2 to -14.2)	0.78 (0.73 to 0.84)
No ACEi/ARB/ARNI	11,766 (35.4%)	561	826	81.7	107.2	-25.5 (-35.4 to -15.5)	0.75 (0.68 to 0.84)
MRA	2052 (6.2%)	145	223	110.4	152.9	-42.6 (-69.5 to -15.7)	0.71 (0.57 to 0.88)
No MRA	31,174 (93.8%)	1535	2130	79.5	96.2	-16.8 (-22.5 to -11.1)	0.81 (0.76 to 0.87)
Loop diuretic	9156 (27.5%)	551	825	96.2	130.6	-34.4 (-46.4 to -22.4)	0.73 (0.65 to 0.81)
No loop diuretic	24,085 (72.5%)	1164	1553	77.7	90.6	-12.9 (-19.2 to -6.5)	0.84 (0.78 to 0.91)
RAASi (ACE/ARB/ARNI/MRA)	22,367 (67.3%)	1194	1642	83.5	98.9	-15.4 (-22.1 to -8.7)	0.82 (0.76 to 0.89)
No RAASi	10,864 (32.7%)	514	744	80.4	105.2	-24.8 (-35.1 to -14.5)	0.76 (0.68 to 0.85)

Favors GLP-1RA ← HR → Favors DPP-4i

Figure 2 | Comparative effectiveness of (a) sodium-glucose cotransporter-2 inhibitors (SGLT-2i) versus dipeptidyl peptidase-4 inhibitors (DPP-4i), (b) glucagon-like peptide-1 receptor agonists (GLP-1RAs) versus DPP-4i, and (Continued)

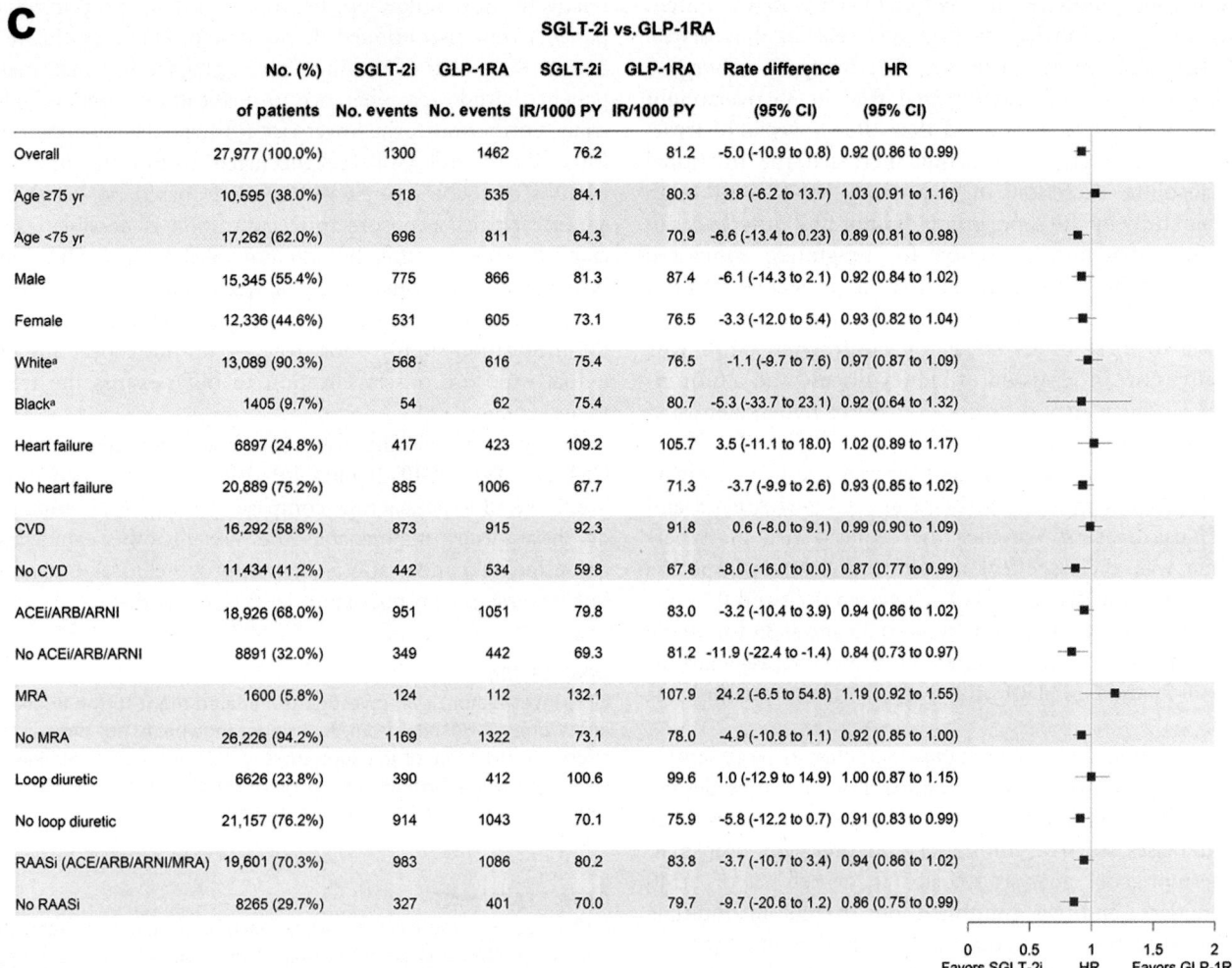

Figure 2 | (Continued) (c) SGLT-2i versus GLP-1RAs on risk of hyperkalemia diagnosis in inpatient or outpatient setting among subgroups after 1:1 propensity score matching. *Only data from Centers for Medicare & Medicaid Services. ACEi, angiotensin-converting enzyme inhibitor; ARB, angiotensin II receptor blocker; ARNI, angiotensin receptor/neprilysin inhibitor; CI, confidence interval; CVD, cardiovascular disease; HR, hazard ratio; IR, incidence rate; MRA, mineralocorticoid receptor antagonist; PY, person-years; RAASi, renin-angiotensin-aldosterone system inhibitor.

because of monitoring protocols, trials have a much higher adherence to drug therapy compared with routine clinical practice; in our population-based study, 61% of participants in routine care discontinued treatment during follow-up. Third, there are differences in the incidence rate of hyperkalemia between the previous meta-analysis of trials and our observational study, likely explained by population differences: among the 6 included trials, the incidence rate for hyperkalemia varied between 1.6 (DECLARE-TIMI [Dapagliflozin Effect on Cardiovascular Events-Thrombolysis in Myocardial Infarction] trial) and 56.9 (DAPA-CKD [Dapagliflozin and Prevention of Adverse Outcomes in Chronic Kidney Disease] trial) hyperkalemia events per 1000 person-years.[17] In contrast, the incidence rate for the primary outcome in our study was higher, between 75.3 and 100.0 hyperkalemia events per 1000 person-years. The difference in incidence rates is likely an underestimate, as the trial relied on serial serum potassium measurements, and our study used claims diagnoses; the findings from our internal validation study suggest that the true incidence rate in our study may be ≈3-fold higher. Fourth, our study provides a head-to-head comparison of SGLT-2i, GLP-1RA, and DPP-4i, rather than placebo. Although SGLT-2i initiators had a lower risk of hyperkalemia compared with DPP-4i, we found only small differences between SGLT-2i and GLP-1RA, and any differences between the latter 2 agents are likely to be small.

The protective association observed for GLP-1RA on the risk of hyperkalemia in a clinical setting has, to our knowledge, not been reported previously. There may be several plausible mechanisms for this finding, although additional research should elucidate the precise mechanisms for our observations. GLP-1RAs regulate water and electrolyte balance in the postprandial state through rapid feed-forward effects on the kidney, and influence tubular handling of electrolytes, including sodium.[20] The increased proximal sodium excretion due to GLP-1RAs may augment potassium secretion by the principal cells in the cortical collecting duct by increasing the electronegative charge.[36] Furthermore, a small randomized trial in 35 overweight participants with T2D showed that after 8 weeks of treatment, the GLP-1RA lixisenatide increased the fractional and absolute excretion of potassium itself,[19] although another study by the same group did not find differences in fractional potassium excretion for liraglutide compared with sitagliptin.[37] We observed that the protective effect of GLP-1RA occurred rapidly (within the first 6 months). In addition to these direct effects on electrolytes, GLP-1RAs may also slow progression of kidney disease and albuminuria,[38–40] which may decrease the risk of hyperkalemia in the long-term.

Our study also had sufficient sample size to investigate single agents within the SGLT-2i and GLP-1RA class and enable us to assess whether the reduced risk of hyperkalemia was a class effect or only observed for specific agents. The consistency of HRs (between 0.72 and 0.77 for single SGLT-2i agents and between 0.75 and 0.86 for single GLP-1RA agents) suggests that the protective associations of SGLT-2i and GLP-1RA on hyperkalemia represent a class effect.

Our study has several strengths, including its large sample size and the use of an active-comparator new user design, which reduces confounding by indication and mitigates time-related biases, such as immortal and prevalent user bias. Furthermore, our analysis adjusted for a rich set of >140 confounders, and we confirmed our results in multiple sensitivity analyses. Our study also has limitations. First, we cannot rule out confounding in our observational study, and we lacked information on dietary habits (e.g., intake of high potassium-containing foods). However, we adjusted for a wide variety of confounders and confounder proxies, including many comorbid conditions, medications, diabetes-specific complications, measures of health care use, and healthy behavior markers, which reflect overall health status.[22] Furthermore, in the subset of patients with available data, we did not observe large imbalances in laboratory measurements that were not included in the propensity score model, including estimated glomerular filtration rate and serum potassium level. Confounding is also expected to be less severe for "unintended effects" or "unexpected outcomes,"[23] such as hyperkalemia, as physicians do not specifically prescribe SGLT-2i or GLP-1RA with the aim to reduce the risk of hyperkalemia.[41] Second, our primary outcome was defined on the basis of claims-based diagnosis codes, rather than serum potassium measurements. In an internal validation study, we found high specificity (>99%) for serum potassium level ≥5.5 or 6.0 mmol/L; thus, relative risks in our study should not be affected. Because sensitivity was low (≈37%), the absolute risk and rate differences represent an underestimate of the true benefit, and SGLT-2i/GLP-1RA will likely have even larger absolute benefits than that observed in our study compared with DPP-4i. Third, our study had relatively short follow-up, because of a high proportion of patients who discontinued the treatment. However, this represents the reality of routine clinical practice in which many patients have lower adherence to medication compared with trials. Furthermore, the lower risk for hyperkalemia observed for SGLT-2i and GLP-1RA occurred within the first few months of follow-up. As in any study based on health insurance claims, exposure misclassification is possible, especially if patients refill, but do not take, their medications; however, in our primary analysis, we censored patients if they did not refill medications within a month following the end of the medication supply; moreover, we do not expect any potential exposure misclassification to differ across the treatment groups.

In conclusion, in this cohort study of US individuals with CKD and T2D, SGLT-2i and GLP-1RAs were associated with a lower risk of hyperkalemia, compared with DPP-4i. Initiation of these drugs may enable the use of other guideline-recommended medications that improve clinical outcomes but increase serum potassium level, such as RASi.

DISCLOSURE

EP is investigator of an investigator-initiated grant to the Brigham and Women's Hospital from Boehringer Ingelheim, not directly related to the topic of the submitted work. DJW reports serving on Data Monitoring Committees for Novo Nordisk, not related to the topic of this work. All the other authors declared no competing interests.

DATA STATEMENT

A data use agreement is required for each of these data sources. Our data use agreements do not permit us to share patient-level source data or data derivatives with individuals and institutions not covered under the data use agreements. The databases used in this study are accessible to other researchers by contacting the data providers and acquiring data use agreements/licenses.

FUNDING STATEMENT

ELF is supported by a Rubicon grant from the Netherlands Organization for Scientific Research. KJL is supported by grants from the National Institute on Aging (RF1AG063381-01 and R01 AG075335). EP is supported by a National Institute of Health grant (K08AG055670), Patient-Centered Outcomes Research Institute grant (DB-2020C2-20326), and a research grant from the US Food and Drug Administration (5U01FD007213). JMP is supported by a National Institutes of Health grant (AR 075117). KB is supported by a grant from the National Institute on Aging (K01AG068365). The funders had no role in the design and conduct of the study; collection, management, analysis, and interpretation of the data; preparation, review, or approval of the manuscript; and decision to submit the manuscript for publication.

AUTHOR CONTRIBUTIONS

ELF and JMP had full access to all of the data in the study and take responsibility for the integrity of the data and the accuracy of the data analysis. Concept and design: ELF, EP, and JMP. Acquisition and analysis of interpretation of data: all authors. Drafting of the manuscript: ELF. Critical revision of the manuscript for important intellectual content: all authors. Statistical analysis: ELF, JM, and AC.

Administrative, technical, or material support: all authors. Supervision: EP and JMP.

SUPPLEMENTARY MATERIAL
Supplementary File (Word)
Supplementary Table S1. Definitions of inclusion and exclusion criteria.
Supplementary Table S2. Outcome definitions.
Supplementary Table S3. Definition of subgroup variables cardiovascular disease and heart failure.
Supplementary Table S4. Full list of baseline characteristics in patients with chronic kidney disease (CKD) and type 2 diabetes, stratified by sodium-glucose cotransporter-2 inhibitor (SGLT-2i) versus dipeptidyl peptidase-4 inhibitor (DPP-4i) initiation in the pooled cohort, before and after 1:1 propensity score matching.
Supplementary Table S5. Full list of baseline characteristics in patients with chronic kidney disease (CKD) and type 2 diabetes, stratified by glucagon-like peptide-1 receptor agonist (GLP-1RA) versus dipeptidyl peptidase-4 inhibitor (DPP-4i) initiation in the pooled cohort, before and after 1:1 propensity score matching.
Supplementary Table S6. Full list of baseline characteristics in patients with chronic kidney disease (CKD) and type 2 diabetes, stratified by sodium-glucose cotransporter-2 inhibitor (SGLT-2i) versus glucagon-like peptide-1 receptor agonist (GLP-1RA) initiation in the pooled cohort, before and after 1:1 propensity score matching.
Supplementary Table S7. Individual sodium-glucose cotransporter-2 inhibitor (SGLT-2i), glucagon-like peptide-1 receptor agonist (GLP-1RA), and dipeptidyl peptidase-4 inhibitor (DPP-4i) agents included in the analysis after 1:1 propensity score matching.
Supplementary Table S8. Follow-up and censoring reasons after 1:1 propensity score matching for (**A**) sodium-glucose cotransporter-2 inhibitor (SGLT-2i) versus dipeptidyl peptidase-4 inhibitor (DPP-4i), (**B**) glucagon-like peptide-1 receptor agonist (GLP-1RA) versus DPP-4i, and (**C**) SGLT-2i versus GLP-1RA.
Supplementary Table S9. Absolute risks and risk differences for the primary outcome at 6-month intervals for sodium-glucose cotransporter-2 inhibitor (SGLT-2i) versus dipeptidyl peptidase-4 inhibitor (DPP-4i), glucagon-like peptide-1 receptor agonist (GLP-1RA) versus DPP-4i, and SGLT-2i versus GLP-1RA.
Supplementary Table S10. Comparative effectiveness of (**A**) sodium-glucose cotransporter-2 inhibitor (SGLT-2i) versus dipeptidyl peptidase-4 inhibitor (DPP-4i), (**B**) glucagon-like peptide-1 receptor agonist (GLP-1RA) versus DPP-4i, and (**C**) SGLT-2i versus GLP-1RA on risk of hyperkalemia diagnosis in inpatient or emergency department setting (secondary outcome) before and after 1:1 propensity score matching.
Supplementary Table S11. Comparative effectiveness of (**A**) sodium-glucose cotransporter-2 inhibitor (SGLT-2i) versus dipeptidyl peptidase-4 inhibitor (DPP-4i), (**B**) glucagon-like peptide-1 receptor agonist (GLP-1RA) versus DPP-4i, and (**C**) SGLT-2i versus GLP-1RA on risk of serum potassium level ≥5.5 mmol/L before and after 1:1 propensity score matching.
Supplementary Table S12. Comparative effectiveness of individual sodium-glucose cotransporter-2 inhibitor (SGLT-2i) and glucagon-like peptide-1 receptor agonist (GLP-1RA) agents compared with dipeptidyl peptidase-4 inhibitor (DPP-4i) on risk of hyperkalemia diagnosis in the inpatient or outpatient setting, after 1:1 propensity score matching.
Supplementary Table S13. Sensitivity analyses: incidence rate differences and hazard ratios for (**A**) sodium-glucose cotransporter-2 inhibitor (SGLT-2i) versus dipeptidyl peptidase-4 inhibitor (DPP-4i), (**B**) glucagon-like peptide-1 receptor agonist (GLP-1RA) versus DPP-4i, and (**C**) SGLT-2i versus GLP-1RA after 1:1 propensity score matching.

Supplementary Figure S1. Overview of study design.
Supplementary Figure S2. Patient flowchart.

REFERENCES

1. Clase CM, Carrero JJ, Ellison DH, et al. Potassium homeostasis and management of dyskalemia in kidney diseases: conclusions from a Kidney Disease: Improving Global Outcomes (KDIGO) Controversies Conference. *Kidney Int*. 2020;97:42–61.
2. Nilsson E, Gasparini A, Arnlov J, et al. Incidence and determinants of hyperkalemia and hypokalemia in a large healthcare system. *Int J Cardiol*. 2017;245:277–284.
3. Acker CG, Johnson JP, Palevsky PM, Greenberg A. Hyperkalemia in hospitalized patients: causes, adequacy of treatment, and results of an attempt to improve physician compliance with published therapy guidelines. *Arch Intern Med*. 1998;158:917–924.
4. Palmer BF. Managing hyperkalemia caused by inhibitors of the renin-angiotensin-aldosterone system. *N Engl J Med*. 2004;351:585–592.
5. Agarwal R, Joseph A, Anker SD, et al. Hyperkalemia risk with finerenone: results from the FIDELIO-DKD trial. *J Am Soc Nephrol*. 2022;33:225–237.
6. Juurlink DN, Mamdani MM, Lee DS, et al. Rates of hyperkalemia after publication of the Randomized Aldactone Evaluation Study. *N Engl J Med*. 2004;351:543–551.
7. Fu EL, Kutz A, Desai RJ. Finerenone in chronic kidney disease and type 2 diabetes: the known and the unknown. *Kidney Int*. 2023;103:30–33.
8. Bandak G, Sang Y, Gasparini A, et al. Hyperkalemia after initiating renin-angiotensin system blockade: the Stockholm Creatinine Measurements (SCREAM) project. *J Am Heart Assoc*. 2017;6:e005428.
9. Desai AS, Swedberg K, McMurray JJ, et al. Incidence and predictors of hyperkalemia in patients with heart failure: an analysis of the CHARM Program. *J Am Coll Cardiol*. 2007;50:1959–1966.
10. Xu Y, Fu EL, Trevisan M, et al. Stopping renin-angiotensin system inhibitors after hyperkalemia and risk of adverse outcomes. *Am Heart J*. 2022;243:177–186.
11. Trevisan M, Fu EL, Xu Y, et al. Stopping mineralocorticoid receptor antagonists after hyperkalaemia: trial emulation in data from routine care. *Eur J Heart Fail*. 2021;23:1698–1707.
12. Lyu B, Sang Y, Selvin E, et al. Pharmacologic treatment of type 2 diabetes in the U.S., Sweden, and Israel. *Diabetes Care*. 2022;45:2926–2934.
13. Harris ST, Patorno E, Zhuo M, et al. Prescribing trends of antidiabetes medications in patients with type 2 diabetes and diabetic kidney disease, a cohort study. *Diabetes Care*. 2021;44:2293–2301.
14. Rossing P, Caramori ML, Chan JCN, et al. Executive summary of the KDIGO 2022 Clinical Practice Guideline for Diabetes Management in Chronic Kidney Disease: an update based on rapidly emerging new evidence. *Kidney Int*. 2022;102:990–999.
15. ElSayed NA, Aleppo G, Aroda VR, et al. 9. Pharmacologic approaches to glycemic treatment: standards of care in diabetes—2023. *Diabetes Care*. 2022;46(suppl 1):S140–S157.
16. Kaze AD, Zhuo M, Kim SC, et al. Association of SGLT2 inhibitors with cardiovascular, kidney, and safety outcomes among patients with diabetic kidney disease: a meta-analysis. *Cardiovasc Diabetol*. 2022;21:47.
17. Neuen BL, Oshima M, Agarwal R, et al. Sodium-glucose cotransporter 2 inhibitors and risk of hyperkalemia in people with type 2 diabetes: a meta-analysis of individual participant data from randomized, controlled trials. *Circulation*. 2022;145:1460–1470.
18. Ferreira JP, Zannad F, Butler J, et al. Empagliflozin and serum potassium in heart failure: an analysis from EMPEROR-Pooled. *Eur Heart J*. 2022;43:2984–2993.
19. Tonneijck L, Muskiet MHA, Blijdorp CJ, et al. Renal tubular effects of prolonged therapy with the GLP-1 receptor agonist lixisenatide in patients with type 2 diabetes mellitus. *Am J Physiol Renal Physiol*. 2019;316:F231–F240.
20. Tonneijck L, Smits MM, Muskiet MHA, et al. Acute renal effects of the GLP-1 receptor agonist exenatide in overweight type 2 diabetes patients: a randomised, double-blind, placebo-controlled trial. *Diabetologia*. 2016;59:1412–1421.
21. Fu EL, van Diepen M, Xu Y, et al. Pharmacoepidemiology for nephrologists (part 2): potential biases and how to overcome them. *Clin Kidney J*. 2021;14:1317–1326.
22. Schneeweiss S, Patorno E. Conducting real-world evidence studies on the clinical outcomes of diabetes treatments. *Endocr Rev*. 2021;42:658–690.

23. Fu EL. Target trial emulation to improve causal inference from observational data: what, why, and how? *J Am Soc Nephrol*. 2023;34: 1305–1314.
24. Carrero JJ, Fu EL, Vestergaard SV, et al. Defining measures of kidney function in observational studies using routine health care data: methodological and reporting considerations. *Kidney Int*. 2023;103: 53–69.
25. Paik JM, Patorno E, Zhuo M, et al. Accuracy of identifying diagnosis of moderate to severe chronic kidney disease in administrative claims data. *Pharmacoepidemiol Drug Saf*. 2022;31:467–475.
26. Hawley CE, Lauffenburger JC, Paik JM, et al. Three sides to the story: adherence trajectories during the first year of SGLT2 inhibitor therapy among Medicare beneficiaries. *Diabetes Care*. 2022;45:604–613.
27. Lash TL, Fox MP, Fink AK. *Applying Quantitative Bias Analysis to Epidemiologic Data*. Springer; 2009.
28. Fu EL, D'Andrea E, Wexler DJ, et al. Safety of sodium-glucose cotransporter-2 inhibitors in patients with CKD and type 2 diabetes: population-based US cohort study. *Clin J Am Soc Nephrol*. 2023;18: 592–601.
29. Kim DH, Schneeweiss S, Glynn RJ, et al. Measuring frailty in Medicare data: development and validation of a claims-based frailty index. *J Gerontol A Biol Sci Med Sci*. 2018;73:980–987.
30. Fu EL, Groenwold RHH, Zoccali C, et al. Merits and caveats of propensity scores to adjust for confounding. *Nephrol Dial Transplant*. 2019;34:1629–1635.
31. Austin PC. Using the standardized difference to compare the prevalence of a binary variable between two groups in observational research. *Commun Stat Simul Comput*. 2009;38:1228–1234.
32. Austin PC. Balance diagnostics for comparing the distribution of baseline covariates between treatment groups in propensity-score matched samples. *Stat Med*. 2009;28:3083–3107.
33. Xu Y, Cheung YB, Lam KF, et al. A simple approach to the estimation of incidence rate difference. *Am J Epidemiol*. 2010;172: 334–343.
34. Putter H, Fiocco M, Geskus RB. Tutorial in biostatistics: competing risks and multi-state models. *Stat Med*. 2007;26:2389–2430.
35. Aetion Evidence Platform (2022). Software for real-world data analysis. Aetion, Inc. Accessed October 2023. http://aetion.com
36. Palmer BF. Regulation of potassium homeostasis. *Clin J Am Soc Nephrol*. 2015;10:1050–1060.
37. Tonneijck L, Smits MM, Muskiet MH, et al. Renal effects of DPP-4 inhibitor sitagliptin or GLP-1 receptor agonist liraglutide in overweight patients with type 2 diabetes: a 12-week, randomized, double-blind, placebo-controlled trial. *Diabetes Care*. 2016;39:2042–2050.
38. Xie Y, Bowe B, Gibson AK, et al. Comparative effectiveness of SGLT2 inhibitors, GLP-1 receptor agonists, DPP-4 inhibitors, and sulfonylureas on risk of kidney outcomes: emulation of a target trial using health care databases. *Diabetes Care*. 2020;43:2859–2869.
39. Xu Y, Fu EL, Clase CM, et al. GLP-1 receptor agonist versus DPP-4 inhibitor and kidney and cardiovascular outcomes in clinical practice in type-2 diabetes. *Kidney Int*. 2022;101:360–368.
40. Sattar N, Lee MMY, Kristensen SL, et al. Cardiovascular, mortality, and kidney outcomes with GLP-1 receptor agonists in patients with type 2 diabetes: a systematic review and meta-analysis of randomised trials. *Lancet Diabetes Endocrinol*. 2021;9:653–662.
41. Vandenbroucke JP. Observational research, randomised trials, and two views of medical science. *PLoS Med*. 2008;5:e67.

clinical investigation

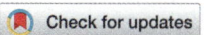

Performance of the European Kidney Function Consortium (EKFC) creatinine-based equation in United States cohorts

see commentary on page 445

Pierre Delanaye[1,2,16], Andrew D. Rule[3,16], Elke Schaeffner[4,16], Etienne Cavalier[5,16], Junyan Shi[6,7], Andrew N. Hoofnagle[7,8,9,10], Ulf Nyman[11,16], Jonas Björk[12,13,15,16] and Hans Pottel[14,15,16]

[1]Department of Nephrology-Dialysis-Transplantation, University of Liège, CHU Sart Tilman, Liège, Belgium; [2]Department of Nephrology-Dialysis-Apheresis, Hôpital Universitaire Carémeau, Nîmes, France; [3]Division of Nephrology and Hypertension, Mayo Clinic, Rochester, Minnesota, USA; [4]Institute of Public Health, Charité – Universitätsmedizin Berlin, Berlin, Germany; [5]Department of Clinical Chemistry, University of Liège, CHU Sart Tilman, Liège, Belgium; [6]Department of Pathology and Laboratory Medicine, University of British Columbia, Vancouver, British Columbia, Canada; [7]Department of Laboratory Medicine and Pathology, University of Washington, Seattle, Washington, USA; [8]Kidney Research Institute, Department of Medicine, University of Washington, Seattle, Washington, USA; [9]Division of Metabolism, Endocrinology, and Nutrition, University of Washington, Seattle, Washington, USA; [10]Department of Medicine, University of Washington, Seattle, Washington, USA; [11]Department of Translational Medicine, Division of Medical Radiology, Lund University, Malmö, Sweden; [12]Division of Occupational and Environmental Medicine, Lund University, Lund, Sweden; [13]Clinical Studies Sweden, Forum South, Skåne University Hospital, Lund, Sweden; and [14]Department of Public Health and Primary Care, KU Leuven Campus Kulak Kortrijk, Kortrijk, Belgium

Estimating glomerular filtration rate (GFR) is important in daily practice to assess kidney function and adapting the best clinical care of patients with and without chronic kidney disease. The new creatinine-based European Kidney Function Consortium (EKFC) equation is used to estimate GFR. This equation was developed and validated mainly in European individuals and based on a rescaled creatinine, with the rescaling factor (Q-value) defined as the median normal value of serum creatinine in a given population. The validation was limited in Non-Black Americans and absent in Black Americans. Here, our cross-sectional analysis included 12,854 participants from nine studies encompassing large numbers of both non-Black and Black Americans with measured GFR by clearance of an exogenous marker (reference method), serum creatinine, age, sex, and self-reported race available. Two strategies were considered with population-specific Q-values in Black and non-Black men and women ($EKFC_{PS}$) or a race-free Q-value ($EKFC_{RF}$). In the whole population, only the $EKFC_{PS}$ equation showed no statistical median bias (0.14, 95% confidence interval [-0.07; 0.35] mL/min/1.73m^2), and the bias for the $EKFC_{RF}$ (0.74, [0.51; 0.94] mL/min/1.73m^2) was closer to zero than that for the Chronic Kidney Disease Epidemiology Collaboration (CKD-EPI$_{2021}$) equation (1.22, [0.99; 1.47]) mL/min/1.73m^2. The percentage of estimated GFR within 30% of measured GFR was similar for CKD-EPI$_{2021}$ (79.2% [78.5%; 79.9%]) and $EKFC_{RF}$ (80.1% [79.4%; 80.7%]), but improved for the $EKFC_{PS}$ equation (81.1% [80.5%; 81.8%]). Thus, our EKFC equations can be used to estimate GFR in the United States incorporating either self-reported race or unknown race at the patient's discretion per hospital registration records.

Kidney International (2024) **105**, 629–637; https://doi.org/10.1016/j.kint.2023.11.024

KEYWORDS: chronic kidney disease; glomerular filtration rate; serum creatinine

Copyright © 2023, International Society of Nephrology. Published by Elsevier Inc. All rights reserved.

Lay Summary

Estimating glomerular filtration rate with serum creatinine remains the most used method in clinical practice. Among different creatinine-based equations recently published, the European Kidney Function Consortium creatinine-based equation has been validated in Europe and Africa, but few data are available from the United States. In this cross-sectional analysis including 12,854 measured glomerular filtration rate and standardized serum creatinine values, we showed that the European Kidney Function Consortium equation was applicable in US populations, also without applying a race correction factor. The European Kidney Function Consortium equation can be a valid alternative to existing creatinine-based equations in the United States.

Correspondence: *Pierre Delanaye, Service de Dialyse, CHU Sart Tilman, Avenue de l'Hôpital 1, 4000 Liège, Belgium. E-mail: pdelanaye@chuliege.be*

[15]These authors contributed equally to this work as last senior authors.

[16]PD, ADR, ES, EC, UN, JB, and HP are members of the European Kidney Function Consortium.

Received 27 June 2023; revised 28 September 2023; accepted 5 November 2023; published online 13 December 2023

Estimating glomerular filtration rate (GFR) remains of high importance in daily practice to assess kidney function and adapting at best clinical care of patients with and without chronic kidney disease.[1] Even if new biomarkers, such as cystatin C, are emerging, creatinine-based equations remain the most used tools worldwide to estimate GFR.[2] Two major innovations have been launched in 2021 regarding such creatinine-based equations. First, a new version of the Chronic Kidney Disease Epidemiology Collaboration (CKD-EPI) equation has been developed that excludes race from the equation. By design, this race-free CKD-EPI$_{2021}$ equation underestimates GFR in Black persons and overestimates GFR in non-Black persons in US people.[3] This race-free equation is recommended for use in the United States by the American Society of Nephrology, the National Kidney Foundation, and the American Association for Clinical Chemistry.[4,5] Patients are effectively not given the option to have their race/ethnicity information used to obtain a more accurate GFR estimate. We developed an approach that empowers patients to decide if they want to self-report their race and, if so, to use that information to, on average, more accurately estimate GFR from their serum creatinine.

A new creatinine-based equation, called the European Kidney Function Consortium (EKFC) equation, has also been developed from a large data set of European participants.[6] This equation is based on rescaled creatinine, using a rescaling factor (Q value) that is the median value for serum creatinine in a normal population of any age, sex, or race. The EKFC equation performs equally well across the whole age and GFR spectrum and has been validated in White European, Black European, and Black African individuals.[7] Validation was limited in non-Black US individuals and absent in Black US individuals.[6,8,9] In the present analysis, we applied US-based Q values to compare this EKFC equation in different US cohorts with a large number of non-Black and Black US participants.

METHODS
Participants
We used data from the following cohorts available from the National Institute of Diabetes and Digestive and Kidney Diseases: Assessing Long Term Outcomes in Living Kidney Donors (ALTOLD),[10] Chronic Renal Insufficiency Cohort (CRIC),[11,12] Consortium for Radiologic Imaging Studies of Polycystic Kidney Disease (CRISP),[13] Diabetes Control and Complications Trial/Epidemiology of Diabetes Interventions and Complications (DCCT/EDIC),[14,15] Preventing Early Renal Loss in Diabetes (PERL),[16] African American Study of Kidney Disease and Hypertension (AASK),[17] and Modified Diet in Renal Disease (MDRD) study.[18] GFR was measured by urinary clearance of iothalamate in CRIC, CRISP, DCCT/EDIC, AASK, and MDRD studies. GFR was measured by iohexol plasma clearance in ALTOLD and PERL studies. Serum creatinine measurements were recalibrated as described in previous publications to be considered as isotope dilution mass spectrometry traceable.[3,11,13,19,20] Serum creatinine was directly measured by an isotope dilution mass spectrometry–traceable enzymatic assay in PERL (Roche Diagnostics).[21] Data are unavailable for ALTOLD regarding the way (standardized or not) serum creatinine has been measured.

Two other cohorts were available from Mayo Clinic (ADR). The first cohort combined data from the Genetic Epidemiology Network of Arteriopathy (GENOA) and Epidemiology of Coronary Artery Calcification (ECAC) studies.[22] The second cohort is based on data from individuals referred to Mayo Clinic, Rochester, Minnesota, to have measured GFR.[23] Only participants having measured GFR and serum creatinine on the same days were considered. In these 2 cohorts, serum creatinine was assayed using an isotope dilution mass spectrometry–traceable enzymatic assay (Roche Diagnostics) and GFR was measured by urinary clearance of iothalamate.[22,23] For the whole database, only 1 GFR result per participant and only adults ($\geq$18 years) were considered. Race was self-reported by participants in most of these studies as previously reported.[3]

Data were anonymized from the source cohorts for the analysis performed at Lund University, Sweden. All procedures involving participants and data were in agreement with the ethical principles for medical research involving human participants established in the World Medical Association Declaration of Helsinki. Written consent had been obtained from the participants of AASK, MDRD, ALTOLD, CRIC, CRISP, DCCT/EDIC, GENOA/ECAC and PERL studies. A waiver of consent was obtained from the Mayo Clinic Institutional Review Board to study patients from the Mayo Clinic Renal Studies Unit database because of the retrospective nature of these clinical data.

Covariates
Sex- and age-specific median creatinine values (Q values) in healthy adults from different populations were previously established (Supplementary Table S1).[6] To establish Q values in White Europeans, we considered a large amount of data from different laboratories in Sweden and Belgium.[24] For US Q values, we used the same type of results published by Shi et al.,[25] also based on laboratory data. These authors collected individual creatinine from patients evaluated at the University of Washington Medicine health care system from January 2018 to August 2019 (creatinine measured using the Jaffe method; isotope dilution mass spectrometry–traceable assay, Beckman Coulter AU system). Q values were 1.00 mg/dl ($n = 10,865$) and 0.73 mg/dl ($n = 9849$) in Black men and women, respectively. Among non-Black (non-Asian) populations, Q values were 0.93 mg/dl ($n = 97,255$) and 0.73 mg/dl ($n = 98,720$) in men and women, respectively. Another source of Q values can also be obtained from the National Health and Nutrition Examination Survey, and the results were similar ($Q = 1.03$ and 0.72 mg/dl for Black men and Black women, 0.94 and 0.70 mg/dl for non-Black men and non-Black women, and 0.99 and 0.71 mg/dl for the race-free Q values; Supplementary Table S1).

We have previously shown that the median creatinine concentration in a healthy adult population, that is, the Q value, could be different in Black and White European populations (whereas the difference between Black Africans and White Europeans is actually low; Supplementary Table S1).[2] There is also evidence for these differences in serum creatinine between White and Black US populations that is independent of GFR.[12] However, there is no evidence for a difference in GFR between White and Black healthy adults.[26] Therefore, we considered 2 strategies: (i) when we accept that there are differences in creatinine generation according to the population, we may consider population-specific Q values (EKFC$_{PS}$, PS = population specific), or (ii) when we omit the difference in creatinine generation, we might use a Q value that is totally race free (EKFC$_{RF}$, RF = race free). In the latter case, we were accepting potential statistical bias in performance when we used a Q value that is the mean of Q values obtained in Black and non-Black populations, that is, 0.97 mg/dl in men and 0.73 mg/dl in women. In the present analysis, both strategies were tested, knowing that differences will be relevant only in male cohorts (as the Q value in Black and non-Black women is the same).[25] The EKFC equations using both

Table 1 | Description of the cohorts

Cohort	Sample size	Age, yr	Measured GFR, ml/min per 1.73 m²	% of women	% of Black participants	% of individuals with urinary clearance
All	12,854	56.0 [42.9; 65.0]	57 [37; 83]	44.3	21.7	93.2
AASK	1844	54.5 [46.0; 62.0]	57 [40; 74]	35.9	100	100
ALTOLD	381	43.3 [33.5; 52.6]	97 [89; 107]	65.1	1.8	0
CRIC	1194	59.0 [48.2; 65.9]	48 [35; 63]	44.4	44.7	100
CRISP	217	34.0 [27.0; 40.0]	93 [78; 112]	59.0	11.1	100
DCCT/EDIC	809	31.0 [27.0; 36.0]	119 [107; 132]	47.8	1.4	100
GENOA/ECAC	1093	66.1 [59.1; 71.2]	80 [66; 93]	56.6	0	100
Mayo Clinic	5069	59.0 [48.0; 69.0]	50 [32; 72]	44.6	2.0	100
MDRD study	1756	51.0 [40.0; 61.0]	36 [24; 53]	39.5	12.4	100
PERL	491	52.0 [44.0; 59.0]	70 [56; 82]	33.6	10.8	0

AASK, African American Study of Kidney Disease and Hypertension; ALTOLD, Assessing Long Term Outcomes in Living Kidney Donors; CRIC, Chronic Renal Insufficiency Cohort; CRISP, Consortium for Radiologic Imaging Studies of Polycystic Kidney Disease; DCCT/EDIC, Diabetes Control and Complications Trial/Epidemiology of Diabetes Interventions and Complications; ECAC, Epidemiology of Coronary Artery Calcification; GENOA, Genetic Epidemiology Network of Arteriopathy; GFR, glomerular filtration rate; MDRD, Modified Diet in Renal Disease; PERL, Preventing Early Renal Loss in Diabetes.
Results are expressed as percentage or median [quartile 1; quartile 3].

strategies were compared with the CKD-EPI$_{2021}$ equation (see description of equations in Supplementary Table S2).

Statistical analyses

All analyses and calculations were performed using SAS 9.4 (SAS Institute Inc.). Data were presented as mean ± SD when the distribution was normal and as median with interquartile range (quartile 1; quartile 3) when not. Normality was assessed using the Kolmogorov-Smirnov test.

The performance of GFR equations was compared with usual metrics: median bias (i.e., estimated GFR – measured GFR) with 95% confidence interval, imprecision (interquartile range), as well as P30 and P20 accuracies (percentage of estimated GFR values within ±30% or 20% of measured GFR) with 95% confidence intervals. The target for statistical bias was zero, but an absolute statistical bias of at most 5 ml/min per 1.73 m² might be considered reasonable. Imprecision should be as low as possible.[27] The target for P30 was to reach >90%, yet P30 > 75% has been considered as "sufficient for good clinical decision making" by the Kidney Disease Outcomes Quality Initiative.[28] A result was considered as better than another one when 95% confidence intervals were not overlapping. Median statistical bias versus age and GFR was graphically presented using median quantile regression with fourth-degree polynomials. Likewise, P30 accuracy was graphically presented versus age and GFR using cubic splines with 3 free knots and using third-degree polynomials. Analyses were performed in the whole population and in the 4 main groups: Black men, Black women, non-Black men and non-Black women.

Stratified analysis in different GFR subgroups was performed according to measured GFR ranges (<15, [15–30[, [30–45[, [45–60[, ≥60 ml/min per 1.73 m²).[1,29] We also performed analyses stratified by age ([18–40[, [40–65[, and ≥ 65 years). These subanalyses were performed in Black and non-Black populations by sex. Finally, a subanalysis was performed per cohort.

Because the characteristics of Black people were different in the various cohorts, notably in terms of GFR levels, we separately matched Black with non-Black using the following matching criteria: age (±3 years), sex (equal), measured GFR (±3 ml/min per 1.73 m²), and body mass index (±2.5 kg/m²). We wanted to investigate whether the performance of the EKFC equations was different in these matching cohorts. For the matched analyses, we considered individuals with body mass index available (n = 4198 non-Black and n = 831 Black). We followed the STROBE (STrengthening the Reporting of OBservational studies in Epidemiology) statement for reporting of observational cross-sectional studies.

RESULTS
Characteristics of participants

Table 1 summarizes the characteristics of the cohorts and Table 2 the characteristics of the 4 main populations (Black men, Black women, non-Black men, and non-Black women). Table 3 presents the performance of the CKD-EPI$_{2021}$ and EKFC equations in the whole population and in the 4 main groups.

Validation in the whole population

In the whole population, only the EKFC$_{PS}$ equation was unbiased, and also the statistical bias for the EKFC$_{RF}$ equation was closer to zero than that for the CKD-EPI$_{2021}$ equation. P20 and P30 were similar (i.e., 95% confidence intervals are overlapping) for CKD-EPI$_{2021}$ and EKFC$_{RF}$, whereas P30 and P20 for EKFC$_{PS}$ were slightly better than those for CKD-EPI$_{2021}$.

Validation in the 4 main populations

In the 4 main groups, the statistical bias for both EKFC$_{PS}$ and EKFC$_{RF}$ was closer to zero than that for CKD-EPI$_{2021}$ in non-Black women and Black men. The statistical bias was also better for EKFC$_{PS}$ than for CKD-EPI$_{2021}$ in non-Black men. Accuracies of the 3 equations were similar in the 4 groups (except P30 for EKFC$_{PS}$, which was better than that for CKD-EPI$_{2021}$ in non-Black men).

The statistical bias and P30 for the 3 equations according to age are shown in Figure 1a and b, respectively, for the whole population and in Supplementary Figures S1 to S4 for the 4 main groups (because women have the same Q values, EKFC$_{RF}$ and EKFC$_{PS}$ are identical in women and merged as EKFC). Results according to age are also presented in Supplementary Table S3 ([18–40], [40–65], and ≥65 years). From Table 3 and Supplementary Tables S3 and S4, it can be seen that performance of the 3 equations was similar in Black and non-Black women (only statistical bias and P30 for non-Black

Table 2 | Clinical and biological characteristics of the main groups

Characteristic	Whole cohort (N = 12,854)	Non-Black men (n = 5459)	Non-Black women (n = 4605)	Black men (n = 1703)	Black women (n = 1087)
Age, yr	56.0 [42.9; 65.0]	57.0 [42.0; 66.0]	55.0 [41.0; 65.0]	54.0 [45.0; 62.0]	55.0 [45.0; 63.0]
Measured GFR, ml/min per 1.73 m^2	57 [37; 83]	57 [36; 84]	61 [37; 89]	57 [40; 74]	49 [34; 67]
% of urinary clearance	93.2	92.3	91.6	97.9	97.8
Serum creatinine, mg/dl	1.30 [0.93; 1.80]	1.40 [1.00; 1.90]	1.00 [0.76; 1.50]	1.60 [1.26; 2.07]	1.35 [1.06; 1.89]
Estimated GFR – CKD-EPI$_{2021}$, ml/min per 1.73 m^2	59 [39; 86]	61 [40; 90]	66 [42; 95]	52 [37; 66]	46 [31; 62]
Estimated GFR – EKFC$_{RF}$, ml/min per 1.73 m^2	58 [39; 82]	61 [41; 86]	63 [41; 88]	53 [38; 67]	45 [32; 60]
Estimated GFR – EKFC$_{PS}$, ml/min per 1.73 m^2	58 [39; 82]	58 [39; 84]	63 [41; 88]	55 [40; 70]	45 [32; 60]

CKD-EPI$_{2021}$, race-free Chronic Kidney Disease Epidemiology Collaboration; EKFC$_{PS}$, European Kidney Function Consortium with population-specific Q values; EKFC$_{RF}$, European Kidney Function Consortium with race-free Q values; GFR, glomerular filtration rate.
Results are expressed as percentage or median [quartile 1; quartile 3].

women was better for both EKFC equations than for CKD-EPI$_{2021}$). In non-Black men, statistical bias was better for EKFC$_{PS}$ in the age groups (where the statistical bias for EKFC$_{RF}$ was similar, larger, or lower than that for CKD-EPI$_{2021}$ in patients aged between 18 and 40, between 40 and 65, and ≥65 years, respectively). In Black men, performance was similar but a better statistical bias for both EKFC equations than that for CKD-EPI$_{2021}$ was observed between 40 and 65 years. From Figure 1 and Supplementary Figures S1 to S4, it can be viewed that both statistical bias and P30 for the 2 EKFC equations were more consistent over the complete age range whereas the CKD-EPI$_{2021}$ equation overestimates GFR in young people (between 18 and 30 years). This observation was especially relevant in non-Black populations.

Table 3 | Performance of the CKD-EPI$_{2021}$ and EKFC equations to estimate glomerular filtration rate

Populations	CKD-EPI$_{2021}$	EKFC$_{RF}$	EKFC$_{PS}$
Whole population (N = 12,854)			
Median bias (95% CI)	1.22 (0.99; 1.47)	0.74 (0.51; 0.94)	0.14 (−0.07; 0.35)
IQR (Q1; Q3)	16.0 [−6.6; 9.4]	15.7 [−7.6; 8.0]	15.4 [−8.1; 7.3]
P30 (95% CI)	79.2 (78.5; 79.9)	80.1 (79.4; 80.7)	81.1 (80.5; 81.8)
P20 (95% CI)	61.6 (60.7; 62.4)	62.4 (61.6; 63.3)	63.7 (62.9; 64.5)
Non-Black population (n = 10,064)			
Median bias (95% CI)	2.78 (2.55; 3.04)	1.93 (1.67; 2.18)	0.85 (0.62; 1.09)
IQR (Q1; Q3)	16.1 [−4.8; 11.3]	15.6 [−6.4; 9.3]	15.6 [−7.6; 8.0]
P30 (95% CI)	78.3 (77.5; 79.1)	79.0 (78.2; 79.8)	80.4 (79.6; 81.2)
P20 (95% CI)	61.4 (60.5; 62.4)	61.9 (61.0; 62.9)	63.3 (62.4; 64.3)
Black population (n = 2790)			
Median bias (95% CI)	−4.01 (−4.44; −3.56)	−3.12 (−3.70; −2.62)	−2.22 (−2.72; −1.83)
IQR (Q1; Q3)	13.9 [−11.6; 2.3]	14.3 [−11.1; 3.2]	14.1 [−10.0; 4.2]
P30 (95% CI)	82.5 (81.1; 83.9)	83.8 (82.4; 85.2)	83.7 (82.4; 85.1)
P20 (95% CI)	62.1 (60.3; 63.9)	64.3 (62.5; 66.0)	64.9 (63.1; 66.7)
Non-Black women (n = 4605)			
Median bias (95% CI)	2.54 (2.20; 2.92)	0.45 (0.08; 0.86)	0.45 (0.08; 0.86)
IQR (Q1; Q3)	16.3 [−5.2; 11.1]	15.7 [−7.9; 7.8]	15.7 [−7.9; 7.8]
P30 (95% CI)	78.9 (77.7; 80.1)	80.9 (79.8; 82.0)	80.9 (79.8; 82.0)
P20 (95% CI)	62.0 (60.6; 63.4)	63.7 (62.3; 65.1)	63.7 (62.3; 65.1)
Non-Black men (n = 5459)			
Median bias (95% CI)	3.01 (2.66; 3.43)	3.09 (2.76; 3.41)	1.14 (0.85; 1.43)
IQR (Q1; Q3)	15.9 [−4.5; 11.3]	15.7 [−5.0; 10.7]	15.6 [−7.3; 8.3]
P30 (95% CI)	77.7 (76.6; 78.8)	77.4 (76.3; 78.5)	80.0 (79.0; 81.1)
P20 (95% CI)	60.9 (59.7; 62.2)	60.4 (59.1; 61.7)	63.1 (61.8; 64.4)
Black women (n = 1087)			
Median bias (95% CI)	−2.98 (−3.75; −2.30)	−3.39 (−4.12; −2.67)	−3.39 (−4.12; −2.67)
IQR (Q1; Q3)	13.6 [−10.7; 2.9]	14.0 [−11.6; 2.4]	14.0 [−11.6; 2.4]
P30 (95% CI)	79.8 (77.4; 82.2)	80.3 (78.0; 82.7)	80.3 (78.0; 82.7)
P20 (95% CI)	60.5 (57.6; 63.4)	60.8 (57.9; 63.7)	60.8 (57.9; 63.7)
Black men (n = 1703)			
Median bias (95% CI)	−4.64 (−5.15; −4.10)	−2.91 (−3.69; −2.30)	−1.35 (−1.97; −0.75)
IQR (Q1; Q3)	14.4 [−12.3; 2.1]	14.4 [−10.7; 3.7]	14.2 [−8.8; 5.4]
P30 (95% CI)	84.3 (82.5; 86.0)	86.0 (84.4; 87.7)	85.9 (84.3; 87.6)
P20 (95% CI)	63.1 (60.8; 65.4)	66.5 (64.2; 68.7)	67.5 (65.2; 69.7)

CKD-EPI$_{2021}$, race-free Chronic Kidney Disease Epidemiology Collaboration; EKFC, European Kidney Function Consortium; EKFC$_{PS}$, European Kidney Function Consortium with population-specific Q values; EKFC$_{RF}$, European Kidney Function Consortium with race-free Q values; IQR, interquartile range; P20, accuracy within 20%; P30, accuracy within 30%; Q1, quartile 1; Q3, quartile 3.
Bias and IQR are expressed in milliliters per minute per 1.73 meter square. P30 and P20 are expressed in percentage.

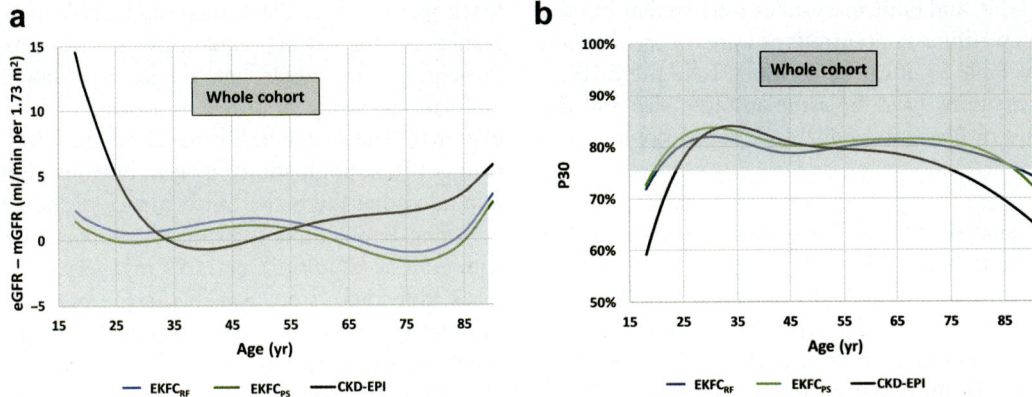

Figure 1 | (a) Statistical bias and (b) accuracy within 30% (P30) for the race-free Chronic Kidney Disease Epidemiology Collaboration (CKD-EPI$_{2021}$), European Kidney Function Consortium with race-free Q values (EKFC$_{RF}$), and European Kidney Function with population-specific Q values (EKFC$_{PS}$) equations in the whole population ($N = 12{,}854$) according to age. eGFR, estimated glomerular filtration rate; mGFR, measured glomerular filtration rate.

The statistical bias and P30 for both equations according to the patients' measured GFR are shown in Figure 2a and b, respectively, for the whole population and in Supplementary Figures S5 to S8 for the 4 main groups. Results according to measured GFR are also presented in Supplementary Table S4 (<60 and ≥ 60 ml/min per 1.73 m^2). Regarding GFR, performance was similar in non-Black and Black women (only in non-Black women with GFR ≥ 60 ml/min per 1.73 m^2, the statistical bias was better for CKD-EPI$_{2021}$ whereas P30 was better for the 2 EKFC equations). In non-Black men with GFR < 60 ml/min per 1.73 m^2, the statistical bias and P20 were better for CKD-EPI$_{2021}$ than for EKFC$_{RF}$ but the statistical bias was lower than for EKFC$_{PS}$. If GFR is ≥ 60 ml/min per 1.73 m^2, the statistical bias for both EKFC equations is further from zero than that for CKD-EPI$_{2021}$. In Black men, performance was similar, expect for a better statistical bias for EKFC$_{PS}$ when GFR is ≥ 60 ml/min per 1.73 m^2.

Validation per cohort

The performance of the 3 equations per cohort is displayed in Supplementary Table S5. The performance of the 3 equations was similar in the CRIC, CRISP, and PERL cohorts. The statistical bias for both EKFC equations was better than that for CKD-EPI$_{2021}$ in the ALTOLD, GENOA/ECAC, and Mayo Clinic cohorts. The statistical bias for the EKFC$_{PS}$ equation was better than that for CKD-EPI$_{2021}$ in the AASK cohort. The statistical bias for the CKD-EPI$_{2021}$ equation was better than that for EKFC$_{RF}$ in the MDRD study cohort and better than those for the 2 EKFC equations in the DCCT/EDIC cohort. Regarding P30, the results are similar in most cohorts, except for a better P30 for CKD-EPI$_{2021}$ than for EKFC$_{RF}$, for both EKFC equations than for CKD-EPI$_{2021}$, and for EKFC$_{PS}$ than for CKD-EPI$_{2021}$ in MDRD, GENOA/ECAC, and Mayo Clinic cohorts, respectively.

Matched analysis

We matched individuals from the Black population ($n = 831$) with individuals from the non-Black population ($n = 1198$). We could identify matching partners for 667 Black participants (80.2%). Individuals without matches were omitted in further analyses. The results of matching according to sex are presented in Supplementary Table S6. As expected, mean age,

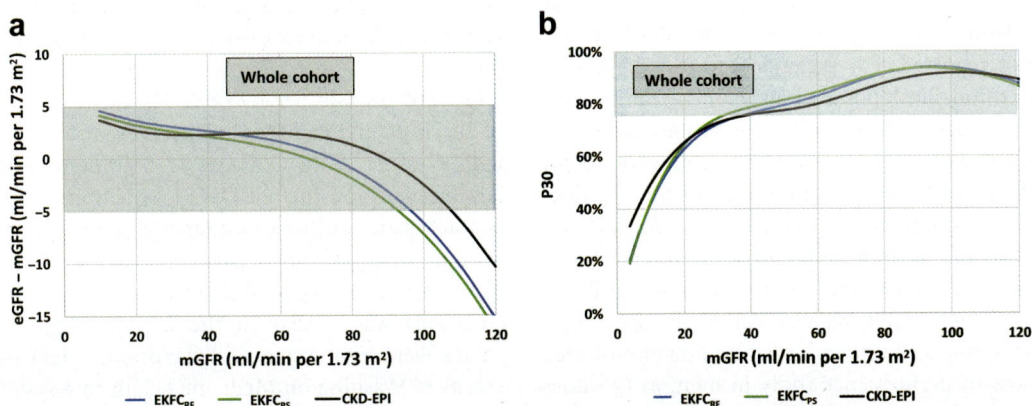

Figure 2 | (a) Statistical bias and (b) accuracy within 30% (P30) for the race-free Chronic Kidney Disease Epidemiology Collaboration (CKD-EPI$_{2021}$), European Kidney Function Consortium with race-free Q values (EKFC$_{RF}$), and European Kidney Function with population-specific Q values (EKFC$_{PS}$) equations in the whole population ($N = 12{,}854$) according to measured glomerular filtration rate (mGFR). eGFR, estimated glomerular filtration rate.

sex, measured GFR, and body mass index were similar but the median serum creatinine concentrations were different. From Supplementary Table S7, it can be seen that both the EKFC$_{PS}$ and EKFC$_{RF}$ equations have the same absolute bias and the same P30 values in Black and non-Black populations.

DISCUSSION

In the present analysis of large US cohorts, we showed that the new creatinine-based EKFC equation is valid with a similar performance to the CKD-EPI$_{2021}$ equation. The EKFC equation has the ambition to be applicable in different populations as long as a Q value, defined as the median "normal" serum creatinine, in the given population is available.[9,30,31] Then, the Q value is used to rescale serum creatinine and can be integrated into the EKFC equation, which has been developed to be accurate in the whole age range.[6] The EKFC equation can also be used with other biomarkers, such as cystatin C (with Q value specifically obtained for cystatin C).[2] Up to now, the equation has been validated in Europe and Africa.[6,9] Preliminary results in Asia are promising,[32–35] but data were limited in the United States.[2,6,8] In the present analysis, we demonstrated that the EKFC equation is as accurate as, and in some subanalyses more accurate than, the creatinine-based CKD-EPI$_{2021}$ equation. Recently, the race variable, frequently used in creatinine-based equations before 2021, has been considered as discriminatory,[4] leading the CKD-EPI consortium to propose the race-free CKD-EPI$_{2021}$ equation.[3] The EKFC equation does not include the variable race because all differences between populations potentially influencing serum creatinine concentration are integrated into Q values. For US Q values, we considered the values published in the literature obtained from a large laboratory database,[25] as we did for European Q values.[24,30] Interestingly, differences in Q values between Black and non-Black populations are relevant only for men but not for women. The similar Q value in Black and non-Black women is a strong argument to assert that the Q value is more dependent on populations than on race. We do not advocate race-based reporting of the GFR estimation result with the EKFC equations. Rather, we would defer to the patient to decide how they self-identify with respect to race: non-Black, Black, or unknown/not reported. For patients who identify themselves as Black or non-Black populations, EKFC$_{PS}$ can be used with specific Q values.[2,25] For patients who choose not to identify themselves as a particular race or as unknown, or for mixed populations, the Q value is the mean of the Q values obtained in Black and non-Black populations, making it race free. Self-reporting of race in hospital registration records can be used to determine the Q value to use without race-based reporting of estimated GFR results. Although there is a slightly more accurate GFR estimation with population-based Q values, the loss of performance (only in men, as Q values are not different by race in women) is quite modest.

More importantly, the EKFC equations have globally the same performance as the CKD-EPI$_{2021}$ equation, with statistical bias being even better for the EKFC equations in non-Black women, non-Black men, and Black men. The performance of the EKFC equations is also more consistent throughout the whole age range, especially in non-Black populations (with a lower statistical bias in young populations). The better performance of the EKFC equation in young Black populations is less obvious, but it must be reminded that the better performance of the EKFC equation in young populations is especially important in individuals with GFR > 60 ml/min per 1.73 m^2. Very few healthy young Black individuals were available in the present cohorts. Also, the analysis per cohort demonstrates that the EKFC equation is performing at least as good as (and sometimes better than) the present CKD-EPI$_{2021}$ equation. The last point is remarkable. Indeed, an equation is always performing better in the cohorts that have been used for its development, and it must be reminded that AASK, MDRD, DCCT/EDIC, and CRIC were used in the development data set and PERL and ALTOLD in the validation data set of the CKD-EPI$_{2021}$ equation.[3] The fact that the EKFC equations are performing as good as (and better than for some cohorts) CKD-EPI$_{2021}$ in these cohorts (except in the MDRD study cohort) was not expected. Moreover, CKD-EPI$_{2021}$ has been developed with iothalamate urinary clearances as a reference method to measure GFR, although the EKFC equation has been mostly developed with GFR measured by iohexol plasma clearances.[3,6] This discrepancy in measuring GFR methods could theoretically disadvantage the performance of the EKFC equation (but eventually it did not). The fact that the EKFC equations are still performing similarly to CKD-EPI$_{2021}$ demonstrates its consistent accuracy.

The strength of our study is the large sample size, which was reached by the inclusion of large cohorts, including both Black and non-Black populations. Our analysis also had limitations. First, the data set did not include children and adolescents. In the seminal article, a major strength of the EKFC equation was the continuity at the transition between adolescent and young adulthood.[6,36] Although there is no reason that this would be different in US populations, this continuity still needs to be demonstrated in US cohorts with children, adolescents, and young adults. Second, our data set is not representative of the general US population. The main limitation is the very few numbers of Black individuals with GFR > 60 ml/min per 1.73 m^2. The fact that the vast majority of Black people included in the present analysis are patients with chronic kidney disease is a limitation shared in the development of the CKD-EPI equations.[37,38] Because the characteristics of Black participants were different, a matched analysis was performed between Black and non-Black populations, which suggested that the performance of the 2 EKFC equations was similar in the 2 populations. Third, US Q values were established with laboratory data from the University of Washington Medicine health care system.[25] It can be argued that these data could not be representative of the United States. However, Q values can also be obtained from the National Health and Nutrition Examination Survey (Supplementary Table S1).[31,38,39] The performance of the

EKFC equations with the National Health and Nutrition Examination Survey Q values is displayed in Supplementary Table S8 and is similar to that obtained with Washington laboratory data. Fourth, cystatin C concentration was not available for analyses in our largest cohort (Mayo Clinic). Still, our main aim was to propose and compare a race-free creatinine-based EKFC equation as it is already known that cystatin C concentration is not influenced by race. Lastly, we must emphasize the absence of an Asian US cohort in our analyses with measured GFR. We can however note that a population-specific Q value for Asian US individuals is available from laboratory data from the University of Washington Medicine health care system (0.93 and 0.67 mg/dl for men and women, respectively).[25]

In conclusion, the creatinine-based EKFC equations can be used in the United States with population-specific Q values. The population, and therefore Q values, can be defined differently (like we did in the present analysis with $EKFC_{RF}$ and $EKFC_{PS}$). We showed a similar performance of the EKFC and CKD-EPI$_{2021}$ equations in US cohorts. The performance of $EKFC_{PS}$ is even slightly better than that of the CKD-EPI$_{2021}$ equation. This result combined with prior observations, showing that the EKFC equation is performing better in Europe, Asia, and Africa than the CKD-EPI$_{2021}$ equation,[6,9,32–34] demonstrates that the EKFC equation with population-specific Q values is applicable worldwide. All equations, however, remain a GFR estimation. If they are useful at the population level, their accuracy might be insufficient for clinical decision at the individual level, and a GFR measurement might still be necessary in some situations.[40,41]

DISCLOSURE
The results presented in this paper have not been published previously in whole or part. PD and EC serve as consultants for Nephrolyx. ES receives honoraria from the National Kidney Foundation and serves as a consultant for AstraZeneca. All the other authors declared no competing interests.

DATA STATEMENT
The short protocol is available to interested readers by contacting Pierre Delanaye at pdelanaye@chuliege.be.

The SAS code is available to interested readers by contacting Hans Pottel at hans.pottel@kuleuven.be.

The data from the Assessing Long Term Outcomes in Living Kidney Donors, Chronic Renal Insufficiency Cohort, Consortium for Radiologic Imaging Studies of Polycystic Kidney Disease, Diabetes Control and Complications Trial/Epidemiology of Diabetes Interventions and Complications, Preventing Early Renal Loss in Diabetes, African American Study of Kidney Disease and Hypertension, and Modified Diet in Renal Disease studies reported here are available on request in the National Institute of Diabetes and Digestive and Kidney Diseases Central Repository. The data from the Mayo Clinic and Genetic Epidemiology Network of Arteriopathy/Epidemiology of Coronary Artery Calcification studies are not publicly available because of the confidential nature of patient information obtained for clinical care. Legal and ethical restrictions prevent public sharing of the data set. Data can be made available for collaborations on request to interested researchers but would generally require a new ethical permission and the permission of each of the data owners.

ACKNOWLEDGMENTS
The Assessing Long Term Outcomes in Living Kidney Donors, Chronic Renal Insufficiency Cohort, Consortium for Radiologic Imaging Studies of Polycystic Kidney Disease, Diabetes Control and Complications Trial/Epidemiology of Diabetes Interventions and Complications, Preventing Early Renal Loss in Diabetes, African American Study of Kidney Disease and Hypertension, and Modified Diet in Renal Disease studies were performed by respective investigators and supported by the National Institute of Diabetes and Digestive and Kidney Diseases (NIDDK). The data from these studies reported here were supplied by the NIDDK Central Repository. This manuscript was not prepared in collaboration with the investigators of the different studies and does not necessarily reflect the opinions or views of these studies, the NIDDK Central Repository, or the NIDDK.

ROLE OF THE FUNDING SOURCE
This study was supported by the Swedish Research Council (Vetenskapsrådet; grant no. 2019-00198). JB has received funding from the Swedish Research Council (VR) to conduct large-scale epidemiological studies linked with registered data from health care. This funding source was not at all involved in design, analysis, presentation, or interpretation of the results from the present study.

SUPPLEMENTARY MATERIAL
Supplementary File (Word)
Supplementary Table S1. Q values determined in different populations.
Supplementary Table S2. Overview of estimating glomerular filtration rate (GFR) equations.
Supplementary Table S3. Performance of the race-free Chronic Kidney Disease Epidemiology Collaboration (CKD-EPI$_{2021}$) and European Kidney Function Consortium (EKFC) equations to estimate glomerular filtration rate according to age.
Supplementary Table S4. Performance of the race-free Chronic Kidney Disease Epidemiology Collaboration (CKD-EPI$_{2021}$) and European Kidney Function Consortium (EKFC) equations to estimate glomerular filtration rate (GFR) according to measured GFR.
Supplementary Table S5. Performance of the equations in different cohorts.
Supplementary Table S6. Patient characteristics of the matched cohorts (Black and non-Black individuals).
Supplementary Table S7. Results of the European Kidney Function Consortium with population-specific Q values (EFKC$_{PS}$) and European Kidney Function Consortium with race-free Q values (EKFC$_{RF}$) equations in the matched cohorts.
Supplementary Table S8. Performance of the European Kidney Function Consortium (EKFC) equations to estimate glomerular filtration rate with Q values obtained from the Washington Medicine health care system (WMS) or National Health and Nutrition Examination Survey (NHANES).
Supplementary Figure S1. (A) Bias and (B) accuracy within 30% (P30) for the race-free Chronic Kidney Disease Epidemiology Collaboration (CKD-EPI$_{2021}$) and European Kidney Function Consortium (EKFC) equations in non-Black women ($n = 4605$) according to age.
Supplementary Figure S2. (A) Bias and (B) accuracy within 30% (P30) for the race-free Chronic Kidney Disease Epidemiology Collaboration (CKD-EPI$_{2021}$), European Kidney Function Consortium with race-free Q values (EKFC$_{RF}$), and European Kidney Function with

population-specific Q values (EKFC$_{PS}$) equations in non-Black men ($n = 5459$) according to age.
Supplementary Figure S3. (**A**) Bias and (**B**) accuracy within 30% (P30) for the race-free Chronic Kidney Disease Epidemiology Collaboration (CKD-EPI$_{2021}$) and European Kidney Function Consortium (EKFC) equations in Black women ($n = 1087$) according to age.
Supplementary Figure S4. (**A**) Bias and (**B**) accuracy within 30% (P30) for the race-free Chronic Kidney Disease Epidemiology Collaboration (CKD-EPI$_{2021}$), European Kidney Function Consortium with race-free Q values (EKFC$_{RF}$), and European Kidney Function with population-specific Q values (EKFC$_{PS}$) equations in Black men ($n = 1703$) according to age.
Supplementary Figure S5. (**A**) Bias and (**B**) accuracy within 30% (P30) for the race-free Chronic Kidney Disease Epidemiology Collaboration (CKD-EPI$_{2021}$) and European Kidney Function Consortium (EKFC) equations in non-Black women ($n = 4605$) according to measured glomerular filtration rate (GFR).
Supplementary Figure S6. (**A**) Bias and (**B**) accuracy within 30% (P30) for the race-free Chronic Kidney Disease Epidemiology Collaboration (CKD-EPI$_{2021}$), European Kidney Function Consortium with race-free Q values (EKFC$_{RF}$), and European Kidney Function with population-specific Q values (EKFC$_{PS}$) equations in non-Black men ($n = 5459$) according to measured glomerular filtration rate (GFR).
Supplementary Figure S7. (**A**) Bias and (**B**) accuracy within 30% (P30) for the race-free Chronic Kidney Disease Epidemiology Collaboration (CKD-EPI$_{2021}$) and European Kidney Function Consortium (EKFC) equations in Black women ($n = 1087$) according to measured glomerular filtration rate (GFR).
Supplementary Figure S8. (**A**) Bias and (**B**) accuracy within 30% (P30) for the race-free Chronic Kidney Disease Epidemiology Collaboration (CKD-EPI$_{2021}$), European Kidney Function Consortium with race-free Q values (EKFC$_{RF}$), and European Kidney Function with population-specific Q values (EKFC$_{PS}$) equations in Black men ($n = 1703$) according to measured glomerular filtration rate (GFR).
Supplementary References.

REFERENCES

1. Kidney Disease: Improving Global Outcomes (KDIGO) CKD Work Group. KDIGO 2012 clinical practice guideline for the evaluation and management of chronic kidney disease. *Kidney Int Suppl*. 2013;3:1–150.
2. Pottel H, Björk J, Rule AD, et al. Cystatin C–based equation to estimate GFR without the inclusion of race and sex. *N Engl J Med*. 2023;388:333–343.
3. Inker LA, Eneanya ND, Coresh J, et al. New creatinine- and cystatin C–based equations to estimate GFR without race. *N Engl J Med*. 2021;385:1737–1749.
4. Delgado C, Baweja M, Crews DC, et al. A unifying approach for GFR estimation: recommendations of the NKF-ASN Task Force on reassessing the inclusion of race in diagnosing kidney disease. *J Am Soc Nephrol*. 2021;32:2994–3015.
5. Miller WG, Kaufman HW, Levey AS, et al. National Kidney Foundation Laboratory Engagement Working Group recommendations for implementing the CKD-EPI 2021 race-free equations for estimated glomerular filtration rate: practical guidance for clinical laboratories. *Clin Chem*. 2022;68:511–520.
6. Pottel H, Björk J, Courbebaisse M, et al. Development and validation of a modified full age spectrum creatinine-based equation to estimate glomerular filtration rate: a cross-sectional analysis of pooled data. *Ann Intern Med*. 2021;174:183–191.
7. Delanaye P, Schaeffner E, Cozzolino M, et al. The new, race-free, Chronic Kidney Disease Epidemiology Consortium (CKD-EPI) equation to estimate glomerular filtration rate: is it applicable in Europe? A position statement by the European Federation of Clinical Chemistry and Laboratory Medicine (EFLM). *Clin Chem Lab Med*. 2023;61:44–47.
8. Levey AS, Tighiouart H, Inker LA. Improving glomerular filtration rate estimation—across the age and diversity spectrum. *Ann Intern Med*. 2021;174:265–267.
9. Delanaye P, Vidal-Petiot E, Björk J, et al. Performance of creatinine-based equations to estimate glomerular filtration rate in White and Black populations in Europe, Brazil, and Africa. *Nephrol Dial Transpl*. 2023;38:106–118.
10. Kasiske BL, Anderson-Haag TL, Duprez DA, et al. A prospective controlled study of metabolic and physiologic effects of kidney donation suggests that donors retain stable kidney function over the first nine years. *Kidney Int*. 2020;98:168–175.
11. Pottel H, Cavalier E, Björk J, et al. Standardization of serum creatinine is essential for accurate use of unbiased estimated GFR equations: evidence from three cohorts matched on renal function. *Clin Kidney J*. 2022;15:2258–2265.
12. Hsu CY, Yang W, Parikh RV, et al. Race, genetic ancestry, and estimating kidney function in CKD. *N Engl J Med*. 2021;385:1750–1760.
13. Rule AD, Torres VE, Chapman AB, et al. Comparison of methods for determining renal function decline in early autosomal dominant polycystic kidney disease: the consortium of radiologic imaging studies of polycystic kidney disease cohort. *J Am Soc Nephrol*. 2006;17:854–862.
14. Ibrahim H, Mondress M, Tello A, et al. An alternative formula to the Cockcroft-Gault and the modification of diet in renal diseases formulas in predicting GFR in individuals with type 1 diabetes. *J Am Soc Nephrol*. 2005;16:1051–1060.
15. de Boer IH, Sun W, Cleary PA, et al. Longitudinal changes in estimated and measured GFR in type 1 diabetes. *J Am Soc Nephrol*. 2014;25:810–818.
16. Doria A, Galecki AT, Spino C, et al. Serum urate lowering with allopurinol and kidney function in type 1 diabetes. *N Engl J Med*. 2020;382:2493–2503.
17. Lewis J, Agodoa L, Cheek D, et al. Comparison of cross-sectional renal function measurements in African Americans with hypertensive nephrosclerosis and of primary formulas to estimate glomerular filtration rate. *Am J Kidney Dis*. 2001;38:744–753.
18. Levey AS, Bosch JP, Lewis JB, et al. Modification of Diet in Renal Disease Study Group. A more accurate method to estimate glomerular filtration rate from serum creatinine: a new prediction equation. *Ann Intern Med*. 1999;130:461–470.
19. Stevens LA, Manzi J, Levey AS, et al. Impact of creatinine calibration on performance of GFR estimating equations in a pooled individual patient database. *Am J Kidney Dis*. 2007;50:21–35.
20. Levey AS, Coresh J, Greene T, et al. Expressing the Modification of Diet in Renal Disease Study equation for estimating glomerular filtration rate with standardized serum creatinine values. *Clin Chem*. 2007;53:766–772.
21. Afkarian M, Polsky S, Parsa A, et al. Preventing Early Renal Loss in Diabetes (PERL) study: a randomized double-blinded trial of allopurinol—rationale, design, and baseline data. *Diabetes Care*. 2019;42:1454–1463.
22. Rule AD, Bailey KR, Lieske JC, et al. Estimating the glomerular filtration rate from serum creatinine is better than from cystatin C for evaluating risk factors associated with chronic kidney disease. *Kidney Int*. 2013;83:1169–1176.
23. Zhang X, Rule AD, McCulloch CE, et al. Tubular secretion of creatinine and kidney function: an observational study. *BMC Nephrol*. 2020;21:108.
24. Björk J, Nyman U, Delanaye P, et al. A novel method for creatinine adjustment makes the revised Lund-Malmö GFR estimating equation applicable in children. *Scand J Clin Lab Invest*. 2020;80:456–463.
25. Shi J, Lindo EG, Baird GS, et al. Calculating estimated glomerular filtration rate without the race correction factor: observations at a large academic medical system. *Clin Chim Acta*. 2021;520:16–22.
26. Poggio ED, Rule AD, Tanchanco R, et al. Demographic and clinical characteristics associated with glomerular filtration rates in living kidney donors. *Kidney Int*. 2009;75:1079–1087.
27. Delanaye P, Pottel H, Botev R. Con: should we abandon the use of the MDRD equation in favour of the CKD-EPI equation? *Nephrol Dial Transpl*. 2013;28:1396–1403.
28. National Kidney Foundation. K/DOQI clinical practice guidelines for chronic kidney disease: evaluation, classification, and stratification. *Am J Kidney Dis*. 2002;39(2 suppl 1):S1–S266.
29. Björk J, Grubb A, Sterner G, et al. Performance of GFR estimating equations stratified by measured or estimated GFR: implications for interpretation. *Am J Kidney Dis*. 2015;66:1107–1108.
30. Pottel H, Vrydags N, Mahieu B, et al. Establishing age/sex related serum creatinine reference intervals from hospital laboratory data based on different statistical methods. *Clin Chim Acta*. 2008;396:49–55.

31. Delanaye P, Pottel H, Glassock RJ. Americentrism in estimation of GFR equations. *Kidney Int*. 2022;101:856–858.
32. Zhao L, Li HL, Liu HJ, et al. Validation of the EKFC equation for glomerular filtration rate estimation and comparison with the Asian-modified CKD-EPI equation in Chinese chronic kidney disease patients in an external study. *Ren Fail*. 2023;45:2150217.
33. Xia F, Hao W, Liang J, et al. Applicability of creatinine-based equations for estimating glomerular filtration rate in elderly Chinese patients. *BMC Geriatr*. 2021;21:1–13.
34. Jeong TD, Hong J, Lee W, et al. Accuracy of the new creatinine-based equations for estimating glomerular filtration rate in Koreans. *Ann Lab Med*. 2023;43:244–252.
35. Ma Y, Wei L, Yong Z, et al. Validation of the European Kidney Function Consortium (EKFC) equation in Chinese adult population: an equation standing on the shoulders of predecessors. *Nephron*. 2023. Published online June 14, 2023. https://doi.org/10.1159/000531030
36. Pottel H, Björk J, Bökenkamp A, et al. Estimating glomerular filtration rate at the transition from pediatric to adult care. *Kidney Int*. 2019;95:1234–1243.
37. Delanaye P, Mariat C, Maillard N, et al. Are the creatinine-based equations accurate to estimate glomerular filtration rate in African American populations? *Clin J Am Soc Nephrol*. 2011;6:906–912.
38. Delanaye P, Mariat C, Cavalier E, et al. The « race » correction in estimating glomerular filtration rate. *Curr Opin Nephrol Hypertens*. 2021;30:525–530.
39. Jones CA, McQuillan GM, Kusek JW, et al. Serum creatinine levels in the US population: third National Health and Nutrition Examination Survey. *Am J Kidney Dis*. 1998;32:992–999.
40. Ebert N, Bevc S, Bökenkamp A, et al. Assessment of kidney function: clinical indications for measured GFR. *Clin Kidney J*. 2021;14:1861–1870.
41. Agarwal R, Delanaye P. Glomerular filtration rate: when to measure and in which patients? *Nephrol Dial Transpl*. 2019;34:2001–2007.

Sodium-glucose cotransporter 2 inhibitors in the treatment of refractory hypomagnesemia

To the editor: I read with great interest the article by Sen et al., showing that 1 of the underlying molecular mechanisms of the kidney-protective effect of sodium-glucose cotransporter 2 (SGLT2) inhibitors in patients with type 2 diabetes is the increment in epidermal growth factor (EGF) expression in the kidney.[1]

EGF acts as an autocrine/paracrine magnesiotropic hormone. EGF stimulates Mg^{2+} reabsorption in the renal distal convoluted tubule via engagement of its receptor on the basolateral membrane of distal convoluted tubule cells and activation of the Mg^{2+} channel transient receptor potential cation channel, subfamily M, member 6 in the apical membrane.[2]

Hypomagnesemia is a frequent finding in patients with diabetes mellitus and provokes glucose intolerance. Meta-analysis of diabetic patients receiving SGLT2 inhibitors has shown reduced hypomagnesemia in patients, with a mean increase in serum magnesium levels of 0.01 to 0.24 mg/dl.[3]

Treatment of severe hypomagnesemia is often challenging. Gastrointestinal absorption limits oral supplementation. The i.v. magnesium infusion enhances urinary magnesium excretion, making serum magnesium level increases transient. Thus, patients with urinary magnesium wasting disorders often have persistent hypomagnesemia.

Several case reports have shown that the use of SGLT2 inhibitors has resulted in improved management in patients with intractable hypomagnesemia.[4] The increased expression and availability of EGF during SGLT2 inhibitor administration could explain the beneficial effect of these drugs in the treatment of refractory hypomagnesemia.

1. Sen T, Ju W, Nair V, et al. Sodium glucose co-transporter 2 inhibition increases epidermal growth factor expression and improves outcomes in patients with type 2 diabetes. *Kidney Int.* 2023;104:828–839.
2. Muallem S, Moe OW. When EGF is offside, magnesium is wasted. *J Clin Invest.* 2007;117:2086–2089.
3. Tang H, Zhang X, Zhang J, et al. Elevated serum magnesium associated with SGLT2 inhibitor use in type 2 diabetes patients: a meta-analysis of randomised controlled trials. *Diabetologia.* 2016;59:2546.
4. Ray CE, Boyd-Shiwarski R, Liu P, et al. SGLT2 inhibitors for treatment of refractory hypomagnesemia: a case report of 3 patients. *Kidney Med.* 2020;2:359–363.

Armando Luis Negri[1]

[1]Instituto de Investigaciones Metabólicas, Universidad del Salvador, Buenos Aires, Argentina

Correspondence: Armando Luis Negri, Instituto de Investigaciones Metabólicas, Libertad 836 1 Piso, Código Postal 1012, Buenos Aires, Argentina. E-mail: armando.negri@gmail.com

Kidney International (2024) 105, 638; https://doi.org/10.1016/j.kint.2023.11.019

Copyright © 2023, International Society of Nephrology. Published by Elsevier Inc. All rights reserved.

Sodium-glucose cotransporter 2 inhibition, epidermal growth factor, and magnesium homeostasis: is there a link?

To the editor: The recent work by Sen et al., "Sodium Glucose Co-transporter 2 Inhibition Increases Epidermal Growth Factor Expression and Improves Outcomes in Patients With Type 2 Diabetes," drew my attention to a possible link between the effect of sodium-glucose cotransporter 2 (SGLT2) inhibitors on magnesium (Mg^{2+}) homeostasis.[1] In their single-cell kidney biopsy studies performed on patients as part of the research, the authors thoroughly demonstrated that SGLT2 inhibitors significantly increased the epidermal growth factor (EGF) mRNA level in the distal convoluted tubular epithelial cells. They were successfully able to demonstrate the link between increased *EGF* mRNA expression, increased urinary EGF/creatinine levels, and improved diabetic kidney outcomes.

Significant data have recently emerged suggestive of the positive impact of SGLT2 inhibitors on magnesium homeostasis as their class effect.[2–4,S1] The mechanism of how SGLT2 inhibitors increase serum Mg^{2+} levels remains an area of

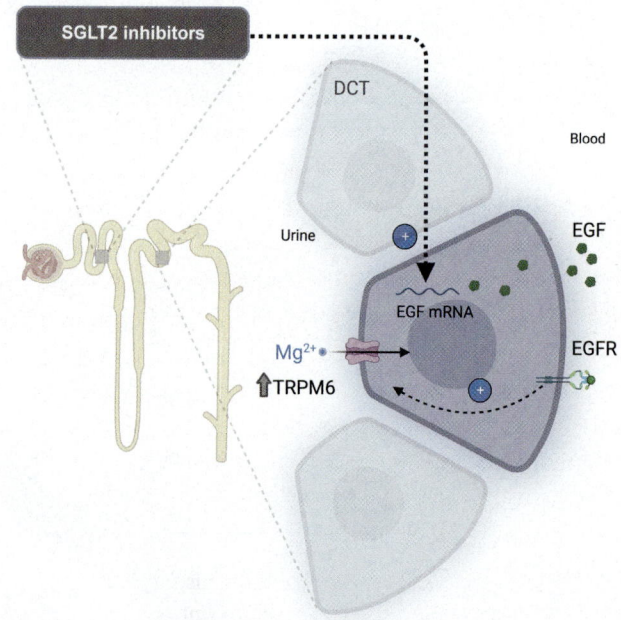

Figure 1 | Sodium-glucose cotransporter 2 (SGLT2) inhibition, epidermal growth factor (EGF), and magnesium homeostasis. SGLT2 inhibitors increase the EGF mRNA level in the distal convoluted tubular (DCT) epithelial cells, resulting in increased production of EGF, which, in turn, can bind to EGF receptor (EGFR), resulting in increased transient receptor potential cation channel, subfamily M, member 6 activity and increased magnesium (Mg^{2+}) absorption.

active investigation. A recent study on animal models showed that dapagliflozin enhanced transient receptor potential cation channel, subfamily M, member 6–mediated transepithelial Mg^{2+} transport in distal convoluted tubular cells.[S2] As EGF is known to increase transient receptor potential cation channel, subfamily M, member 6 activity,[S3] I believe this study provides a promising link between the effect of SGLT2 inhibitors and magnesium homeostasis, potentially via its effect on the EGF pathway in the distal convoluted tubular cells (Figure 1). I appeal that further studies examining such a direct link are highly desired to improve our understanding of the effect of SGLT2 inhibitors on magnesium homeostasis and to examine whether SGLT2 inhibitors can become a novel class of medicines in treating hypomagnesemia.

ACKNOWLEDGMENTS
Figure 1 was created with BioRender.com.

SUPPLEMENTARY MATERIAL
Supplementary File (PDF)
Supplementary References.

1. Sen T, Ju W, Nair V, et al. Sodium glucose co-transporter 2 inhibition increases epidermal growth factor expression and improves outcomes in patients with type 2 diabetes. *Kidney Int.* 2023;104:828–839.
2. Tang H, Zhang X, Zhang J, et al. Elevated serum magnesium associated with SGLT2 inhibitor use in type 2 diabetes patients: a meta-analysis of randomised controlled trials. *Diabetologia.* 2016;59:2546–2551.
3. Gilbert RE, Mende C, Vijapurkar U, et al. Effects of canagliflozin on serum magnesium in patients with type 2 diabetes mellitus: a post hoc analysis of randomized controlled trials. *Diabetes Ther.* 2017;8:451–458.
4. Toto RD, Goldenberg R, Chertow GM, et al. Correction of hypomagnesemia by dapagliflozin in patients with type 2 diabetes: a post hoc analysis of 10 randomized, placebo-controlled trials. *J Diabetes Complications.* 2019;33:107402.

Chintan V. Shah[1]
[1]Division of Nephrology, Hypertension and Renal Transplantation, University of Florida, Gainesville, Florida, USA

Correspondence: *Chintan V. Shah, Division of Nephrology, Hypertension and Renal Transplantation, University of Florida, College of Medicine, 1600 SW Archer Rd, Room CG-98, Gainesville, Florida 32610, USA. E-mail: shahc@ufl.edu*

Kidney International (2024) **105**, 638–639; https://doi.org/10.1016/j.kint.2023.10.032
Copyright © 2023, International Society of Nephrology. Published by Elsevier Inc. All rights reserved.

The authors reply: We thank Shah for his interest and valuable insights[1] regarding our recent work.[2] The suggestion that the effect of sodium-glucose cotransporter 2 (SGLT2) inhibitors on magnesium levels may be mediated through the epidermal growth factor (EGF) signaling pathway in distal convoluted tubular 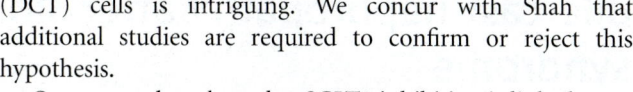 (DCT) cells is intriguing. We concur with Shah that additional studies are required to confirm or reject this hypothesis.

Our recent data show that SGLT2 inhibition is linked to an increase in *EGF* transcription in DCT cells in patients with type 2 diabetes. This insight may also advance our understanding of how SGLT2 inhibitors positively affect magnesium homeostasis. Analysis of the gene expression data sets from our study, which was not included in the original publication, demonstrates an increased *TRPM6* expression in DCT cells of patients treated with SGLT2 inhibitors. Nonetheless, more in-depth studies are needed to elucidate the molecular relationship between SGLT2 inhibition in proximal tubular cells, the increase in EGF, the activation of EGF–EGF receptor–transient receptor potential cation channel, subfamily M, member 6 (TRPM6) pathway in DCT cells, and the overall regulation of magnesium homeostasis.

The growing access to detailed molecular and clinical phenotyping data from clinical studies, including multi-omics information from noninvasive biofluids and from kidney biopsies at both the tissue and single-cell levels, offers substantial prospects for future research, as highlighted in our study. These investigations will improve our understanding of the pathophysiology of diabetic kidney disease and the mechanistic underpinnings of current and novel interventions. Furthermore, they might reveal promising new avenues for treatment.

1. Shah CV. Sodium-glucose cotransporter 2 inhibition, epidermal growth factor, and magnesium homeostasis: is there a link? *Kidney Int.* 2024;105:638–639.
2. Sen T, Ju W, Nair V, et al. Sodium glucose co-transporter 2 inhibition increases epidermal growth factor expression and improves outcomes in patients with type 2 diabetes. *Kidney Int.* 2023;104:828–839.

Wenjun Ju[1,2], Hiddo J.L. Heerspink[3,4], Matthias Kretzler[1,2] and Petter Bjornstad[5,6]
[1]Division of Nephrology, Department of Internal Medicine, University of Michigan, Ann Arbor, Michigan, USA; [2]Department of Computational Medicine and Bioinformatics, University of Michigan, Ann Arbor, Michigan, USA; [3]Department of Clinical Pharmacy and Pharmacology, University of Groningen, University Medical Centre Groningen, Groningen, the Netherlands; [4]The George Institute for Global Health, University New South Wales, Sydney, New South Wales, Australia; [5]Section of Endocrinology, Department of Pediatrics, University of Colorado School of Medicine, Aurora, Colorado, USA; and [6]Division of Renal Diseases and Hypertension, Department of Medicine, University of Colorado School of Medicine, Aurora, Colorado, USA

Correspondence: *Hiddo J.L. Heerspink, Department of Clinical Pharmacy and Pharmacology, De Brug 50C-1-011, AP50 University Medical Center Groningen, PO BOX 30001, 9700 AD Groningen, the Netherlands. E-mail: h.j.lambers.heerspink@umcg.nl*

Kidney International (2024) **105**, 639; https://doi.org/10.1016/j.kint.2023.10.033
Copyright © 2023, International Society of Nephrology. Published by Elsevier Inc. All rights reserved.

Bile cast nephropathy after sinusoidal obstruction syndrome

Toshiki Terao[1,2], Kyosuke Horikawa[3] and Ken-ichi Matsuoka[1]

[1]Department of Hematology and Oncology, Okayama University Hospital, Okayama, Japan; [2]Department of Hematology, Oncology and Respiratory Medicine, Okayama University Graduate School of Medicine, Dentistry and Pharmaceutical Sciences, Okayama, Japan; and [3]Department of Pathology and Oncology, Okayama University Graduate School of Medicine, Dentistry, and Pharmaceutical Sciences, Okayama, Japan

Correspondence: *Toshiki Terao, Department of Hematology and Oncology, Okayama University, 2-5-1 Shikata-cho, Kita-ku, Okayama 700-8558, Japan. E-mail: tarao.toshiki.0127@gmail.com*

Kidney International (2024) **105,** 640; https://doi.org/10.1016/j.kint.2023.08.027

Copyright © 2023, International Society of Nephrology. Published by Elsevier Inc. All rights reserved.

A 25-year-old male patient was transferred to our hospital for the treatment of refractory acute myeloid leukemia. Despite undergoing an initial allogeneic hematopoietic stem cell transplantation 2 months before hospital transfer, his acute myeloid leukemia remained unresponsive. Despite receiving salvage chemotherapy, including venetoclax, his acute myeloid leukemia continued to progress. The conditioning regimen for his second hematopoietic stem cell transplantation consisted of fludarabine, melphalan, and low-dose total body irradiation, with post-transplant cyclophosphamide administered for graft versus host disease prophylaxis. On the day of the second hematopoietic stem cell transplantation, laboratory studies revealed a white cell count of 40/μl with 90% myeloblasts, a hemoglobin level of 6.3 g/dl, a platelet count of 10,000/μl, a total bilirubin level of 3.5 mg/dl, and a serum creatinine level of 0.29 mg/dl. On day 6, the patient developed sinusoidal obstruction syndrome, initiating continuous hemodiafiltration due to acute kidney injury and oliguria. Despite receiving intensive supportive care, the sinusoidal obstruction syndrome and acute kidney injury did not resolve. On day 20, after the second hematopoietic stem cell transplantation, his acute myeloid leukemia relapsed, and he ultimately

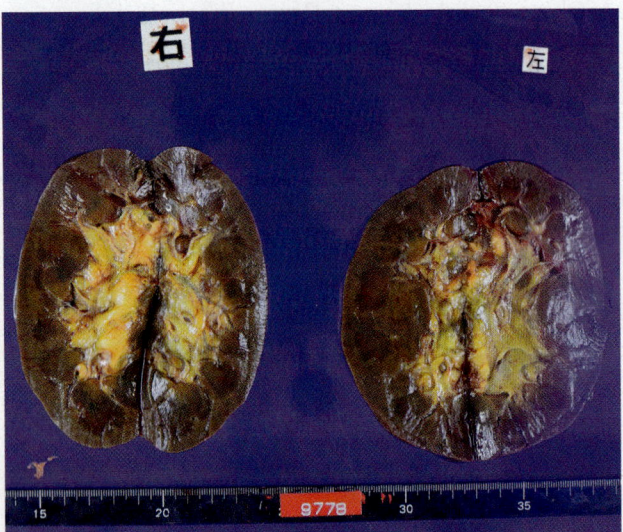

Figure 1 | Cross-section of the kidney. The kidney cortex is altered in yellow, suggesting bilirubin deposition. The characters above the kidney indicate "right" and "left" in Japanese.

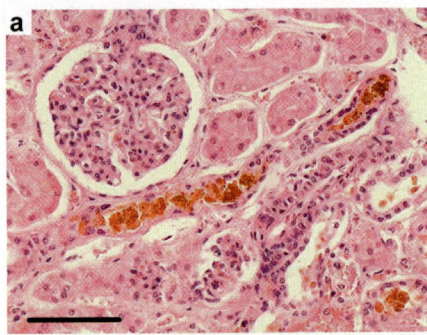

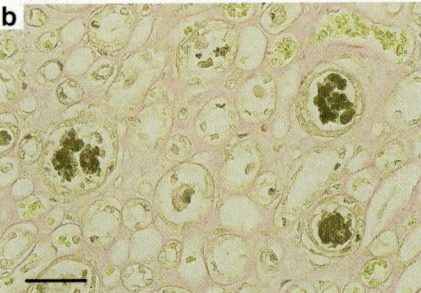

Figure 2 | (a) The pathology section showing the presence of bile casts and pigments in the distal tubules (hematoxylin and eosin staining). Original magnification ×200. (**b**) Hall stain showing the bile casts and pigments in green and yellow. Original magnification ×400. To optimize viewing of this image, please see the online version of this article at www.kidney-international.org.

succumbed on day 31. His total bilirubin level before death was 19.7 mg/dl. Postmortem examination revealed a grossly yellow kidney (Figure 1), whereas histologic analysis revealed numerous brown pigments and casts in the distal tubules (hematoxylin and eosin stain in Figure 2a; bar = 100 μm). Hall stain highlights these pigments and casts in green and yellow (Figure 2b; bar = 50 μm), leading to the diagnosis of bile cast nephropathy. No significant changes were noted in the glomeruli and interstitial. This illustrative case shows that renal impairment accompanied by sinusoidal obstruction syndrome can be attributed not only to abnormal fluid distribution but also to bile cast nephropathy resulting from hyperbilirubinemia.

ACKNOWLEDGMENT

We thank Dr. Wakako Oda (Department of Pathology, Okayama City Hospital, Okayama, Japan) for Hall stain. The authors did not receive financial support from any organization for the submitted work.

Cardiac tamponade diagnosed on nephrologist-performed point-of-care ultrasonography

Aisha Batool[1] and Abhilash Koratala[1]

[1]Division of Nephrology, Medical College of Wisconsin, Milwaukee, Wisconsin, USA

Correspondence: *Abhilash Koratala, Division of Nephrology, Medical College of Wisconsin, 8701 W Watertown Plank Rd, Room A 7633, Wauwatosa, Wisconsin 53226, USA. E-mail: akoratala@mcw.edu*

In recent times, point-of-care ultrasonography (POCUS) has become an integral component of physical examination, and the realm of nephrologist-performed POCUS is expanding beyond kidney ultrasonography. A 59-year-old man with a history of untreated hypothyroidism presented with lower extremity swelling and shortness of breath. Laboratory testing revealed a significantly elevated level of thyroid-stimulating hormone of 43 mIU/ml (reference, 0.5–5 mIU/ml) and undetectable free T3 and T4. A chest radiograph showed an enlarged cardiac silhouette. A transthoracic echocardiogram demonstrated moderate to large circumferential pericardial effusion without echocardiographic signs of tamponade and severely reduced left ventricular systolic function. The patient began to receive i.v. levothyroxine. The hospital course was complicated by circulatory shock presumed to be of mixed septic and cardiogenic cause, requiring vasopressor therapy. Nephrology consultation was sought for oliguric acute kidney injury. Urine microscopy revealed muddy brown casts suggestive of acute tubular necrosis. As assessing hemodynamics is a vital component of acute kidney injury evaluation, we performed POCUS, which revealed a plethoric inferior vena cava and a large circumferential pericardial effusion. Right ventricular diastolic collapse was clearly demonstrated (Figure 1, Supplementary Figure S1, and Supplementary Video S1), suggestive of tamponade physiology. The patient underwent emergent pericardiocentesis with removal of 450 ml of fluid, resulting in a significant decrease in the requirement for vasopressors and an improvement in urine output. Teaching points: (i) Although tamponade is traditionally considered a clinical diagnosis, the distinction is blurry in the era of POCUS, and it is crucial to promptly address any concerning sonographic findings. Moreover, it is well recognized that the sensitivity of conventional physical examination findings (such as the Beck triad) is low for the diagnosis of tamponade. (ii) Hemodynamics are dynamic. Having a recent formal echocardiogram does not obviate the need for POCUS. (iii) The presence of urine microscopy findings indicative of tubular injury should not deter us from assessing ongoing hemodynamic insults.

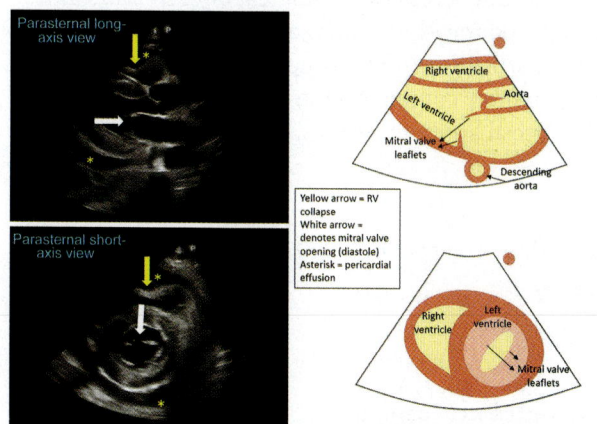

Figure 1 | Parasternal long- and short-axis views of the heart, demonstrating pericardial effusion and right ventricular collapse. Illustration is licensed from Vecteezy. RV, right ventricle.

DISCLOSURE
All the authors declared no competing interests.

FUNDING STATEMENT
AK reports research funding from KidneyCure and the American Society of Nephrology's William and Sandra Bennett Clinical Scholars Grant.

STATEMENT OF HUMAN AND ANIMAL RIGHTS
This clinical image complies with the ethical standards outlined in the journal. This case study is not formal research involving human participants or animals.

SUPPLEMENTARY MATERIAL
Supplementary File (JPG)
Supplementary Figure S1. Top panel: Subxiphoid 4-chamber view demonstrating pericardial effusion. Arrow points to the right ventricle. Bottom panel: Parasternal long-axis view after pericardiocentesis, demonstrating resolution of the effusion and right ventricular collapse. Illustration is licensed from Vecteezy.
Supplementary File (MP4)
Supplementary Video S1. Ultrasonography clips of various standard cardiac views, demonstrating pericardial effusion and signs of cardiac tamponade.

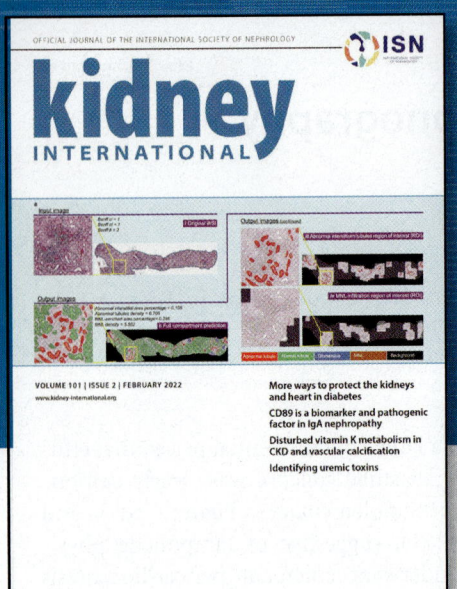

kidney INTERNATIONAL

The Official Journal of the International Society of Nephrology

Publishes 12 times per year
ISSN: 0085-2538

Members of the International Society of Nephrology receive *KI* as a benefit of membership.

For ISN membership information, please contact:

Angélique De Smet
ISN Membership Coordinator
Email: membership@theisn.org

2020 Journal Impact Factor: 10.612
2020 Citescore*: 14.4
Journal Citation Reports® (Clarivate Analytics, 2021)

Editor: Pierre Ronco, MD, PhD

Kidney International Supplements, an official journal of the International Society of Nephrology, is one of the most cited journals in nephrology and is widely regarded as the world's premier journal on the development and consequences of kidney disease. *KI* publishes original research in both basic science and clinical medicine covering renal physiology, biochemistry, pathology, immunology, morphology and more. It aims to inform the renal researcher and the practicing nephrologist on all aspects of renal studies, including basic and clinical research, emerging therapeutics, and novel diagnosis.

KI Online for Members and Subscribers!

Subscriptions to *Kidney International* include access to the online version of the journal, with instant access to the full text of each issue as it publishes. *KI's* website (kidney-international.org) offers exclusive online-only content, such as articles-in-press, supplementary data, and topical collections. Complimentary content on the website includes select articles, editorials, special announcements, and special features.

Access KI!
On the web: www.kidney-international.org
On Twitter: @Kidney_Int

Submit Your Article!
https://mc.manuscriptcentral.com/ki

Your subscription to KI includes the companion journal, *KI Supplements*.

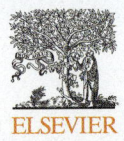
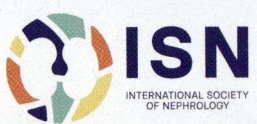

make your diagnosis

The Case | A patient with skin rash, monoclonal gammopathy, and proteinuria

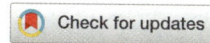

Justyna Fryc[1] and Beata Naumnik[1]

[1]1st Department of Nephrology and Transplantation With Dialysis Unit, Medical University of Bialystok, Bialystok, Poland

Correspondence: *Justyna Fryc, 1st Department of Nephrology and Transplantation With Dialysis Unit, Medical University of Bialystok, Zurawia 14 Street, 15-540 Bialystok, Poland. E-mail: justyna.fryc@umb.edu.pl*

Kidney International (2024) **105**, 643–644; https://doi.org/10.1016/j.kint.2023.10.010 Copyright © 2023, International Society of Nephrology. Published by Elsevier Inc. All rights reserved.

A 67-year-old female European-American patient was referred for evaluation of proteinuria and a diagnosis of monoclonal gammopathy. The patient reported a 4-year history of recurrent and nonpruritic urticarial rash, weight loss of 10 kg in the past year, and pain and swelling in the lower extremities. Physical examination findings revealed erythematous, annular, and maculopapular lesions, ranging from 0.5 to 7 cm in diameter and distributed over the trunk and extremities (Supplementary Figure S1A). These skin changes were less edematous than those seen in typical chronic urticaria. They developed and partially resolved within 24 to 48 hours without scarring. Skin biopsy results revealed interstitial neutrophilic infiltrates (without vasculitis) characteristic of neutrophilic urticarial dermatosis (Supplementary Figure S1B).

Laboratory findings included an estimated glomerular filtration rate of 56 ml/min per 1.73 m² and nephrotic-range proteinuria (9.7 g/24 h). Serum immunofixation showed a monoclonal IgM κ band. Additional test results revealed an elevated white blood cell count (13.8×10^3/mm³) with neutrophilia (10.37×10^3/mm³), elevated C-reactive protein (73 mg/l), erythrocyte sedimentation rate of 118 mm/h, thrombocytosis (504×10^3/mm³), and mild anemia (hemoglobin, 11.5 g/dl; mean corpuscular volume, 82.4 fl). Procalcitonin, lactate dehydrogenase, and complement components C3 and C4 values were normal. Bone marrow biopsy results showed no abnormalities. Autoimmune test results were normal, including antinuclear

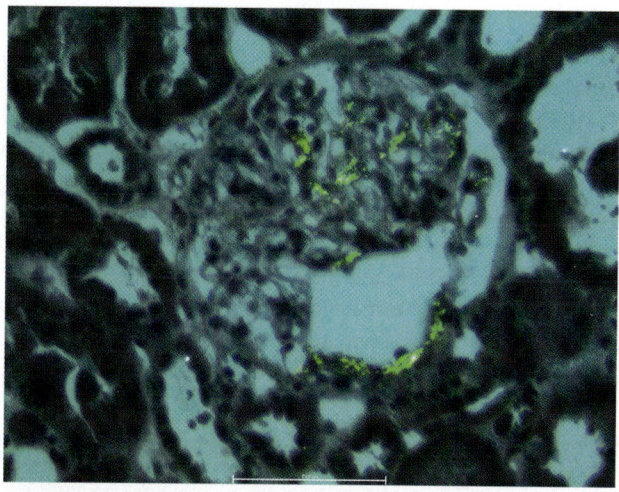

Figure 1 | Glomerulus. Congo red staining showing green birefringence under the polarized light (light microscopy, original magnification ×400). To optimize viewing of this image, please see the online version of this article at www.kidney-international.org.

antibodies, anti-neutrophil cytoplasmic antibodies (ANCA) (both anti-proteinase 3 ANCA and anti-myeloperoxidase ANCA), rheumatoid factor, and cryoglobulins. Additional test results excluded viral infections, Lyme disease, and tuberculosis. Colonoscopy, gastroscopy, and computed tomography of the chest, abdomen, and pelvis showed no significant abnormalities. A kidney biopsy was performed (Figure 1).

What is your diagnosis?

SEE NEXT PAGE FOR ANSWERS

The Diagnosis | Amyloid A amyloidosis associated with Schnitzler syndrome

The kidney biopsy result showed mesangial and segmental capillary wall staining of amyloid deposits (Figure 1). Immunohistochemistry for amyloid A was strongly positive in glomerular amyloid deposits (Supplementary Figure S2A). Electron microscopy revealed randomly arranged amyloid fibrils in the vessel wall (Supplementary Figure S2B).

According to the Strasbourg classification criteria, the patient was diagnosed with an autoinflammatory disorder, Schnitzler syndrome. This classification includes 2 obligatory criteria: urticarial rash and monoclonal gammopathy (usually IgM, less often IgG). Minor symptoms include neutrophilic urticarial dermatosis on skin biopsy, elevated levels of inflammatory markers, recurrent fever, and abnormal bone remodeling, with or without bone pain. A definitive diagnosis of Schnitzler syndrome is made when the 2 mandatory criteria and 2 minor criteria (in the case of IgM gammopathy) or 3 minor criteria (in the case of IgG gammopathy) are present.[1,2] In addition to these criteria, patients may present with myalgia, arthralgia, weight loss, lymphadenopathy, and hepatosplenomegaly.

A urticarial rash is usually the first manifestation, but neutrophilic urticarial dermatosis is not specific to Schnitzler syndrome. The differential diagnosis includes other autoimmune or autoinflammatory diseases, including cryopyrin-associated periodic syndrome, adult-onset Still disease, or lupus erythematosus. In Schnitzler syndrome, the rash affects the trunk and extremities, with rare head and neck involvement. The palms and soles are never affected. The frequency of rashes varies from daily to a few times a year.

The patient was treated with an interleukin-1 antagonist (daily s.c. injections of 100 mg anakinra), resulting in the resolution of the skin lesions within 48 hours and reduced inflammatory serum markers. However, deterioration of kidney function (estimated glomerular filtration rate, 30 ml/min per 1.73 m^2) and increased proteinuria (18 g/24 h) were observed 6 months later.

This patient presented with a constellation of classic symptoms suggestive of Schnitzler syndrome, but the diagnosis had been delayed for many years, and the onset of amyloid A amyloidosis caused irreversible renal damage.

Schnitzler syndrome is a rare and poorly understood cause of amyloid A amyloidosis. Frequent delay in diagnosis is due to its rarity and low symptom specificity, similar to other autoimmune or hematologic diseases. Only 300 cases of the syndrome have been reported, mostly in European-descent adults.[3] Molecular characterization of amyloid deposition in monoclonal gammopathy is essential because of the differences in clinical course and treatment between light chain (AL) and amyloid A (AA) amyloidosis. Lack of awareness of this late-onset autoinflammatory syndrome delays the correct diagnosis and implementation of effective treatment with interleukin-1 inhibitors (anakinra, rilonacept, or canakinumab) to prevent the development of amyloid A amyloidosis. This case report highlights the need for increased care and knowledge of Schnitzler syndrome, as effective treatment strategies are available.

DISCLOSURE
All the authors declared no competing interests.

ACKNOWLEDGMENTS
We are grateful for editorial assistance by Dr. Jeffrey B. Kopp from the National Institute of Diabetes and Digestive and Kidney Diseases, National Institutes of Health. We thank Prof. Lech Chyczewski, Dr. Grzegorz Zalewski, Dr. Beata Szynaka, and Dr. Agata Piłaszewicz-Puza for their help in interpreting the pathomorphologic images; and Dr. Ewa Wiesik-Szewczyk for enrolling our patient in the Polish National Treatment Program for Autoinflammatory Diseases.

SUPPLEMENTARY MATERIAL
Supplementary File (Word)
Supplementary Figure S1. (**A**) Skin lesions. Urticarial rash. (**B**) Skin lesions. Histopathologic analysis showing neutrophilic urticarial dermatosis. In the s.c. layer, visible clusters of neutrophils (arrows) are located mainly near blood vessels. Scattered neutrophils are visible throughout the s.c. layer (hematoxylin-eosin [H&E] staining).
Supplementary Figure S2. (**A**) Immunohistochemical stain shows amyloid amyloid A deposits within the glomeruli (original magnification ×400). (**B**) Deposits containing randomly arrayed amyloid fibrils (7 to 12 nm in diameter) in the vessel wall and around the vessel in the renal stroma (electron microscopy, original magnification ×25,000).

REFERENCES
1. Simon A, Asli B, Braun-Falco M, et al. Schnitzler's syndrome: diagnosis, treatment, and follow-up. *Allergy*. 2013;68:562–568.
2. Gusdorf L, Asli B, Barbarot S, et al. Schnitzler syndrome: validation and applicability of diagnostic criteria in real-life patients. *Allergy*. 2017;72:177–182.
3. de Koning HD. Schnitzler's syndrome: lessons from 281 cases. *Clin Transl Allergy*. 2014;4:41.

kidney INTERNATIONAL supplements

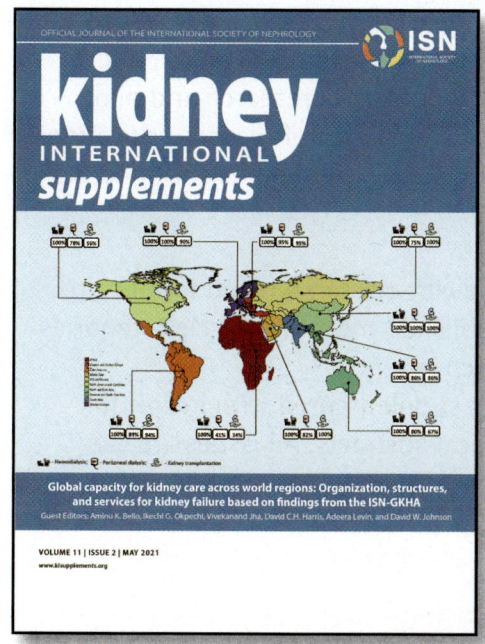

2020 Journal Impact Factor: 10.545
2020 Citescore*: 24.0

Journal Citation Reports® (Clarivate Analytics, 2021)

Kidney International Supplements is the Official Journal of the International Society of Nephrology

Editor: Pierre Ronco, MD, PhD

Kidney International Supplements is published on behalf of the International Society of Nephrology (ISN) and comes complimentary as part of a subscription to *Kidney International*. *Kidney International Supplements* is a peer-reviewed journal whose focus is sponsored, topical content of interest to the nephrology community.

Access *KI Supplements*!
On the web: www.kisupplements.org
On Twitter: @Kidney_Int

Members of the International Society of Nephrology receive *KI Supplements* as a benefit of membership.

For ISN membership information, please contact:

Angélique De Smet, ISN Membership Coordinator
Email: membership@theisn.org

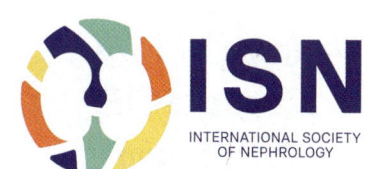

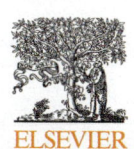

Your subscription to *KI* includes the companion journal, *KI Supplements*.

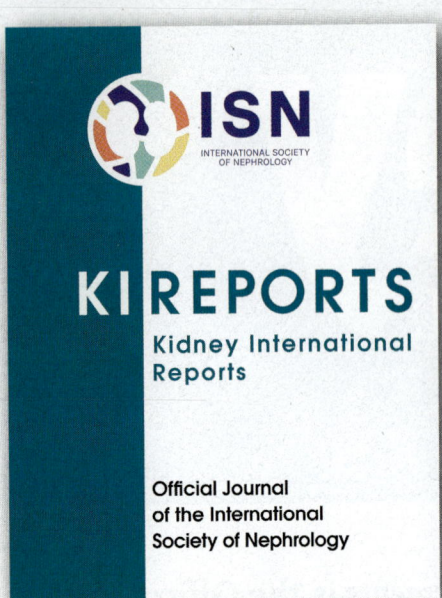

Find the leading clinical and translational research in kidney disease at *Kidney International Reports*

Editor-in-Chief:
Jai Radhakrishnan, MD, MS
Columbia University
New York, NY

Deputy Editor:
Sumit Mohan, MD, MPH
Columbia University
New York, NY

Open Access

An official journal of the

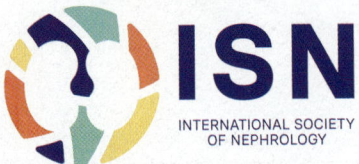

Indexed in PMC, Scopus, SCIE, DOAJ, and Google Scholar

Kidney International Reports is a peer-reviewed, online open access journal publishing clinical and translational research related to kidney disease from across the globe. Of particular interest are submissions related to clinical trials, epidemiology, systematic reviews (including meta-analyses), outcomes research and pilot studies of novel therapies. An additional area of focus is educational content, including teaching cases, society guidelines and meeting reports.

With the rapidly increasing worldwide readership and interest in *KI Reports,* the journal is now published monthly. Article categories include full length articles, research letters and reviews. Original research is supplemented with insightful expert commentaries and graphical abstracts. All issues are available for free at www.kireports.org.

Access KI Reports!
On the web: www.kireports.org
On Twitter: @KIReports

Submit Your Article!
https://mc.manuscriptcentral.com/kir

| 2020 Journal Impact Factor*: 4.164 | 2020 Citescore: 4.3 |

Journal Citation Reports® (Clarivate Analytics, 2021)

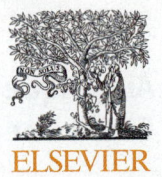